MW00744070

# The Clinical Care of the Aged Person

# The Clinical Care
# of the Aged Person

*An Interdisciplinary Perspective*

*Edited by*
David G. Satin, MD
Harvard Medical School

*with*

Barbara A. Blakeney, RNC, MS
Jennifer M. Bottomley, MS, RPT
Margot C. Howe, MS, OTR, EdD
Helen D. Smith, MS, OTR

*New York    Oxford*
OXFORD UNIVERSITY PRESS
1994

WT
30
C641
1994

Oxford University Press

Oxford   New York   Toronto
Delhi   Bombay   Calcutta   Madras   Karachi
Kuala Lumpur   Singapore   Hong Kong   Tokyo
Nairobi   Dar es Salaam   Cape Town
Melbourne   Auckland   Madrid

and associated companies in
Berlin   Ibadan

Library of Congress Cataloging-in-Publication Data
The Clinical care of the aged person : an interdisciplinary perspective /
edited by David G. Satin, with Barbara Blakeney ... [et al.].
p. cm.   Includes bibliographical references and index.
ISBN 0-19-505290-0
1. Geriatrics. 2. Aged — Medical care. 3. Aged — Health and hygiene.
I. Satin, David G. II. Blakeney, Barbara A.
[DNLM: 1. Health Services for the Aged — organization & administra-
tion. 2. Health Policy. 3. Geriatrics.   WT 30 C641 1994]
RC952.C534   1994   362.1'9897 — dc20
DNLM/DLC for Library of Congress                           93-38279

9 8 7 6 5 4 3 2 1
Printed in the United States of America
on acid-free paper

# Preface

Concern with the enlarging population of aged in all developed and industrialized countries has been with us for some time now and has increased the interest in geriatrics — the health problems and care of the aged. Courses, specialized education programs and centers, and subspecialization in various health disciplines have developed. It was striking, then, that both faculty members and students in a broad range of health disciplines complained about the lack of a training program that covered the gamut of geriatric issues. People also commented on the lack of a program that brought together the full range of disciplines — and both students and teachers — that contribute to the health of the aged, though this is rare in all health education. The idealistic sought such a comprehensive, integrated, and interdisciplinary geriatric education program. The pragmatic were resigned to learning and practicing on their own.

The 1960s and 1970s were characterized by enthusiasm and practical support for community-oriented, nontraditional service and education programs, as well as by innovation in professional identities and roles. In 1979 a group of schools and departments training health professionals responded to this need for comprehensive, clinical, and interdisciplinary education in geriatrics and to encouragement from the U.S. National Institutes of Health (NIH) to submit a grant proposal for a research and demonstration project in interdisciplinary education in geriatrics. The goal was to study contemporary education for the care of the aged of clinicians in various disciplines, as well as the process and product of developing interdisciplinary education to this end. However, by the time the grant proposal was submitted, the NIH review committee that was to address this application was being phased out. Its review criteria had become unclear, and its membership was substantially changed, having no experience with such projects. This reflected a developing shift in societal interests away from liberal challenge, change, and social activism, and toward conservative academic study and institutional stability. Thus the committee that had originally encouraged the research and demonstration grant almost unanimously now rejected it.

Undaunted, the interdisciplinary faculty planning group was still committed to the project and decided to implement at least the core didactic program. And so *The Clinical Care of the Aged Person: An Interdisciplinary Perspective* has been taught ever since. It is still the only comprehensive, clinical, interdisciplinary course in geriatrics in the region, and national surveys have suggested it is the only truly interdisciplinary education program in the nation. The students and faculty have represented the disciplines of administration, anatomy, anthropology, business, engineering, ethics, law, medicine, nursing, nutrition, occupational therapy, pharmacy, physical therapy, psychiatry, psychology, public health, religion, social work, and sociology.

In the process of teaching, we have sought reading materials and a textbook that would provide factual and theoretical depth to the seminar exercises. This search has clearly demonstrated the paucity of broad, interdisciplinary materials. Although there is a continuing flow of textbooks in geriatrics, almost all address one discipline (e.g., medicine, nursing, or social work), focus on a narrow aspect of the aged (e.g., the biology of aging, maximizing the functional capacity of the aged, the history of health care policy relating to the aged and what its future should be, the ethics of care of the aged, or images of aging in popular culture), or are nonclinically oriented (e.g., stress research, public policy and economics, or theory). Therefore, the core and guest faculty of our educational program have documented and expanded their areas of expertise in compiling this textbook of clinical geriatrics.

The goals of this text are three:

1. To provide substantive information on aging, the health problems of the aged, and health care for them.
2. To present a comprehensive, integrated approach to health care for any population or health need as demonstrated in the care of the aged.
3. To teach the theory and practice of an interdisciplinary approach to health issues as exemplified in work with the aged.

To achieve the first goal of teaching substantive information, the bulk of the text is devoted to chapters on individual health care issues. The chapters are grouped into parts on clinical issues for the individual, interpersonal and societal issues, theoretical issues of interdisciplinary education and practice, and the integration of the issues in interdisciplinary care.

To achieve the second goal of integrating the issues of health care of the aged, the first chapter presents a discussion among a panel of aged persons, who present their naturally integrated life experiences of aging, health concerns, and care needs. Part introductions bring to bear the perspectives of several disciplines. Then, throughout the text, many of the same issues are addressed from different persepectives in different chapters. Finally, in the last chapter, a large panel of professionals working with the aged engages in a case conference treating all health-related factors for a sample individual.

To achieve the third goal of teaching an interdisciplinary approach, the introductions to each of the four parts of the text give interdisciplinary perspectives on the respective subject areas: Barbara Blakeney (a nurse clinician), Jennifer Bottomley (a physical therapist), Margot Howe (an occupational therapist specializing in mental disabilities), David Satin (a physician and psychiatrist), and Helen Smith (an occupational therapist specializing in physical disabilities) make complementary and contrasting contributions. More specifically, each chapter, written by those with primary expertise in its subject matter, acknowledges the contributions of other disciplines and the ways in which these disciplines relate to one another. The first chapter documents the need for an interdisciplinary approach to naturally integrated geriatric issues. Subsequent chapters specifically address the theory of interdisciplinary working relationships and the practice of team development and maintenance. Finally, the last chapter empirically illustrates the interdisciplinary approach.

This volume is meant as a teaching tool and a source book for those working with the aged or teaching others how to do so. It supplements experience and organizes theory and practice into perspectives and strategies for action. The text can stand alone, but it can also serve (as we use it) to support didactic and practicum education, by putting experience into context and freeing class or supervision time for exploration and application. All this can be useful to clinical practitioners and students who need to prepare for direct care. It is also useful to policy makers, planners, and administrators who need to understand the complexities of clinical life in order to prepare a regulatory, resource-allocation, and institutional context that will support the health and function of the aged and their clinical care.

We certainly recognize that we are presenting one among many approaches to geriatrics, and one that stands in contrast to traditional and common thinking and practice. Our basic purpose is to inform those interested in the aged of this alternative so they may apply it in appropriate situations. Indeed, we expect to be *model* rather than *modal*: It is essential that the comprehensive, integrated, interdisciplinary approach to geriatrics be available to those interested in the health of the aged.

Newton Centre, MA                                                           *David G. Satin*
October 1993

# Contents

Contributors  xiii

1. The Aged View Their Health Care  3
*Masie Eaton, Elizabeth B. Lindemann, Cecilia Menard, Alford and Evelyn Orwig, Max and Elaine Siegel, and Fay Salmon; with Jennifer M. Bottomley and David G. Satin*

*Précis:* A panel of aged persons—articulate, and dealing with various health issues and life settings—provide their perspectives through discussion with one another and with sympathetic health care professionals. They discuss aging and the life of the aged, family and other supports, religion and church as resources, experiences of illness and treatment, perspectives on the health care system, and death and suicide.

## I  Clinical Issues for the Individual  23

2. Physical Health Problems and Treatment of the Aged  27
*Terrence A. O'Malley, Barbara A. Blakeney*

*Précis:* Physical illness and treatment in the aged are contrasted with those in younger people. The physical health problems that appear differently in the aged or to which the aged are more prone are described. Treatment is discussed.

3. Emotional and Cognitive Issues in the Care of the Aged  62
*David G. Satin*

*Précis:* Psychiatric illness and treatment among the aged are contrasted with those among younger people. The various etiological factors—life experience, genetics, noxious physical influences, and social and cultural environment—are explored. The relative frequency of these problems is discussed, and the most common ones are described, along with their causes and appropriate treatment. The effects of health care, long-term care institutions, and dying are addressed.

4. Oral Health and Treatment of the Aged  108
*Athena S. Papas, Maureen C. Rounds*

*Précis:* The importance of dental and oral function to the aged person is explored. The connection of dental problems to physical, emotional, nutritional, and social health is examined, as are the effects of problems in these other areas on dental structure and function. The adaptation of dental treatment to the special needs and circumstances of the aged is presented.

### 5. Drug Therapy in the Aged Patient  137
*Joseph M. Scavone*

***Précis:*** Concepts are presented — therapeutic, toxic, side, and hypersensitivity effects; and absorption, distribution, chemical action, storage, and excretion. The effects of aging are detailed. The medications most commonly used by the aged are described in terms of the above concepts. The interaction of medications with other medications, foods, and disease processes is discussed. Prescription and use patterns of medication are explored in relation to their effects on health and treatment.

### 6. Nutritional Concerns and Problems of the Aged  193
*Johanna T. Dwyer*

***Précis:*** The importance of nutrition generally and that of specific nutrients for the aged person are described. Minimum and maximum intake standards and the process of standardization are detailed. Natural diet and supplemental sources of nutrients are discussed. The nutrients most important to the aged are presented individually, in terms of their actions, daily requirements, and sources.

### 7. Principles and Practice in Geriatric Rehabilitation  230
*Jennifer M. Bottomley*

***Précis:*** A philosophy of respect for the aged as people and optimism as to their capacity to regain physical and social skills underly specific discussions of the meaning of disability, impairment, and handicap; evaluation and treatment planning techniques; and methods of recovering and supporting function. The presentation of various disabilities integrates physical function and the activities of daily living. Prevention and maintenance are emphasized.

## II  Interpersonal and Societal Issues  281

### 8. The Ageing Family  285
*Frances L. Portnoy*

***Précis:*** The significance of family to the aged is explored. Patterns of family relationship are described, with the benefits and problems they present. Helping interventions in family relationships and methods of supplementing family resources are detailed.

### 9. Work, Productivity, and Worth in Old Age  294
*Margot C. Howe*

***Précis:*** In Western culture social worth and self-esteem are tied to work and productive activity. The participation of the aged in the work force and their patterns of activity are described. The relationship of these facts to the social status and social acceptance of the aged and their mental health is explored. Therapeutic activity approaches that benefit the sense of satisfaction, mental health, social integration, and functional capacity of the aged are described. Avocational and volunteer activity is highlighted.

### 10. Ethical Issues at the End of Life: Death, Dying, and the Care of the Aged  311
*David Barnard*

***Précis:*** Ethical considerations, recognized and unrecognized, permeate the health care of the aged. Issues of values, cultural patterns, personal styles, and general individual freedom and dignity are involved in the actions of patients, health professionals, health institutions, and health policy. These issues are illustrated, and ways of recognizing and dealing with them are discussed. The student is helped to address these issues realistically and honestly, rather than being given formulas for categorization and action.

## 11. Legal Issues in the Care of the Aged  329
*Thomas F. O'Hare*

**Précis:** Statutory and case law affect the health care of the aged. The concepts of responsibility, freedom, restraint, compulsion, and substituted judgment are presented. The law, precedents, and legal procedures in these matters are described, with notes made of variation in different jurisdictions. Financial and estate planning is addressed.

## 12. Disability Trends and Community Long-Term Health Care for the Aged  346
*Alan M. Jette*

**Précis:** Long-term health care affects almost all of the aged, in the form of long-term health care for chronic diseases, supportive services for impaired function, adaptive equipment and modifications in the environment for disabilities, and institutional care for the dependent aged. The place of long-term care in the lives and health care of the aged is explored, as well as the economics and administration of long-term care systems. Models of effective long-term care, and the technology and professional practice necessary to them, are presented. Expectations and recommendations for the future are addressed.

## 13. The Economics of the Health-Care System: Financing Health Care for the Aged Person  362
*Glenn S. Koocher, Diane S. Piktialis*

**Précis:** The political and financial history of health care for the aged is reviewed, including private care, voluntary agencies, and government. Current laws, agencies, and programs are described, including their interrelationship and the areas they do and do not cover. These are then related to the individual aged person's needs and care. The relationship of intent to practical effect is highlighted, in view of the practice of professional caregivers and the health care the aged receive.

# III  Theoretical Issues of Interdisciplinary Education and Practice  389

## 14. The Interdisciplinary, Integrated Approach to Professional Practice with the Aged  391
*David G. Satin*

**Précis:** Many programs and texts use the term "interdisciplinary" loosely. A conceptual framework and range of models of disciplinary working relationships are presented. The interdisciplinary mode of working relationship, the resources required for it, and its benefits and costs are detailed. The integrated, comprehensive approach to the aged and their health care is contrasted with the more usual fragmentation of training and care according to isolated health specialities and health problems.

## 15. Developing the Interdisciplinary Team  404
*Benjamin S. Siegel*

**Précis:** The principles of team function and the working relationship between the health professions are detailed. Practical issues that practicing professionals and teams must deal with are addressed, with methods for forming, maturing, and maintaining effectively functioning interdisciplinary teams. Finally, methods for teaching team principles and function are provided.

## 16. Attitudes, Values, and Ideologies as Influences on the Professional Education and Practice of Those Who Care for the Aged  426
*Lisa Gurland*

*Précis:* In addition to theory and technology, the perspectives and practices of health care professionals contribute significantly to the health care that the aged receive. The personal and professional backgrounds of these health care providers are analyzed, and commonalities and differences among the various disciplines are identified. The effect of these factors on the kinds of health care to be found in different health care agencies is described. Finally, improved training of health professionals, their choice of practice sites, and referral of aged persons for care to settings appropriate to their needs are suggested to improve both the health care of the aged and the effective practice of health care professionals.

# IV   The Interdisciplinary Care of Aged Persons — An Integration of the Issues  449

## 17. An Interdisciplinary Case Conference  451
*David G. Satin (ed.)*

*Précis:* All of the chapter authors take part in a case conference, which illustrates (1) the contributions their various disciplines make to diagnosis and treatment; (2) the comprehensive and integrated understanding of the aged person that emerges from these contributions; and (3) the process of interdisciplinary planning and action.

Index  487

# Contributors

*Note:* Institutional affiliations are given for identification purposes only. The perspectives and opinions in this text are those of the individual authors only and do not reflect those of the institutions listed, the publisher, or the editors.

**David Barnard, MA, MTS, PhD:** Professor and Chairman, Department of Humanities, College of Medicine, The Milton S. Hershey Medical Center, Pennsylvania State University; President, Society of Health and Human Values, 1991–1992

**Barbara A. Blakeney, RNC, MS:** Principal Public Health Nurse, Homeless Services and Addiction Services, Department of Public Health, Department of Health and Hospitals, City of Boston

**Jennifer M. Bottomley, MS, RPT:** Area Rehabilitation Coordinator, Outside Rehabilitation Services, The Hillhaven Corporation; former Lecturer, Program in Physical Therapy, MGH Institute of Health Professions; former Clinical Supervisor for Physical Therapy, Cushing Hospital, Framingham, MA

**Johanna T. Dwyer, MS, MSc, DSc:** Professor of Medicine (Nutrition) and Professor of Community Health, Tufts University School of Medicine; Director, Frances Stern Nutrition Center and Dietetic Internship, New England Medical Center Hospitals

**Marjorie Glassman, OTR, MSW, LICSW:** Former Director, Services for Older People, Family Service Association of Greater Boston

**Lisa Gurland, MEd, LCSW, RN, PsyD:** Consultant and Trainer, AIDS Program, Massachusetts Department of Public Health; specialist in community mental health and care for the caregiver, consulting to community organizations; Board of Directors, North End Community Health Committee, Inc., Boston

**Margot C. Howe, MS, OTR, EdD:** Professor *emerita,* Tufts University–Boston School of Occupational Therapy

**Alan M. Jette, RPT, MPH, PhD:** Senior Research Scientist, New England Research Institute; Lecturer, Harvard School of Dental Medicine

**Glenn S. Koocher, AB, MPA:** Legislative Representative for New England, American Association of Retired Persons; Associate Editor, *Hospital Managed Care and Direct Contracting*; former Senior Program Consultant, Health Programs Development Area Program Manager, and Director of Medicare Beneficiary Education, Blue Cross and Blue Shield of Massachusetts, Inc.

**Thomas F. O'Hare, JD:** Private practice of law specializing in mental health law

**Terrence A. O'Malley, MD:** Instructor in Medicine, Harvard Medical School; Assistant Physician, Massachusetts General Hospital

**Athena S. Papas, DMD, PhD:** Associate Professor, Department of General Dentistry,

Tufts University School of Dental Medicine; Co-Head, Division of Geriatric Dentistry, Tufts University School of Dental Medicine; Director, Geriatric Outreach Program, Tufts University School of Dental Medicine; Director, Oral Medicine Service, Tufts University School of Dental Medicine

**Diane S. Piktialis, MA, PhD:** Vice-president for Elder Care, Work/Family Directions, Inc., Boston; former Director of Policy and Program Development, Blue Cross and Blue Shield of Massachusetts, Inc.; former Assistant Secretary, Massachusetts Executive Office of Elder Affairs

**Frances L. Portnoy, RN, MS, MA, PhD:** Professor, College of Nursing and College of Public and Community Service, and Senior Fellow, Gerontology Institute, University of Massachusetts—Boston

**Maureen C. Rounds, MEd, RDH:** Clinical Professor, Department of General Dentistry, Tufts School of Dental Medicine; Registered Dietician, Frances Stern Nutrition Center, New England Medical Center Hospitals

**David G. Satin, AB, MD, FAPA:** Assistant Clinical Professor of Psychiatry and Member, Division on Aging, Harvard Medical School; Assistant Visiting Physician, McLean Hospital; President, Geriatric Health Resource, Inc.

**Joseph M. Scavone, BS, MS, PharmD:** Professor and Division Head, Division of Clinical and Administrative Pharmacy, College of Pharmacy, University of Iowa; Assistant Clinical Professor of Psychiatry, Tufts University School of Medicine; Adjunct Assistant Professor of Community Medicine and Socio-Medical Sciences, Boston University School of Medicine

**Benjamin S. Siegel, MD:** Professor of Pediatrics and Psychiatry, and Director of Medical Student Education in Pediatrics, Boston University School of Medicine; Senior Pediatrician, Primary Care Training Program, Boston City Hospital

**Helen D. Smith, MS, OTR:** Professor of Occupational Therapy, Tufts University–Boston School of Occupational Therapy

# The Clinical Care of the Aged Person

# 1

## The Aged View Their Health and Care

Masie Eaton, Elizabeth B. Lindemann, Cecelia Menard, Alford and
Evelyn Orwig, Max and Elaine Siegel, and Fay Salmon
with
Jennifer M. Bottomley and David G. Satin

Students of geriatrics have asked that they not only learn *about* the aged but *from* them.
This is reasonable, since clinical education should be based on clinical reality and prepare students for clinical practice (although this principle is too often honored in the
breach rather than the observance). Therefore, we recruited a panel of aged people representing a range of functional capacities: community dwellers, participants in structured
activity programs, and residents of long-term care facilities. We asked these people to
present their experiences and ideas about aging, health problems, and health care. A
group discussion took place in the nursing home in which one of the panel members
lives, and essential portions of the discussion are presented here. The panel members
have reviewed and amended the results to ensure that their experiences and thoughts are
accurately represented.

Masie Eaton is 83 years old, lives with a companion in an independent apartment, and
has written poetry. Elizabeth Lindemann, 75 years old and widowed, is a semiretired
social worker who has remained very active in community, church, and organizational
affairs. Cecelia Menard, who is 87 years old, lives in a chronic disease hospital because
of chronic illness. Alford Orwig is 81 years old, retired, and in precarious health. He
lives in an independent apartment with his wife, Evelyn Orwig, who is 79 years old and
healthy. Max Siegel, 75 years old, is a retired attorney and supermarket owner. He and
his wife, Elaine Siegel, a retired nurse aged 76, live in their own house, are active in
elderly affairs advocacy groups, and serve as a community blood pressure screening
team. Fay Salmon, 85 years old and divorced, is a former concert pianist and piano
teacher, who entered a nursing home after suffering a stroke. An active member in and
representative of the resident council, she was the hostess for this panel discussion.

AGING AND LIFE REVIEW

JENNIFER M. BOTTOMLEY: How does it feel to get old?
FAY SALMON: Well, it's all a matter of how you feel, and it's up to you. Of course, age
    and attitude are the most important things to think about. Age isn't only numbers;

3

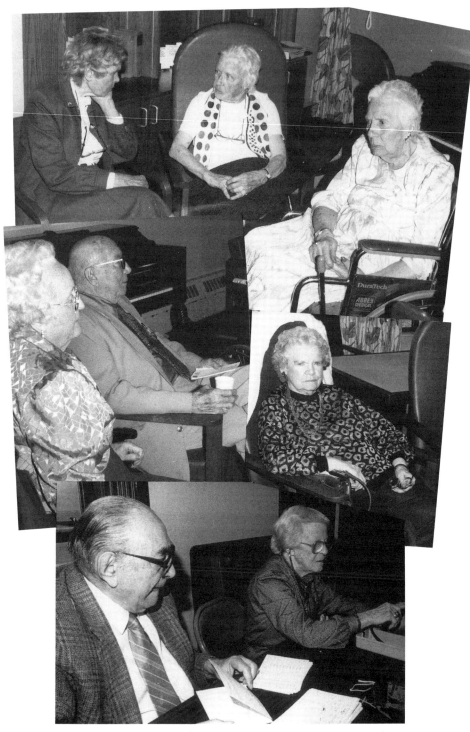

The panel *(clockwise from top left)*: Elizabeth B. Lindemann, Masie Eaton, Fay Salmon, Cecelia Menard, Elaine Siegel, Max Siegel, Evelyn Orwig, and Alford Orwig.

attitude makes it a different story. Alright, so I'm getting gray hair. I don't need gray hair! So I have it rinsed to a white mink, which is much better than gray hair. And everybody loves it and I love it too. So there you are: It's not important that you're getting older and then learn to think that you are dying — that's sad if you learn to look at things that way. What's important is the attitude that your hair isn't good. Think of the things you have. I have my family: I just became a grandmother. A great-grandmother! Twice now! I have a little boy of 2 and a little one was just born. I like living to see that. Isn't that something?

ALFORD ORWIG: That's great! I think there are many advantages to growing old. There are disadvantages as well, as we're all well aware. But there are so many advantages: First of all, my wife and I have a good life, and I think that's important. We've been happily married for 56 years and have one child, a daughter, who's half my age. And when I think of all the things that she is going to enjoy in the next 40 years, it's very rewarding.

SALMON: Sure. That's a fulfillment.

A. ORWIG: Yes, I think we have the best of it really, because we've gone through a lot of good times. We've had tough times, too. And there are so many things that have happened in our lifetime that I think, if we look back on it, we can be very happy that we lived to this age. As I look at the world today and see some of the disadvantages, I think that we are very, very fortunate to have had the experience of our times. And then, of course, it is a matter of your attitude.

EVELYN ORWIG: That's the main thing.

A. ORWIG: It's a matter of accepting what you have to go through. I never thought I'd live to be 80 or 81. I never thought about it, really. They say you live a day at a time, and that's true. You live a year at a time and time pases so quickly that, before you know it, here we are older people. Not old yet, but older. So I think that it's wonderful to be old as long as you are not bedridden and helpless.

SALMON: I agree.

BOTTOMLEY: Mrs. Lindemann, do you want to talk about what it's like to get old?

ELIZABETH LINDEMANN: I don't know, because I haven't gotten old yet! I'm only 75, but I think I'm certainly preoccupied with the idea of what it will be like to be old. Lately, I have a great feeling of pressure to get the things done that I still want to do because I don't know what can happen. Anything can happen any day. I had two parents who had cardiac problems. That's better than some things I can think of, but it can come on you pretty fast. And so I'm working quite hard right now on finishing the things I want to finish.

E. ORWIG: I think that aging is as much a state of mind as it is a state of health and body. I have come to the place where I try to accept things that I can't change. I have often said I have a strong Christian faith and I believe that when my time comes there's not going to be any problem. I feel like if I have lived my life as well as I can and have done as much as I can, then when I go I have no fear whatsoever for the future. I don't fear death at all, and I can say that honestly. I feel that we're in God's hands, and He's the one who determines when we're born and He's the one who determines when we go. I was just thinking: I don't know how many of you enjoy game shows on television, but there's the game show *Jeopardy*. They are having senior citizens on this week. I thought this was rather interesting, because just yesterday they had two women and one man on and they answered the questions and did very well for senior citizens. It was one of the women who won. And in the next game we had two men and one women, and who do you think won? It was the woman. She was way far ahead of the men. I don't know why and I'm not putting down the men, but it was the woman who won, and I wondered if women don't keep their minds more occupied and more active than some men do. This is a question that I've kind of kicked around myself. I think the more active we keep our minds the better we are. We don't think about our bodies if our minds are active. I've had a number of operations and I don't want to have any more. They cut my back twice and I have diverticulitis, so it isn't like I don't have anything wrong with me. I have some problems, but there are other things in life besides that to worry about.

A. ORWIG: Me.

SALMON: And you're together. Isn't that wonderful?

E. ORWIG: It's one of the greatest things of all. I mean, if we have each other and we help each other. You won't believe the things he does for me! He treats me like I'm a little kitten on a cushion and says I mustn't do this and tells me I mustn't bend and I mustn't strain myself.

SALMON: You have something very good. You've got a gift from God to have your husband.

E. ORWIG: Yes, I have a gift from God. I also have a twin sister. She is not married. She is a retired nurse. We are going to be 80 years old next month. If she has said it once she's said it 20 times: "Do you realize we're going to be 80 years old next month?" I never even think about how old I'm going to be. It's very important to her. She never felt old before, but all of a sudden we're going to be 80! My husband and I were married for 17 years before God gave us a child, and He gave us our daughter. She's a missionary in Cameroon, West Africa, and she's in this country on furlough right now. She's away from home because she has so many speaking engagements. On Mother's Day she sent my sister a Mother's Day card, and on it it said, "To my other mother." So my husband always says he married twins. We are sort of a trio. When he takes me out to eat he takes my sister too. We have a really fine, happy relationship. I have so much to be thankful for. So much to be happy about. I'm very, very thankful.

SALMON: Sure, because most people have lost their mates.

E. ORWIG: Yes.

SALMON: Things have happened and these people are alone. Alone.

E. ORWIG: There are a lot of things I can't do because of this back. It used to get me down, but it doesn't anymore because, by comparison, there are other people who are so much worse off than I am. You just have to look around you.

Before we came to Massachusetts to retire we lived in Richmond, Virginia, and we had our home. We had seven rooms and three bathrooms, a large yard, and all of this. And then suddenly our daughter leaves home and here we are. Then my husband got Bell's Palsy and he had other problems and had to retire. Here we are with this big house but spending time traveling around. Then we make the adjust-

ment when we moved from this great big house where we have room to put everything to an apartment with two and a half rooms. It's hard to try to condense the
things that belong to you and that you don't want to give up. That was a very traumatic experience for me to try to give up our home that we'd worked hard for and
then have to get rid of our belongings because we just didn't have room for them.
To adjust at our age to a small place was very, very difficult. I must confess that.
However, we've survived, and again I say you have to accept things that you can't
change. We are making the best of it.

SALMON: But isn't it easier for you not to have to worry about all the big rooms and
cleaning? I think you should be happy.

E. ORWIG: Yes, I'm very happy. My husband does the cleaning, he does the laundry, he
does everything.

A. ORWIG: Aren't you lucky!

E. ORWIG: I certainly am.

A. ORWIG: I'm priceless, darling. As a man I'm also severely outnumbered here.

MASIE EATON: Well, I have such an extraordinarily large family that I hardly know
where to begin telling you how I feel about being old. I just had my 12th great-
grandchild. I feel as if I were somewhat like confetti. I love them all and I keep in
touch with them all as much as I can. Then I have three children of my own: one
son and two daughters. Most of my life seems to be my interest in what they're
doing. I do love young people very much. I think they all seem to get along with
me. I'm thankful that I'm not bringing up teenagers right now. There are teenagers
in my family and they are all great. It's a great, great responsibility bringing up
teenagers. I find that I don't have much time to think about growing old except
when I fall down, as I did recently but only broke one finger. I don't dread the
future, really. I think the trouble I have found is that you come all of a sudden to
find yourself where you are and you think, "Oh my goodness! Is this me?" I'm 84
now and I just think, "Goodness, I never thought I'd get here and still be able to
walk!" I'm so absorbed in my grandchildren and great-grandchildren, and interested in their lives that it keeps me feeling young, really. I was thinking of something really quite extraordinary: Of all these children and grandchildren and great-
grandchildren that my husband and I had, there are 24 babies born from our
marriage and every single one of them has been perfect until the last one, who is a
Down's baby. That, of course, is sad, very sad. But the whole approach to Down's
Syndrome now is so wonderful and people know so much more about it. That little
girl is going to be loved and cherished and taken care of, and there are so many
good things that can happen. It can bring a family together. I think the thing I feel
as I'm growing older is that there is a big hole in front of me. One seems at the edge
of a precipice somehow. I've always been able to look beyond the present. For most
of us, when we begin as children we go from one grade to the next, we go to
school, we go to college, get married, get a job or whatever it might be, and we
have our children. There's always something that's going to be next. And then this
comes along. I think that when you get to be the age all of the people here are, there
isn't any next step. You're just there. If you want to know what will happen next,
nobody can tell you. No one knows.

A. ORWIG: It's all in the Bible, if you really want a source of information, Mrs. Eaton.

SALMON: Wait a minute. Age has nothing to do with it. I'm 86 and I'm shooting for 90, and they tell me the way I'm going I may shoot for 102! So one never knows. Age has nothing to do with it. Eight-four isn't old today. Women in their 80s are young.

EATON: Well, it really depends on how you feel.

SALMON: Attitude again.

EATON: And you can be awfully lonely if you don't have people whom you love and whom you can care about. I don't have anybody living with me, but I know they're available somewhere if I want and need them.

CECELIA MENARD: Well, I don't say that I'm old. I volunteer, you know, and do a lot of different work, visit the patients from room to room in the hospital where I live. I work in the chapel and volunteer for all sorts of things in the hospital.

A. ORWIG: One of the reasons that I'm glad I'm at this age and have lived most of my life already is that things are changing so desperately morally in our country and all over the world. I think that the kids are the ones to be concerned about. We have formed the habit of blaming the administration or the president for everything. I wouldn't want to be president for a million dollars. The guy can't win. I don't know why anybody wants to be president any more. At any rate, the children today are victims, they're neglected, and if they are turning out bad, it's not the fault so much of the kids themselves as it is of their parents and the system. When you think that before they are teenagers, the children are subject to so many things. Parents find it necessary for both of them to work for one reason or another. So the kids are either put in the hands of a babysitter or a day-care center or something like that. What the children really need is parental love and care. So many of them are missing that today. So when you think about growing old, you can just be glad that you didn't have to go through that. What would have happened to us? So now should not we, the elderly, pitch in and do what we can to help to the extent that we have the capability and opportunity?

While my wife and I are not grandparents — and it looks as though we may not be in our lifetime because we have a single daughter who's 40 years old — we have many, many who call us grandma and grandpa, because we love children. And we can just see what's happening to some of them. I just think that instead of worrying so much about the elderly, we ought to worry about our kids and our families. That's where the problem is today. I'm glad that you professional folks are concerned about us. I'm not ungrateful. But I'm just saying that the big problem I see in the country today is the way our children are. We just throw them aside and let them wander around, do drugs, and so forth. The family influence is what we've had the benefit of. So many of the children don't have it today.

SALMON: I think a lot of it is the way we raised our children. What they see, that's how they are going to be. Surroundings, the parents, the genes. Nine times out of 10 you do your best, although even your best sometimes is no good. As far as women going out to work today, they just don't want to stay home to take care of babies. They want it all. They want to have the children and they want to go out. I have a granddaughter: She just had the second great-grandchild and she had a very good job. Now she's waiting for the little one to be able to get on his feet and then, when the children are about 2 or 3 years old, she'll go back to work. She knows a very good nurse, a woman who loves children and knows how to take care of them. They pay for it though — they have to pay high for it — but that's how they're arranging it. Women don't want to sit home.

MENARD: Well, I think that some mothers have to work today.

SALMON: That's a different story for sure.

MENARD: Mothers don't want to leave their children, but they've got to work. Everything is so expensive that even when there's a salary coming in, it's not enough to take care of the family. That's why I think the children are not getting the care, but you can't blame some of the mothers. They've got to work to make both ends meet.

SALMON: I had to do it. I got married, had my one son, and I went out teaching music. One time I came home and the sitter said, "I'm not going to take care of him — he kicked me. I won't come here again." So I thought, "Oh my goodness." His grandmother on the other side — she was a good soul — she took care of my son. That was when he was 4 or 5 years old. As he grew older, I went to live with my sister in a nice home. The surroundings were good. He began to develop good friends and he also got very heavy. I said, "You don't like getting that way, darling. Why don't you let me get you to a good doctor?" I did. He took him under his wing. He wanted my son to take up medicine and my son didn't want medicine. I thought maybe he'd take music. My son didn't want music. He found his own way. He used to sit in his room and say, "Now, if anyone comes into my room, I don't want to be bothered." And we wouldn't dare; he had to study. He got a scholarship to City College of New York, he got a scholarship to Harvard. So you see, it's what's in the children and what they have behind them. If they see parents who are going to drink and smoke and use crack and pot, they're not going to turn out good. They're either going to be despondent and not care or they're going to waste a long life. That's my story.

E. ORWIG: I had a very fine position as an executive of a corporation, and yet when my daughter Carol was born, I resigned and took care of her myself until she started school at age 5. Then when she was in school, I volunteered to do some secretarial work at our church, but I was always at home when she returned.

BOTTOMLEY: Mrs. Siegel, what does it feel like to get old?

ELAINE SIEGEL: Every day is a new day. Some days I get up feeling good, some days I don't feel good, but I keep busy. We do free blood pressure screening with the elderly. That keeps us occupied. I play bridge once a week, go to the library, and take walks whenever the weather is good. We take care of the house and the yard, see the children. Keeping busy is important. Yes, when I look in the mirror I feel old. I know I'm old. I wake up with these aches and pains every day, but they go away. I am 76. Some days I feel 50; nothing younger than 50 or 60. I can do as many things as I could in those days, it just takes me longer to do things.

SALMON: Age has nothing to do with it. Age is irrelevent. I'm going to be 86. I don't feel like it. I have a good family to enjoy; two great-grandchildren. I want to live. So why should I consider the age 86? It's just a state of mind. I don't go by years. Eight-six is only old if you're going to make it old. Eight-six is how you feel. If I want to enjoy my family and my home, people, or my music — which is life to me — then I'm not old until I die. Everybody thinks I'm getting old because I'm 86, but I feel good and I'm going to shoot for 90.

E. SIEGEL: You'll live longer than that. I had a little 5-year-old granddaughter visit me last week. She hadn't seen me for a while. She said, "You're old, grandma!" You can expect that from a 5-year-old. My other grandchildren don't say that and they know how old I am.

A. ORWIG: I feel 81 today. That's how old I am. The reason I feel 81 is that it's raining and my arthritis is bothering me. But other than that I don't really feel 81. I think we've discussed this: Everything is relative, and if you accept your age and the vicissitudes of life that so early befall us, I think you get used to it. It's a way of life. And while I gimp around a little bit and I can't do a lot of the things that I'd like to do, still and all I'm enjoying life. I'm enjoying being married to this sweetheart. Every morning when I get up I look in the mirror and I say, "Are you still here?" And then I say, "Thank you for another day." I think that's an attitude that you develop. You can complain about everything that bothers you and you'll be miserable. You can be thankful for what you still have and be happy. Maybe I'm an optimist.

SALMON: I lost the thing that was most important to me when I lost my left eye. And I only have the right hand now. My music was most important to me. You get over that too if you fight it long enough. What do we live for? For our families and for our great-grandchildren.

A. ORWIG: I'm reminded that I had Bell's Palsy: That's the paralysis of one side of your face. It's kind of like a stroke in its effect. I lost half of my smile. I can't whistle at the girls any more. One day Evelyn had to go to the dentist and he gave her three shots of novocaine for a root canal proposition, and she was looking at herself in the mirror and she only had half a smile. She called me over and she said, "Look! Smile!" So between the two of us we had a smile.

E. ORWIG: Telling this to our only daughter, whom we don't see very often, she said, "Never mind, Daddy, you do more with half a smile than a lot of people do with a whole one." I thought that was rather clear. I can't believe I'm as old as I am. I'll be 80 next month. How old I feel depends on what the day is. If my back is bothering me, then I feel older than I do when I'm feeling very good. I would say that normally I feel like a woman in her 60s . A woman in her 80s has slowed down. It takes longer to do things. Of course, I have a handicap with my back. But I think your attitude has a great deal to do with how you feel. I wouldn't want to be very young. I'd rather be as old as I am than be a child again.

A. ORWIG: You miss too much.

E. ORWIG: I've been a child. It's just not real. In reality I can't even imagine being a child. Life has been good to me. I feel that you get out of it every day what you put into it. I try to stretch my mind a little bit. I read. I think you stagnate if you don't keep your mind real active.

E. SIEGEL: When you get older, you feel as though you are more dependent on your children, and if you have a husband you are lucky: He'll take care of you in different situations. You feel things differently when you are old. You're afraid of being ill and having to go into a hospital. You worry about if you are going to make it through.

SALMON: You don't have to worry about it if there's someone to take care of you. I have a very devoted son, thank God. But if you have nobody when you get older, then that's a different story.

A. ORWIG: We don't know what's going to happen economically. We were married in 1931. We didn't have two nickles to rub together. It was just a question of the times back then.

E. ORWIG: There were bread lines in New York. We were living in New Jersey. I had a job and a lot of people didn't. The company my father was working for closed down — they went bankrupt — so my father had no job. He had always wanted to have a chicken farm, so he decided to come up to Hopkinton, Massachusetts, where my older sister lived, and start a chicken farm. He bought a few chickens and started them, and then he had a heart attack and died. He never did have his chicken farm. There was no money. Al and I were keeping company. He had only some part-time work, so I couldn't very well move to Massachusetts and give up my job. So we got married. It was convenient: Two could live as cheap as one, you know. Besides, we were helping our parents. I guess I was making about 30 dollars a week.

MAX SIEGEL: Boy, that was a lot of money! Most of the men were making maybe 5 or 6 dollars a week. It was enough just to get by. If two people were working at 10 dollars a week, you could get by in the 1930s.

E. ORWIG: I was a very good secretary. I couldn't afford to give up my job. We had kept company for 3 years before we decided to get married in my father's house. That was the last day I saw him alive. Since that day, it's been step by step. God's taken care of us and I expect He'll continue to do so.

MENARD: I'm 86 years old. I wish I could be just 40. It's a hard life. I keep busy all the time. I have a strong faith in God. I come from a family of 10 children. My mother passed away at 45 and I had to take over and become a mother. The youngest one was 5 years old. I took care of them and brought them up. And fortunately there's 9 of us living and many children. It's wonderful. We weren't rich; in fact, we were poor. I had to give up school in the seventh grade to help my family. At my last position I worked at a hospital in central sterilization. That was quite an experience.

EATON: In June I'll be 84. I feel about 50.

LINDEMANN: I'm 75. It's difficult to tell how old I feel inside. All of a sudden you realize that you're slowing down and you can't always do what you used to do. Sometimes I feel like a hand-me-down, too old to be useful for anything. Right now I feel 102. I still think it would be nice to be younger again, even as young as a child. When I am with small children, I forget my age and enjoy the same things they are enjoying.

M. SIEGEL: I'm 75. Today I feel about 80. Yesterday I felt about 40.

E. SIEGEL: I'm 9 months older than he is. I feel about 60. That's a good age.


FAMILY AND OTHER SUPPORTS

SATIN: How do older people handle illness and disability? Whom do they turn to?

E. SIEGEL: I have two sons. One lives in Washington and one lives here. The one that lives in Washington always says, "Don't worry, Ben will take care of you. He's nearby." It seems that sons are always busy with their own families. I don't think that we should infringe on them with our illnesses or bother them because they really have their own lives to live and they have their own children. I thought it would be so nice to have a daughter. I sometimes think that daughters are closer than sons, show more concern, and willingly provide more care.

SALMON: Don't daughters have their own families too? They want to go out and be on their own, and they're busy too. At least you have somebody to rely on. To just get old and have nobody. . . .

M. SIEGEL: You can always fight with your daughter, but you can't fight with your daughter-in-law. There's a difference there. She is not your child. With your child, if you feel like reprimanding them or agreeing with them, you can. With your in-laws you have to bite your tongue and measure every single word.

MENARD: Oh, I wouldn't say that. I have a daughter-in-law. She's so nice she's like a daughter to me. I have my own daughter, but she has emphysema and has to have oxygen at all times, so I don't see her very much. I'm very sad. I feel very bad for her.

SALMON: My son is a very busy man, but he finds the time to call me from an airplane and say, "I'm just boarding and I'll be with you there." He has time and he always knows where I am. I don't bother him always. I'm well taken care of, but there are just some things you'd like to share when you are going through them.

E. SIEGEL: Oh, I understand. We have Ben, but we don't want to bother him sometimes. If you need them, you call.

EATON: I think that my three children and my family help. When I need them, they're all there as much as they can be. I don't belong to any church, but always went to church with my father and my mother. We would go there quite often. I haven't found the church helpful to me — I'm not a church person — but, as I said, my grand-children have been very supportive.

M. SIEGEL: How do you feel about burdening them?

EATON: I don't allow myself to burden them.

M. SIEGEL: When you have to become a burden to them . . . that's the thing that bothers me.

EATON: I think that's a state of mind. If you think you are going to become a burden on your children, then you're probably right.

M. SIEGEL: That's what I think ahead about. It's something to think about. I think we all think about it too: becoming a burden to our children. And we don't know what the answer is.

EATON: Well, I never feel as if I'm going to be a burden to them. I don't mind them say-ing to me, "Don't talk about nursing homes or anything else. When the time comes we'll talk about it, but not now." Of course I don't want to be a burden to them, but if I become more of a burden than I can talk about, what am I going to do? They won't let me leave my home until the health-care system provides much better long-term care than it does now. Until then the family's all together. That's the way it works for me.

SALMON: I'm most certainly not a burden to my children because they are living their lives the way they want to. And I'm at a very good nursing home. If I were home, would they stay home with me? They don't have the time and they probably wouldn't want to do it. I wouldn't be given the care I'm given here. When they have the time, they seek me out. I don't seek them out but I see them regularly.

M. SIEGEL: You're very lucky. Because economically your children can afford to keep you in your nursing home. I've seen some homes that are really disastrous. Yours is a nice place. That's why I'm saying you're lucky.

SALMON: I don't deny that. All the homes aren't like mine. I came from a home that wasn't quite as good. We got good care, but my children couldn't see me.

E. ORWIG: We are fortunate enough. The reason we came to Hopkinton is because I have a large family. My sisters and brothers have a lot of children. We have nieces and grandnieces and great-grandnieces now, and they are all around us. And that was the reason we came. It was at their insistence that we moved back to Hopkinton, where they can keep an eye on us. I had to have back surgery twice. We were away and we didn't have anybody, just the two of us. And the doctor said, "You should be around family where they can help you and they always can keep an eye on you." So, we're very fortunate that way. We have burial arrangements and all of that taken care of. And we have our God who loves us and cares for us. I'm not concerned about burdening my family.

A. ORWIG: We live it a day at a time. We originally had a little money set aside. We thought we had our lives taken care of. But with medical expenses and all, we had to pay our own way, so we don't have a lot of money set aside any longer. I think that there are so many variables. How do you know what tomorrow's going to bring? And why should we worry ourselves sick — sicker than we are — about "what happens if . . . ?" Running up big expenses is the thing that really concerns us, but what can we do about it? I'll tell you one thing I'm not going to do is, I'm not going to go down to the garage and turn the car on. That would violate my faith in God and be contrary to the teaching of the word of God, the Bible.

E. ORWIG: That's not my solution either. Everybody to his own taste.

A. ORWIG: I don't anticipate that our daughter is going to be in any position to bail us out. She doesn't make any money. She's dependent on other people to pay her way because she's not on a salary. So she's not in a position where she could possibly give up what she's doing. She's educated: a teacher by profession. I don't look to her to take care of me in my old age, although she would be willing to do so. Now, she's very much concerned about us, including being happier when we moved to Hopkinton. Believe it or not, I have something like a hundred in-laws living around Hopkinton. Like Evelyn, I put my faith in the Lord. He has taken very good care of us so far, so why not trust in Him to work it out for the future?

E. ORWIG: If one of the family won't take us, another one might.

A. ORWIG: They've been very solicitous of our welfare.

E. ORWIG: We might have to let them take us in. But we don't know what might happen and we don't want people worrying about us. Anything could happen.

MENARD: The way I look at it is, I put my life in the hands of the Lord. I came to the chronic disease hospital because Dr. Kay was my doctor at the community hospital. He was afraid that if I went home I'd get the same illness that I had. I really can't depend on my children. The way I look at it, they have problems that I don't need. My daughter is an invalid. She used to smoke and 8 years ago she had to stop. She developed emphysema and now she has to be on oxygen for the rest of her life. So I can not get any help from her. I wish I could help her.

EATON: We all fear that we might become a burden to our children. I grew up in a family where we never had to really deal with that. I've always been in a family that had older people living with them. My great-grandmother and my grandmother were always a part of the family. My grandmother took care of her mother for 10 years before she died. My mother lived with us for 5 to 6 years before she died. In my time both my daughters and my son say to me, "You'll never be a burden to us. Never. We love you, and if the time comes that we need to take care of you, we will." I guess that's what caring is all about. I never have the feeling that I'll be a burden to them, but I could be wrong. My family always says, "We'll take care of the situation if it comes along." They love me and will take care of me, regardless. We can work things out. It's always been surprising to me when my friends say, "Oh, you don't want to be a burden to your children, do you?" Had all the people experienced what it is like living with your mother and grandmother while growing up, they'd surely have no question about what they would want for their parents. The family is always there. If you don't have that family there, then you need to talk about it.

M. SIEGEL: You said something about burdens. My history is my father got sick and had his leg amputated and went through a whole lot of different kinds of illnesses. I distinctly remember he was at our house and my wife had to give him shots of Novocaine and morphine for pain. And he used to say to me . . . I'm at a loss now. That's something that I always remember, and I never want my kids to go through that. I remember when he was dying. It was at the Jewish Memorial Hospital. Elaine and I stayed by his side until he actually died. No one else in the rest of the whole family did that. Okay, so she may tell me to be quiet, but it seems we always have the burden. And I know that in everybody else's family there always is one that seems to have the burden of taking care of the elderly in that family. It isn't fair! That's why I say that I don't want to be a burden to my children. I wished the same thing with my mother. She went through a lot of disability. If you're lucky, you can wake up dead. Then you're lucky. You're not bothering anybody. Now the bother of needing care and of being a burden is something I don't want to think about.

## RELIGION AND CHURCH

SATIN: What about the church as a resource? What part does religion or the church or God play in your lives?

EATON: One of my granddaughters just had a third child, and she's a Down's baby. All the people at the parents' church — which is a Mormon church — have been just wonderful; supportive and helpful in every way. It's a very outstanding community. How they rally around those who don't have as much! They've all helped in ways that one can hardly express. They have offered love to her and to her family.

E. ORWIG: I turn to the Lord when I need help. I long to say that. It's amazing how the Lord has taken care of me, and I give the Lord the credit. My family was poor. We came over from England, a large family. We lived on a farm in Canada. We had nothing. As children we were lucky to survive. And if you were lucky, you'd go to business college and get a job, and sometimes I'd wonder how I was going to manage when I got older and couldn't support myself. I'd think about that a lot: What am I going to do when I get old? And I live it one day at a time. We do not have a lot of money. We're not as fortunate as some other people. We depend on our Social Security and we each have a small pension. I'm amazed at the way we can live and enjoy our lives! We don't need a lot of money. We have enough to live. I don't worry about my daughter. She's a missionary and she's still got her life ahead of her; she's just 40 years old. They have an organization that she's working for where she's a linguistics expert. The organization that she's with has a retirement plan, but she's going to have to depend on the Lord too. We all have to depend on Him for our next breath. We can't take our next breath unless the Lord wills it.

MENARD: I believe in God and I come from a religious family. God was always there to help me. Now that I am old, God is even closer and is still my best friend. Going to church brings me a great deal of joy. I am not afraid of death because I know I shall see God in heaven. If you don't have faith, you have nothing. People don't believe like they did years ago and the way the world is going is sad. The world is in a mess.

SALMON: I know there's a God. It's probably not the same God that you believe in. Its wonderful being Jewish. It's wonderful being able to depend on religion. I could be alone if I wanted to, but I don't feel alone. I feel like I'm with somebody who favors me. God has blessed me with my son, and that is my life. I am older than I feel and I've had a good life. It doesn't matter if your skin is white or yellow or black, there will always be a God for you.

E. SIEGEL: I was brought up in a Jewish home, in a synagogue. My family had a lasting place in the church. It was important to be Jews and live as if we were Jewish. I've been comforted by my faith and I've lived by my faith's rules and all. It's always been there when I needed that strength.

M. SIEGEL: It seems to me it's healthy to be involved in the church, and my wife and I have always done that. We've been out there helping people for the last 10 years. We've been traveling throughout Greater Boston doing free blood pressure screening for the elderly. We not only take care of them when we see them, but we also check up on them to make sure if they need any medical help, they get it. Religion teaches that you're supposed to help one another. We pray for them and, though Elaine won't say it, it's motivation for us.

LINDEMANN: I have difficulty with the way the church exists now. I have difficulty with the concept of God. All religions worship somebody. Perhaps it's not the same God, but they all believe in some higher being. From the Mormons to the Baptists, they all teach the same thing. But I don't often see a lot of learning going on. I view the church more as a community. It should be based in the community, helping each other, living for the betterment of mankind, because within that community we find strength. I have found that in the Quaker church people are not totally concerned with theology. There's a fellowship and people are there for each other. They believe in God and practice what the fellowship offers: love for all people. In order to develop an unquestioning faith, you'd have to ignore the more practical side of living, that is, reality. I go to church on a regular basis and I go for one thing, and that is the community my church offers. I need the strength of that community. When I look to the youth who have no belief in themselves and certainly not in a God, I am worried about their futures. There are many problems that the young need to face today that were never even a consideration for those in my generation. I think the youth in this day and age would benefit from the strength of the community the church has to offer.

M. SIEGEL: I am my brother's keeper.

EATON: This may sound somewhat unconventional, but I question the existence of God. I have very deep faith in something that might be God, faith that there is a higher being that is managing this all. We don't know what kind of being it is or what we'd like to call it. We don't even know if there is a being at all. But I feel very confident that there is something over and above and beyond. I know that it's watching over us. But I can't put it in words. I can't agree with God as such or the church as such, but I can feel this wonderful power that is there when we need it. I don't know about finding that strength. I think it's something that comes from within you. I can't quite conceptualize the presence of a God. But if there is a God, He is surely that power that we feel inside and not some unseen creature in the sky. The word "God" bothers me because it does not inspire anything in me. If you say "God," then I don't believe in it.

E. ORWIG: Did you go to church or Sunday school when you were a child?

EATON: I went to a Sunday school with my friends for about a year and pasted pictures in books. My father and mother used to go to church all through my growing-up years. My father grew up in a family where his mother was Catholic and his father was Protestant. My father said that never was he going to direct his children as to which church, if any, they wished to join. I don't think he attached much importance to belonging to any particular church. I never joined any church. All my friends say to me, "Why don't you come to church?" But I don't feel the need to. It doesn't help me. I respect people's visions of God, but it doesn't help me to put a face on God. There is a power there that I recognize. But it isn't the church, as far as I'm concerned. However, I confess I was pressured by a friend to join a church some years ago. I went for a while and then stopped.

A. ORWIG: I fell and injured my face, and had a lengthy hospitalizaton with treatments for my injuries and a heart problem I didn't know I had. In the end I had excellent care and a good recovery. I feel God's hand in this. First, I did not know I had a heart problem. I was not driving the car at the time. Had I been and blacked out, it could have been a disaster. Second, I was at a very convenient place when I fell and smashed my nose. Help was available immediately. Police and ambulance were there in no time at all. My wife was notified I was going to the hospital, but just as she was going out the door our doctor called and told her I was being transferred to the second hospital. Coincidence, luck, or God's provision? I prefer the last.

## ILLNESS AND TREATMENT

SALMON: I have two sisters, and I think I am better off than they. Though I have one eye, one arm, and one leg, I'm better off. One sister is two years older than I, and my sister is what you'd call a manic-depressive. She says OK, how are you, and she doesn't care and she doesn't know. You know what I mean? Well, that's not living. And then I have another sister. We had a condominium together for 12 years. Since I got the stroke she's still living there and she's had the whole place fixed up. The piano is still there, but there's no Fay to play on it; it's just a piece of furniture. But she has Parkinson's disease, and that isn't good either. You see now I can enjoy more, and she seems sort of worried about it. She says she has no control over her feet. Well, I have control of one foot and I can go all around, even if I'm in a wheelchair. Am I an optimist? Yes, I'm an optimist, but your health and your attitude are everything. It isn't how you look, it isn't what kind of hair you have but how you look at it. I walk out of the dining room even after breakfast, with my earrings and my makeup because the better you look the more people respect you. And I respect myself. And then they say, "You look so beautiful," and that helps too!

A. ORWIG: As long as you can have a measure of health. Now there are those who are less fortunate than we, or bedridden, or whatever, with not much that they can do. They are just waiting for their time to come, to go into eternity.

BOTTOMLEY: What does it feel like to need institutionalization?

SALMON: Any illness changes your life. When I first came here to the nursing home, I looked around at my room and said, "From now on this is going to be my home." Music and art go together, so I looked around and I started coordinating my colors. I have my television and my tapes and my cassette case. I'm not antisocial, but in a place like this there are so many people that you like and don't like that you have to pick. You're not that free. Bricklaying, well, that's just not my speed; music was my thing. Then there are personalities. I have only one good friend. Now that this renovated dining room is opening, we must sit together, but there was so much confusion down there today that we were parted. I said, "Don't worry, Elsa, I will see that we get together." So you see, in a place like this you can be lonesome and you can be otherwise. It's according to how you go about it.

MENARD: I lived at the elderly apartments. And when I first started there, I got very depressed. The first doctor they took me to wanted to put me in a mental hospital, and my son said, "No, you're not going to a mental hospital." He finally got me into the community hospital. I didn't know when they took me to the hospital and I had a psychiatrist. I was in the hospital for 4½ months. While I was at the hospital, I developed ulcers on my heels and they thought they'd have to amputate. My son and daughter-in-law said, "No," so they performed surgery. They couldn't stitch it up; it had to heal by itself. So why did I come to the chronic disease hospital? It was Dr. Kay, my family doctor. He was on the council of the hospital and he advised me to stay at the hospital. He didn't want me to go back to housekeeping again, because he was afraid I'd get the way I was before. When I arrived at the chronic disease hospital I was on the sick ward, oh, maybe 3 or 4 months. Then I went to the rehab ward. One of the doctors gave me the wrong medication and I went down again. They had to feed me and dress me and everything. I told the doctors and the nurses, but they wouldn't listen. Finally, Dr. Kay came from the community hospital to visit me and I told him that they were giving me the wrong medication. So he took me right off of that medicine. There was a great change in me: You can ask Jennifer. Then I started to improve a little, but I had to start to walk all over again.

Isn't that right, Jennifer? And that's why I'm at the chronic disease hospital. That's my home.

SALMON: When you consider it, it's amazing how this nursing home is really a hospital. I don't say they operate here. If illnesses are serious, they take residents to the hospital. But we have a very good doctor here — an excellent doctor. They have meetings, and all the nurses and the supervisors get together and are told up to the minute how each person is. I think it's natural to want your privacy and to want to go out if you can, but if you're too sick you can't go out here just like in a hospital.


## THE HEALTH CARE SYSTEM

BOTTOMLEY: What do you think about the medical system these days? Does it serve the needs of the aged?

MENARD: I don't think so. The president has cut down so much on Medicare and so forth.

SALMON: Long-term care needs a lot of money, money, money.

LINDEMANN: I realize that it's a complicated challenge to devise a health-care system that is fair to everyone, but, with the experience of other nations to guide us, it should be possible. I see medical care in the USA in a state of transition in which competing trends leave a part of the population underserved. Brilliant cures take precedence over basic, primary care and prevention. Medical practice is sometimes conducted as a business rather than as a profession, so that every minute spent with a patient is reckoned in terms of its monetary cost. This is especially hard on the elderly, who come to doctors expecting that they will make time available to hear their complaints and explain the results of their tests in words they can understand.

MENARD: I think they should have the kind of health care they have in England and Canada. I think people would be better-off — at least the elderly. In fact, all people would be better-off.

E. ORWIG: Like socialized medicine?

MENARD: Yes.

A. ORWIG: I don't quite agree with that.

MENARD: No? I had an uncle who lived up in Winnepeg, Manitoba. He was the reverend monsignor. We were talking about the health plan in Canada and he said, "That's the best plan." I've heard several people from Canada and different places talk about that health plan. They're all for it.

SALMON: What does it entail?

E. ORWIG: Well, there are two sides to it. I was born in England. They have socialized medicine there. Of course, I haven't lived there since I was a child. America's my country. But I have relatives in England, and I know that sometimes when people need operations they have to wait up to 6 months before they can even get into hospitals. There are so many demands on them, and they don't have the facilities and the services we get here in this country. Medicare doesn't cover everything. That's not what was promised. But it's better than nothing. And Social Security? We wouldn't be able to live without that.

MENARD: How much does it cost to go to a doctor these days?

E. ORWIG: Forty-five, 55 dollars.

A. ORWIG: But there again you do have something in Medicare. It takes care of a large part of that. Let me give you an example of what Medicare plus Blue Cross/Blue Shield did for me in July of 1987: I suddenly gained 30 pounds of fluid in 2 weeks. Upon consulting my doctor, he had me hospitalized for a series of tests to determine the cause and have me dried out. The specialists consulted finally came up with a malfunctioning kidney — nephritis — and, after 80 years of ignorance, I learned that I never had but one kidney. This somewhat hindered some of the usual procedures for treatment. The culprit that had caused the confused kidney to send certain products into the urinary system instead of the blood was a prescribed medicine I had been taking for arthritis. Various medicines and careful monitoring took care of the problems, and after 2 weeks I was permitted to go home. The hospital bill alone was $6,600. Medicare and Blue Cross took care of all but $3.91, which I gladly paid. In addition to that were the doctors' bills, lab work, and so forth. The doctors were all cooperative. Medicare and Blue Cross paid most of these costs, leaving a reasonable amount for me to handle. Conclusion: Medicare and Blue Cross are still doing a great job for the elderly.

MENARD: What if a person doesn't have Medicare?

A. ORWIG: Well, that's your own fault if you don't have Medicare for doctors' bills.

MENARD: Oh no, I don't agree with that!

A. ORWIG: Well, you had an opportunity to be under Medicare for doctors' bills when you turned 65. I think that we are very fortunate in having as much protection as we do with Medicare and whatever supplement we have to it because the costs are so prohibitive these days. We know that we spent an awful lot of money of our own for one reason or another before Medicare was effective. Going back just a little while, we had insurance programs. I worked as a salesman for a company that had insurance on all the employees. I worked there a couple of years after I became 65. And the first thing that happened when I got to be 65 was that the other insurance companies started issuing endorsements, endorsing me out, removing some of the benefits that I had before because, theoretically, I was going to have Medicare. Medicare, too, has gone through some changes so that we don't have as much as we formerly had. But we do have something. And it's not all that expensive for the portion that Medicare takes care of. The only problem that we have is that Medicare and the doctors and the hospitals don't seem to agree on what's a fair amount of compensation, and we pick up the difference.

I have had another evidence of the goodness of the Lord and the benefits of Medicare and Blue Cross/Blue Shield: I was grocery shopping, took the groceries to the car, then went back to select some geraniums that were outside on the sidewalk. As I reached for a particular one, I stumbled, fell flat on my face, and gouged a big hole in my nose, which bled profusely. They called an ambulance and rushed me to the hospital emergency room, where it was discovered that I also had a fluctuating heartbeat. At my request, I was then transferred to another hospital's cardiac care unit, where my heart was monitored, a plastic surgeon put my face together, and I eventually had a pacemaker installed. After 5 days I was discharged. I had the best of care — top specialists in their fields — all of this based on showing Medicare and Blue Cross/Blue Shield cards. The hospital bill alone was over $13,000. This does not include doctors' and other miscellaneous bills to come. However, the doctors are all filing with Medicare and Blue Cross. The point is, Medicare and Blue Cross coverage will bear the brunt of the expense. Another boost for Medicare!

M. SIEGEL: Medicare, as set up today, doesn't help any of the adults of our age for long-term care. That's one of the sad parts of socialized health care. I think that a lot of people think that if they have Medicare and Medicare supplement insurance they are all set, but they are only set for acute happenings. They are not set for long-term care. If we get sick, we have to spend down all our money before we can get any help from the government. I won't say it isn't fair, because that's the system. But this is the only uncivilized country — or should I say, civilized country that's uncivilized as far as health care goes. Only the United States and South Africa do not care for their elderly. I was reading what a wonderful system they have up in Canada. From cradle to grave. Europe has the same system. There's no reason in the world, I think, that we shouldn't have the same system. What more can I say?

A. ORWIG: Now I agree with our friend Mr. Siegel that we need some kind of catastrophic care and some kind of long-term-care insurance, because the two of us could barely survive now if we had to pay the bills that would accumulate if we have a serious or prolonged illness.

E. ORWIG: It doesn't have to be prolonged. Two weeks and it's $6,000.


## DEATH

SALMON: Do you think of death a lot? Do you think about dying? How do you think about dying?

LINDEMANN: Well, the process of dying I find rather uninteresting. I think when I get to the point of dying, somebody else is going to have to worry about it, because by that time I probably won't know what's happening. If I do know, I don't think it will scare me. I mean, anyone who's lived through a few operations and has had an anesthetic knows what it's like.

SALMON: When people are very sick they want to go, but I cling to life as much as I can. I like life. I love to see the flowers and the sky. I don't like to think of dying at all.

LINDEMANN: Well, when you say, "think of dying," you mean, "think of not being here" or "not knowing who's going to be president next" or "what my grandson is going to choose for his vocation"? Now that bothers me because I want to know what's going on, and the idea of just being pushed out of the world so that other people know what's going on and I don't, that's hard to take.

SALMON: I know exactly what you are saying. That's just how I think.

M. SIEGEL: When the time comes that I feel that I have outlived my usefulness, I'm going downstairs in the garage and then I'm going to turn the car on. We're going together — my wife says that she'll join me. We've spoken about it, too. Really. That's the way I feel, and I'm not kidding. I told my children this maybe 10 years ago. And I'm of sound mind.

E. SIEGEL: We haven't put it in writing.

LINDEMANN: I just wonder how the kids will feel. I would not have liked my parents to have done that. It would take at least 6 months to tie up all the legal stuff. That is, from the perspective of the survivors, death is a long-term proposition. I have one thing very much in common with Mrs. Salmon: If I didn't have money in the bank I don't know what I'd do. I think I'm lucky. I've been planning ahead and in a few years I will go into a place like Mrs. Salmon's, so my children will not have to worry and I won't make such a mess.

SALMON: You talk of old age as if we were all dying, and it doesn't have to be like this. It would be a shame to take your own life if you could go on living. You have to keep on living. I wouldn't want to give up life for a minute. Even if it's just to wheel down the hall of the nursing home for a cup of coffee and know we'll all be laughing and talking and telling jokes. And you feel that your fellow residents become your family, so your family is always near. If they told me I only have an hour to live, I'd want to have that hour.

## CONCLUSION

SATIN: It seems to me that we need at least another 2 hours, maybe another 2 years, to discuss all of these issues. I hope that people will think these issues over and add any additional ideas and thoughts.

BOTTOMLEY: Remember, this is going to be a chapter in a textbook used to teach people to *be* health-care professionals for the aged.

SATIN: This book will be read by nurses, social workers, occupational therapists, physical therapists, pastoral counselors, ministers, physicians, administrators, planners, and others. You all, as older people, need to tell these students how to prepare themselves to care *well* for older people. So give your ideas and your advice to them about what they need to know, how they need to learn, and how they need to prepare. In our course at Harvard, "The Clinical Care of the Aged Person: An Interdisciplinary Prespective," we ask each of the students to rate each of the sessions: evaluate how good and helpful it is. Meeting with you and hearing from you has always been rated as the best, most educational session of the course.

BOTTOMLEY: Thank you all for educating us all. Thank you for giving us your time.

SATIN: We hope to see you all again next year.

M. SIEGEL: The Lord willing.

# I
# Clinical Issues for the Individual

Part I of the text addresses the health problems of the aged as individuals — the influences of the aging process, illnesses, treatments (including prevention, acute care, and rehabilitation), and the sick role — and assesses the impact of social, economic, and institutional factors.

In Chapter 2, Physical Health Problems and Treatment of the Aged, Barbara Blakeney, a nurse clinician and specialist in geriatric nursing, and Terrence O'Malley, a primary-care internist, explore the major physical health changes that accompany aging and the diagnosable illnesses more commonly found in this population group. In describing both preventive and acute-care treatment, the authors emphasize the importance of a vigorous and optimistic approach to the health care of the aged. Significantly, they demonstrate the complementary contributions of physicians and nurses — the pathophysiology, diagnosis, and medical treatment of the physician on one hand, and the patient education and functional support of the nurse on the other — and thereby illustrate, on a small scale, the benefits of the interdisciplinary approach.

Chapter 3, Emotional and Cognitive Issues in the Care of the Aged, is written by a psychiatrist with both geriatric and community mental health backgrounds. Thus, it presents an unusually broad perspective on the biological, intrapsychic, interpersonal, and socioeconomic issues affecting the well-being of the aged. In explaining the normal changes that occur in the lives of the aged, the reactions and adjustments they must make to expectable life crises, as well as diagnosable pathology, David Satin also addresses the reactions of the surrounding community and society (including the health care system itself) to the aged and their effects on the morale and functioning of these people. Throughout the chapter, the aged are depicted as functioning members of the community interacting with their environments.

The subject of Chapter 4, Oral Health and Treatment of the Aged, is often underemphasized and undervalued in the study and treatment of the aged. Athena Papas, a geriatric dentist and nutritionist, distinguishes the effects of normal aging on oral health from those of common neglect and discusses the influence of dental illness in other body systems. She stresses the benefits of preventive care and treatment informed by current research, including innovative approaches to tooth and gingival diseases and home care. She brings to our attention the opportunity the aged have for maintaining oral health and function far beyond what negative stereotypes suggest.

In Chapter 5, Joseph Scavone, a clinical pharmacist and pharmacologist, applies a clear, clinical approach to Drug Therapy in the Aged Patient. He explores the interaction of physiologic function, illness, and drug treatment. Included among the topics he addresses are: the interaction of multiple illnesses and treatments; the effect of nutritional status and the influence of foods on drug absorption and utilization; and such social factors as cost, custom, and convenience.

Chapter 6, Nutritional Concerns and Problems of the Aged, investigates another subject often overlooked in both clinical education and practice. Johanna Dwyer, a nutritionist teacher and researcher, presents the basic nutritional needs of the aged and their usual nutritional status, based on current research. She addresses the limitations of current knowledge due to biases in available research data and the paucity of data on the nutritional physiochemistry and behavior of the aged themselves. There is growing sentiment that this area is important to the etiology and treatment of illnesses other than simple malnutrition, as well as to longevity and the promotion of good health in general.

Chapter 7, Principles and Practice in Geriatric Rehabilitation, examines a field of new interest to geriatrics and gerontology. It is customary to think of the aged as deteriorating and therefore in need of intensive care for acute illnesses and custodial care for inevitable disability. Jennifer Bottomley, a physical therapist, calls attention to the functional capacity and resilience of the aged and argues for the practicality of care aimed at resuming a functional state. She presents the concepts and terminology of disability and rehabilitation and describes detailed rehabilitation techniques and protocols for some of the most important geriatric disabilities.

Crucial to an interdisciplinary perspective on clinical issues for the individual is David Satin's medical and psychiatric view that the disabilities and disease discussed in Part I are exceptions to normal aging. Although such disabilities and disease become more frequent as people age, older people who seek health care are functioning individuals who simply experience an interruption, distortion, or limitation of function. Caregivers must focus on helping the aged to return to their usual health and activities. Therefore, it is important for caregivers to know about the range of healthful life-styles and functioning aged people can experience. Barbara Blakeney supports this argument from the nursing perspective: We have to remember that the word *disease* means "dis-ease" — a state of discomfort and dysfunction. Disease, whether in old or young people, is not a normal state, and it is no more appropriate for clinicians to accept disease in old people than in young people. A reaction such as, "Well, what do you expect? You're eighty!" stereotypes the aged. Unfortunately, we clinicians easily fall into this attitude if we don't realize that the aged people we treat come to us because they are not feeling well and are seeking treatment to restore them to health. Clinicians must realize that most of the aged function very well for long periods of time and that being old is not — or should not be — equated with being ill. We need to appreciate how great an adaptive reserve the aged have. Jennifer Bottomley confirms that, from the point of view of a physical therapist, the aged are very resilient. Much of what is diminished by illness can be regained with proper rehabilition services. Our attention should be not only on disease but rehabilitation.

Blakeney also contributes the perspective of nursing in focusing on the way human systems change as they age. Each of the chapters in Part I helps us understand how particular diseases affect the function and adaptation of systems that are, themselves, changing. We must also recognize that systems change at different rates and that aged people vary accordingly in their ability to recuperate from trauma or illness. Ultimately, we need to understand that this should inform the way we clinicians apply technical procedures and general caregiving to the aged. Helen Smith adds that, from an occupational therapist's perspective, the gradual pace of change with age in the functional systems gives people a chance to adapt gradually to decreased function. The aged have the opportunity to modify the way they interact with the environment, modify the environment itself, change their styles of living, and gradually adapt their activities of daily living. Blakeney observes that this means, over time, that people can adapt and adjust to changes that are far greater than they could deal with if they happened more abruptly. Satin views this process of adaptation as reciprocal compensation: as one system decompensates, another is mobilized to compensate.

Both occupational therapists, Margot Howe and Helen Smith, agree that this adaptation and rehabilitation may be largely unconscious: People, like the systems within them, can automatically adapt to aging and loss of function when it occurs gradually. Howe stresses that it takes time and expertise to look at all the systems within individuals and comprehend the patterns of strengths and vulnerabilities in order to assist them, which supports the need for a multiplicity of services and treatment disciplines.

Satin points out that any primary caregiver must address not only disease and adaptation but also the effect on health and function of the helping interventions, professionals, and health care system. Health care interventions must be sensitive both to impairments and coping, and therefore must be adaptive rather than maladaptive. Unknowingly, helping interventions may interfere with coping. Howe expands on this: Over time, the aged have developed strategies for coping with life and disabilities. These can be very difficult to understand, and helping professionals may not be aware of them. Therefore, to plan treatment clinicians have to be patient and get to know their clients. Bottomley points out that, aside from treatment, prevention also plays a role in caring for the aged. An important and almost universal factor in aging is inactivity, or "hypokinetics," and thus one thing we health professionals should do is encourage continued activity. Most preventive programs involve exercise, nutrition, dental care, and healthful habits and lifestyles.

Satin encourages clinicians to help the aged themselves not to be "ageist." Even the aged need to be educated about viewing themselves as healthy and functional. On the other hand, clinicians and the aged must not be unrealistic and deny the effects of age, disability, and illness. Howe thinks that, since must of the information we have about the disease and health problems of the aged come from clinical observation and judgment that have not been rigorously researched, we need to recognize that what we "know" starts out tinged by clinicians' expectations about the aged. They are judgments rather than hard facts. Blakeney agrees that, because we don't yet have enough solid research on aging, we are influenced by our clinical experiences and our cultural and social expectations of aging. We have to be acutely aware of how expectation and experience interact.

# 2

# Physical Health Problems
# and Treatment of the Aged

Terrence A. O'Malley
Barbara A. Blakeney

## INTERDISCIPLINARY CARE: A COMPREHENSIVE,
## INTEGRATED, AND HUMANE APPROACH

Ideally, the treatment of physical health problems in the aged is guided by the wishes of an informed patient who can determine the limits of treatment, if any, on the basis of likely outcomes and risks. The impressive and expanding armamentarium of modern health care is of little value unless patients can regulate it for their benefit. The aged are no different from other members of society in valuing their autonomy. Their choices for or against treatment are based on the value they place on extending their lives, avoiding pain, maintaining independence, forestalling financial hardship, making it "easy" for other family members, having a "good death," and other personal reasons.

Perhaps the greatest difference between the aged and the rest of society is the relatively lower value they place on extending life at the potential cost of independence and comfort. It is important for the health-care team to be aware of the patient's goals and primary reasons for choosing a particular course of treatment so that the term's responses will be consistent with the will of the patient.

Comprehensive intervention involves all the necessary disciplines in the development and implementation of the treatment plan. Certain clinical problems lend themselves to predictable courses of treatment, using specific disciplines. Home care and long-term care, in particular, rely heavily on medicine and nursing. However, treatment is often incomplete without recourse to other disciplines. This is especially true in the case of conditions that impair or have the potential to impair function. Mental health services, social services, and restorative services can help return function to the most independent level possible. In the interdisciplinary team model, multiple perspectives from multiple disciplines are guided by the common goals of treatment established by the patient.

Interdisciplinary teams make many important contributions to the care of the patient. One of the most significant is to help the individual cope with the chronicity of illness and disability. Crucial to this purpose are team stability and consistency, which makes possible long-term relationships between patients and their caretakers. Clinicians who know their patients and their patients' families well are better able to respond to changing needs over time and to focus on concrete interventions that help patients maintain as much function as possible as long as possible in spite of the often inevitable advancement of disease.

The health-care team must be prepared to address problems of all kinds: physical, financial, environmental, psychological, and spiritual. Team members must often serve as a source of energy for the patient, who is exhausted from disability, and for the primary caretaker, who bears the responsibility of providing care. In addition, team members must find the time to support and energize each other so that each can continue to enhance the skills and energy of the team as a whole.

### Extent of Care

Explicit goals of treatment are essential in formulating a plan of care. Three commonly pursued goals of intervention are (1) the improvement of function, (2) the prolongation of life, and (3) the enhancement of comfort and prevention of suffering. All three may be appropriate for an individual at different times in the course of an illness.

The process by which treatment goals are established is as important as the resulting plan. Treatment goals represent a consensus reached by the patient, family, and clinicians about the costs and benefits of different treatment options. These goals may remain unaltered despite changes in the patient's condition, but, more commonly, they evolve to take into account changing prognoses and the development or resolution of complicating illnesses. The goal of prolonging life may be replaced by that of maintaining comfort and dignity when modes of treatment become more painful or less successful or unappealing to the patient or family.

The ethical issues raised in the process of developing a course of treatment are often difficult. The most appropriate role for clinicians is to provide patients and their families with the most realistic prognosis possible and with an accurate description of the treatment options available, their benefits, and their risks. It is not appropriate to establish treatment goals unilaterally. This denies patients the ultimate authority to determine their plan of care based on criteria important to them and their families.

It is also critical that all the members of the interdisciplinary team be aware of and feel able to support the treatment decisions made by the patient, family, or guardian. The inability of clinicians to support legally available options of treatment or nontreatment supported by the patient may require them to withdraw from the patient's care. What constitutes "extraordinary means" to one member of the team may not to another. The clinician who defines hydration as "basic" may find that belief challenged by those who feel it is "extraordinary" intervention. It is important that team members share a common understanding of such issues. They must support each other as well as the patient and family if they are to stay together over time.

Some patients pose distinctive challenges. Treating the depressed patient, for example, requires special care as well as attention to the issue of autonomy. It is possible to undertreat a depressed individual who appears competent but who is acting inappropriately because of depression. Before agreeing to withhold further treatment at the request of a depressed patient, it is essential that the depression itself be discounted and the wider context of comfort, dignity, and prognosis associated with existing conditions be considered independently of the patient's expressed wishes. This is not to imply that depressed patients do not have the same right to determine their own care as nondepressed patients do. However, clinicians must be careful not to become unsuspecting participants in a patient's self-distructive behavior.

Incompetent patients are another group whose care is especially difficult. In particular, their problematic care raises the issue of substituted judgment. Formal and informal mechanisms exist by which appropriate treatment goals can be established when a patient is unable to participate in their formulation. Often clinicians deal in an informal way with the family. A spouse or other close relative provides an interpretation of what the incompetent patient would want done if able to express a preference. The assumption underlying this approach is that the family member has the best knowledge of the patient's previously stated wishes. However, there are circumstances in which financial gain, fatigue, depression, and other personal reasons drive the family member's decisions. In cases where close family ties are absent or consensus is not possible, the courts, through formal proceedings, can appoint a guardian to make decisions on the patient's behalf. Indeed, guardianship allows incompetent patients to have treatment recommendations refused on their behalf, thereby sparing them from procedures that competent individuals have a right to refuse. For a more extensive discussion of guardianship, see Chapter 11, Legal Issues in the Care of the Aged.

Treatment goals should be established for elderly patients while they are most able to participate in the process. In a growing number of states, hospitals and primary-care providers are required to furnish their patients with the opportunity to establish health-care proxies and identify individuals who would make decisions on the patients' behalf in the event of their incapacitation. Clinicians must spend time with their elderly patients to help them choose a proxy and to discuss their views on various treatment options. The attention paid to these issues while the patient is mentally alert will assist everyone as the illness progresses.

Once clarified, the patient's wishes must be made known to all concerned caretakers. This is particularly true for nursing-home patients who have access to a level of care exceeding that of elderly persons living at home and who are usually more ill and functionally impaired. We have found it useful to establish five operational levels of care each of which defines what is referred to as the patient's treatment status. The following scale could serve as a guidepost for management of nursing-home patients.

*Status 4:* The patient is to be hospitalized for any treatments that exceed the nursing home's capabilities and that are necessary to prolong life or maintain comfort. Such treatments are to include resuscitation and surgical intervention.

*Status 3:* The patient is to be hospitalized for any treatments that exceed the nursing home's capabilities and that are necessary to prolong life or maintain comfort. Such treatments are not to include resuscitation. Surgical intervention is limited to conditions with a high probability of a successful outcome.

*Status 2:* The patient is not to be hospitalized but is to be treated in the nursing home and to receive all interventions necessary to promote comfort and a successful resolution of illness. Such interventions are limited by their availability in the nursing home but include diagnostic tests, hydration through nasogastric tube feedings, IV fluids if available, and IM or IV antibiotics.

*Status 1:* The patient is to be treated only in the nursing home and is to receive interventions to promote comfort and empirical treatments for presumed infection that are limited to oral medications. No diagnostic testing is to be performed, nor NG-tube feedings.

*Status 0:* The patient is to be treated only in the nursing home. Interventions are limited to ensuring comfort. No treatments are to be given beyond those necessary to relieve or prevent pain.

These levels of care serve as approximations in determining the initial management of emergent problems. It is essential that the treatment status for each patient be established by means of discussion with the patient and family. A status should not be imposed unilaterally by the health-care team. Because these levels are approximations, they need to be restated and clarified as conditions change. The treatment status derives from the clearly stated goals of treatment and, as such, helps the team to focus on the specifics of care. The most recent treatment status should be noted clearly in the patient's record and all team members by some method alerted when the status changes.

Articulation of the goals of treatment facilitates the choice of interventions. Often, impairment of function is an even more important result of illness in the aged than is shortened life, so generally clinicians address both function and disease, choosing certain interventions to interrupt the pathophysiological process of disease, and others to enable the elderly patient to function as independently as possible. Frequently, the latter interventions are the most clinically significant because of the irreversibility of many chronic illnesses, such as stroke, dementia, advanced cancer, and end-stage cardiac, renal, and pulmonary disease. Also, many diseases result in a "final common pathway" of disability for which generic interventions directed at functional status are most appropriate. Functional status — the ability to perform the activities of daily living — often serves as a useful benchmark for choosing the type and intensity of interventions. (See Chapter 9, Work, Productivity, and Worth in Old Age.)

Interventions to augment functional status have benefits beyond their impact on the patient. They also help support the primary caretakers and maintain the elderly patient's informal support network. These interventions include personal-care services (e.g., homemakers, home health aids, and meal service), transportation services, restorative care services (i.e., physical and occupational therapy, adaptive devices, and modification of the physical environment), medical and nursing care, and supervisory services (i.e., guardianship, conservatorship, and the power of attorney). Interventions targeted specifically at reinforcing the support network include the provision of respite services, support groups, counseling, and access to the health-care team for ongoing advice and information regarding the prognosis and the anticipated needs of the patient.

In the following section, we review the common physical problems of the elderly in a brief and limited way, simplifying a number of concepts and omitting discussion of many conditions, in order to acquaint the other members of the interdisciplinary team with the basic issues involved in the medical treatment of the elderly. We have organized our discussion according to the general organ systems, offering a brief description of their function and physiology and the associated changes that occur within each system as the result of normal aging. In addition, we describe the more common illnesses associated with each system and discuss their incidence, their significance, and their impact on functional status. Finally, we examine appropriate interventions.

This format does not lend itself to the discussion of several significant problems of the elderly that involve multiple organ systems — for example, incontinence and falls. The reader is referred to the references at the end of the chapter for definitive reviews of these issues.[1-4]

## THE CENTRAL NERVOUS SYSTEM

The central nervous system (CNS) processes information from the senses and controls movement, cognition, and behavior. Injury to parts of this system result in significant functional impairments, including reduced strength, inability to stand or walk, and poor coordination of the fine movements required in dressing, meal preparation, and personal hygiene. Even more significant impairments include altered perception, cognition, and behavior. Substantial behavioral changes, such as confusion, poor memory, altered judgment, deteriorated social skills, paranoia, and decreased ability to engage in social relationships, can create needs for supervision and personal-care services that exceed the capabilities even of long-term care facilities. Because it is so difficult to provide adequate care in the home setting to such cognitively impaired individuals, dementia is the leading cause of placement of the elderly in long-term care, having a devastating impact on the family as well as on the aged individual. CNS impairment is a primary cause of functional disability in the aged.

### Normal Aging

The process of normal aging results in a gradual decrease in the size and number of cells in many locations within the CNS. Autopsies and computerized tomography, or CT scans, have shown that the size and weight of the brain decline with age. Metabolic activity, as measured by oxygen consumption and blood flow, slows, and the rate of conduction of the peripheral nerves declines steadily. However, although there is a continual diminution of the components of the CNS over time, there is no associated neurological deficit that can be ascribed solely to aging. Despite the many physical changes in the CNS and the peripheral nervous system, normal aging does not result in significant neurological impairment or in impaired function.

The functional impairments resulting from CNS dysfunction can be severe. They can be categorized according to changes in cognition (affecting, for example, judgment, comprehension, and memory), changes in sensory input (producing, for example, blindness, deafness, and neuropathy), and changes in the ability to execute actions (leading, for example, to paralysis, gait disorders, loss of coordination, incontinence, and aphasia). Reduced capacity in any of these spheres can be the consequence and cause of alterations in psychiatric performance as well.

Many diseases can lead to CNS impairment. Some are preventable, and early medical intervention is essential. Others are relentlessly progressive, and because they do not respond to disease-specific interventions, they call for interventions directed at achieving the individual's maximum functional level.

Following is a brief and greatly simplified survey of the more common types of neurological disease in the aged. More extensive discussions are available in general textbooks of neurology.

## The Senses

Communication with the external world occurs through the senses: The ability to see, smell, taste, touch, and hear are the primary means by which one remains aware of and interacts with one's environment. Although the senses often function in concert, it is only recently that they have been studied together. Because the senses are not yet viewed as a single area of clinical specialty, the interrelationship among them is often not understood.

The senses age differently. Some, such as the sense of touch, do not decline, if at all, until extreme old age. Others, such as hearing and vision, begin to decline as early as midlife, with significant changes occurring by the age of 65. Impaired sensory capabilities can contribute to depression, confusion, dementia, anxiety, and poor self-concept.

HEARING. Sounds provide the major means of communication between people, allowing certain forms of intimacy, sharing of concerns, and closeness. Significant losses in hearing will thus severely impact social interaction, independence, and environmental safety. Hearing impairments constitute the largest chronic physical disability in the United States, where an estimated 6 million people suffer from some kind of hearing impairment severe enough to produce a level of social handicap. Among the aged the most common cause of auditory loss is presbycusis, the progressive bilateral loss of high-tone hearing, which occurs because of degenerative changes in the auditory system.

The loss of high-tone hearing in presbycusis leads to a progressive inability to understand speech. Parts or whole words are lost because they are made up of high tones or because of interference from background noise. Hearing aids and surgical implants provide some relief, but often the hearing loss can be only partially ameliorated because of mixed etiology, which in fact characterizes most cases. The clinical focus should be on improving and maintaining as much hearing capability as possible and assisting the aged person and the family to adapt to its limitations by substituting forms of communication or environmental stimuli that will compensate for the hearing loss that remains. The clinician needs to be mindful of the effects of hearing loss on all aspects of the aged person's life. Failure to consider these effects when evaluating depression, confusion, possible attention span deficits, and a variety of other clinical problems, may lead to less than adequate clinical intervention.

VISION. Our society depends heavily on visual cues. Much of our communication is through visual images such as the written word and television, and the nonverbal communication of facial expressions and body language. Vision allows for the identification of much that is in one's environment. It is essential for environmental safety, independence, and mobility.

With aging, several structural changes occur in the eye that result in the decline of visual acuity. Many of these changes begin at age 40 and progress steadily over time. The characteristically slow progression allows for gradual accommodation to declining function. However, the cumulative effects of the process of decline can result in loss of independence and mobility.

The lens ages early so that, by the age of 50, most people will exhibit some signs of degeneration. The normally clear lens becomes discolored, opaque, and rigid. In addition, certain ligaments and muscles that control the movement of the lens relax, limiting the ability of the lens to focus on near objects. Gradually the lens becomes rigid and flat, a condition known as presbyopia, resulting in a lessening of visual acuity and constriction of the visual field.

As the lens ages, the risk of cataracts increases. Because the lens is clouded, light rays entering through the lens scatter, causing glare, which can be very disorienting. Also, as the lens thickens, the anterior chamber becomes more shallow, increasing the risk of acute angle-closure glaucoma.

With increasing age, less light reaches the retina. As a consequence, more light is needed to be able to see, and more time to adapt to sudden changes from bright to diminished light. Age also affects color vision. Discoloration of the lens leads, for example, to filtering of blues and greens. The decline in color vision may affect any part of the color spectrum.

Over time, atrophy of orbital fat produces some recession of the eye. This leads to the characteristic sunken-eye appearance known as enophthalmos, which is often accompanied by a deepening of the upper-lid fold and slight obstruction of the peripheral fields. The skin of the upper lid also tends to relax, causing the upper lid to drop onto the lashes; this results in some restriction of the lid and leads to an upper-lid ptosis, or drooping. When severe, such a condition will limit vision for objects above eye level, such as traffic lights and stop signs.

Tear production also declines with age. If there has been sufficient relaxation of the lid, the direction of the tear duct will change as well. Normally, the direction is inward, toward the eye itself, but with relaxation, the direction is changed so that it is focused away from the eye and exposed to the air, causing excessive tearing. This condition, if pronounced enough, leads to senile extropion, in which the lower lid is separated from the lower protion of the globe, and to chronic irritation of the conjunctive. Entropion, or the turning in of the lower lid, may also occur, resulting in irritation of the cornea and conjunctiva. Sever cases of either entropion or extropion require plastic surgery for correction.

Retinal detachment, vitreous hemorrhage, macular degeneration, and glaucoma are all more common in the aged and can result in severe visual impairment. Laser and surgical techniques are available to correct these conditions or delay further impairments in some patients.

TOUCH. The act of touching provides important information about one's environment and is an important means of communicating. The aging process often leads to a general decline in tactile sensitivity. This is discussed more fully in later sections.

SMELL. A close association exists between the sense of smell and human behavior. Olfactory memory is very powerful and can elicit strong emotions. The effects of aging alone on the sense of smell are minimal, although, with age, there is a marked decline in the number of nerve fibers to the olfactory bulb. Eating is perhaps the most directly affected activity when olfactory acuity declines. Because the flavor of food cannot be detected without the sense of smell, the aged person suffering a loss of smell may complain that food is tasteless. For the person with olfactory loss, the taste of hot foods is more easily perceived than that of cold foods. As with all of the senses, smell serves to promote safety by signaling potential danger, such as exposure to smoke, toxins, or contaminated food. Methods to compensate for the loss of smell include the use of smoke detectors, careful labeling, and the removal of all hazardous chemicals from the environment.

TASTE. The sense of taste is closely associated with those of smell and vision. How food looks and smells enhances or detracts from its taste.

Taste buds located in different areas of the tongue are responsible for perceiving four basic flavors: bitter, salty, sweet, and sour. Any pathology affecting the tongue also affects the sensory capacity of the affected areas and hence the perception of certain flavors. Sensitivity of taste also declines with age. For those who smoke cigarettes, their habit is a factor in that decline. Partial compensation for the loss of taste can be achieved by serving food that is more visually appealing, serving foods hot, increasing the use of herbs and spices to enhance taste, creating an enjoyable social and physical environment, and maintaining good oral hygiene.

## CNS DISEASE

### Organic Brain Syndromes

Cognitive disorders of all types account for nearly two thirds of nursing home admissions and affect a significant majority of the aged who are incapacitated by illness.[5–6] Severe cognitive dysfunction may not reduce an individual's longevity, especially if meticulous attention is given to treatable complicating illnesses. As a result, the aged with cognitive dysfunction make up the largest group of functionally disabled individuals. The conditions producing alterations in cognitive function – called organic brain syndromes – can be divided into several groups on the basis of reversibility and chronicity.[7]

DELIRIUM. Acute cognitive dysfunction with rapid onset, without underlying damage to brain tissue, carries the best prognosis for recovery. Such dysfunction results from toxic or metabolic derangements that affect the normal functioning of the brain, causing the acute confusional states known as delirium. Susceptibility to toxic/metabolic delirium is not limited to the aged; however, the more limited metabolic reserve of the aging brain makes the aged more sensitive than younger persons to minor stresses.

Confusion, restlessness, agitation, poor attention span, reversal of sleep-wake cycles, hallucinations, and paranoia can all be manifestations of delirium. Because subtle changes due to correctable toxic/metabolic abnormalities can persist for extended periods before they are recognized as resulting from potentially reversible causes, approximate interventions are frequently delayed. It is particularly important for these reversible conditions to be identified by the health-care team, because failure to intervene in a timely manner can result in permanent cognitive dysfunction. Equally important is the risk that

Table 2.1    Common Causes of Toxic/Metabolic Organic Brain Dysfunction

Drugs
  Alcohol
  Psychotropics (tranquilizers, antipsychotics, antidepressants)
  Over-the-counter sleep, cold, and allergy medications
  Analgesics
  Antihypertensives (alpha methyl dopa, clonidine, reserpine)
  Beta-blockers (propranolol)
  Antiparkinsonian medications
  Anticonvulsants (phenobarbital, phenylantoin, carbamazepine)
  Digoxin
  $H_2$ blockers (cimetadine)
  Amphetamines

Metabolic abnormalities
  Hypoglycemia
  Hyponatremia
  Hypocalcemia
  Hypothermia
  Hypothyroidism
  Hypoxia
  Vitamin $B_{12}$ deficiency
  Cortisol deficiency

  Hepatic failure (elevated ammonia)
  Renal failure (elevated blood urea nitrogen, or BUN; elevated creatinine)
  Elevated cortisol
  Pulmonary failure (elevated carbon dioxide)
  Hypercalcemia
  Hyperthyroidism
  Hyperglycemia
  Hypernatremia
  Hyperthermia

Mixed
  Multiple abnormalities from above list

inappropriate treatment will result in further functional impairment or a greatly increased risk of injury. Organic brain dysfunction resulting from toxic/metabolic causes usually has a good prognosis for recovery when the underlying abnormality is corrected. Table 2.1 lists the more common causes of toxic encephalopathy in the elderly.

Interventions are directed at identifying and correcting the underlying metabolic abnormality. Although the prognosis for return to baseline CNS function is usually good with correction of the abnormality, the patient's overall prognosis is often determined by the underlying disease causing the metabolic abnormality rather than by the degree of brain dysfunction. However, during a confusional state the individual is more prone to accidental injury; complications such as aspiration pneumonia; and further cognitive dysfunction due to inappropriate use of sedatives, which may aggravate rather than relieve the agitation. The occurrence of any of these complications may worsen the overall prognosis for recovery. Acute toxic/metabolic delirium may coexist with chronic, progressive forms of organic brain dysfunction.

DEMENTIA. Dementias are characterized by the slow onset of increasing intellectual impairment, including disorientation, memory loss, diminished ability to reason and make sound judgments, loss of social skills, and the development of regressed or antisocial behavior. Frequently, depression is superimposed on dementia as a reaction to the perceived loss of intellectual skills, which lead to further cognitive impairment. (See Chapter 3, Emotional and Cognitive Issues in the Care of the Aged.) Although dementias cause a progressive decline in intellectual function, often factors contribute to cognitive dysfunction, such as depression or drug-induced confusion, that are reversible and whose correction results in improved function.

Alzheimer's disease and multi-infarct dementia are the two most common forms of irreversible dementia. Each has a fairly characteristic pattern of onset. Alzheimer's disease usually progresses slowly and begins insidiously. It is not associated with focal neurological deficits or abrupt changes in severity. Patients typically begin with short-term memory deficits, which progress to severely regressed behavior, inability to learn or remember new tasks, and loss of ability to perform the activities of daily living. Multi-infarct dementia is usually of more rapid onset, occurs in younger individuals, and progresses in a step-wise fashion with abrupt worsening and subsequent plateaus of function. Frequently, there are focal neurological deficits, such as paresis and paresthesia. Often, the individual is male, hypertensive, diabetic, and shows evidence of generalized atherosclerosis.

It is important to distinguish between these two types of dementia because the prevention of recurrent cerebral infarction may arrest the progression of multi-infarct dementia, which has as its pathophysiological basis irreversible brain damage resulting from repetitive ischemic injury caused by emboli or bleeding. Normalization of blood pressure is the most effective intervention known. Other reversible dementias, such as those resulting from hypothyroidism, vitamin $B_{12}$ deficiency, and normal-pressure hydrocephalus, can become "fixed" and unresponsive to treatment unless identified and treated at an early stage. Early identification of these "correctable" dementias is essential. Unfortunately, no such therapeutic imperative yet exists for Alzheimer's disease, which is of unclear etiology and without treatment at this time. The identification of an abnormal protein, beta amyloid, which is increased in Alzheimer's patients, may provide a therapeutic approach in the future.

Initial evaluation of an individual with chronic cognitive impairment includes screening for hypertension, atherosclerotic vascular disease, and associated focal neurological deficits, laboratory tests for thyroid function, evidence of syphilis, vitamin $B_{12}$ level, folate level, and cranial computerized tomography.

Once the reversible causes of dementia have been ruled out, the main tasks of the clinical team are to minister to the patient's emotional needs, assist in the act of grieving for lost function, alter the environment so that the patient's remaining skills can be used, augment the patient's capacity to successfully undertake the activities of daily living, educate the family, provide emotional and physical support for the family and caretakers, and provide the patient and family with a realistic prognosis. Any superimposed illness can cause a rapid and prolonged decline in mental status, which may totally resolve as the illness is treated. This decline in function with illness is to be expected and needs to be explained to the family. It should not lead the health-care team to abandon therapeutic plans prematurely.

The cognitive deficits of dementia create functional deficits that require careful anaylsis and intervention if accidental injury or iatrogenic illness is to be avoided. Frequently encountered problems in the later stages of dementia include incontinence, agitation, wandering, and potentially unsafe behaviors such as smoking, cooking, and stair climbing. Progressive inability to swallow can lead to aspiration or malnutrition. Assistance with finances, transportation, shopping, meal preparation, housekeeping, and supervision of potentially unsafe behaviors needs to be instituted early in the course of dementia. The overriding philosophy guiding these interventions is to permit the individual the greatest degree of personal autonomy, consistent with mutually agreed-upon goals of care and safety. These issues are best negotiated with the patient and the patient's family or support system, because it is usually the adequacy of the support system and its ability to tolerate the changing functional impairments that determine the degree of autonomy enjoyed by the patient. The inability of the patient's support system to meet the physical, emotional, or psychological demands of caring is the single greatest determinant of institutionalization and its associated loss of autonomy.

The interdisciplinary team has a key role to play in the maintenance of the patient's support system. It is of course much easier to maintain a support system than it is to create one or to reestablish one that has fallen apart. The guiding principle is to "support the supports," without whom there is no support system. The health-care team can further this goal by easing the burden on the support system. They can do this by reducing the need of the aged for physical care. Being careful to address problems with vision, hearing, dentition, and nutrition, they can promote the patient's maximum level of function. They can lessen physical impairments through physical therapy, occupational therapy, adaptive devices, and environmental changes, which partially compensate for the patient's loss of function. The team must also anticipate new or increasing needs and coordinate the timely planning and implementation of strategies to meet them.

An essential part of case management is to include in planning the individuals who make up the support system so that they are kept aware of the trends and pace of caretaking. This helps the caretakers to feel recognized and sustains their commitment. Emotional support and guidance are particularly important, as are the recognition of burnout in any of the caretakers and the setting of realistic limits on the extent of appropriate care. Recourse to respite care can provide essential release from the burdens of caretaking and help the primary caretakers extend the time they are able to tend to the patient. The care of the patient with dementia is extremely demanding, requiring constant involvement on the part of the entire health-care team.

## Cerebrovascular Diseases

In contrast to the dementias, which result in "global" brain dysfunction, cerebrovascular disease more commonly results in focal brain dysfunction. There are several different types of cerebrovascular disease, each with a different pathophysiological mechanism, prognosis, and treatment. Clinically, it is important to distinguish among them in order to identify those with effective therapies and effective preventive interventions. Early intervention in certain types of cerebrovascular disease can prevent devastating neurological impairment.[8]

The pathophysiology of cerebrovascular disease is characterized by the interruption of blood flow to brain tissue, with resultant cell damage or death from ischemia. Decreases in the heart's ability to pump blood can lead to ischemia, as can blockage of the blood vessels to or within the brain, caused by atheromatous plaques, emboli, or inflammation of the lining of the blood vessels. Uncontrolled hypertension, diabetes mellitus, smoking, and elevated cholesterol contribute to cerebrovascular disease directly by their effects on the brain's blood vessels or indirectly by affecting the heart. It is essential to identify the pathophysiological process by which brain tissue is being damaged so that further injury can be prevented if possible. This process may include the rupture of small blood vessels because of hypertension; the abrupt blockage of vessels by emboli from the heart or by atheromatous plaques in the large arteries leading to the brain; or the spontaneous formation of blood clots within the blood vessels because of local increases in coagulability.

Interventions must be specifically directed at the underlying pathophysiology. Hypertension can be controlled by medication and diet. The prevention of emboli usually requires the use of anticoagulants such as aspirin or warfarin. The risk of bleeding, both into the brain and into other organs, increases with the use of these agents and often limits their use in certain patients. Emboli resulting from cardiac arrhythmias can be prevented by a return to normal sinus rhythm through the use of electrical cardioversion or antiarrhythmics such as quinidine, procainamide, and digoxin. Because of the heightened risk of intracerebral bleeding, anticoagulants are avoided in the presence of hypertension and in strokes resulting from bleeding into brain tissue. On the other hand, abrupt lowering of blood pressure in thrombotic strokes can result in extension of the area of ischemia and further impairments. Despite cranial computerized tomography, angiography, and echocardiography, it is sometimes difficult to determine the exact cause of a new neurological deficit.

Recurrent, small strokes can result in "multi-infarct" dementia, which is second only to Alzheimer's disease as a cause of global cognitive dysfunction. More commonly, however, limited areas of the brain are damaged, which produces "focal" disabilities. These can include loss of motor or sensory function over the right or left side of the body; alterations in vision and speech; and alterations in the ability to interpret sensory input. The extent of the deficit following a stroke depends on the location and function of the injured part of the brain, the degree of damage, and the availability of unaffected regions of the brain that can assume the lost function. Residual effects can be so subtle as to be functionally negligible or so extensive that only the most basic brain functions, the control of respiration and blood pressure, are preserved.

Between these extremes, rehabilitative services are used to prevent further functional impairment. By maintaining abilities that are not affected, preventing the loss of limb motion in spite of paralysis, and motivating patients to take an active role in their rehabilitation, physical therapy prevents further loss of function. By retraining patients in the use of their limbs, teaching them the use of adaptive devices, and improving body mechanics, physical therapy improves functional capacity. Small changes can make a large difference in an individual's autonomy. The ability to drive a car may depend on the development of adequate upper-body strength to permit independent transfer from a wheelchair to the car. The ability to move independently from the bed to a commode may be sufficient to allow an aged person to remain at home. The participation in most self-care may enable the aged person to function at the "extended care facility" level of care rather than at the "skilled nursing facility" level.

The goal of poststroke rehabilitation is to permit the individual to function at the highest level possible. The end point of therapy varies with the extent of the underlying injury and the potential for reversing or compensating for the lost function. What may appear to be small or inconsequential gains from the standpoint of functional ability may be essential to the psychological well-being of the poststroke patient. Loss of control, loss of function, and loss of self-worth usually have a devastating impact on the aged stroke victim. The rewards of even small gains in autonomy should not be underestimated. (See Chapter 7, Principles and Practice in Geriatric Rehabilitation.)

### Parkinson's Disease

Parkinson's disease is a progressive degenerative disease of unknown cause. *Parkinson's syndrome* is the term used to describe the same constellation of anatomical, motor, and intellectual deficits that characterize the disease but that result from exposure to specific agents. The syndrome can be postencephalitic (von Economo's disease), posttraumatic (boxer's parkinsonism), or toxin induced (following ingestion of MPTP), or it can result from the use of neuroleptics or reserpine.

With few exceptions, parkinsonism is a syndrome of the aged. When fully developed, it is characterized by increased limb rigidity; stooped posture; shuffling gait; decreased mental acuity; difficulty in initiating movement; and a tremor, usually symmetrical and rhythmic, that is abolished by intentional movement. Early in its course, however, parkinsonism may produce an asymmetrical tremor, a slight increase in muscle tone with associated decrease in spontaneous movement, immobile facies with loss of spontaneous expression, and generalized stiffness. As these restrictions on voluntary movement progress, they result in significant functional impairment. Associated incontinence and constipation further complicate the management of afflicted individuals.

Benign familial tremor is often mistaken for Parkinson's disease early in its course. Characteristically the tremor is more rapid (7–9 tremors per second) and increases with action. As a result, patients complain of an inability to lift a spoon or cup without spilling its contents. There is no associated hypokenesia or gait disorder. Alcohol, sedatives, and beta-blockers (such as propranolol) effectively reduce the amplitude of the tremor.

In parkinsonism, drug treatment and intensive physical therapy are frequently helpful; however, these interventions do not change the relentless progression of functional impairments. Drug therapy is directed at the amelioration of symptoms at the lowest effective dose. Drugs are of three general classes: those that are anticholenergic, those that mimic the effects of dopamine (such as bromocryptine), and those that replenish dopamine (L-dopa). Anticholenergic drugs, such as amantadine, diphenhydramine, trehexyphenidyl, procyclidine, and benztropine methanesulfonate, are effective in most patients. The side effects include dry mouth, blurred vision, constipation, urinary retention, confusion, sedation, and delirium. They frequently limit the choice of agent and dosage. Bromocryptine has a direct dopaminelike effect and shares the same side effects as L-dopa.

Because the response to L-dopa, the most effective agent, diminishes over time, its use is reserved for the later stages of the disease and is administered at the lowest possible dose. Frequent side effects include postural hypotension, nausea, and the development of dyskinesia and akethesia. Drug treatment is highly empirical and often requires frequent changes in dose, schedule, and drug to achieve the greatest functional benefit with the fewest side effects.

Experiments involving transplantation of fetal tissue into dopamine-depleted areas of the brain have shown promising early results but have not been well enough established to be offered as treatment. The other nonmedical treatment of parkinsonism is intensive physical therapy to maintain strength, avoid contractions, and maintain activity. Despite the progressive nature of this illness, many patients can maintain full function for several decades with a combination of physical therapy and drug treatment.

Two other reversible gait disorders in the aged are normal-pressure hydrocephalus and cervical spondylosis. Although they are relatively uncommon, both are potentially reversible through surgery. If not identified and corrected early in their courses, both can result in irreversible damage.

### Normal-Pressure Hydrocephalus

Normal-pressure hydrocephalus (NPH) presents with the clinical triad of dementia, a slow shuffling gait, and urinary incontinence. Dilation of the ventricles with hydrocephalus is thought to affect the function of the surrounding brain tissue, which controls leg motion and bladder function. CT scans of the head can establish the presence of ventricular enlargement but cannot determine whether it is due to atrophy of brain tissue or enlargement of the ventricles. However, in selected cases that have shown clinical improvement after repeated removal of cerebrospinal fluid, placement of a surgical shunt from the ventricle to the peritoneum occasionally results in resolution of the dementia and gait disorder.

### Cervical Spondylosis

Cervical spondylosis is caused by the impingement on the cervical spinal cord of bony spurs resulting from severe degenerative arthritis. Patients usually develop a clumsy, spastic, and stiff gait, incontinence, and diminished sensation in the legs. Cervical CT scanning, myelograms, magnetic resonance imaging (MRI) can establish the location and extent of spinal cord impingement. Surgical decompression of the spinal cord can frequently interrupt the progression of this condition and its associated severe disability.

### Peripheral Neuropathy

With aging, the number and size of the peripheral nerve fibers diminish with a concomitant decrease in conduction velocity. There is often a clinically insignificant decrease in touch and the ability to perceive vibration. The peripheral nerves, however, are easily affected by nutritional deficiencies, toxins, and endocrine disorders. The resulting neuropathies can cause marked loss of position sense, with resulting instability and falling, chronic pain, and dyesthesia. The list of causative agents is extensive.

The common nutritional deficiencies that lead to neuropathy are insufficient folic acid, as a result of poor diet or folic acid antagonists such as diphenylhydantoin and sulfonamides; inadequate vitamin $B_{12}$, the malabsorption of which can cause pernicious anemia; and alcohol-related deficiencies of thiamine, pyridoxine, and other B vitamins. Toxic neuropathies can result from exposure to heavy metal (such as lead and arsenic), from medications (nitrofurantoin, disulfiram, and diphenylhydantoin), or from uremia. Replacement of the deficiency and removal of the toxin are the cornerstones of therapy.

Diabetic neuropathy can take several forms. A distal sensory polyneuropathy affects the hands and feet, causing diminished sensation and burning pain; a proximal motor neuropathy results in proximal muscle wasting and weakness; and a diffuse autonomic neuropathy results in orthostatic hypotension, neurogenic bladder, constipation, and bowel immotility. In addition to these diffuse forms of neuropathy, single nerves can be affected. The resulting mononeuropathies can cause loss of ocular muscle function and painful nerve-root and branch dysfunction. Treatment is symptomatic and may involve analgesics, physical therapy, and splinting. Relief from painful dysesthesias may be obtained in some cases with the use of diphenylhydantoin, amitriptylene, or carbamazepine. Tight control of the blood sugar appears neither to prevent nor lessen diabetic neuropathy. Rarely, another endocrine disease, hypothyroidism, can present with neuropathy. It responds to thyroid hormone replacement. Other causes of neuropathy in the aged include amyloid and paraneoplastic syndromes, (resulting from tumors of the lung or ovary, and from multiple myeloma).

## THE MUSCULOSKELETAL SYSTEM AND MUSCULOSKELETAL DISEASE

The musculoskeletal system is comprised of the bony skeleton, muscles (with their tendons), and joints (including ligaments and cartilage). The individual experiences gradually decreasing strength, control, and mobility as the components of this system age.

### Muscle

Muscle alterations with aging are complex and poorly understood. The composition of muscle changes over time as myofibrils are replaced by fat, collagen, and scar tissue. Individual muscle fibrils also change as water, sodium, and chloride increase with age. Blood flow to the muscles decreases with age, which reduces the amount of nutrients and energy available to the muscle. Strength declines. This process begins early in life and accelerates rapidly after the fifth decade. By age 60, the total loss represents 10–20% of the maximum muscle power attained at age 30.

### Myopathy and Myositis

Muscle dysfunction in the aged is usually the result of toxic or metabolic factors acting on muscle rather than any intrinsic disease of the muscle. Symptoms suggesting myopathy include weakness in the hip-girdle muscles, making it difficult to rise from a chair, and the development of a waddling gait or shoulder-girdle weakness, manifested by the inability to lift objects above shoulder level. Muscle soreness is not a usual finding with myopathy and is more common with myositis, in which there is infiltration of the muscles by inflammatory cells. Polymyositis can be ideopathic or related to the presence of an underlying carcinoma. Myositis usually responds to steroids or other anti-inflammatory agents.

Muscle weakness can result from several correctable causes, including hyperthyroidism, alcoholism, adrenocortical steroid excess (as a result of Cushing's disease or the administration of steroids), and hypokalemia (from diarrhea or the use of diuretics). Correction of the underlying cause usually results in resolution of the weakness.

## Bones

Aging brings many complex and poorly understood changes in bone structure. Until about the age 45, bone mass increases in both men and women. Over the next 25 years, both show a progressive decline in bone mass, with women losing about 25% and men approximately 12%. Although bone growth continues into old age, reabsorption of the interior of the long and flat bones increases until reabsorption occurs at a greater rate than the formation of new bone. As a result, bone strength and stability decline. This is particularly true of trabecular bone, which is found in the highest proportions in vertebral bodies, wrists, and hips. This correlates with the clinical observation of increased incidence of fractures at these sites with age.

## Osteoporosis and Osteomalacia

Osteoporosis results when the production of new bone mass is exceeded by the reabsorption of old bone. The result is that bone becomes structurally weakened. The greater the bone mass attained at the time resorption exceeds the creation of new bone, the more time is needed before significant structural changes result. This in part accounts for the higher incidence of clinically significant osteoporosis in women than men, because men have greater bone mass. The reasons for the differential rates of demineralization of bone between men and women are in fact not understood, but several factors appear to have a role in the process.

Malabsorption of calcium leads to poor bone mineralization, or osteomalacia, a condition that affects both sexes. Negative calcium balance can result from many factors, such as calcium deficiency in the diet, malabsorption, and accelerated loss. Impaired absorption of calcium from the intestine can be due to insufficient vitamin D because of diet or renal or hepatic disease. Intestinal malabsorption syndromes, such as sprue and regional enteritis, can affect calcium absorption. Endocrine disorders affecting calcium balance include hyperthyroidism; excess corticosteroids, as in Cushing's disease or steroid administration; hyperparathyroidism, which leads to excessive calcium resorption; and hypoparathyroidism, which results in poor absorption. Estrogen deficiency occurring with menopause leads to accelerated bone loss, which can be partially reversed by replacing estrogen.

Immobility for any reason and at any age can lead to marked negative calcium balance. When a limb is immobilized, localized osteoporosis occurs. Thus, for the elderly, decreased mobility for any reason adds to the already abundant factors present for the development of osteoporosis. The presence of osteoporosis requires a thorough review of potentially treatable causes. Treatment consists of a judicious balance of exercise, medication, and dietary manipulation.

## *Joints*

Degenerative changes in the joints begin as early as the second or third decade and after age 40 progress more rapidly. These changes occur mainly in the weight-bearing joints, such as the knees, hips, and lumbar spine. By age 30 the cartilage that composes the weight-bearing surfaces of these joints begins to crack, shred, and fray. Over time, deep vertical fissures appear, and the cartilage-producing cells die or become less active. Ultimately, the cartilage layers erode, exposing the bone beneath to direct contact with opposing bone. This contact causes pain and produces crepitus, or grinding, when the joint is moved. New bone formation is stimulated, but the bone growth is irregular and often interferes with joint mobility as the resulting ostephytes enlarge.

The synovial membranes that surround and protect the joints also exhibit changes due to aging. The synovial lining thickens, and the synovial fluid becomes more viscous. Other changes include the shrinkage of the intervertebral discs in the lumbar spine because of loss of water content in the discs. Coupled with vertebral body collapse, disc shrinkage can produce a significant loss of height.

## *Degenerative Arthritis*

Arthritis is an inflammation within the joint space which causes pain, loss of mobility, and deformity of the joint. There are several different types of arthritis, but many lead to a common final pathway known as degenerative joint disease (DJD), or osteoarthritis. Recurrent joint trauma results in intra-articular bleeding and the release of proteolytic enzymes, which sets up a cycle of increased cartilage damage, bleeding, and the release of further destructive enzymes. Over time, cartilage is eroded and new bone growth stimulated, and the joint gradually loses its ability to respond to trauma, thus becoming more susceptible to additional trauma and damage. Pain develops because of irritation of the periosteum and the joint capsule and because of spasm of the peri-articular muscles. Unlike rheumatoid arthritis, the synovial membrane in osteoarthritis is not primarily involved in this process. However, over time it can become fibrotic as a result of the primary degenerative process.

The joints most often affected by DJD are those of the hands, knees, hips, and the lumbar and cervical spine. DJD is manifested clinically by stiffness and pain, which increase with use of the joints. Impaired mobility makes it difficult to accomplish the routine activities of daily living.

## *Rheumatoid Arthritis*

Rheumatoid arthritis can occur at any age and is characterized by the abrupt onset of symmetrical joint swelling, erythema, and pain. Inflammation of the synovial membrane results in the release of proteolytic enzymes, which perpetuate inflammation and joint damage. Morning stiffness is more pronounced and of longer duration than in DJD. The involved joints tend to be the small joints of the hands and feet, the wrists, shoulders, elbows, and ankles. Eventually deformities occur, affecting mobility and the basic activities of daily living. As rheumatoid arthritis is a systemic disease, multiple signs and symptoms are often present. These include fever, fatigue, malaise, poor appetite, weight loss, nutritional deficiencies, weakness, anemia, enlarged spleen, and lymphadenopathy. Response to therapy is usually quite good. Given the ease with which the aged develop muscle atrophy with disuse, aggressive physical therapy is essential to maintain strength and range of motion.

### Gout

Gout is a form of arthritis that usually affects only a few joints. Needlelike crystals of uric acid are deposited in the joints, tendons, and bursae, inciting a rapidly progressive inflammatory reaction. The result is an abrupt onset of severe pain and the development of an acutely tender and inflamed joint, which can incapacitate the individual very quickly. In middle age gout is episodic, but in later years it tends to occur with greater frequency and in more joints. Gout affects men more than women. It occurs spontaneously or as a result of other illnesses or treatments. Some diuretics used to treat congestive heart failure or hypertension may cause gout because they interfere with the secretion of uric acid from the kidney, thereby causing an elevated uric acid level. Other causes of gout include rapid tissue turnover such as that seen in lymphoma, leukemia, thalassemia, psoriasis, and pernicious anemia. Acidosis of any cause, resulting from diabetes, alcohol ingestion, or renal failure, can also precipitate gout. The treatment is medical, and if treatment is undertaken early in the course of chronic gout, the prognosis for preventing permanent joint deformity is good.

### Temporal Arteritis and Polymyalgia Rheumatica

Inflammation of the small and medium-sized arteries that arise from the aortic arch give rise to a condition called giant-cell arteritis, or temporal arteritis (TA). It is part of a spectrum of conditions which include that of polymyalgia rheumatica (PMR), which is only seen in individuals over the age of 50. Neck and hip-girdle stiffness and pain, an elevated sedimentation rate, low-grade anemia, fever, weight loss, elevated globulins, and rapid response to steroids are the characteristic signs of PMR. Of greatest clinical significance is the high incidence of sudden monocular blindness that can result from the obliteration of the opthalmic artery by arteritis. This potential outcome requires that early and aggressive evaluation and treatment be made of anyone suspected of having PMR/TA. Diagnosis is established by biopsy of the temporal artery to look for evidence of arteritis. The biopsy is positive in approximately 50% of cases; however, a negative result on biopsy does not exclude the presence of PMR/TA. It is a relapsing, systemic disease that usually responds to steroids and resolves over 1 to 2 years. It is one of the most common preventable causes of blindness in the aged.

The development of effective anti-inflammatory medications and improvement of surgical interventions in joint disease has changed the current management of end-stage

DJD. Joint replacement can be very effective in restoring function and limiting pain. Joint fusion and anti-inflammatory medications are often effective in pain control. However, for individuals who are not surgical candidates or who cannot tolerate the side effects of medication, progressive arthritis can be overwhelming at any age. The focus of care for these individuals is on the management of pain and the preservation of mobility and function. As the arthritis progresses, the attention of the health-care team must shift to assisting the individual to cope with new restrictions and limitations on function. The sense of frustration and helplessness that accompanies severe arthritis becomes a major focus of intervention.

## THE KIDNEYS AND RENAL DISEASE

The kidneys are the major modulators of the amounts of water, sodium, and potassium found in the extracellular fluid of the body. They also are a primary route of drug excretion and are important in maintaining an appropriate blood pressure. Alterations in renal function can have profound effects on all of these essential functions.

With age, the amount of blood that can be filtered by the kidneys shows a steady decline. This is in part due to a decline in the amount of blood arriving at the kidneys because of heart disease or narrowing of the blood vessels. It is also due in large part to a decrease in the number and size of the glomeruli, which are the areas of the kidney that filter plasma. The ability of the kidney to reabsorb water and solutes from the filtered plasma also declines. Although these reabsorptive capacities remain, they operate at a significantly lower level in the aged and help to account for the decreased capacity of an aged person to excrete excess water or to retain water in the event of dehydration.

There are eight commonly encountered problems in the aged to which altered renal function contributes: too much or too little water, too much or too little sodium, too much potassium, drug intoxication, and acute and chronic renal failure. All of these dislocations of body homeostasis can result in altered mental status and can be life threatening. All require prompt medical management.

### *Sodium and Water Balance*

The aging kidney has a diminished capacity for excreting large amounts of water because of its inability to excrete a very diluted urine. The water excess that results leads to a dilution of serum sodium, which in turn results in fatigue, lethargy, nonspecific weakness, and confusion. In extreme cases, seizures and coma can result. The use of hypotonic solutions during intravenous therapy frequently causes retention of excess water. Retention may also result from the syndrome of inappropriate antidiuretic hormone secretion (SIADH), which causes the kidneys to excrete a concentrated urine. Head trauma, stroke, pneumonia, and certain drugs can cause SIADH. Several commonly used medications can also induce hyponatremia, including aspirin, haloperidol, chlorpropamide, acetaminophen, barbiturates, and amitriptyline.

Regardless of the mechanism, the results of low-serum sodium can be life threatening and require immediate intervention to reverse the decline in sodium. Since the problem is usually one of excess water rather than decreased sodium, treatment usually consists of restricting free water or promoting the excretion of dilute urine. The addition of sodium through the use of hypertonic solutions is reserved for the most severe cases.

At the other extreme of water balance, dehydration, the aging kidney has a diminished capacity to conserve water by making a more concentrated urine. The consequence of this deficit is that the aged individual is much more susceptible to dehydration in the presence of fever. Because of the concurrent changes in mental status, the effect of fever and mild dehydration may be enough to initiate a vicious cycle in which the aged person, having grown confused and having lost the thirst mechanism, becomes progressively dehydrated and disoriented. Significant dehydration is often an associated finding in elderly persons presenting with illnesses such as pneumonia, urinary tract infections, and strokes. The inability to maintain adequate hydration is often the deciding factor precipitating the admission of these persons to a hospital. Intravenous fluid replacement is often required to regain fluid balance. Frequently, the changes in mental status resulting from dehydration and elevated serum sodium last long after the fluid imbalance has been corrected.

Increasing the amount of sodium presented to the aging kidney results in retention of sodium because the excess load cannot be as effectively excreted as it is by younger organs. Because water retention occurs with sodium retention, an increased sodium load causes expansion of the total extracellular fluid compartment. This results in congestive heart failure, edema, and elevated blood pressure.

Alternatively, the aging kidney cannot correct for a decrease in the amount of sodium presented to the kidneys. The aging kidney loses sodium and therefore is less able to maintain homeostasis when limited sodium is presented to it. What results is a steady decline in the total extracellular fluid compartment, with associated hypotension, dizziness, weakness, and falling.

The reduced functional reserve of the aging kidney makes it less able to correct for alterations of water and salt that would not stress the younger individual. The resulting abnormalities of sodium and water content frequently accompany other illnesses, increasing both morbidity and mortality in the aged.

### Potassium Balance

Excess potassium, or hyperkalemia, can cause fatal cardiac arrhythmias. It is more common in the aged because of several age-related changes in renal function. Aldosterone is the hormone responsible for maintaining potassium balance through its effects on the kidney. It causes potassium to be exchanged for sodium in the urine, with the net result that potassium is excreted and sodium retained. With age, the amount of aldosterone diminishes and so does the kidneys' capacity to excrete potassium. The presence of potassium-sparing drugs or diabetes amplifies these effects. With dehydration, there is both decreased renal blood flow and acidosis, resulting in a marked decrease in the excretion of potassium and a significant shift of potassium from within the cells into the extracellular space. The resulting severe hyperkalemia can cause life-threatening arrhythmias.

### Drug Intoxication

The kidneys are one of the major routes of drug detoxification and excretion. Progressive decline in renal function results in lower clearances for many different types of drugs. Higher serum levels are reached and maintained longer in the elderly than in younger individuals using the same amount of a drug. For many compounds this means that standard adult dosages result in toxic blood levels in the elderly. As a consequence, many of their drug dosages need to be adjusted downward. Among the most important drugs their kidneys retain are digitalis, several types of antibiotics, and oral diabetic agents.

### Acute and Chronic Renal Failure

Acute cessation of renal function can occur at any age, but the diminished blood supply of the aging kidney renders it more susceptible to injury. Hypotension is the usual precipitating cause and can result from dehydration, overmedication, surgery, or sepsis. Acute injury from certain antibiotics or from the contrast dye used in radiology can also result in acute renal shutdown.

Acute renal failure is associated with the rapid buildup of toxic waste products and drugs, fluid overload, and elevation of serum potassium. Any of these complications can be fatal if not managed correctly. In addition, the immune system is impaired; and patients with acute renal failure frequently die as a result of infections.

Chronic renal failure is marked by slow deterioration of renal function and is usually detected when the presence of another illness stresses the renal system and when an elevated BUN (blood urea nitrogen), hyponatremia, or increased fluid retention warrant an evaluation of renal function. The functional effects of chronic renal failure result primarily from anemia and congestive heart failure. Patients with renal disease severe enough to cause significant chronic changes in mental status have a poor prognosis and often require dialysis or kidney transplantation.

### THE RESPIRATORY SYSTEM AND RESPIRATORY DISEASE

The respiratory system functions to ensure the exchange of oxygen and carbon dioxide between the air and the blood within the lungs. This system can be thought of as having several related but separate mechanisms: movement of air into and out of the lungs, the exchange of oxygen and carbon dioxide, and the defense of the lung from infection. Changes with age affect every aspect of the respiratory system.

The chest wall becomes a less efficient bellows with age. The anteroposterior diameter of the chest increases and the rib cage becomes more rigid as progressive curvature of the spine, calcification of costal cartilage, and osteoporosis limit the compliance of the chest wall. The chest muscles atrophy with age and also contribute to the gradual decline in the efficiency with which air is moved into and out of the lungs. The collapse of small airways because of the loss of elasticity in lung tissue with age results in increasing resistance to air flow. As a result, the amount of physical effort that must go into breathing increases by 20% between the ages of 20 and 70.

Although the bronchi are not usually affected by normal aging, the surface area of the alveoli decreases by 4% with each decade of life. The alveolar wall is also thinner and contains fewer capillaries for the delivery of blood. With the loss of elasticity and recoil, the size of the alveoli increases. It is the loss of recoil that creates an increased susceptibility to airway collapse, the major factor contributing to the altered distribution of air within the lungs.

Ideally, each area of the lung where blood is available for gas exchange would be ventilated, thereby giving a perfect match of ventilation and perfusion. With age, larger areas of the lung are perfused but not ventilated because of airway collapse and redistribution of blood flow. This results in the return of unoxygenated blood to the general circulation and decreased efficiency of the respiratory system. Pulmonary circulation may also decline with age, further reducing the capacity of the system to respond to the demand for an increased supply of oxygen to the tissues.

Changing mechanics within the lung and the chest wall also make the lung more susceptible to infection with age. The gag reflex is diminished, which increases the risk of aspiration. Concurrently, the cough reflex is also diminished and the effectiveness of the cough reduced because of reduced chest wall compliance and chest muscle strength. Ciliary action, which normally moves secretions up and out of the lungs, also declines, particularly in smokers. These factors combine to compromise the lung's ability to defend against infection.

Some drugs play important roles in depressing the respiratory system. Sedatives and analgesics, such as alcohol and narcotics, are known to depress respiration and dull the cough and gag reflexes, thus predisposing the elderly person to the risks of hypoxia and aspiration pneumonia.

The two most common types of disease affecting the respiratory system are pneumonias, which compromise gas exchange and serve as a source of sepsis, and diseases that affect the amount of air flow in the lungs, such as chronic obstructive pulmonary disease (COPD) and asthma.

### Pneumonia

Pneumonia is the most common infectious cause of death in the elderly and the most common infection requiring hospitalization. Patients with other serious conditions, such as diabetes, cancer, stroke, congestive heart failure, dementia, and renal failure, often die of pneumonia. The high incidence of pneumonia results in part from the weakening of the local pulmonary defenses with age. However, the high mortality of pneumonia is largely due to its more subtle presentation in the elderly. Typical symptoms, such as a productive cough, fever, and pleuritic chest pain, are frequently absent. More subtle symptoms, such as confusion, alteration of sleep-wake cycles, increased congestive heart failure, anorexia, and "failure to thrive," are the rule. Misdiagnosis and late diagnosis are common and contribute to the high mortality of penumonia.

Successful treatment of pneumonia requires early recognition and institution of proper antibiotic therapy. The identification of the causative bacteria in the examination of a sputum sample is the single most important diagnostic test for determining initial antibiotic therapy. Unfortunately, such samples are often difficult to obtain in a dehydrated and uncooperative elderly patient. As a result, therapy is often empirical and not as specifically directed or effective as possible. Hydration, nutritional support, chest physical therapy, and treatment of complicating illnesses, are often required in addition to antibiotics.

### Obstructive Lung Disease

Conditions that cause obstruction to air flow within the lungs are called obstructive airway diseases. They share the common characteristic of increased resistance to air flow within the airways. Asthma is a reversible obstructive airway disease characterized by episodic increases in airway resistance because of spasm and the narrowing of airways in response to infection, allergic reactions, and environmental conditions. Chronic obstructive pulmonary disease (COPD) denotes conditions of increased airway resistance that are irreversible because of permanent structural damage from cigarette smoking, infections, or toxic exposures.

*Emphysema* is a term used to describe the condition deriving from the permanent destruction of alveoli, and the resulting expansion of the remaining alveoli. In emphysema, the reduction of the area in which gas exchange can occur results in perfusion/ventilation mismatch and hypoxia. Emphysema is associated with increased airway resistance, which is caused by the collapse of small airways.

Chronic bronchitis is a disease process in which chronic inflammation of the small airways leads to increased mucus, airway plugging, and destruction of small airways. As a consequence, airflow is reduced because of the permanent narrowing of the small airways. Often a reversible component of the airway obstruction is superimposed on the chronic changes. Cigarette smoking, the leading cause of chronic bronchitis, multiplies the deleterious effects of other environmental agents, such as asbestos, silica, coal dust, and fibers. Frequently, emphysema and chronic bronchitis coexist.

Patients with obstructive airway disease usually manifest disabilities that result either from hypoxia, hypercapnia, or dyspnea. Both hypoxia and hypercapnia can cause confusion, fatigue, and progressive heart failure. Breathlessness, or dyspnea, is usually the most limiting symptom of COPD. Functional impairment due to COPD can be severe, and COPD is often fatal. Over half of the patients die within 2 years of their first episode of respiratory failure. These patients require extensive therapeutic and supportive interventions.

The treatment goal for individuals with COPD is to prevent smoking and to maintain optimum functioning for as long as possible. This usually involves medication, oxygen therapy, and environmental changes designed to reduce exertion. The depression that accompanies chronic illness of all types can be particularly significant in COPD patients, many of whom feel that they have brought it on themselves by smoking. Because of its complexity, COPD is an excellent example of a health problem that requires an interdisciplinary approach.

## THE SKIN AND SKIN DISEASE

The largest organ of the body, the skin functions to protect the interior of the organism from the effects of pathogens, toxins, environmental extremes, trauma, and ultraviolet irradiation. With age, and often as the result of the accumulated effects of repeated injury, the skin changes. It grows and heals more slowly. It becomes more sensitive to most toxins and is less able to resist injury. It becomes less effective as a barrier to infections. The specialized appendages, such as sweat and the sebum glands, pressure and touch sensors, and hair follicles, atrophy, resulting in dryness, decreased ability to alter body temperature through sweating, and loss of hair. The small blood vessels in the skin diminish with age, a change that contributes to its lessened effectiveness as a barrier to infection, diminished reserve for repair, and altered ability to assist in thermoregulation.

Several skin diseases that are common in the aged can have significant effects on function. These include malignant tumors, herpes zoster, and decubitus ulcers.

### Malignant Tumors

The three most important malignant skin tumors in the aged are basal-cell carcinoma, squamous-cell carcinoma, and malignant melanoma.

Basal-cell carcinomas arise in areas of sun-exposed skin and increase with the intensity and duration of sun exposure. Genetic background is also an important risk factor. The prevalence of these tumors increases with fair skin and decreases with more intensely pigmented skin. The most common sites are the face, tops of the ears, neck, anterior chest, arms, and hands. Treatment is virtually always successful in eradicating basal-cell carcinomas unless there has been extensive local invasion of muscle and bone. These tumors rarely metastasize but can be locally invasive and deforming if not treated soon enough. Fortunately, they grow slowly and seldom get large enough to be more than a cosmetic problem.

Squamous-cell carcinomas arise from chronically irritated skin. Sun damage is the most common cause, but other irritants include tobacco (affecting the lips and mouth), snuff (affecting the nose), coal tar, soot, and X-rays. Chronically traumatized scars following burns or surgery are other sites of predilection. These cancers are locally invasive and frequently metastasize to regional lymph nodes, brain, and lung. Early detection and excision result in higher cure rates. Extensive surgery with excision of all regional lymph nodes and radiation therapy are frequently employed to cure these tumors. They respond poorly to chemotherapy.

Malignant melanoma is also the result of sun damage. In the elderly, lentigo maligna melanomas are most common and present as flat areas of increased pigmentation. Because the prognosis for survival with melanoma is related to the depth of skin invasion at the time of excision, these melanomas have a good prognosis if removed early. The same principle applies to the other forms of melanoma found in the elderly. Melanomas metastisize early and extensively to the brain, lungs, liver, and bone.

### Herpes Zoster

Herpes zoster results from the reactivation of a dormant varicella virus (chicken pox) that has been sequestered in a sensory nerve root. The result is an intensely painful and pruritic eruption over the area inervated by the sensory nerve root. Immunocompromised hosts, such as those on steroids or with chronic diseases that alter the immune response as do cancer, HIV infection, and renal failure, have a greater incidence of zoster. However, normal individuals also get zoster: The reasons for its reactivation are obscure.

Two types of disability result from this infection. First, the eruption itself requires local care to prevent superinfection by bacteria. The associated pain inhibits mobility, appetite, and sleep. Second, there is a high incidence of postherpetic neuralgia in the aged. Severe burning pain can persist for months, long after the local eruption has resolved. Although some medications can lessen the severity of the initial pain, the patient with postherpetic neuralgia usually requires narcotics for relief. The development of effective antiviral agents such as acyclovir has lessened the morbidity of zoster.

### Decubitus ulcers

Decubitus ulcers result from pressure-induced damage to the skin. They are most common in situations in which there is forced immobility because of illness or injury; diminished response to pain because of altered sensorium or the inability to move; and altered nutritional status, which is usually the result of some other illness or injury. Rarely seen in otherwise healthy elderly persons, decubitus ulcers are secondary to other illnesses and are not simply a consequence of aging or a by-product of the altered healing properties of aging skin.

It takes less than an hour of unrelieved pressure exceeding that of the capillary blood flow to induce pressure necrosis. Bony prominences such as those over the coccyx, lateral hips, heels, ankles, elbows, and scapulae are frequently subjected to pressure high enough to cause ischemic injury. Malnutrition and diminished cutaneous blood flow contribute to the genesis and the perpetuation of these ulcers.

The best intervention is prevention, which requires meticulous attention to potential pressure areas and the development of treatment strategies to ensure that pressure is distributed widely and not left long on any one spot. Once a pressure sore develops, it must be kept free from any further pressure in order to heal. This may result in new pressure sores developing because fewer positions are available in which to place the patient and pressure is thereby concentrated on fewer areas.

Treatment of decubitus ulcers includes debridement of any dead skin, either surgically or through dressing changes designed to remove necrotic tissue. In order for an ulcer to heal, the base of the ulcer must be free of necrotic debris and bacteria and provide a suitable environment for the growth of new skin. It must be kept pressure free. Furthermore, the patient must receive adequate nutrition, including trace elements and vitamins such as zinc and vitamin C. Surgical closure is sometimes required. Given the intensity and duration of treatment required to heal a decubitus ulcer once it has been established, every effort should be made to prevent the occurrence of pressure sores through careful positioning and frequent turning of the patient, air and water mattresses to distribute pressure, and attention to nutrition.

## THE ENDOCRINE SYSTEM AND ENDOCRINE DISEASE

The endocrine system encompasses a diverse group of organs and specialized glands that produce hormones. Hormones are chemical messengers that instruct cells with complementary receptors to perform a specific metabolic act. The thyroid gland elaborates thyroxine, which in turn modulates the overall metabolic rate of cells and the organism. Parathyroid glands elaborate parathyroid hormone, which is central to the regulation of calcium metabolism. The islet cells of the pancreas produce insulin, which helps regulate glucose metabolism. Three hormones help modulate the fluid and electrolyte balance of the body: the posterior pituitary gland makes antidiuretic hormone, the kidneys produce renin, and the adrenal glands produce aldosterone.

Although many other hormones exist, excess and deficiency of the previously listed hormones account for most of the clinically significant endocrine diseases encountered in the aged. With aging there appears to be a reduction in the sensitivity of the target cells to the hormone messenger. This is due, in some cases, to a lessening of the number of hormone receptors found on the target cells.

### Thyroid Disease

Clinically significant disease can result from both excess and deficiency of thyroid hormone. In both hyper- and hypothyroidism, the presentation of the syndrome can be very different in the aged than it is in younger patients. As is the rule in most illnesses in the elderly, the presentation is usually more subtle and the symptoms and signs less specific.

Hypothyroidism is common in the aged and results from failure of the thyroid gland to elaborate sufficient thyroid hormone despite maximum stimulation of the gland by thyroid-stimulating hormone (TSH). Vague symptoms abound: dry skin, chronic muscle and joint pains, lethargy, confusion, weight gain, edema, depression, apathy, sensitivity to sedatives, and cold intolerance. Patients with severe hypothyroidism may develop life-threatening hyponatremia, fail to develop a febrile response to infections, have prolonged hypoglycemia, develop hypothermia, and have cognitive dysfunction resembling dementia. These "hypofunctions" are seen most commonly in the hospitalized patient who experiences the stress of surgery or other acute illness. More subtle abnormalities, such as pseudodementia, depression, and lethargy, are more common in the ambulatory patient.

Untreated hypothyroidism places the individual at increased risk of death from concurrent illness. Treatment involves the gradual replacement of thyroid hormone on a daily basis until the TSH level becomes normal. This usually requires dosage adjustments monthly for several months.

In the aged, hyperthyroidism results most commonly from an excess of thyroid hormone released from a multinodular goiter. Although many symptoms of hyperthyroidism in the aged are similar to those in the younger patient, they are usually more subtle. Common manifestations include the new development of glucose intolerance, as in diabetes mellitus; congestive heart failure; atrial fibrillation; muscle weakness; weight loss; diarrhea; and agitation. However, there is a small group of the aged with "apathetic hyperthyroidism," in which the presentation of disease is diametrically different from the usual. These individuals show depression, apathy, failure to thrive, and constipation. Although their symptoms are similar to patients with hypothyroidism, correction of the elevated thyroid hormone level abolishes the symptoms.

Surgical ablation of the thyroid gland is rarely done and is usually reserved for situations in which the enlarged gland compromises the patient's airway. The use of radioactive iodine, which is selectively concentrated in the gland, produces the most lasting reduction in hormone levels. It is so effective that virtually all patients treated with this modality develop hypothyroidism requiring hormone replacement. Medications, such as propylthiouricil, which block the production of thyroid hormone, are an effective alternative to radioactive iodine. Their use is complicated by the development of bone marrow suppression and a significant relapse rate when the medication is withdrawn. However, in the majority of cases both types of treatment produce excellent results.

## Glucose Metabolism

The number of insulin receptors found on cell membranes decreases with age. Reflecting this change, the incidence of glucose intolerance increases with age, reaching nearly 25% at age 85. In the aged, it is important to identify glucose intolerance not only to prevent the complications of untreated diabetes (neuropathy, retinopathy, nephropathy, and accelerated atherosclerosis), but, even more, to identify those individuals at risk for non-ketotic hyperosmolar coma (NKHC) or severe hyperglycemia, which can be precipitated by infection, dehydration, or other physiologic stress.

Nonketotic hyperosmolar coma is exclusively a disease of aged diabetics. It is characterized by extremely high blood sugars and osmolarity, or hyperosmolarity. Patients present with mental status changes that range from lethargy to coma. They are severely dehydrated and frequently hypotensive. It is often easy to overlook the precipitating event (e.g., pneumonia, urinary tract infection, or myocardial infarction) because the severity of the neurological changes suggests a primary neurological event.

Dehydration and hypotension are more significant clinical problems than hyperglycemia. Treatment consists of fluid replacement and low-dose insulin therapy to slowly bring down the elevated blood sugar. This syndrome can be prevented by identifying the diabetic patients who are slipping into the cycle of infection, decreased oral intake, dehydration, increased blood sugar, and the resulting acceleration of dehydration through the forced excretion of water when the kidney cannot reabsorb all of the glucose presented to it. Rehydration and treatment of the primary illness will usually prevent the development of NKHC.

## Antidiuretic Hormone

Antidiuretic hormone (ADH) increases the reabsorbtion of water from the kidney. The release of ADH is stimulated by a decrease in circulating fluid volume or an increase in osmolarity. It is an important part of the endocrine system that maintains fluid balance. Under certain circumstances, the pituitary makes excessive amounts of ADH, which results in the syndrome of inappropriate ADH secretion (SIADH). Several intracranial processes, such as stroke, meningitis, and subdural hematoma, and intrathoracic conditions, such as pneumonia, tuberculosis, and bronchiectasis, can cause SIADH. Recurring episodes of SIADH precipitated by acute viral illness have been reported as well.

SIADH causes excess water retention, which in turn causes a severe dilution of serum sodium. This results in lethargy, confusion, and seizures. SIADH can be intermittent or chronic. It usually responds to restricting free water and correcting the precipitating factors.

### Parathyroid Disease

Parathyroid hormone maintains calcium balance by stimulating the absorption of calcium from the intestine, reabsorption from the urine, and mobilization from bone. The amount of circulating parathyroid hormone increases with age because of age-related decreases in the amount of calcium absorbed from the intestine. Part of this decrease results from lower levels of calcium and vitamin D (essential for the absorption of calcium) in the diet and from less sunlight-mediated conversion of vitamin D than the more active forms.

A decrease in the circulating levels of ionized calcium triggers the release of parathyroid hormone. In situations such as renal failure, serum calcium levels decrease because of binding with retained phosphates normally excreted in the urine. The resulting decrease in calcium triggers the release of parathyroid hormone and often raises its level out of the normal range. This is called secondary hyperparathyroidism. Parathyroid hormone levels usually return to normal when the stimulus for lowering calcium is removed. Occasionally, however, the parathyroid glands continue to overproduce the hormone even after the stimulus is removed. As a consequence, the autonomously hyperfunctioning parathyroid glands raise the serum calcium level and produce clinically apparent hyperparathyroidism.

A more common cause of hyperparathyroidism is the development of a single parathyroid adenoma that produces excess hormone. In either situation, the elevated calcium level causes profound mental status changes, including confusion, lethargy, and coma. Elevated calcium is a reversible cause of altered mental status in the aged. Osteomalacia, renal stones, and peptic ulcer disease are also associated with hyperparathyroidism. However, in the aged they are less common than mental status changes.

Parathyroid surgery is an effective treatment. Conservative management using high-sodium diets, phosphate supplements, and diuretics such as furosemide is also effective in patients who cannot tolerate surgery. Hypoparathyroidism can result from surgery or develop spontaneously. It is rare, and the main symptom, tetany, can usually be prevented by calcium supplements and agents, such as hydrochlorothiazide, that retard calcium loss by the kidneys.


## THE CARDIOVASCULAR SYSTEM AND CARDIOVASCULAR DISEASE

### Cardiac Disease

The heart is the pump that drives the circulation of blood through the arteries throughout the body. Although there are no clinically significant effects on heart function that can be solely ascribed to aging, the aging heart is more likely to have been impaired by one of the four basic types of cardiac disease: cardiomyopathies, ischemic heart disease, conduction system diseases, and valvular heart disease. The result is that the aging heart is less effective as a pump and usually has less reserve to meet unusually high demands for output. As the severity of heart disease increases, the functional abilities of the individual become more restricted.

CARDIOMYOPATHY. Cardiomyopathies are conditions in which the heart muscle is altered so that cardiac function is impaired. In some types, the muscle weakens because of poor nutrition, toxins, infections, or genetic factors, and the heart dilates as a result. Congestive heart failure may occur if the heart cannot contract strongly enough to empty a sufficient amount of blood into the circulation to meet the body's needs. In other types of cardiomyopathy, the heart muscle hypertrophies because of hypertension, outflow obstruction, or genetic factors. In this situation, several different mechanisms act to impair function. The hypertrophied heart is stiff and does not easily fill with blood. As a result, the heart contracts vigorously, but there is little forward circulation to show for the effort, and the body's needs for circulation are not met. In other forms of hypertrophic cardiomyopathy, abnormally contracting muscle obstructs the outflow of blood from the heart. The more strongly the heart contracts, the greater is the obstruction. Treatment is directed at correcting or ameliorating the pathophysiology of the underlying cause of the heart failure.

In dilated cardiomypathies, the heart is not strong enough to move blood against the pressure in the blood vessels. As a result, fluid builds up in the pulmonary circulation, causing pulmonary edema, difficulty in breathing, low blood oxygen, and further stress on the metabolic needs of the body. Treatment is directed toward strengthening the heart muscle through such medications as digoxin. More effective emptying of the heart can be achieved if the pressure against which the heart has to move blood is decreased. This is called afterload reduction. Agents that reduce afterload include nitrates, peripheral vasodilators (e.g., prazocin and hydralazine), and other blood pressure-lowering agents. Diuretics that reduce the amount of fluid being sent to the heart, producing what is called preload reduction, also help to decrease pulmonary edema and improve cardiac function.

In hypertrophic cardiomyopathy, the problem is to fill the heart adequately with blood and to keep the heart muscle from contracting so vigorously that it obstructs the outflow of blood. *Diastolic dysfunction* is the term used to describe the inability of the heart to fill adequately during its relaxation phase, diastole.

Although each of these cardiomypathies can cause congestive heart failure, treatment must be appropriate to the underlying pathophysiology. Modification of the patient's environment to reduce metabolic demands, reverse hyperthyroidism, and maintain physical fitness are applicable to every case of cardiac disease.

ISCHEMIC HEART DISEASE. Ischemic heart disease, also called coronary artery disease (CAD), results from blockage of blood flow to the heart muscle. This can cause death of muscle cells—that is, myocardial infarction, or "heart attack"—if the loss of blood flow occurs rapidly and lasts 30 to 60 minutes. Ischemia can be reversible and the muscle cells gradually regain their ability to contract as circulation is restored. Ischemic heart muscle functions poorly and can result in congestive heart failure if enough of the heart muscle is affected. Furthermore, muscle deprived of its blood supply becomes prone to chaotic and unregulated contractions that can result in life-threatening arrhythmias.

Early intervention in ischemic heart disease takes several forms. The most important is to reduce the "risk factors" that predispose individuals to the development of CAD. Risk factor interventions that have proved effective include cessation of cigarette smoking, reduction of elevated blood pressure, and lowering of serum cholesterol. Secondary prevention of heart attacks once CAD has been established requires, in addition to reducing risk factors, the use of aspirin, to prevent platelet aggregation that may initiate obstruction of a coronary artery, and beta-blockers, which appear to limit the extent of muscle injury.

Management of symptomatic CAD is similar in all age groups and consists of medical and surgical interventions. Since the pathophysiology of CAD is the mismatch between the metabolic demands of the heart muscle and the ability of the coronary arteries to supply blood, interventions are directed at decreasing the metabolic needs of the heart muscle or increasing the ability of the coronary arteries to carry blood. The metabolic demands of the heart muscle can be reduced by lowering the pressure against which the heart has to push blood, by reducing the rate at which the heart contracts, and by reducing the overall metabolic demands of the body by correcting hyperthyroidism, anemia, low oxygen, or elevated temperature. Calcium channel blocking agents and beta-blockers reduce the metabolic demands on the heart muscle, and nitroglycerine reduces the pressure against which the heart has to pump blood.

Surgical intervention is directed at increasing the capacity of the coronary arteries to provide blood to the heart muscle. Critically narrowed sections of the arteries can be identified by means of cardiac catheterization and angiography. They can be circumvented by grafts (i.e., coronary artery bypass grafts, or CABGs) or removed by transluminal angioplasty if the narrowing occurs in larger branches of the coronary arteries. The results of CABG surgery and angioplasty are determined more by the preoperative function of the patient's heart than by the patient's age. In the absence of other severe coexisting disease, the aged are good candidates for cardiac surgery.

The treatment of acute heart attacks in the aged runs the gamut from infarct reduction using clot-dissolving agents (such as t-PA or streptokinase) and emergency angioplasty to comfort measures only. The determination of where in the spectrum of care the individual is most appropriately treated is a decision made jointly by the patient, physician, and family. Intervention often requires critical decisions to be made rapidly in the middle of a medical emergency. There are appropriate limits to treatment that are often lost sight of in the attempt to apply the latest technology. Further, ethical discussion of this important issue is presented in Chapter 10, Ethical Issues at the End of Life.

The rehabilitation of patients who have suffered myocardial infarction is an interdisciplinary task, involving nutritionists, to reduce dietary risk factors; physical and occupational therapists, to help patients achieve maximal functioning; nurses, to supervise medications, teach patients about their condition, and monitor family dynamics; psychiatrists, on occasion, to help resolve issues of grief and depression; and medical practitioners, to monitor therapy and educate patients about their appropriate level of functioning.

CONDUCTION SYSTEM DISEASE. Conduction system diseases are those that affect the rate and rhythm of the heart's contractions. The propagation of the electrical wave that results in the coordinated contraction of the heart muscle is initiated in the two pacemaker sites in the heart and carried initially along specialized pathways that spread the wave widely throughout the conduction system of the heart. These pacemakers and pathways can be damaged by many different agents, including those that result in cardiomyopathies and myocardial infarctions. The most common consequences of pacemaker dysfunction are extremely rapid (tachycardic) contractions, poorly coordinated (dysrhythmic) contractions, or extremely slow (bradycardic) contractions, which are less effective in moving blood and result in diminished cardiac output. Low cardiac output can result in confusion, fatigue, poor exercise tolerance, and congestive heart failure. Rapid reductions in cardiac output can cause syncope.

Tachycardias and poorly coordinated rhythms, such as atrial fibrillation, are usually treated with medication to control the rate of contraction and convert the rhythm back to normal. Occasionally, electrical cardioversion is required. Bradycardia is usually managed by surgical implantation of an artificial pacemaker, which can be set to trigger a heartbeat at a predetermined rate. Age, per se, is not a contraindication to pacemaker therapy; the surgery is minor and well tolerated.

VALVULAR HEART DISEASE. In addition to its muscle, conduction system, and blood supply, the heart has valves that function to keep the blood flowing in one direction. Defects of the heart valves are of two types: stenosis, or narrowing, which causes the forward blood flow to be restricted; and insufficiency, or regurgitation, which results in the backward flow of blood, which then must be pumped again. Both defects increase the heart's work load and reduce the effectiveness of the pumping action. The two valves most frequently involved are the mitral and aortic valves, both on the left side of the heart, which moves blood into systemic circulation.

Rheumatic valve disease, which results from previous episodes of rheumatic fever, is the most common cause of mitral stenosis and insufficiency in the aged. Congestive heart failure, arrhythmias, and embolization of blood clots from the heart to the brain and other organs are the most common complications of mitral valve disease. These conditions require attentive medical management, which includes the use of anticoagulants to prevent emboli, diuretics to control congestive heart failure, and digitalis or other medications to control the heart rate. Nutritional support is often required to ensure compliance with a low-sodium diet. Because of the potentially serious side effects from too much anticoagulant (i.e., bleeding and hemorrhagic stroke) and too much digoxin (a cause of arrhythmias), their narrow range of effective dosages, and the deleterious effect of inadequate dosage, compliance with medications is a significant issue. Patients' failure to take the correct dosage often results in iatrogenic disease.

Surgical intervention to correct mitral stenosis must be timed to avoid the development of fixed pulmonary hypertension and right-sided heart failure. To effect valve replacement or valvulotomy, whereby the valve is widened but not replaced, open heart surgery is necessary. Transluminal valvulotomy, in which the valve is widened by using catheter-guided balloons, offers a significantly lower operative risk in selected patients. Almost all patients continue to require medication for control of heart rate, prevention of emboli, and treatment of congestive heart failure.

Aortic valve disease, which is not uncommon in the aged, results from rheumatic valve disease, increasing damage to a congenitally misformed valve, or the progression of age-related injury to an otherwise normal valve. The gradual buildup of scar tissue and calcium on the valve leaflets is in fact part of the normal aging of the valve. The most clinically significant lesion is stenosis of the aortic valve. This results in a progressive increase in the resistance to the flow of blood out of the heart. As a result, the heart must pump blood against increasingly greater afterload. Patients can experience angina without coronary artery disease, because even normal coronary arteries are unable to deliver sufficient blood to meet the metabolic demands of the overtaxed heart muscle. As the stenosis increases, transient decreases in cardiac output because of arrhythmias or ischemia result in syncope. Finally, when the heart is no longer able to compensate by hypertrophy for the increasing resistance to flow, congestive heart failure supervenes. Unlike previously discussed situations in which congestive heart failure occurs and is amenable to medical treatment, congestive heart failure in aortic stenosis carries a grave prognosis and can be effectively managed only by surgical replacement of the damaged valve.

Endocarditis, an infection of the heart valve, is a rare but significant illness in the aged. This is due not only to its potential for causing death or severe disability, but also to its subtle presentation. Lethargy, fatigue, anorexia, "failure to thrive," anemia, worsening congestive heart failure, worsening renal failure, low-grade fever, embolic stroke or transient ischemic attack, worsening control of diabetes, and development of a new heart murmur are all potentially caused by bacterial endocarditis. Early and intensive antibiotic therapy can be lifesaving.

### Vascular Disease

HYPERTENSION. Hypertension is another common condition affecting the cardiovascular system. It is clear that the aged with systolic blood pressures above 160 mmHg and diastolic pressures above 90 mmHg are increased risk for stroke, congestive heart failure in the form of hypertensive cardiomyopathy, and renal failure. Isolated systolic hypertension carries a similar risk. Treatment to lower pressure significantly lowers the risks of developing these complications. Medical and dietary management are the mainstays of treatment. Compliance with medication and the early identification and avoidance of drug-induced side effects, such as dizziness, hypokalemia, depression, syncope, and confusion, are the major challenges to the health-care team.

PERIPHERAL VASCULAR DISEASE. Peripheral vascular disease is frequently the result of untreated hypertension, cigarette smoking, diabetes mellitus, and elevated cholesterol. When early intervention to reduce risk factors is unsuccessful, management is through the modification of diet to reduce weight and cholesterol, medications to enhance blood flow and reduce blood pressure, and behavior modification to reduce cigarette consumption. Surgical intervention is effective in cases of symptomatic peripheral vascular disease, which results in pain at rest, claudication, or nonhealing ulcers. As in coronary artery disease, partial obstructions of peripheral arteries, most commonly in the legs, can be treated with bypass grafting or by dilating the obstructed sections of the arteries using transluminal angioplasty.

Amputation may be required for the relief of pain and to stop the spread of infection in patients for whom other surgical procedures are impossible. Because a patient's ability to ambulate is greatly affected by the level at which the amputation is performed, the most distral site is preferred. However, the amputation must be performed at a level at which there is sufficient blood supply to ensure adequate healing. Blood supply usually improves as one goes proximally. Reoperation is usually required if the amputation is below the area of adequate blood supply and the incision does not heal, with the result that the patient is exposed to the risks of surgery again.

The loss of a limb is a traumatic event. Often the process of grieving must begin before the actual surgery and is helped by contributions from social services, psychiatry, nursing, and rehabilitative services. Depression is a major impediment to the successful rehabilitation of these patients and must be addressed if intensive nursing and physical therapy are to be successful.

## THE GASTROINTESTINAL SYSTEM AND GASTROINTESTINAL DISEASE

The gastrointestinal system includes the oral cavity, esophagus, stomach, liver, gallbladder, pancreas, and the small and large intestines. The role of the system is to facilitate the ingestion, breakdown, and absorption of food. Age-related changes in function are more apparent in some portions of the system than in others. For example, the loss of dentition and diminution of salivary gland activity with age impair mastication and deglutition, thereby affecting the overall function of the system. There are no other significant age-related changes in bowel function that can be ascribed solely to aging.

However, the aging gastrointestinal system is more susceptible to cancer, vascular insufficiency, and chronic degenerative conditions. Common gastrointestinal problems encountered in the aged include: dysphagia; ulcer disease; pernicious anemia; cancer of the pancreas, stomach, and large intestine; constipation; and cholelithiasis. Gastrointestinal complaints are extremely common in the aged, and gastrointestinal disease accounts for over a quarter of hospital admissions.

### Dysphagia

Dysphagia, or difficulty in swallowing, commonly results from neuromuscular disorders such as stroke, Parkinson's disease, diabetes, and other neuropathies. Malnutrition results from decreased intake of food, and aspiration of oral contents is a common accompaniment that frequently results in pneumonia. Carcinoma of the esophagus usually presents with dysphagia and the sensation of food "hanging up" in the esophagus. It has a poor prognosis for cure and usually requires extensive palliative treatment. Hiatus hernia, another cause of dysphagia, is increasingly common in the aged: few cases are symptomatic and medical management with antacids and $H_2$ blockers is effective.

### Ulcer Disease

Ulcer disease is common in the elderly, and the presentation is often atypical. Complications of obstruction, bleeding, and perforation are more common in the aged than in younger individuals. Emergency surgical treatment for bleeding in the elderly carries up to a 20% mortality. Medical management is effective in uncomplicated cases and rests on the use of antacids, the avoidance of salicylates and other nonsteroidal anti-inflammatory agents, and the administration of $H_2$ blockers such as cimetidine. Cimetidine-induced confusion is a common complication in the aged and its avoidance requires a reduced dose.

## Pernicious Anemia

Pernicious anemia results from a common age-related decline in the absorption of vitamin $B_{12}$. This usually occurs with chronic inflammation of the lining of the stomach, called atrophic gastritis. Not only can impaired $B_{12}$ absorption cause significant disease (i.e., dementia, neuropathy, and anemia) but it is associated with a higher incidence of carcinoma of the stomach. The replacement of vitamin $B_{12}$ through monthly injections effectively prevents or corrects the deficiency. However, this treatment has no effect on the risk of gastric cancer.

## Cancer

Gastrointestinal malignancies are second only to lung cancers as the cause of deaths by cancer. The esophagus, stomach, pancreas, and large intestine are the most common cancer sites. Cancer of the stomach is more common with advancing age, has its peak incidence in the eighth and ninth decades, and has a poor 5-year survival rate. Cancer of the pancreas has a similar 5-year survival rate, but its peak incidence is in the sixth decade. Late diagnosis because of atypical, vague, or misleading symptoms, such as depression or altered mental status, is the rule. Cancer of the colon accounts for half of all gastrointestinal malignancies. Because they are usually less "clinically silent" than the other malignancies, intervention is usually earlier and more successful. Rectal bleeding, anemia, weight loss, and altered bowel habits are the common presenting complaints. However, weakness, depression, fatigue, anorexia, and decreased functional competence are also early "nonspecific" clues to colon cancer. Unless the elderly person's condition makes it likely that they will soon die from some other cause. surgery is often required for cure or to prevent intestinal obstruction. Five-year survival rates vary widely, depending on the extent of the tumor at the time of intial treatment, but complete cures and long remissions are possible.

## Constipation

Constipation is increasingly common with advancing age. Although bowel transit times are normal in otherwise healthy adults, many other age-related factors can contribute to having fewer than three stools per week. Inactivity, inadequate dietary fiber, inadequate fluids, the side effects of drugs (i.e., narcotics, iron, sedatives, and anticholinergics), oversedation, confusion, and prior laxative abuse can all contribute to constipation. Alterations in the intestine that are due to local disease, such as hemorrhoids, strictures, diverticulitis, and cancer, can also contribute to constipation. Correction of the contributory factors, improved diet and increased exercise as tolerated, use of regular periodic laxatives when needed, and patient education are usually effective. For those patients who are too confused to respond to the urge to stool, regular disimpaction is important.

## Biliary Tract Disease

The incidence of gallstone disease, or cholelithiasis, increases with age, occurring, in nearly one third of those over the age of 70. Although most gallstones are "silent," infection and biliary obstruction due to stones are increasingly common in the elderly. Emergency surgery for cholecystitis in the elderly carries a 25% mortality rate. This has spurred some to advocate "prophylactic" gallstone removal, or cholecystectomy, in the elderly with multiple small stones, which pose the highest risk for passing and for causing obstruction. Nonoperative techniques are being developed such as endoscopic papilotomy, in which the bile duct is widened from within the intestine by use of an endoscope. This technique is useful for the elderly who would otherwise not tolerate anesthesia and surgery. The use of lithotripsy to shatter gallstones with sound waves, instillation of chemicals to dissolve stones, the development of oral medication to dissolve or prevent the recurrence of stones, and laparoscopic surgery will play increasingly important roles as these techniques are perfected.

Many other conditions can affect the elderly: appendicitis, ischemic bowel disease, inflammatory bowel disease, and acute and chronic pancreatitis, to name a few. Each carries a higher mortality and morbidity rate in the elderly than in younger patients, partly because of atypical presentation and late diagnosis. In gastrointestinal disease, as in all facets of illness in the elderly, early diagnosis requires that the health-care team be alert to symptoms and ever willing to evaluate new symptoms.

This brief review of health problems in the elderly should be supplemented with reference to standard textbooks for discussion in greater depth.

## REFERENCES

1. Gryfe, C. I., Amies, A., & Ashley, M. J. (1977). A longitudinal study of falls in an elderly population: 1. Incidence and morbidity. *Age and Aging, 6,* 201.

2. Lepsitz, L. A. (1988). Falls and syncope. In J. W. Rowe & R. W. Besdine (Eds.), *Geriatric Medicine* (pp. 208–218). Boston: Little, Brown.

3. Tinetti, M. D., William, T. F., & Mayewski, R. (1986). Fall risk index for elderly patients based on number of chronic disabilities. *American Journal of Medicine, 80,* 429.

4. Resnick, N. M. (1988). Urinary Incontinence — A treatable disorder. In J. W. Rowe & R. W. Besdine (Eds.), *Geriatric Medicine* (pp. 246–265). Boston: Little, Brown.

5. Katzman, R. (1986). Alzheimer's disease. *New England Journal of Medicine, 314,* 964.

6. Kay, D., & Bergman, K. (1980). Epidemiology of mental disorders among the aged in the community. In J. Birren & B. Sloane (Eds.), *Handbook of Mental Health and Aging.* Englewood Cliffs, NJ: Prentice-Hall.

7. Besdine, R. W. (1988). Dementia and delirium. In J. W. Rowe and R. W. Besdine (Eds.), *Geriatric Medicine* (pp. 375–401). Boston: Little, Brown.

8. Cutler, R. W. P. (1984). Cerebrovascular diseases. In Rubenstein and Federman (Eds.), *Scientific American Medicine* (Vol. 2; pp. 1–12). New York: Scientific American.

# 3

# Emotional and Cognitive Issues in the Care of the Aged

David G. Satin

## DEFINITIONS OF OLD AGE

The cognitive and emotional issues of old age are important in the care and treatment of the aged. Crucial to the discussion of these issues are both the aged person's self-image and society's perception of the aged, individually and as a group.

Everyone knows what old age is, or has ideas on the issue, but almost everyone has a different concept. The most common definition — at least in this society — is age 65 years or more. This, in fact, is part of a politico-economic definition of old age: The logic is that, at least in earlier times, workers were too disabled by age to be functional after age 65 (on the average), and that this standard retirement age made them eligible for release from labor and for whatever material supports the society offered its unemployables. It may also be seen as a mechanism for facilitating the advancement of younger workers by removing older incumbents in higher positions. There is also the legend of Otto von Bismarck (Chancellor of Prussia in the late nineteenth century, who is associated with pioneering European social welfare policies) who schemed to set 65 years as the universal retirement age so that he could remove some of his political opponents from power.

A second definition of old age is based on the time of transition in a vocational role. Thus, the time when people no longer perform their primary vocational roles is when they become old. This naturally makes old age relative — to the nature of the vocational role (some roles can be carried on into older age than can others) and to the individual's capacity (some people remain competent longer than others). For example, housewives and mothers become old in this vocational sense and may substantially retire from their work when they have passed their childbearing years and their children are independent and have left home. Those employed outside the home, in contrast, become old when they are retired from their jobs by reason of whatever policies and criteria are relevant — 20 years of active service for the military; age 65 or 70 for school teachers; when no longer able to serve effectively for household domestics; or by their own choice for Supreme Court judges. This definition of old age raises several interesting issues: as people retain their functional capacities longer because of changes in nutrition, environmental hazard controls, and medical care, old age may come later in life. Also, as jobs change with the development of new industries and with the growing technological assistance available to workers in the form of automation and robotics, the demands of work change, leading to longer sustained competence (as less physical labor and precision are required) or earlier obsolescence (as newer learning and relearning or more sustained attention and precison are required). Thus, old age may come earlier in some industries and later in others. Finally, post-retirement vocations are advocated by geriatricians and gerontologists. If people take on second jobs (for pay, as volunteers, or as hobbies), they may become "young" again, in a vocational sense and, perhaps, in a mental health sense as well.

Old age may also be defined in terms of functional capacity. A panel of septuagenarians was discussing the positive aspects of old age, and these individuals were observed to refer often to "those old people." When asked who "they" were, in contrast to the panel members themselves, a definition of old age emerged that included four factors: not a part of an active social network, no productive activity, dependence on others for care, and major physical disability. The panelists and the audience agreed that, by this definition, one can be old at age 35 and not old at age 85. None of the panelists was old, because they included a neuropsychiatrist who was still active in his academic department and in writing pursuits, a case manager in a home-care program for the aged, and a community activist who was busy taking the pulse of her neighbors, in terms of political and human services needs, and advocating for them with governmental and political offices.


## THE LEGITIMACY OF GERIATRICS AND GERIATRIC PSYCHIATRY

As we have looked critically at the aged, so we should also look critically at those who offer health care to the aged. How is the health, illness, and treatment of the aged different from that of younger people, and what is the difference between geriatricians and other health care professionals?

It may be asserted categorically that the aged have no illnesses that younger people do not have, and are not immune to any of the illnesses that younger people have. Younger people have dementia (e.g., perinatal brain damage, heavy-metal encephalopathies, and ruptured congenital intracerebral aneurysms), arthritis (e.g., both rheumatoid and degenerative), arteriosclerotic cardiovascular disease, and impairments of special senses (e.g., lenticular cataracts and otosclerosis). The aged are subject to pneumonia, bone fractures, psychoneuroses, and drug and alcohol abuse. The only health-related problem that is unique to the aged is being labeled "old." This stereotyping is often associated with a nihilistic attitude: pessimism and disinterest in treating illnesses, and the assumption that disability, discomfort, and unhappiness are normal in old age. This raises the old dilemma of "Is she sick because she is old, or is she old because she is sick?"

"Ageism," as this negative stereotyping is labeled, is a reflection of the youth bias of Western, industrial and post-industrial societies. Chapter 16, Attitudes, Values, and Ideologies as Influences on the Professional Education and Practice of Those Who Care for the Aged, speaks to the thinking behind health care planning and practice generally, and the effect it has on the aged and their care in particular. The value placed on change, novelty, and technological mastery, and youth, speed, and flexibility as characteristics associated with these valued activities, inherently devalues the aged throughout the culture. For example, as Lisa Gurland (1985) has pointed out:

> The idea that "quick is good" is exemplified by the test battery often used to diagnose clients with cognitive and emotional problems. On intelligence scales the examinee is given credit for accomplishing tasks quickly. Thus, the faster one performs tasks correctly, the more intelligent one is supposed to be. Projective tests are also timed, and the amount of time one takes to respond is considered meaningful from a psychodynamic perspective. Little attention is paid to the age of the client. Thus it is no wonder that the aged are so quickly written off as demented. To judge an entire section of the population by standards and values inappropriate to their developmental level is both prejudicial and unethical.

The real differences between the aged and younger groups in health and illness are quantitative, not qualitative. In the aged some health problems are more common, such as Alzheimer's and multi-infarct dementia, degenerative joint disease, and lenticular cataract. Some health problems are less likely to appear for the first time, such as schizophrenia, multiple sclerosis, and allergic disorders. The aged have less physiological reserve in several areas, because of accumulated damage or degeneration. Kidney function may be one quarter of that of a young adult, liver function one third, and lung function one half, and the number of nerve cells in the central nervous system decreases steadily from early adulthood. For a variety of reasons, the aged do not show signs of illness as vividly as do younger people. For instance, they may not raise as high a fever with an infection, show as much infiltrate on a chest X-ray with pneumonia, have as much pain with a heart attack, or be as sad with a depression. For some of the above reasons, the aged are more sensitive to the effects and interaction of medications and other treatments; illnesses and impairments; nutrition and other health maintenance factors; and the emotional, social, and physical environment within which they live.

What is it, then, that geriatricians have or can do that differentiates them from other health care professionals? On the positive side, those who are interested in the aged and focus their work on them can develop an understanding of and sensitivity to the quantitative differences that may make a crucial difference in their care. They may be attentive to the health maintenance factors that are important to the aged. They may be alert to the muted and idiosyncratic signs of illness. They are expected to understand the modification of treatment approaches that are essential to be of more help than risk to the aged. And they should have a broad perspective on the complex and sensitively interactive constellation of factors that affect the health of the aged and that must be attended to when health care intervention is necessary. All these things geriatricians should know, respect, and incorporate in their professional practices. They should demonstrate them to other health care professionals who treat the aged and teach them to professionals and nonprofessional caregivers alike. But the most important precept is, perhaps, the most ineffable and hard to teach: the geriatrician must respect, like, and be sympathetic with the aged, and be able to develop a rapport with them.

On the negative side, the establishment of specialties and subspecialties in the health care professions can serve to narrow perspectives and spheres of competence both within and without the specialties. The establishment of geriatrics and geriatric psychiatry (or "geropsychiatry," as it is sometimes streamlined) should not encourage an in-group isolation of communication and collaboration. It should not reserve clinical care, education, and research relating to the aged to an elite group. The academic and professional tendency to manufacture empires for the efficient winning of funds, fame, power, and career advancement for the incumbents should be strenuously resisted. The experience, knowledge, skill, and facility in working with the aged comes from those who work with them and are best contributed by these front-line workers. To claim that those attributes reside only in the specially initiated is to distort reality. To divert these resources for other purposes (such as academic research or political struggles between professional guilds) is to pilfer scarce, badly needed resources and deprive the aged themselves.

The argument has been made that gerontology is a distinct field of theory and study, and geriatrics a distinct field of applied professional practice. This is institutionalized in the burgeoning number of professional societies focused on the aged. Clinically, geriatrics is recognized as a subspecialty through academic degrees and professional credentials offered by the disciplines of internal medicine and family practice, nursing, social work, and psychiatry. Also, in the United States, research, training, and clinical services focused on the aged are supported by several branches of the Federal Department of Health and Human Services, the Veterans Administration, some universities, and various projects sponsored by private foundations. Therefore, real or illusory, aging is a field of endeavor with concrete representation in the current society.

## THE PLACE OF EMOTIONAL AND COGNITIVE ISSUES
## IN PROFESSIONAL PRACTICE

Not all health care professionals are mental health professionals (psychiatrists, clinical psychologists, psychiatric social workers, psychiatric nurses, mental-disability occupational therapists, pastoral counselors, etc.). Not all geriatric clinicians are geriatric mental health professionals. How are psychiatric issues relevant to the education and practice of nonpsychiatric professionals who have more than enough education, responsibility, and work in their own specialties?

Emotional and cognitive issues affect nonpsychiatric health both directly and indirectly. Emotions can directly increase or maintain a physical disorder, or may play a role in causing it. Let us look at some examples of this.

- A 66-year-old woman has had chronic, progressive rheumatoid arthritis for many years. Not only has it become difficult for her to walk, but she has withdrawn from volunteer activities and social contacts with friends, and has become depressed, pessimistic, and negativistic toward her husband. She feels that an old, crippled woman has nothing much to look forward to. Her rheumatologist adjusts her medications and gives some attention to other physical treatments, but spends time regularly talking about her hopelessness, low self-esteem, and bitterness, and gently encourages her to resume the hobbies and social contacts she enjoyed. Her mood improves and she is able to walk and use her hands with much more facility and less pain than before. The prognosis is for a much slower progression of her continuing arthritis.

Emotional problems can increase focus and emphasis on independent physical problems, as illustrated in the following case.

- A 75-year-old widow is found to have intractable leg pain even when her mild bursitis is treated as vigorously as the rheumatologist dares. When it is discovered that she suffers from chronic depression and withdrawal since her husband's death, this is treated with supportive psychotherapy, involvement in social activities, and antidepressant medication in small, geriatric doses. The depression disappears, she becomes more friendly and outgoing, and the pain becomes too negligible to require treatment.

A concern for the emotional and cognitive significance of health care will influence the choice of treatment approaches and the way the health care professional approaches the patient.

- An 85-year-old man is barely coping with the pain and stiffness of osteoarthritis, the loss of his ability to walk for pleasure and self-care, his lowered self-esteem as a more dependent person, his diminished dignity in the eyes of those he has to ask for help, and his waning hope for recovery. Because his growing panic presages a major depression, his dentist decides against extracting his damaged teeth, as she would normally do. Instead, she allies herself with the patient in determining to save the teeth by any means possible.
- A 73-year-old widow with a paranoid personality is hospitalized because of deepening depression and angry feelings of abandonment. She is found to have early carcinoma of the breast. To everyone's surprise, she impulsively elects the most self-mutilating form of treatment — radical mastectomy. The geriatric psychiatrist and the surgeon agree that this choice represents angry self-destructiveness, and treatment is delayed while the patient is asked to think about the loss of body parts and disfigurement she faces. By confronting her with the anger and despair this choice represents, the psychiatrist and surgeon demonstrate that they want kinder and more protective treatment for her than she is choosing for herself. She is helped to elect a more self-preservative and equally effective treatment: removal of the local tumor followed by X-ray therapy, which will leave negligible scarring.

It is well known that only a small proportion of the population is in contact with mental health professionals. A much smaller proportion of the aged population is, since the aged were educated in an era when mental illness was shameful and psychiatric treatment brutal and hopeless. Mental health professionals, in turn, often look upon the aged as normally deteriorated and unable to benefit from treatment. Thus primary-care physicians, visiting nurses, local clergy, dentists, pharmacists, and others are much more likely to encounter emotional and cognitive issues. This puts them in a crucial position to identify needs, which constitutes case finding, and to be the first source of help, which constitutes preventive intervention. There may be no one else available, since the aged may refuse referral to mental health professionals both out of fear of those professions, and out of trust and investment in the nonpsychiatric professionals they have already chosen and come to know.

Health professionals have an obligation to deal with the emotional and cognitive problems of their patients to the extent they are able. When clinical professionals assume clinical responsibility for patients, they assume responsibility for whole people. This realization is essential to making correct diagnoses and choosing appropriate treatment, which takes into account all the incidental and side effects of prescribed care. This view also implies an ethical responsiblity to patients, who look upon a health professional as learned and capable in general and not only limited to one specialty. In fact, the aged tend to be socially isolated and may not have access to other professionals or even other interested and trustworthy people. Thus, if they are turned away by the professionals they happen to face, they may have no one. To address only the organ or disease of one's specialty is to be an academic. To address only the diagnostic or treatment procedure is to be a technician. Only by addressing the whole person is one a full health professional.

## NORMAL CHANGES WITH AGING

As noted above, loss of abilities and happiness should not be tolerated as a normal part of aging. But this is not to say there are no normal changes with aging. It is crucial to distinguish between normal and pathological changes, because the former require reassurance and adaptation, and the latter require concern and correction. The aged themselves are liable to share societal prejudices against aging and the aged, since they have shared the same acculturation and the same lack of empathy for the aged it entailed. Now they are the objects of their own prejudices, and suffer a special anguish from this predicament. Consequently, the aged as well as their families, neighbors, and professional caretakers, need to understand and deal appropriately with the normal changes that come with aging.

The first thing to note about the aged is that they have lived a long time. Aging thus implies much experience with life events, the evolving life cycle, and coping with tasks and problems. The aged have accumulated knowledge, skills, and (in those who are thoughtful) perspective. Thus, they may be resources to those who are less experienced and shorter-sighted. In fact, the combination of experience, perspective, and judgment may amount to wisdom, which increases with age in those who are alert and interested.

The personal experience the aged have had with past events, environments, cultures, and values are of special interest. This may give them insight into the roots and context of current conditions that those brought up in the present cannot have. They may also be a link to younger people's heritage, giving a sense of stability and meaning that may be missing from the hurly-burly of current practical affairs. The aged may be looked upon as walking archives of history and tradition that are as valuable to those locked in the battle for achievement or survival, as they are to historians and cultural anthropologists.

Some concrete things change with age. Learning, remembering, thinking, decision-making, and responding become slower. It is essential to distinguish this slowing from the impairment of cognitive processing that comes, for instance, with dementia. This is one of the opportunities to misinterpret aging as pathology, and to treat all the aged as defective. The normal aged require more time and less distraction, and they must not be overburdened with multiple simultaneous tasks; under suitable conditions, they can demonstrate quite effective ability to learn, remember, and deal with responsibility. This should be borne in mind when examining an aged person to avoid misinterpreting delayed or confused responses.

"With advancing age people remain like themselves, only more so" is another geriatric axiom. There is a continuity in personality throughout life. In old age people become free of the diplomatic inhibitions that limit them while they are employed and ambitious for the future. They also become impatient with falsity and delay. These characteristics make them freer in expressing their personalities and more outspoken in their opinions. Emotions may become muted. The aged do not exult or despair as easily as younger people do, perhaps, in part, because they have learned through long experience that nothing is so good or so bad that it will not pass and be survived. This is not to say that the aged are not gratified or hurt, but they may be more subdued in their reactions. On the other hand, some aged persons may be more emotionally labile, responding sensitively to the supports and losses in their environments. This is related to a greater need on their parts for other individuals and resources as their own abilities, resources, options, and remaining time wane. They are more vulnerable to dependency, anxiety, insecurity, and mistrust, and show this either as a fleeting response to changes in their circumstances or as a pervasive emotional coloration of their outlooks on the world.

Knowledge and skill become outmoded. This is not peculiar to the aged: With the accelerating pace of technological change, younger workers must be retrained or become obsolescent every 5 to 10 years. The aged, too, can learn, but at an ever-slower pace, and sooner or later either fall behind or give up the race and become obsolete. However, judgment is not lost with age, and may remain as a special resource in coming to terms with changed conditions.

Values are much more difficult to change. They are learned, not as relative to circumstances and goals, but as eternal and taking precedence over practical affairs. Thus, it is in the area of morality, ethics, and priorities that the aged are most likely to be viewed as old-fashioned — as, literally, they are. It is in this area that they are most likely to feel alienated from the world and least tolerant of changes in the people and practices around them. And it is in matters of values that disgust and despair are most likely to be aroused. A good deal of insight and good will are necessary on the part of young and old alike to come to some *modus vivandi* of mutual respect and cohabitation.

The most obvious changes with aging may be physical. The special senses — vision, hearing, taste, and smell — are impaired by a number of normal deterioration processes. Strength and endurance decrease. Change in hair color; loss of hair; loss of elasticity in the skin, leading to wrinkling and sagging; and loss of muscle mass and fat deposits, cause characteristic changes in appearance. Secondary sexual characteristics — body contour and sexual organs — lose their distinctiveness, which is closely tied to ideas of beauty and social desirability. And sexual function is more limited and muted, though many studies have demonstrated that it continues into extreme advanced age, remaining a sense of much meaning and satisfaction.

The normal loss of anatomical and physiological function and the accumulation of injuries result in decreased physical functional capacity, as mentioned previously. Illness and disability limit mobility, access, and the comfort and energy to participate in activities. The decreased relevance of knowledge, skills, and values alienates the aged from their younger communities. The loss of important relationships isolates the aged socially, as children grow independent, relatives and friends move away, and elders and contemporaries, who once formed key social relationships, die. In addition, the aged are the poorest age segment of the population, having lost their earning capacity and living on fixed incomes. For all these reasons the aged are less capable, more vulnerable to increasing functional loss through further impairment and lack of resilience and reserve, and ever less autonomous. The realistic appreciation of this inexorable regression sets a tone of existential loss and limits for the aged.

A major criterion for identity, status, and a sense of worth, work and productivity are of great importance in this Western culture (see Chapter 9, Work, Productivity, and Worth in Old Age). As mentioned earlier, loss of work is a marker for old age, making people socially nonfunctional. Correspondingly, retirement undermines a sense of identity and self-esteem. Their absence of material productivity and acquisition is an important source of the devaluation of the aged in our culture. Certainly their lot is not improved by the debates over the burden of the growing population of nonproductive aged people on the shrinking population of younger workers, and the need to stem the drain of money into social and medical support for the aged. For these reasons, those approaching retirement and old age should prepare themselves for this dangerous life transition by preparing structured activities for the future. Physical health and economic security are not sufficient to ensure a sense of self-esteem and social worth. A respected and meaningful role in life is necessary for good mental health. This is no less true in old age, but more difficult to realize.

There are many routes to this meaningful social role. Recent statutory prohibitions against mandatory retirement ages in some industries have ameliorated the problem by delaying retirement. Older people have found second jobs and even careers after retirement, sometimes serendipitously, through finding work that matches their interests and talents, being recruited by an employment program for the aged, or by joining a social or political cause. Sometimes older people intentionally plan and prepare a second career for themselves, so that retirement provides the freedom and time to expand an old hobby or a new interest. A third alternative, available in certain societies, is heightened family or community status. The bearer of cultural education, the honored veteran of a long life, the honorary chief, or the ultimate social arbitor are, for example, prescribed roles in the Italian, Chinese, and African cultures. Finally, retirement in the sense of freedom from any obligation may be welcomed by some of the aged: to indulge in hobbies, to travel, to gain an education purely for intellectual enjoyment, or to defy all rules and schedules.

Family relationships shift with old age (see Chapter 8, The Ageing Family). In the best circumstances, there is a leveling between generations as the relationship of adult to child shifts to one of adult to adult. With increasing disability, insecurity, and loss of self-confidence, the aged may become more dependent and their children assume more caretaking and decision-making responsibilities. The theory of "role reversal" between parent and child has been criticized. The psychological pattern of the parent-child relationship and the social distinction between generations are rarely obliterated; rather, the younger generation assumes practical functions, sometimes in grateful repayment for past caretaking, sometimes with resentment, feeling them a burden. The shifts in family relationships may stir up old feelings and conflicts, often exacerbating nostalgia for what has been lost, sad longings for what never was, or anger for what has been suffered. The result may be closeness and sharing, more or less painful exploration, sometimes reconciliation, or else endless, bitter conflict. In any case, the family is the most intimate and meaningful social unit in which people — including the aged — live.

Self-image changes with old age. As mentioned previously, the aged are members of a particular society and share its attitudes toward old age. If these are negative, as is often true in Western society, old age may be a time of loss of self-respect and dignity. If old age has its own roles and honors, it may be comfortable and even welcomed — as the philosopher Giorgio de Santayana anticipated, a permanent relief from the turmoil of youth. One's life accomplishments may lead to satisfaction with achievement and honor, or to disappointment with failure and rejection. Finally, self-image is also determined by one's personal adjustment, in the sense of Erik Erikson's developmental stage of ego integrity versus despair.

Individuals are conditioned by their cultural and social environments, and their opportunities and limitations are determined more by what is permitted than by what is physically possible. Some societies include the aged in their structures and values; in these societies the aged have a place and a purpose in their own minds and in those of their communities. In others they are nonfunctional, intruders physically and economically. Until recently in the modern United States, the aged have made up such a small proportion of the population that they have represented an anomaly. As life expectancy increases, the aged population grows (see Chapter 12, Disability Trends and Community Long-Term Health Care for the Aged). At first, the aged were viewed as an increasing burden that had to be dealt with efficiently. More recently, the combination of their increasing political influence and the dawning recognition that they have constructive capacity is stimulating a more fundamental change in the cultural perspective on the aged. They may yet win a place of function and honor in a restructured society.


EMOTIONAL PROBLEMS OF THE AGED

Emotional problems are, in part, the outcome of past and current experiences and patterns of perception and reaction. In addition, they are a maladaptive use to which brain functions are put, and may also result from impairment of brain, metabolic, and/or endocrine structure and function. Emotional problems encompass mood, pace of thought and behavior, content of thought and behavior, organization of thought, social relationships, and reality orientation.

Emotional problems may be judged from various perspectives. A *normative* approach posits healthy or correct function, judges specific cases in relation to that standard, and attempts to bring individuals or groups as much as possible into conformity with the standard. This is sometimes labeled as the "medical model." A *developmental* perspective posits a process of progression from more immature, simple, lower functioning to more mature, complex, higher functioning, again in a prescribed order. An *adaptational* perspective looks upon people as coping with opportunities, options, and demands, and working out some way of functioning in relation to them. Here there is less prescription of what is right, but more of what is effective. Finally, a *phenomenological* perspective accepts a more universal spectrum of feeling, thinking, and behavior without imposing standards of propriety or preference.

In the discussion that follows, we will be guided somewhat more by the normative perspective because this is most often encountered in clinical work with the aged and is the one our clinical colleagues most often use. However, reference will be made to old age as a developmental stage, and to the aged as coping with the changed opportunities and losses of their conditions.

### Depression

Depression (Major Depressive Episode, Major Depression, and Dysthymic Disorder— Depressive Neurosis, in the various diagnostic systems) is the most common emotional problem in the aged. Surveys indicate that 12% to 25% of those in the community show signs of clinical depression or significant unhappiness. Recent epidemiological studies by such workers as Dan Blazer suggest that different cohorts (groups born at different times) show different prevalences of depression—a relatively lower percentage of people born prior to 1925 exhibited depression than did those born around the turn of the century or those born more recently. This suggests that old age is not the only cause of depression, but that early life learning and experiences contribute resistance or predisposition to the conditions met late in life.

Depression in the aged may present in very different ways:

The *apathetic* type is the most common, characterized by withdrawal, unresponsiveness, disinterest, confusion, and loss of social and self-care activities. This is the depression that makes up a large proportion of what is termed "pseudodementia," because it is most likely to be mistaken for dementia or senility.

The *agitated* type is characterized by overactivity, perpetual worry and doubt, clinging and pleading for help and reassurance, distractability and poor concentration, along with anorexia and insomnia. Delusions of guilt, punishment, catastrophe, or blame are not uncommon.

The *somaticizing* type focuses on physical symptoms and fears of illness, whether by misinterpreting real bodily sensations, exaggerating manageable physical illnesses, or creating the conviction of illness out of fears or others' experiences. A major danger is that health care professionals may overevaluate or overtreat these symptoms, thus reinforcing the hypochondriacal delusions and, not unlikely, creating real physical problems through the effects of medication or surgical procedures.

*Paranoid* flavoring may be incorporated into any type of depression, in the form of resentment of family, friends, or workmates for failing to appreciate and help the afflicted person. Health care professionals who try to help may be treated with suspicion and rejection for not showing enough sincerity, competence, or availability.

An *existential* depression may account for the significant proportion of the aged who are not happy and active, and those who commit suicide without showing the classic signs of sadness, despair, deterioration of behavior, anorexia, and sleep disturbance. These are the people who have decided, coolly and thoughtfully, that life no longer is worth living. This may stem from loss of people or roles that made life worthwhile, or from overwhelming burdens such as physical disablity, poverty, social isolation, or fatal illness. Such people are alert, sensible, competent . . . and determined.

The *depressive personality* (Cyclothymic Personality, Depressed) is a way of describing those who have a persistently unhappy, dissatisfied, pessimistic attitude throughout life. When they become aged, this personality orientation continues, finding focus and justification in the circumstances, losses, disabilities, and rejections of old age. In some cases, interestingly, they take the real insults of old age more in stride than do those whose more positive outlooks are disappointed: The depressive personality is used to and expects disappointment. However, Weisman and Worden have described people who seem to have lost their reasons for living and do not survive adversity or illness as well as others. These people are more likely to die under the stress of severe and fatal illness.

SUICIDE. Suicide is a significant concern in the aged. The U.S. Public Health Service finds the highest rate (cases per 100,000 population) among the oldest white males:

| Age | White Males | White Females | Nonwhite Males | Nonwhite Females |
|---|---|---|---|---|
| 15–19 | 6.7 | 2.1 | 4.8 | 2.4 |
| 35–39 | 21.0 | 10.2 | 12.6 | 3.6 |
| 55–59 | 37.6 | 12.1 | 14.6 | 4.4 |
| 85+ | 59.0 | 4.3 | 23.9 | 3.3 |

In the aged, suicide attempts are much more likely to be successful. The ratio of attempts to successes under age 40 is 7:1; at age 60 it is 1:1; at ages 63–69, it is three times the population average; and at age 85 and over, it is five times the population average. The methods used in suicide attempts are much more lethal in the aged than in younger groups: cutting, shooting, jumping from high places, drowning, and hanging. One must also consider occult forms of suicide in the aged, such as refusal to eat, refusal of medical care, withdrawal, and loss of vitality. The impression is that the desire to die prompts suicides among the aged whereas the desire to manipulate ambivalent relationships prompts suicide among the young.

The risk factors for suicide in the aged include marital divorce and separation, widowhood (especially the first year), living alone, alcoholism, organic brain disease (especially that with poor judgment), unemployment, poverty, and poor health. It is interesting to note that males and those in higher socioeconomic groups have higher rates of suicide.

Losses — of people, of competence, of status, of health, of autonomy — seem to be an important precipitant of suicide, especially when the aged people lack the judgment and self-control with which to deal with these losses. Sadness is a much more common contributor than psychiatric, neurological, or physical illness. Life seems to become unbearable or worthless:

> The tide goes out, little by little; the tide goes out and whatever is left of us lies like a beached ship, rotting on the shore among all the other detritus — empty crab shells, clam shells, dried seaweed, the indestructible plastic cup, a few old rags, pieces of driftwood. The tide of love goes out. Anna is now one with Alex and all the others, hardly distinguishable. I can say of them all, "I loved you once, long ago." And what is left of you? A lapis lazuli pin, a faded rose petal, once pink, slipped into the pages of this copybook.

But, ironically enough, I, Caro, am still here. I still have to manage to die, and whatever powers I have must be concentrated on doing it soon. I want my death to be something more like me than slow disintegration. "Do not go gentle into that good night" . . . the words, so hackneyed by now, come back to me like a command from somewhere way down inside, where there is still fire, if only the fire of anger and disgust. (Sarton, 1973, p. 121)

TREATMENT. The treatment of depression is a subject of much current debate, with biological explanations and treatments much in vogue. In fact, treatment should be related to the causes of depression, its manifestations, and the available resources. In the overwhelming majority of cases, the aged are depressed about something, whether this be the loss of a spouse, decreasing competence and satisfactions, impending danger or death, or the lack of a satisfying role. Therefore, this human response requires a human response: a person or persons who care, provide support and companionship through the ordeal, and can be the links to new resources, activities, social relationships, and perspectives on self and the world. Erich Lindemann was the first to describe this "bridging relationship" in his studies on grief work and preventive intervention from 1939 to 1954.

It may be necessary to explore in more depth people's preexisting perception of the self and the world, expectations of what they will offer, and response patterns for dealing with the perceived reality. This requires analytic and insight psychotherapy of one form or another, to become aware of the burdensome feelings; to recognize the underlying patterns of thought, feeling, and action; to find alternative perspectives and actions; and, finally, to change behavior and relationships. The world with which the aged contend may have to be changed, as much of the stress and limitation on them derive from it. Those with appropriate expertise may be needed to relieve problems, such as ill health, limited mobility, social isolation, inadequate living arrangements, or poverty. The aged often need advice, training, and encouragement to change their own skills and behavior patterns, and caretakers may have to make the environment more supportive, structured, and supervised in special ways to compensate for the limitations of the aged, either by supplementing the environment in which they already live or by transferring them to more supportive environments (see Chapter 9, Work, Productivity, and Worth in Old Age, and Chapter 12, Disability Trends and Community Long-Term Health Care for the Aged).

Antidepressant medications may be necessary to enhance concentration and provide the optimism and energy that allow the aged to deal effectively with their internal and external environments. These medications have proliferated in recent years, so there is a wider range of therapeutic effects and side effects from which to choose. The mechanisms of action are still not well understood, however, despite much research and theoretical speculation. Justification for the use of antidepressants rests on empirical grounds. Much thought must be given to the risks and benefits of using them, since the aged are exquisitely sensitive to medication dosage, side effects, and interactions with other illnesses and treatments. Although some people judge the degree of geriatric psychiatric care by the degree of drug therapy, health care practitioners are admonished to heed the caution against overtreatment.

Our discussion of depression would not be complete without a discussion of electroconvulsive therapy (ECT). This is one of the older and more controversial treatments for depression. In the past it was draconian, producing much discomfort, risk of injury, and disabling aftereffects. In recent years this treatment has been much softened and controlled, and patients protected against injury, so that risks and aftereffects are minimal. Even those aged fragile because of cardiac, skeletal, or vascular vulnerability can be treated with reasonable safety. ECT is effective in about 80% of the aged selected as appropriate for it (as compared with 70% to 75% of the aged selected for antidepressant medication). And the depression responds more quickly, on average. Despite ECT's persisting bad reputation among some who had experience with it in the distant past and with certain consumer advocacy groups, it is surprisingly well accepted by many of the aged and their families who have suffered the prolonged misery and frustration of severe depression.

### Anxiety

Anxiety is the second most common emotional problem in the aged as in the rest of society. A general feeling of insecurity and vulnerability may color the outlook of a sizable proportion of the aged, as mentioned in the discussion of changes brought about by normal aging. Acute demands on the aged or, equally, the loss of capacities or resources is likely to sharply increase anxiety, apprehension, or panic (Panic Disorder or Anxiety Reaction, in the various diagnostic systems). Because of the eroding sense of robustness and flexibility, this crisis state may abate much more slowly than in younger people. Some of the aged do not recover very well, but are left permanently impaired in their range of function, ability to relate to others, and capacity for autonomy (Generalized Anxiety Disorder). As is true with depression, people may bring abiding anxiety to their old age. Those who are chronically anxious (Anxiety Reaction), repeatedly panicked (Panic Disorder), or focus their anxiety on specific situations or objects (Phobic States or Reactions) will be so when they are aged. When their resources and vigor dwindle in old age, anxiety is likely to be the mode of their reactions. The focus tends to be on people, conditions, situations, and objects in their current environments, which may be more restricted because of aged people's disabilities or restricted resources.

TREATMENT. Treatment addresses both the causes and symptoms of the anxiety. Certainly, every effort should be made to reduce the anxiety-provoking stresses, through reducing or pacing demands and changes. Coping resources should be strengthened by providing information, help in planning, and support in taking action to deal with the stressors. Arranging for a trusted, sympathetic, and competent helper is one of the most effective interventions. Antianxiety medications and, perhaps, nighttime sedatives may be necessary to enable the aged to gather their attention and energies to collaborate effectively in the coping process and resume effective functioning thereafter.

### Situational Reactions

Situational reactions may become more common among the aged, because of increasing stresses and decreasing internal and external resources.

The *Acute Confusional State* is a stress reaction more common in the aged than in other age groups. This is a condition of passivity, mild restlessness, withdrawal, poor attention and concentration, insomnia, mild to moderate anxiety and perplexity, and disorganization and incompetence. It comes on over a period of hours or days in response to the demands or changes that overwhelm aged people's ability to cope. Of course, the more formidable the stress and the more limited people's coping capacities, the more likely acute confusional states will occur.

TREATMENT. The treatment of stress reactions is to recognize and give help in coping with demands. Recovery is prompt, taking a period of hours or days. Again, the aged are at risk of being labeled demented or senile if found in this state of nonfunction, and of being treated custodially (i.e., the condition is not treated). Lack of treatment can result in demoralization, loss of skill in carrying out the activities of daily living, atrophy of physical vigor, and depression. A temporary condition can thus be turned into a chronic and eventually irreversible one. This is one of the best illustrations of the need for active and accurate work with the aged; the assumption of deterioration and hopelessness becomes a self-fulfilling prophecy.

### Paraphrenia

Paraphrenia is a major mental illness most often found in the aged. Its manifestations are a fairly well developed delusional system, centering on suspicion, mistrust, and fear of specific individuals, behaviors, and settings. Unlike paranoid schizophrenia, thinking and behavior remain organized and the person competent. Unlike paranoid psychosis, the rest of the person's thinking and relationships are normal.

One major contributor to paraphrenia seems to be a situation of loneliness, social isolation, an impoverished life, and loss of past relationships and hopes. Often people focus their anger, fear, sense of loss of control, and fascination on a half-real, half-fantasied person as a way of expressing their feelings in a concrete and yet manageably limited way. Impairment of communication because of a vision or hearing defect, limited locomotion, or cultural isolation, inhibits the ability to test and correct these misapprehensions. Cognitive deficiencies, through delirium or dementia (discussed later) further impairs the ability to comprehend and cope flexibly with the unhappy situation.

TREATMENT. Treatment addresses both the symptoms and the cause of paraphrenia. Small and carefully titrated doses of carefully chosen antipsychotic medications may help to reduce the vividness and intrusiveness of the paranoid thinking. Building a trusting and understanding relationship breaks into the loneliness, angry feeling of abandonment, and lack of reality testing. Redressing the social isolation, limited function, sense of loss and abandonment, and sensory impairment (with hearing aids, cataract surgery, improved lighting, etc.) often results in the gradual fading of the compensatory symptomatology by making it unnecessary.

### Paranoid State

Paranoid thinking is probably somewhat more common among the aged than in other age groups. In the paranoid state there is a general attitude of suspicion, disbelief, hostility, and pessimism. It seems that any given event, situation, or relationship is an excuse for venting these feelings rather than a cause of them. Any chance justification for disappointment is treated as no more significant than a neutral or successful event, and there may even be a surprising tolerance of negative experiences. New relationships — such as those with health professionals — may be welcomed as a relief from the (reportedly) dastardly and disastrous ones in the past, but the new ones, too, soon turn sour and fall into place with the rest. This is not to say that the paranoid aged ask for nothing; their sense of entitlement continues, and they may be amazingly effective at getting attention and resources, though no response satisfies them.

The paranoid aged often were demanding, perfectionistic, wary, and socially distant in their younger days. As disappointments accumulate, hopes for change fade, social and occupational connections are lost, and the future itself grows short, the most self-protective adjustment is one of refusal to hope or to attempt rewarding relationships. Only cynical insight into the unworthiness and hopelessness of people and life offers a measure of (negative) control and safety.

TREATMENT. The treatment of the paranoid aged must avoid any attempt to disprove the mistrust and pessimism, or for the health professional to become an exception to the long line of incompetents and malevolents in the past. The key is to avoid being drawn into the paranoid battle. Simplicity, directness, openness, politeness, and sticking strictly to business is the stance of choice. This will help the paranoid aged to get as much help as possible without sabotaging themselves with diversionary relationship issues. In the end, health professionals who take this tack may come to be much more trusted and the relationship with patients much more durable; treatment will ultimately be more successful than if an overly considerate and intimate relationship is attempted.

In some cases appropriate doses of antipsychotic medications may "sweeten" the personality, making patients more sociable than they have been in decades. Health professionals must take care to maintain patients' tolerance for this foreign intervention, paying special attention to side effects. It is not necessary that paranoid patients understand or even take it voluntarily at first (sometimes it is started in settings of psychotic crisis and involuntary treatment). Respect for strong authority of health professionals may simply guide patients, who may also simply appreciate the easing of tension afforded by the medication.

### Other Emotional Problems

Emotional problems appear in the aged as in other age groups. Though not unknown, schizophrenia and mania are less likely to start in old age. Generally, younger people with these illnesses as well as with personality and psychosomatic disorders carry their problems with them into old age. In general, the symptomatology of emotions, like that of physical disorders, is more muted and less energetically acted out in the aged than in younger individuals. When symptomatology is more extreme, the aged tend to become confused, withdrawn, and easily exhausted, regressing toward a common core of overload and helplessness: a confusional state.

TREATMENT. Treatment is based on that for emotional disorders in younger people. Here, again, medication dosages must be tailored to the metabolic tolerance of the aged and to the context of other physiological impairments and treatments. Support and care for the person and for other problems must form a comprehenaive treatment program.

## SUBSTANCE ABUSE

### Alcoholism

Alcoholism is more common in the aged than is recognized. One source is younger alcoholics who become aged alcoholics. In addition, people who have always behaved properly become lonely and frightened in old age. When elderly individuals haven't family or a cohesive community to turn to, they may turn to the solace of an alcoholic haze. These are solitary drinkers, who drink in the privacy of their homes because they are ashamed and deny their dependence on alcohol. The signs of this type of aged alcoholism are an unaccountably fluctuating "dementia," poor self-care (slovenly dress, grooming, and housekeeping), repeated self-injury (from falls), withdrawal from people and activities, malnutrition (as appetite and funds are expended on alcohol), and poor health care (untreated illnesses). Health care professionals often do not consider alcohol abuse as a possibility and are ashamed to ask nice little old ladies/gentlemen about such misbehavior. Such questioning and further investigation through family, friends, and neighbors is essential to effective health care, and is usually accepted realistically by the aged — whether guilty or innocent.

TREATMENT. Treatment for the aged who have carried alcoholism — and the behavior pattern and personality disorder associated with it — from past life into old age follows the approaches for alcoholism in general. Such people are very likely to be familiar with self-help groups such as Alcoholics Anonymous, treatment facilities such as detoxification units, the medical complications of alcoholism (gastritis, cirrhosis of the liver, esophageal varices, pancreatitis, peripheral neuritis, dementia, withdrawal states and delirium tremens, etc.), and the treatment for them. Disulfiram ("Antabuse") should be used with caution: It is primarily effective as a threat of catastrophic reaction if alcohol is imbibed, and those who can use this threat to bolster their resistance to drinking need not deal with the reaction itself. However, the aged alcoholic who is impulsive or self-destructive enough to drink despite disulfiram treatment should be evaluated medically for risk from the peripheral vasodilation, hypotension, vomiting, and syncope of the reaction. Those with cardiac disease, cerebral vascular disease, seizure disorder, gastric ulcer, osteoporosis, and so forth, are not good candidates for this modality of treatment.

The aged who develop alcohol abuse out of depression, loneliness, and anxiety require a different treatment approach. They are exquisitely sensitive to shame and rejection, from which they already suffer, and would be further wounded and alienated by the harsh confrontation and behavior control of treatment for entrenched alcoholic personality disorder. The treatment of choice is, first, sympathetic recognition and support for their plight. In patients, understanding and respect must replace the bewilderment and disgust with which they treat themselves for having so violated their previous self-images. Help for medical problems and material deprivation should be obtained, without demanding self-help from people whose energy and resources are too depleted for this. When self-esteem, a sense of competence, and trust have been reestablished, patients should be embarked on a program of restructuring and enriching their lives; both the effort and successful results promote a positive self-image. In all of this, psychotropic medication plays little or no part. It is an inadequate substitute for self- or others' care, and the debilitated aged are especially vulnerable to toxicity and side effects. Only if treatment for alcohol withdrawal or associated psychiatric disorders (anxiety, depression, insomnia) is needed, should carefully regulated doses of medications be applied.

## Drug Abuse

Drug abuse also occurs in the elderly; sometimes it is preexisting, but sometimes we see newly acquired forms. Young drug abusers become old drug abusers, though the frenzy to obtain drugs and their effects tends to die down as an individual ages, and more judgment and self-care are exhibited. Those who are heedless probably die young. Many aged people misuse therapeutic drugs, whether prescribed or over-the-counter.

However, not all aged individuals who have problems with drugs abused drugs when they were younger. Because health concerns are a high priority among the aged, they are always interested in and willing to experiment with treatment approaches to ailments that are often chronic and can only be incompletely relieved. The aged will shop among health practitioners (physicians, nurses, pharmacists, podiatrists, dentists, chiropractors, etc.) for alternative diagnoses and treatments, and alternate and combine them in ways that seem promising. They will save medications obtained from past illnesses and apply them to new ones that seem similar. They will exchange experiences and medications with their peers who seem knowledgeable or helpful. And many health professionals are inaccurate in their diagnosis and prescription for diseases of the aged. This uncontrolled drug availability and use, combined with the sensitivity of the aged to drug effects, makes for a great potential for misuse. One consequence can be drug dependency and withdrawal reactions.

Dependency on the psychological effect of drugs is associated with the use of tranquilizers and sedatives, which are among the drugs most commonly (and, often, thoughtlessly) prescribed by medical practitioners focused on relief of psychological problems that consume inordinate time in the office. Loosening of prescription laws has made low-potency sedative preparations available over the counter for "simple nervous tension," premenstrual syndrome, insomnia, colds, and so forth. Bromine preparations, which used to be favored for these purposes, are still available and may be used out of habit by the aged. Pain medications present another set of problems, and make narcotic addiction quite possible.

Dependency for physiological effects is especially characteristic of bowel and stomach control medications. Habitual use of these medications may result in the loss of physiological reflex patterns and self-regulation. There is also risk of nutritional impairment due to interference with the absorption of essential nutrients, and risk of dehydration due to excessive water excretion.

TREATMENT. The treatment for drug abuse is largely preventive. Education of the aged about the proper diagnosis, prognosis, and treatment of their various ailments is the first line of defense. Non-pharmacological treatment, through exercise, diet, and physical measures, should be explored. Appropriate consultation with competent authorities can be advocated. It is then incumbent on health care practitioners to have competent authorities available, that is, health professionals trained both in the health problems and treatment of the aged, and in effective communication and working relationships with them. Interest in and patience with chronic diseases and rehabilitative/palliative treament are also important. All sources of medication should be involved, physicians and pharmacists most of all. Withdrawal of the aged from drugs on which they have become dependent requires support of vulnerable metabolic, physiologic, and nutritional systems. But a cure will not last if the needs that prompted the unwise search for relief through drugs are not met. Bad health care should be replaced by good health care, which will alleviate both the physical problem and the emotional discomfort and fear. Again, this means competent, caring health professionals (see Chapter 16, Attitudes, Values, and Ideologies as Influences on the Professional Education and Practice of Those Who Care for the Aged).

## COGNITIVE PROBLEMS OF THE AGED

Cognitive problems result from impairment of brain structure or function. Cognitive impairment may affect alertness, attention, concentration, orientation, memory, mental control, abstract thinking, judgment, insight, and grasp of current events, and may also influence emotional phenomena.

### *Delirium*

Delirium is an acute and usually reversible disorder of brain function. It has a rapid onset (a matter of hours or days) and is characterized by a fluctuating state of alertness, confusion, disorientation, impairment of both recent and remote memory, anxiety, apprehension, agitation, disordered sleep-wake pattern, and visual (much more often than auditory) illusions and hallucinations.

There are several sources of acute disorder of brain function. The most common is drug effects, and the most common of these is prescribed medications. In fact, it may be said that when sudden change in thinking and behavior is observed in the aged the first examination to be undertaken is that of the medicines that are being taken. As mentioned previously, dosages may be too high for the aged physiology to cope with, the physiology may be impaired by old or new injury and thus less tolerant, side effects may be more prominent, combinations of medications have enhanced or unintended effects, and the interaction of drugs and illnesses may produce brain function impairment.

Of course, other toxins must also be considered. Alcohol and therapeutic drugs are a possible source of cognitive deficit, as are heavy metals, neurotoxins in insect and rodent poisons, and other toxins.

Infectious diseases also pose risks of cognitive impairment. The toxic condition itself, fever, and the consequent dehydration and malnutrition are hazards. Direct infection of the brain in meningitis, encephalitis, and abscesses, and metastatic infection from other sites (e.g., in bacterial endocarditis) produce functional consequences.

Malnutrition and dehydration from other sources are of concern, such as poverty; weakness; physical incapacitation; fear of being attacked; and emotional and cognitive disorders that impair judgment, attention, realistic thinking, memory, or social contact. The aged are vulnerable to physical illnesses that impair their intake or retention of nutrients and fluids: for example, diarrhea, painful mouths, dental defects (not enough teeth to deal with the food available, poor and uncomfortable dentures, painful gums, etc.), obstruction of the gastrointenstinal tract (by tumors or an obstructing peptic ulcer), diseases of the liver, gallbladder, or stomach, and impairment of gastrointestinal motility (as in paralytic ileus). Severe constipation may be one of the most common digestive diseases of the aged that affect cognitive function, and those caring for aged who are unable to understand or communicate their needs are well aware of this source of impairment of alertness and behavior.

Failure of the major organ systems affects brain function, as in congestive heart failure, renal failure, and liver failure. Anemia, stemming from nutritional deficiency, blood loss, or disorders of the blood-forming organs, can significantly impair cognitive function.

Endocrine and metabolic disorders produce characteristic emotional and cognitive syndromes, reflecting the close interaction of the nervous and endocrine systems. Overactive thryroid function (Graves' disease) produces anxiety, confusion, and hyperactivity, insomnia, and sometimes acute mania or a paranoid state; in the aged it may produce depression, anxiety, and agitation. Underactive thyroid (myxedema) produces depression, apathy, weakness and lethargy, poor attention and concentration, and apparent memory defect—a pseudodementia. Sometimes this is associated with a paranoid state, the "myxedema madness" of past eras. Abnormalities of the adrenal cortex can result in paranoid delusional states, poor judgment, confusion, and disorganized thinking. Pituitary hyperactvity (Cushing's disease), with increased levels of adrenocorticotropic hormone and consequently elevated cortisone, produces depression, irritability, and sometimes agitation and anxiety. Diabetes mellitus, with periods of high or low blood sugar level, can produce states of confusion, disorientation, irritability, slow response, and weakness. Depression is the earliest sign of pernicious anemia (poor absorption of vitamin $B_{12}$ with resultant anemia and spinal cord damage), and is found in 20% to 60% of those with Parkinson's disease.

Major physical insults to the body almost always produce a delirious state of one degree or another. Myocardial infarctions ("heart attacks"), cerebrovascular accidents (strokes), and major operations (especially heart surgery) result in periods of confusion, disorientation, agitation, panic, and depression. Some of this is caused by the brain's being deprived of oxygen and nutrients to some degree. The changed treatment and environment of the intensive care unit, the medications and alterations in nutrition and hydration (from decreased feeding, increased intravenous hydration, and artificial substitute replenishment) are other important factors. Fear, uncertainty, and loneliness in the midst of professional hustle and bustle are major contributors.

Paraneoplastic syndrome—the indirect effects of malignancy on parts of the body not directly touched by the cancer—besides fever, skin reactions, and other abnormalities of organ function, may produce confusion, disorganization, disorientation, overactivity, delusional and fantasy thinking, restlessness, and fluctuating levels of consciousness, mixed with clear and rational mental functioning.

Finally, we must mention the acute confusional state. Noted earlier as one consequence of overwhelming emotional and decisional burdens, especially in the aged, it can also be the result of physiological burdens that overtax the brain's and body's coping capacity, and lead to the disorganized, erratic, and incompetent functioning of a delirious state.

TREATMENT. Treatment ultimately involves correction of the toxic, nutritional, metabolic, infectious, endocrine, and physiologic causes of the delirium as promptly as possible. However, temporary supportive measures may help the aged weather this stress. Human reassurance, support, and simple companionship (ideally from known and trusted people) are basic. An atmosphere of low stimulation from light, sound, activity, and extremes of temperature, avoids taxing the system. Gentle orientation by means of adequate light; unchanging setting and staff; and reminders of the situation, place, and identity of the aged themselves will minimize confusion and delusions. Activity should be limited to prevent aged patients from being hurt or lost. Personal supervision is preferable, but physical restraints are often necessary. Again, psychotropic medication should be minimized to avoid complicating the already compromised biochemistry and physiology of the aged, but antianxiety or sedative medication may be necessary to reduce apprehension, restlessness, and combativeness, and to help with acceptance of nutrition and rest. When they can be comprehended, information and reassurance help allay fear and misunderstanding.

## Dementia

The term *dementia* is usually reserved for slowly developing, irreversible defects in cognitive function. Some are stable, and some progressive. Dementias may affect any combination of cognitive functions, depending on the location and nature of the structural or biochemical damage. Overall, only about 5% of the aged show clinically significant dementia, and only one fifth of these require institutional care.

ALZHEIMER'S DISEASE. Senile dementia or Alzheimer's disease (the traditional "senility") accounts for 50% to 60% of dementias in the aged. It consists of an abnormal loss of nerve cells in various parts of the cerebral cortex, with characteristic signs of the deterioration of these cells (e.g., neurofibrillary tangles and senile plaques). The location of the cell loss helps account for the specific cognitive functions that deteriorate in any given case. The age of onset of the disease may be as early as the late 40s or early 50s; it is increasingly frequent with advancing age, affecting some 40% of those over age 75. The disease is progressive, ending eventually in death. The speed of progression varies widely, from 6 months to 20 years, but often is in the range of 3 to 5 years. It is often helpful for the patient, family, and caretakers to gauge the rate of future progression by the past rate.

Despite increasing research on etiology, the cause or causes of the disease are unknown.

Recent evidence suggests a hereditary component in some cases. Also, other dementias have been found to be combined with senile dementia, for example, Parkinson's disease and Down's syndrome. Studies of toxicity (e.g., aluminum), viral infection, abnormality in neurotransmission (i.e., in enzymes and receptor sites), nutritional components, and so forth, have not been proven as yet.

Symptoms start with difficulty in naming objects (dysnomia). This is followed by impairment of recent memory, of new learning, and of the ability to change topics or cognitive sets. At this stage, the aged are often aware of changes in themselves and react with puzzlement, apprehension, depression, and/or despair. Then labile mood, depression, irritability, and narrowing of interests appear, and insight and care about their conditions fade. The next stage is callousness in social relations, negligence in self-care, loss of understanding and skill at physical tasks (buttoning, operating household appliances, games, etc.), disorganization (in dressing, daily routine, and self-care), shallowness of thought and emotions, and concrete thinking. Suspiciousness, paraphrenia, and a paranoid psychosis are possible. Finally, speech and physical control are gradually lost, as is long-term memory. With this come incontinence, inability to care for routine needs (i.e., feeding, dressing, bathing, and toileting), disorientation, agitation and erratic crying out, inability to recognize family and friends, and loss of understanding of personal needs and wishes. The severity of impairment can vary from hour to hour and day to day. Localized symptoms, which depend on the sites of great nerve cell loss, may include seizures, impairment of vision, early impairment of language function (i.e., speaking, understanding of spoken communication, reading, writing), and localized weakness or paralysis. In the end there is mental and physical inertia, loss of strength, wasting, decreasing alertness, and death from some chance disease or general deterioration.

MULTI-INFARCT DEMENTIA.  Multi-Infarct dementia accounts for another 20% to 25% of dementias in the aged. The cause is repeated brain damage (cerebral infarcts) due to loss of blood supply to local areas through hemorrhage or thrombosis. There is a stepwise progression in symptoms as a blood vessel is lost. The brain suffers from temporary impairment because of stress reaction, then some function returns as the reaction subsides and nearby blood vessels can expand to take over part of the lost supply. However, some brain tissue dies from inadequate supply and its function is permanently lost. A period of stability follows until the next blood vessel is affected. The steps may be large or small, depending on the size and location of the blood vessel(s) affected. As succeeding infarcts occur, the residual brain damage is cumulative. If cerebral vasculature and consequent brain damage are arrested — as when hypertension is controlled, vascular disease is cured, or the brain is protected against emboli with special intravascular shields — the disease may not be progressive, though the impairment already sustained is permanent.

TRANSIENT ISCHEMIC ATTACKS.  Transient Ischemic Attacks (TIA's) should be mentioned. These are temporary compromises in cerebral vascular supply that produce temporary impairment of brain function that mimic small infarcts. Factors that contribute to these events include the narrowing of arteries that supply the brain, medications that lower blood pressure, anemia, heart failure, and cardiac arrhythmias. The symptoms, which include giddiness or fainting, focal or general weakness, slurred speech or loss of speech, blindness, confusion, and partial or complete seizures, are entirely transitory if no significant portion of brain tissue is permanently damaged. Otherwise, an infarct produces some residual damage and impairment. In any case, the symptoms serve as a warning of vulnerability to permanent brain damage.

Repeated cerebral blood vessel damage may be due to any disease process that affects blood vessels elsewhere. The most frequent causes are hypertension and arteriosclerosis — high blood pressure ruptures atherosclerotic plaques or the blood vessels weakened by them. Diabetes mellitus aggravates both conditions. Cerebral hemorrhage may be caused by rupturing of congenital or acquired aneurysms; cerebral arteritis; or head trauma. Embolisms may be due to endocarditis; heart valves or linings damaged by rheumatic fever; artificial heart valves on which thrombi collect; irritation or narrowing of major arteries supplying the head and brain (usually through arteriosclerosis), leading to critical reduction of the blood supply and sometimes emboli; or blood vessel disease in other parts of the body that produces irritation and thrombosis formation.

The symptoms, which depend entirely on the functions of the areas of the brain that have been damaged, may include paralyses, loss of sensation, impairment of vision, deficiency in the processing of language, memory loss, confusion, loss of impulse control and social skills as a result of frontal lobe damage, and seizures.

MISCELLANEOUS CAUSES. Other diseases produce dementia. Parkinson's disease, in which the control of muscle function is impaired by a loss of nerve cells in the substantia nigra area of the brain, resulting in inadequate supply of the neurotransmitter dopamine, produces dementia in about 30% of the cases. There is debate as to whether this constitutes a distinct dementia or overlaps with senile dementia both in symptoms and in brain appearance. An additional 80% show impairments of attention and visual-spatial function with little of the senile dementia brain findings. It is noteworthy that the medications used to treat Parkinson's disease may produce recent memory defect (anticholinergic drugs) or attention deficits (levodopa, or L-dopa).

Normal-pressure hydrocephalus has received attention, probably more because of its clear signs and treatment than because of its frequency. The triad of dementia, gait disturbance, and incontinence is the hallmark of this disease. Cerebrospinal fluid accumulates, causing pressure on and eventually damage to brain tissue. The treatment is surgical placement of a shunt that drains excess fluid from the cerebral ventricles to the abdomen, heart, or a major blood vessel. This can halt the progression of the dementia and reverse at least the gait disturbance and incontinence.

Other causes of dementia are relatively rare. They include one or more large cerebrovascular accidents that damage the cognitive areas of the cortex; collections of blood on the surface or within the substance of the brain that are large and long-lasting enough to leave permanent damage; encephalitis; traumatic injury (auto accidents, gunshot wounds, etc.); tumors that destroy cerebral tissue by infiltration or pressure; and the rarer degenerative and metabolic diseases, such as Kreutzfeld-Jakob's and Huntington's.

Again, it is well to be alert to pseudodementia. Depression, delirium, acute or chronic intoxications, the hyper- or hypoglycemic states of diabetes mellitus, and acute confusional states may bear some resemblance to dementia. The fate of aged people suffering from these conditions and the responsible practice of health professionals may hinge on avoiding the presumption that cognitive changes in the aged betoken senile dementia, and on carefully exploring in every case the nature, cause, and possible treatment of the disabilities.

TREATMENT. Treatment for dementia is basically humane and should take into account the fact that the demented aged, their families and colleagues, and their caretakers share the prolonged and tragic struggle. The aged look to a future of indefinite length, devoted to an earned rest from work, to devotion to long-deferred hobbies and social relations, or to the accomplishment of some valued task, only to find prospects turned into one of insidious, inexorable destruction. Their independence and control of their lives and relationships will be steadily eroded to helplessness and subordination to others.

Sympathy, honesty, respect, and dependability are the cornerstones of treatment. The goal is to resurrect a sense of self-worth independent of the accidental loss of skills and activities. It is important to tolerate the self-deception, rage, blame, despair, apathy, and other reactions with which the progressively demented aged will fight back at varying levels of sophistication, depending on the competences available to them. One or several constant, intimate relationships are the vehicles for the achievement of these goals.

The aged, including those in the early stages of dementia, do benefit from psychotherapy. The opportunity for life review to reconfirm personal worth and valuable accomplishments can counterbalance the impending loss of life in this group, as in others with terminal diseases. The urgency of the task and the limited time available make these and other aged very motivated patients. Old conflicts can be cleared up, relationships reconciled, and emotional perspective and tranquility gained. Energy and determination can be marshaled to deal with the implacable march of dementia

A second major therapeutic objective is to support the capacitities that are available at any stage of dementia. This means, most importantly, using them so that skills are retained (once lost they may not be recoverable because of waning learning capacity) and so that the demented and those about them recognize these positive attributes. Cognitive and physical aids will gradually be needed to support decreasing abilities: Often making notes and adhering to stable activity schedules make up for memory and learning defects, and labeling or color coding things and places is helpful. Increasingly attendants will be needed to help accomplish tasks such as travel, social contacts, dressing, and bathing. In more advanced stages it is very helpful to limit the pace of events, stimuli, and change in environment to accommodate the limited processing capacity of the demented.

As judgment and impulse control deteriorate and agitation and negative reactions increase, responsibility must be transferred to others. Legal conservatorship over property and guardianship over the person are necessary so that decisions can be made and resources marshaled for prudence and safety (see Chapter 11, Legal Issues in the Care of the Aged). The decision to place the dementing aged in professional care is complex and difficult. It is addressed at greater length in a later section, The Emotional and Cognitive Effects of Nursing Homes, and in Chapter 12, Disability Trends and Community Long-Term Health Care for the Aged. The demented aged probably function better cognitively and behaviorally in the familiar surroundings of their homes and without the demands of learning a new environment, daily routine, and social network entailed in moving to a long-term care facility. However, the demands on caretakers and the technology needed are tremendous, and seem to require a Thirty-Six Hour Day (Mace and Rabins, 1981). Pragmatically, it is rare that families can adequately care for dementing aged members when behavior is hard to control, as their physical care is a heavy burden. Not possessing the needed professional skills and technical equipment, and finding the emotional reactions intolerable, families ultimately decide on placement in a long-term care facility.

Physical, emotional, and behavioral control of the patients may become necessary for the safety of all concerned, and also to keep them acceptable by family, fellow-patients, and the long-term care institutions on which they and their families rely. Ideally, good management by nursing and recreation staff and by family should be the primary control. Reassuring and orienting companionship, activities of the appropriate cognitive level and duration, and reinforcement of satisfying and safe behavioral patterns, can handle many needs. Physical controls are often used too routinely. Posey restraints (fabric or mesh vests with long belts that tie around chair backs or bed headboards), geri-chairs (with high arms and trays that lock the patient into the chair), and padded belts (that can be tied to fixed objects) are becoming standard items in admission orders for aged patients in nursing homes or hospitals even if dementia is not one of their diagnoses. The reason given is "for safety," though more often it is the prejudice of the staff, convenience in the management of demanding behavior, and concern for the perceived legal risks to the institution and staff that encourage the use of such restraints. In fact, they are necessary to some degree, but their use should be minimized, since they increase frustration, fear, resentment, and shame. Medication, too, is resorted to routinely for "chemical restraint" as often as for relief of emotional and behavioral symptoms. Used selectively and with care, it can help. Appropriate doses of antipsychotic medications can help control agitation and paranoia, and can reduce severe anxiety. Short-acting antianxiety medications can reduce anxiety, restlessness, and insomnia. The depression in reaction to the recognition of the slow dissoluton of one's being and the depression that is a symptom of the dementia itself may respond to antidepressant medications. Sedatives for sleep have limited effectiveness and should usually be avoided, as they produce more confusion and loss of behavioral control during the night hours, when these are already problems. In all, medications, judiciously handled, can increase comfort, attention, and impulse control, and make available the functional capacities that the demented retain.

The family faces a catastrophic assault. A member — often a senior and key member — is removed, leaving much reparative work to be done. A person who is known well and is, perhaps, emotionally important, is changing in awful ways, producing shock, revulsion, and sadness. Old feelings, relationships, and conflicts are disinterred, and may be reenacted in the distorted form of old bitterness, guilt, gratitude, or unexpressed love. A crushing emotional and physical burden grows, producing dedication, obligation, resentment, and exhaustion. The struggle to handle these changes, burdens, and feelings is immense. The family needs perspective, strength, patience, and skill in sorting out and dealing with these multiple tasks. These resources may be inherent in the family members and the family as a whole. Sometimes the family is drawn together and latent capacities are realized. At times, professional intervention can mobilize inherent strengths or supplement them with information, insight, and practical help. Certainly, helping professionals should broaden their attention and ministrations to encompass families as well as the demented aged. Family meetings are almost always indicated to make overt the understanding family members have of dementia, their feelings about the increasingly demented aged, and their conflicting loyalties and obligations — to the aged, the rest of the family, themselves, and the plans that have been intruded upon. When specific conflicts or inability to acknowledge reality and feelings, or obstructed communication with the demented aged or among family members is identified, continued family therapy or individual therapy may be indicated. This should be handled more informally than in other circumstances, to avoid the feeling that another burden is being piled on top of the dementia. This working-through may help prepare family members for dealing effectively with later losses, including their own aging, losses of function, and deaths. Meetings of family and demented aged members also open communication and strengthen relationships. Meetings between family and staff are often helpful and sometimes rescue the care of the demented from ruin through misunderstandings and polarized conflict.

The helping professionals dealing with the demented aged have much to contend with, too. As people they are frustrated, repelled, frightened, and angry, at least to some degree. They have varying degrees of knowledge and skill, and the organizational context within which they work may not be supportive enough to them in their work and their personal struggles. Education in the causes, courses, and care of dementia may be needed. Case-centered consultation on the management of individual cases — including that of the families of patients — may enhance professional performance and on-the-job learning. And consultee-centered consultation or even formal or informal psychotherapy may help resolve personal prejudices and emotional conflicts and open the way to personal and professional growth. Program and staff consultation to institutions can provide administrative and program enhancement of the functions of all involved.

## EMOTIONAL AND COGNITIVE ASPECTS OF PHYSICAL ILLNESS

Physical illness, much more frequent in the aged than in younger groups, has different practical consequences and meanings for the aged. It is, in itself, a sign of aging, and thus resented and feared. It intrudes upon the fragile continuation of effective functioning or further burdens people already staggering under multiple disabilities. Even getting help for physical illness adds another burden on people already struggling with the illness itself. The administrative and financial aspects of illness and treatment are yet another complication, which will be addressed in Chapter 13, The Economics of the Health-Care System: Financing Health Care for the Aged Person. The need to make decisions about health and maintenance programs and caregivers in an era when the aged and their needs are big entrepreneurial business would tax the doughtiest at any age. The observation is apt: "Old age ain't for sissies."

The loss of physical competence is a threat to autonomy and to self-image. People who have worked since childhood, prided themselves on their hardiness and skills, been responsible for workers or clients in their vocations, and cared for other family members now find themselves limited in their capacities, dependent on others, and even facing invalidism. They are different people: not young and vigorous, but old and sick. They also occupy different roles in their homes and communities. No longer are they vigorous and independent, achievers, the helpers of others. Now they are the limited, the observers, and those whom others help. Closely allied with this is the change in relationship to family, colleagues, and neighbors, as others occupy the roles of initiative and authority, those with a future. Finally, there are implications for survival. Illness and impairment bring a threat to security. The ill aged may not be able to keep up their houses or apartments, shop or prepare meals for themselves, or care for their business affairs. In some cases they bear essential responsibilities to others, such as the care of dependent adult children (retarded, mentally ill, alcoholic), or child care for working relatives.

TREATMENT. Treatment of the emotional and cognitive consequences of physical illness includes, importantly, effective physical health care. Disabilities may be minimized, comfort increased, and vigor returned. What is required is comprehensive diagnosis, removal of the disablties that are reversible, and rehabilitiation and supports to minimize irreversible residual disability. All of this depends on an optimistic and sympathetic view of the aged, and the integrated, interdisciplinary treatment approach advocated in this book. Obviously, health care professionals need these attitudes, but the aged themselves and their families must share them in order to collaborate in comprehensive health maintentance, treatment, and rehabilitation.

Beyond this, the aged must maintain (or regain) self-respect and hope. The initial shock of disability may produce despair or bitterness, as well as fear of anything related to illness. They may avoid or fight treatment procedures, health professionals, and information about their conditions, because these arouse panic. Alternatively, they may surrender to a hopelessness that is out of proportion to reality and prepare for helplessness and even death. It may take persistence and diplomacy to gain their attention and trust. Sheer loyalty and dependability may gain the caretaker respect. Appreciating the shock and upset the ill aged feel will establish rapport. Gradually offering factual information about disabilities, treatment, and realistic outlook with different courses of action may correct misapprehensions based on misinformation and past esperiences with tragedy and loss. And giving as much control and choice as possible may help reestablish dignity and initiative. Bear in mind, however, that people vary in the initiative vs dependence they are comfortable with. Some need to know findings and conditions at all times, decide action, and sanction treatment and treaters; health professionals are truly health advisers to these people. Some want to have general updates periodically and know that trusted people are in charge; beyond this, they delegate decisions and actions to others. And at the other extreme, there are those who cannot bear to know and take responsibilty but who are used to leaving remedial action to family authorities, the doctors, or God. It is important to give people what is comprehensible and helpful to them — not what is theoretically "healthy" or what attending clinicians would want for themselves.

In the case of physical illness, as with dementia, past conflicts and unhappy relationships may resurface, stimulated by the general stress situation or by such factors as the specifics of the illness, dependence on family or professionals, loss of the defenses that strength and autonomy may have represented, or strains in relationships precipitated by the physical illness and treatment. Here, as in the case of other life crises, the opportunity may arise to recognize these unresolved problems and deal with them while they are accessible. Insight psychotherapy — often focused because of the crisis and distraction of the illness and treatment — may be productive, as may marital and family therapy.

Psychotropic medications should play a very limited role. The physically ill aged, already disabled by impaired organ function, nutrition, and metabolic function, are coping with other medications and are thus at increased risk of toxic effects and side effects. Behavioral problems should be dealt with through effective nursing management (orientation, support, information, distraction, activity, limited stimulation, etc.). If it is necessary to control behavior that poses a danger to the aged themselves, other patients, or staff, or if this behavior is dangerously compromising medical care, then the least dangerous medications should be considered — often the older ones, such as paraldehyde and chloral hydrate, that have been supplanted by more sophisticated (and intrusive) ones. At times paranoia, hallucinations, and extreme agitation call for antipsychotic medications. In these cases, minimal doses of effective drugs should be introduced carefully and monitored continuously by nursing as well as physician staff, since their effects may vary continually in response to changes in other treatments and physical condition.

Some of the same family and staff issues that arise in cases of dementia may apply to the physically ill aged. Families must be kept informed of the physical illness and treatments so that they can understand patients' symptoms and the treatment that is given or avoided. Both families and staff need information about emotional and cognitive reactions to illness and treatment, in order to be more tolerant of them and prepared to act helpfully.

## EMOTIONAL AND COGNITIVE ASPECTS OF LONG-TERM CARE

Transfer to long-term care institutions and the life there have major emotional and cognitive effects.

### Adjustment Period

A period of adjustment must be distinguished from other problems the aged bring with them to or develop in long-term care. The change from living at home to "being put in a nursing home" is major, carrying overtones of being "old" (in the pejorative sense), of being diminished socially and in terms of worth, and of having lost control of one's life. The change has implications — whether faced or not — of being abandoned, either by those who are present but do not respond in time of need or by those who are not present but whom one should have been able to call upon in crisis. No matter what the reality is of the care needed, what the past intentions and efforts of caretakers were, or what the virtues of the long-term care facility might be, the specters of loss, fear, and abandonment loom.

Some of the aged "do not go gentle into that good night . . . [but] rage against the dimming of the light," as Dylan Thomas advised. They deny their physical or mental disabilities; are outraged at suggestions that they give up their long-standing roles and environments; and fight the transition not only vocally, through appeals to cultural duty and family tradition, but physically, and legally if necessary. These are the "difficult cases," and their "irrationality" is liable to be attributed, again, to old age and senility.

Others appear to be "reasonable," acknowledging their needs, appreciating the alternative care that has been tried and found inadequate, evaluating and choosing the long-term care facility, and preparing for the move. It comes as a surprise that a few days, weeks, or even months after a pleasant admission and happy adjustment, residents become panicked, depressed, angry, and critical, or else apathetic and regressive. The reasoning and preparation of the past may be forgotten or denied, or they may not be able to explain their changes of heart. In any event, they become "psychiatric cases."

Still others appear to accept realistically the change in their abilities and needs and the relocation that is required. But they, too, acknowledge the sadness, sense of loss, and surrender to change that have been visited upon them.

The key to dealing with the adjustment period is to expect and accept it as a classic example of a life crisis (Lindemann, 1956). It is not an extraordinary problem that betokens weakness in the aged, or mismanagement in their families, or failure in caretaking professional staff; it is something that all must expect to deal with as a concomitant of disability and relocation. To respect their travail, the institutionalized aged must be treated with sympathy and support, but with an air of calm to counteract panic and instill confidence that this can be handled. During this period it is advisable to have family visit often — at least those who can tolerate the strong and ambivalent emotions — as this reassures the aged of the continued caring and availability of those they fear lost. Caretakers should encourage the aged to ventilate their experiences and feelings, taking pains to review with them both the positive and negative ones and gently providing reality orientation when emotion becomes destructively distorted. Thus, it is important to allow enough time to work through this stage of the adjustment process, lest feelings go unrecognized and unresolved and remain a lasting burden and block.

When the pressure abates and the aged have the energy to begin to look realistically about them, it is time to introduce them to the people and activities of their current environment. It may be helpful to remind them that this is their home, in fact as well as in name, and that they can look to it for companionship, understanding, activity, and satisfaction. It is helpful for families to reduce their visiting at this time to allow the aged to stop thinking of the facility as a temporary intrusion into their old home and family lives and start looking to it for their resources. Insightful reinstatement of old interests, activities, and roles (e.g., gardening, teaching, child care, and crafts) can aid in restoring initiative, confidence, self-respect, and optimism.

Here again, medication plays a limited role in dulling only the severest symptoms. It may well be ineffective, because a very real and inescapable trauma must be dealt with. Also, the aged in long-term care institutions are likely to be already compromised with physical illnesses or dementia and thus especially vulnerable to toxic and side effects of psychotropic medications. Antianxiety drugs (short-acting to avoid cumulative toxicity) are most likely to be useful and the least dangerous. At times, a major depression has been developing prior to institutionalization, either as a reaction to declining competence and independence or as one of the causes of inability to function outside professional care. In other cases, the depression is precipitated by the catastrophe of institutionalization. In these cases antidepressant medications can help alleviate withdrawal, anergy, and despair; almost never sufficient in themselves, they serve to supplement the support, resocialization, and psychotherapy mentioned above. Antipsychotic medications should be resisted, both because of their risk of debilitation and because they reinforce the habit of dealing with the problem of adjustment as a defect in the aged rather than as a task for all involved.

### Life in Long-Term Care

Long-term care can be hell or a modestly satisfying earthly existence, depending on whether it is seen as the loss of a previous life or the start of a new one. There are many changes to be dealt with in the new "home." The physical environment is different, and the aged, who learn slowly even without dementia, will be disoriented and mourning for their lost homes at first. The routines are different, representing another learning task. It may not be recognized that new routines violate behaviors that have special importance for the aged. These behaviors may be long-standing habits, such as waking early to get tasks done or because parents taught "early to bed and early to rise" as a virtue. They may be reminders of past relationships or activities, such as getting breakfast for a spouse who had an early job. They may be defenses against emotional problems, such as pacing around the building checking doors and windows to allay anxiety or even a touch of paranoia. The people are different, and often of community and ethnic backgrounds the newcomers are not used to. Besides aggravating the sense of loss of both family and cultural heritage, this represents a social learning task the aged may have avoided even when they were at home. And the food is likely to be different, carrying a special preverbal, direct emotional impact that increases the sense of alienation.

On another plane, people's roles and statuses are changed in long-term care facilities. In all but the most sensitive and creative settings, mothers, fathers, neighbors, church elders, master artisans, and so forth, become uniform "residents." Women who used to rule their own households are now in a group subordinate to other women who are in charge. Adding insult to injury, the supervisors are often young women of their daughters' or granddaughters' ages. Rules and discipline are determined by strangers from a strange culture, who relegate the aged to the inherently inferior status of patient.

If one considers the major dislocation and cultural and psychological disorientation the aged must face in addition to the impairments—physical, cognitive, emotional, social, and/or economic—that forced them to move out of their homes and into long-term care, it is clear that great courage, flexibility, and energy indeed are needed to adapt. Essentially, these people must acculturate themselves and develop new identities and roles.

TREATMENT. Treatment emphasizes functional and spiritual rehabilitation. The first consideration is restoring in the institutionalized aged a sincere interest in and appreciation of their former selves, so that they can feel that they have enough worth to preserve themselves. The second consideration is developing a program, physical setting, set of values and goals, and staff that are adaptable enough to recognize and make a place for the individuality of the many residents of the facility. The third consideration is discovering and nurturing the talents, interests, experiences, and personality style of each aged person for whom the institution is now home (see Chapter 9, Work, Productivity, and Worth in Old Age). Treatment of psychopathology, through psychotherapy, expressive therapy, milieu therapy, and/or pharmacotherapy, will prove to be a minor part of the effort.

This may appear to be an impossibly complex and burdensome task. However, with creativity, flexibility, and commitment, it can be interesting and rewarding. In collaborating with the aged in understanding and realizing their value and individuality, the potential for learning about the richness and adaptability of people is tremendous. The task of creating community environments that allow for the flowering of these people together is a microcosm of the effort to structure a humane world. Administrators, social scientists, and politicians have much of the knowledge and skill that are relevant (see Chapter 12, Disability Trends and Community Long-Term Health Care for the Aged). Mental and physical health professionals can contribute insights into the interface of individual and social organisms. The challenge is not to subordinate the individual to an inflexible social/administrative system, as often happens, or fail to make the institution viable while attending to the individual's rights or pathology.

## Family in Long-Term Care

Families of the institutionalized aged also require attention. Families, too, undergo the destruction of old relationships and adjustment to new roles and cultures (see chapter 8: The Aged and Their Families). As families see their aged members change in competence, appearance, and role, they must assume new roles *vis-à-vis* the aged and reassess their own identities without the former contributions of these aged. It may be that, in some sense, children become adults only when their parents can no longer function in parental roles. Crises of self-doubt and insecurity about the future are one result.

Families must take responsibility for the comfort, support, and companionship of their aged in long-term care institutions. This can be a labor of love or an onerous burden reluctantly assumed. This is another juncture at which past relationships between the aged and the caretaking families may be reactivated. Gratitude, prescribed duty, disappointment, a sense of being inadequate and unwanted, revenge, and so forth, may all be acted out as families deal with the placement in long-term care of their aged members. Guilt for failing to prevent the deterioration of the aged and care for them in the family context is a frequent reaction, especially in cultures such as the Italian and Chinese, which prescribe filial dedication to parents.

The projection of feelings and needs onto the professional staff is almost universal. These will be the loving caretakers that the families could not be—the angels of mercy who fulfill the families' obligations but who may also be reminders of their failures. These may also be the scapegoats for the families' guilty failures and the objects of demands, mistrust, and complaint. And these may also be the confessors, comforters, and advisers for the families themselves, who are as bereft and bewildered as are the aged.

TREATMENT. Treatment includes consultation and education for the families, who may lack understanding of the disabilities, treatment, and outlook for their aged members.

This may be a result of the failure of health professionals to provide this information, as the professionals confine their responsibilities to the aged patients. Families may also resist or distort understanding, as they cling to unrealistic hope or unrealistic despair. Information about the aged relatives, the treatment process, and the identities and roles of the treating professionals are the basis for realistic understanding and participation.

Positive roles must be found for the families. They have the right to responsible participation in the care of their aged relatives. Their cultural or family traditions may require them to participate — as in Italian and Chinese families, where filial obligations are strong. And they have much to contribute, in terms of their intimate understanding of the aged long-term care patients, their positive influence on them, their commitment, and their supplementation of the caregiving manpower pool. A first step in defining such roles is for families and professionals to learn about one another. A second is to gain an appreciation of everyone's interest in and contributions to the aged. A third is to develop effective lines of communication for gaining and providing information, voicing concerns and complaints, and obtaining redress of grievances and failures. When suspicion, hostility, and conflict develop between families and professionals, family-staff conferences must be held to correct misunderstandings, voice concerns, and replan goals, methods, and roles. If this is impossible, it is doubtful whether good long-term care can be accomplished, and some change in participants or placement should be seriously considered.

In long-term care as in other aspects of the lives of the aged, the needs of families must be considered as equal to those of the aged. Families may have mental health problems that need attention. These can be addressed in family therapy (with or without the aged relatives, as indicated by the issues and the ability of the aged to participate), in marital therapy, or in individual therapy for family members. Whether this takes place at the long-term care facility depends in part on the facility's definition of its interest in and responsibility for families as well as for aged residents. In part it depends on the families' needs for confidentiality and for relief from the burdens of long-term care. Thus, familial issues can be attended to as part of a community process in the long-term care program or attended to outside it.

The emotional and cognitive issues of staff in long-term care are also important. They will be addressed later in the section on professional health care for the aged.


DEATH AND THE AGED

### Attitudes toward Death

The aged know death, as all people do from the age of 4 or 5. The aged have had extensive experience with death through the natural catastrophes, wars, and loss of colleagues and family they have encountered over long lives. They often have come to expect it, and are less surprised and frightened by it than are younger people. They may accept it as appropriate or welcome it as a rest from worry, responsibility, sickness, and effort. Their sense of the limits of life make them more serious and responsible about finishing tasks, achieving goals, fulfilling responsibilities, and being sincere in and demanding sincerity from relationships.

Cultural beliefs determine the meaning of death and the ways of controlling it and incorporating it into life (Johnson and McGee, 1986). It may mean a terrible accounting, a welcomed return to peace and acceptance, an exciting opportunity for a new beginning, or a feared dissolution of being. Social structure determines the sense of belonging in life and of continuation after death through identification with a group (e.g., a political party), personal relationships (e.g., living on in the memories of those whose lives have been touched), or accomplishments (e.g., a book one has written, a disease discovered and named after oneself, a park dedicated to one's work on behalf of the community). Personal attitudes determine a sense of security, trust, optimism, control, aggressiveness, and so forth. For the aged, all these factors are reflected in the meaning of death and their reaction to it.

Weisman and Worden's study of the factors that affect survival in cancer is illustrative. Patients lived longer who were angry and demanding of attention without alienating others; who were indifferent to or denied death, thus making others more hopeful; and who were seen by staff as cooperative and, therefore, given more support. Patients died sooner who had experienced the absence of parents for extended periods of time early in life; had poor social relationships; were depressed and hopeless, felt death was inevitable, and wanted to die; and were not fearful of death, but discussed it openly.

### Care in the Normal Experience of Dying

POSITIVE WORK. Positive work with the dying aged is sometimes overlooked in the nihilism that follows the terminal prognosis. But the dying still live, and live in especially precious life space. Of basic help is an attitude toward them of respect, loyalty, dependability, and open communication. This preserves their participation in the world. Often the dying are written off or shunned by those who do not know of help they can offer.

Active interventions include enabling the dying to vent their feelings, which gives them an opportunity to explore, share, and develop awareness of their experience.

Support; orientation; information about their conditions, treatment, and outlooks; and participation in decisions about their lives and illnesses maintain the dying as dignified and responsible participants in their lives. This dignity and responsibility are often taken from them as they are transformed into objects of treatment or pity, or are no longer of interest in the world of the living.

Life review is valuable in clarifying the integrity, meaning, and value of the lives that the dying are soon to lose . . . or complete. This can, in turn, help them to find interests, tasks, and priorities to occupy the remainder of their lives, and to achieve those new goals. Much of great value may be accomplished in the short lives of the terminally ill: reconciling with estranged family, settling practical affairs, completing projects, and preparing the future of those who will be left alive.

INFORMATION SHARING. Information sharing is an important aspect of the dying process. As mentioned above, both the dying and their families have a right to information about medical condition, available treatment, and the future with and without various interventions (see Chapter 11, Legal Issues in the Care of the Aged). Sharing this information also opens communication and collaboration among the dying, family, and caretakers; no one is favored or excluded. In particular, it facilitates the dying aged's responsible participation in treatment, family affairs, and worldly responsibility — roles of vitality that are too often taken from them unnoticed through the customary authoritarian or paternalistic process of medical care and "protection" by the family. Participating in these roles makes it possible for the dying aged to experience fully not only the last of life but also death. In mental health terms, this full and honest participation helps to prevent confusion, self-doubt, and mistrust of family and health professionals. The prescription is to treat the dying aged as responsible, competent collaborators. An insightful exploration of their preferred ways of coping with problems, dangers, and decisions will indicate what they can do and what they will look to others to do. Sensitive attention to the questions they ask or avoid asking and to the information they attend to or ignore (or "do not understand" or "forget") will indicate what they want to know. The task is fourfold: (1) to offer information and participation; (2) to help the dying aged to be as active as possible, not to force on them more than they will or can assume; (3) to find others who can assume the roles the dying aged themselves choose not to assume; (4) to respect their styles of dealing with death, whatever they may be, and appreciate them as people.

DECISION MAKING.  Decision making should include the dying aged as responsible participants. This principle is a matter of law. It also recognizes that the dying aged have capability that other participants do not have — a knowledge of their own values and priorities. Only the dying can judge whether life is more important than pain or whether the husbanding of finances for the heirs is more important than their own comfort. This principle acknowledges the capacity of the dying aged and their families to bear discomfort and to deal with decision making. And it is an essential part of a collaborative view of health, illness, and treatment: Health professionals are medical advisers to and collaborators with the dying aged and their families in conceptualizing and dealing with health problems. This contrasts with an authoritarian view, whereby patients put themselves in the hands of healers, health professionals direct the cure, patients comply, and families offer support and comfort. Alternatives should be discussed with the dying aged in respect to treatment, placement, goals, and limits to prolongation of life, and decisions should be made jointly. The dying aged should be helped to participate maximally, not left to blunder in confirmation of some prejudice about their incompetence. Their wish to delegate decisions to family or professionals should be honored, with sensitivity to their preferences and needs and with frequent invitations to resume more active participation.

The roles of families differ in different families. In some cases families take over or maintain their power, having always directed the lives of their now-dying aged members. In some cases the aged and the family think, feel, and act jointly. In some the families are in the background with advice and support. And in some the families have no role, either because of the extreme autonomy (or tyranny) of the aged members, or because of alienation and exclusion. In every case, it is important to explore and respect the family roles and to apportion the information sharing and decision making according to the family style.

The rights and needs of health professionals should not be overlooked. They do have expertise. They must be able to practice competently. They have ethical standards that they are expected to uphold and that they revere. There are legal responsibilities that they are held to under penalty of law. And they come to the human service field because of a concern for people. In the current contest between professional authority and consumers' rights, a mutual respect for one another's rights and contributions can be lost. It may be unusual to suggest that health professionals be full participants, not dictators and not servants, in the processes of information sharing and decision making. This indicates frequent review by the patient, family, and staff and meetings for planning, with decisions made by consensus.

RELIGION. Religion as a support and structure for death has fallen into disrepute. Although religion may no longer be central to the social and institutional life of this society, it is still capable of providing structure and meaning in times of life crisis. The theology or dogma provides meaning to unexpected upheavals. The liturgical ceremony provides a sense of control and participation in experiences that might otherwise feel overwhelming. The morality, or prescriptions for behavior, provides reassurance that justice and propriety prevail in times of arbitrary burdens and losses. The religious community, or congregation, provides fellowship and support in otherwise lonely struggles. Finally, the variety of beliefs in life after death provides a sense of continuity and survival in the face of the fragility of life. This age-old source of comfort, developed by society over time to cope with mortal vulnerability, should not be overlooked either by the dying aged or those concerned about them, even though the impulse to religion may have lain dormant through most of their lives.

It is wise to ask the dying about the importance of religion in their lives, and what the tenets of their religions are in terms of sin, virtue, death, afterlife, and the part supernatural beings play in helping, protecting, and determining outcomes. Unless they adamantly reject religion, the dying should be encouraged to consider the comfort and help it can offer. Clerics and religious ceremony should be made available if these hold promise for them. Health professionals should be comfortable in exploring religious beliefs and acknowledging their own (without evangelizing) to aid the dying in using this resource.

### Care of Emotional and Cognitive Problems in Dying

CARE OF APPREHENSION AND ANXIETY. For the dying aged and their families, the sources of anxiety reside in the reality situation, including health problems, their effects on the functioning of the aged and their families, and finances; in the lack of information about health problems, treatment, and prognosis; in the lack of control over oneself and the situation; in the effects of the diseases and treatments; and in previous personality or psychiatric problems.

The various treatments for anxiety derive logically from these sources. Information about the illness, treatment, and prognosis substitutes reality, which is almost always more manageable than the fantasies and dread that people are prey to because of ignorance. Orientation to setting, time, and activities helps those who feel lost in the close atmosphere and rigid regimens of their institutionalized settings. Support and comfort from human companionship is irreplaceable. By this is meant person-to-person interaction, which responds to the need for personal validation and function; for this, professional treatment, artificial activities, and entertainment technology (television, high-fidelity sound systems, games, etc.), though valuable each in its own way, are no substitute. Light and sound at all times — especially during the dark and lonely night hours, when stimulation and distraction are minimal — may provide comfort and maintain personality organization.

Psychotherapy, practiced with humanity, is a vehicle for human contact and self-affirmation. It can also explore the anxiety and its sources, both recent and remote; clarify the current situation; and help strengthen or find coping skills and resources.

Comfort for the dying aged should not be skimped on. When used with awareness of their benefits, risks, and side effects, and the special adaptations needed for the aged, medications can help dull the anguish of the dying (see Chapter 5, Drug Therapy in the Aged Patient). Antianxiety medications can relieve tension, apprehension, and sleeplessness. Short-acting ones (e.g., alprazolam, oxazepam, lorazepam, or clonazepam) that can be adjusted flexibly are preferred. Antipsychotic medications in small doses may be indicated for agitation, severe panic, and psychotic decompensation with confusion and misinterpretation of reality. Here high-potency drugs (e.g., perphenazine, trifluoperazine, haloperidol) are preferable to low-potency drugs (e.g., thioridazine and chlorpromazine) in that they interfere less with alertness and carry less risk of cardiac, gastrointestinal, and other toxicity. Sedatives have both advantages and disadvantages: They may help sleep and counteract agitation, but they may also increase confusion and loss of cognitive and behavioral control, especially if these are already compromised by disease or emotions. Here again, short-acting drugs that can be used flexibly are preferable: Chloral hydrate, diphenhydramine, and triazolam are examples of these. Beware of drug interactions with analgesics, antiemetics, muscle relaxants, and other sedatives used to treat the physical health problems of the dying aged.

CARE OF ANGER AND OPPOSITIONALISM. Anger and oppositionalism may result from feelings of helplessness, fear, and disappointment in the failing of strengths previously relied upon, as well as from previous personality and psychiatric problems. Help consists in reinstilling in the dying aged a sense of acceptance and validation of themselves as respected and competent people. Reassurance and clarification of the reality situation may be useful. Giving control and/or finding surrogates whom the dying aged can trust can reverse panic.

Psychotherapy may be possible when the dying aged can put aside their travail and trust enough to develop rapport. After an acceptance of and respect for the valiant battle they are waging has been gained, the sources of anger can be identified and a collaboration with staff — as well as with the disease and life — can be negotiated. Setting limits to destructive behavior, in conjunction with constructive assertiveness, may be important. Antianxiety and antipsychotic medication may be helpful in reducing emotional pressure and impulsivity.

In cases of critical medical care or decisions, moral and legal rights and obligations may have to be carefully considered and allocated — to the dying aged, their families, or court-appointed guardians.

CARE OF DELIRIUM AND CONFUSION. Delirium and confusion can be a consequence of the fatal disease itself (cardiac decompensation, uremia, liver failure, etc.), the cerebral effects of the disease (paraneoplastic syndrome, cerebral metastases, infection, etc.), intercurrent disease (infection, fever, etc.), medications (for pain, sleep, inflammation, agitation, antineoplastic chemotherapy, etc.), malnutrition and dehydration, and the emotional consequences of illness (e.g., anxiety, isolation, pain, and exhaustion).

Again, human reassurance and support are helpful in themselves and as mediators to other treatments. Also useful is reality orientation, achieved by means of the company of people, light at all times, and cues such as calendars, clocks, signs, and the mass media (e.g., radio, television, and the newspapers). The treatment of the primary disease and its consequences, along with a careful review and revision of noxious medications, gets at the source of delirium and confusion, while posing the least risk. Antipsychotic medication can be helpful too (see Care of Apprehension and Anxiety, and Care of Anger and Oppositionalism).

CARE OF DELUSIONS AND HALLUCINATIONS. Delusions and hallucinations may be the result of metabolic abnormalities secondary to the following conditions: the terminal illness or complications; brain damage due to malignancy; paraneoplastic syndrome; the overwhelming emotional stress of the illness, treatment, impending death, or pain — stress that produces a condition similar to that of the acute confusional state; malnutrition or dehydration; sleep deprivation; or exacerbation of preexisting psychosis. These factors cumulatively undermine reality orientation and control of fear and fantasy. Dementia makes the dying aged cognitively more vulnerable, mental retardation makes them intellectually more vulnerable (in that they are less capable of using more sophisticated defenses, such as paranoia, obsessions, or rationalization), and preexisting psychosis makes them emotionally more vulnerable.

A primary treatment is to identify and correct the metabolic abnormality or malnutrition/dehydration, or treat a neoplasm underlying the paraneoplastic syndrome. A therapeutic relationship or counseling aimed at support, ventilation of feelings, gaining control over unmanageable feelings, and reinforcing reality orientation, can strengthen the defenses against the assaults on the ego that these physiological and emotional stresses pose. More structured psychotherapy is sometimes feasible to gain insight into and resolution of preexisting problems (e.g., fear of vulnerability, guilt and expectation of punishment, and mistrust of helpers). This makes it possible to see the current situation more realistically and to cope with it more constructively. Sedatives and antianxiety medications may help remove ego-weakening psychological states. Antipsychotic and antianxiety medications are often indicated to reduce delusions, hallucinations, agitation, and panic. Such medications increase comfort and make it possibe to provide medical treatment and health maintenance (feeding, sleep, bathing, exercise, etc.).

CARE OF DEPRESSION, WITHDRAWAL, AND APATHY. Depression, withdrawal, and apathy are very likely to stem from the reality situation of disability, discomfort, and impending death. Lack of human companionship, warmth, and open communication with family and caretaking professionals is another source. Concern about dealing with the present and the future (e.g., with personal care, finances, loss of relationships, etc.) may overwhelm the dying aged and their loved ones and produce feelings of hopelessness. Previous personality orientation or psychiatric problems may color or determine reactions to the reality situation.

Here as much as in any of the problems of the dying aged, it is important to become acquainted with the people themselves and to gain an understanding of their experiences, values, views of their current predicaments, and customary ways of coping. This will inform the caretaking professionals about how to promote ventilation of pent-up feelings, self-acceptance, validation of feelings, and reexamination by the dying aged of their views of the situation and their ways of coping with it. Sheer support and companionship may be the most important things — perhaps the only things — that the caretaker has to offer. As in dementia, life review may be healing, allowing virtues and accomplishments, persisting abilities, interests, obligations, and work projects to be completed. This can reawaken a sense of self-worth and vitality and permit a reinvestment in life.

The treatment of depressed, withdrawn, and apathetic individuals requires caring, a capacity for empathy, and time on the part of health professionals — resources that may be strained in health care systems that are often busy and technology oriented. Do health-care professionals and systems possess the requisite expertise? Can they afford the necessary expenditures of staff and time? Indeed, the question is: Can health professionals and systems care for these aged and their needs? (See the later section, Emotional and Cognitive Aspects of Professional Health Care, and Chapter 16, Attitudes, Values, and Ideologies as Influences on the Professional Education and Practice of Those Who Care for the Aged.)

There is often an expectation that psychotropic medications — antidepressants or other less specific ones — are applicable. In fact, they are of little use here. The dying aged are dealing with a depressing reality, and medications cannot make them happy about it. Also, the coexisting physical illnesses, dislocations, and treatments increase the risk of side effects and toxic effects. However, antianxiety and sedative medications can help the dying cope with the realities of their situation by reducing depressive symptoms.

### The Role of Families, and Working With Them

Families have older and more natural relationships with the aged members than do health professionals. This truism needs emphasis in an age when the care of disabilities is delegated to experts, and the dying aged tend to be sequestered in institutions. The experts and institutions have a tendency to focus on their own cultures and staff; patients are incorporated as the objects of health care, but there is little place for their families. In fact, in administering to the needs of the dying aged, families have always been a normal part of decision making, sanctioning of care, and technical consultation. There is a mutual emotional attachment between the aged and their families that finds expression in physical closeness, communication, and the provision of material care. Thus, it should be expected that space and time will be devoted to these family functions, and families should be recognized as fulfilling caretaking roles along with the health care professionals and institutions.

Family members express their own attitudes and feelings. They will communicate their fear of death, feelings about illness and treatments, and attitudes toward health professionals to the aged, other patients and families, health professionals, and health-care institutions. Their particular relationships with and feelings toward the dying aged will color their behavior. Culture and family tradition will structure the roles families take in relation to the dying aged. If the roles are respected, these family members can be helpful liaisons between their families and health care programs; if the roles are blocked, conflict and destruction of health care may well ensue.

- A 77-year-old, widowed, Italian-born woman was hospitalized for terminal breast carcinoma. Her children, nieces and nephews, and grandchildren would visit her in groups at erratic times of the day. A middle-aged man among them would stand on the periphery of the treatment team as they made rounds and examined and discussed this woman. The staff members were surprised, uncomfortable, and angry at this intrusion of a layman and relative into the confidential and technical meetings of medical professionals. Resentful and sarcastic remarks were made in private, and he was asked to remove himself until he was given appropriate information at some unspecified time. He became loud and demanding that he be told about his mother's condition and treatment. In a private meeting with one of the physicians, this man informed the physician that he was the dying woman's oldest son, and that in this Italian family it was his responsibility to report back to the family his mother's condition, and to see to it that she got the best treatment; if he failed in this duty, the family would be very angry with him. He asked that the physician help him fulfill his duty; in this way intrusion and conflict could be avoided. Thereafter the physician made it a point to keep this son fully informed, and conflict and hostility ceased completely.

As demonstrated by this account, the family's composition, cultural heritage, constellation of relationships, and attitudes should be understood so that they and the health care professionals can fill appropriate roles. Where information is lacking, education about illness and treatment and human relationships is needed, or relationships or behavior require changing, these issues should be addressed. Then the families can perform their appropriate roles as full participants in care, as consultants to the dying aged and/or health professionals, as interested parties, or as uninvolved bystanders.

### Contributions and Needs of Health Professionals

Health care professionals have their own professional responsibilities and rights that serve to maintain a high level of function, identity, and respect and that determine their roles with the dying aged. Many of these professionals see themselves as cure agents. They feel failure and resentment at the dying aged who have defied their curative efforts, so they tend to feel uncomfortable and helpless around these people and avoid them.

Health professionals need group support, planning, and evaluation to deal with the dying aged. This potentiates their joint efforts through mutual understanding and respect, recognition of areas of overlap of expertise, consultation and education, coordination, and flexibility of roles (see Chapter 14, The Interdisciplinary, Integrated Approach to Professional Practice with the Aged).

Hospice is a special professional approach to the care of the dying aged that has emotional and cognitive significance. It offers specifically palliative care: symptomatic relief, psychosocial support, work with both patient and family, and an interdisciplinary team approach. Its goal is to maximize the quality and meaningfulness of life rather than cure disease or prolong life. Hospice specifies a setting of the patient's choice, rather than a setting dedicated to the work of professionals. Terminally ill patients value most hospice services, but especially medical control of symptoms, home nursing, and psychological counseling. Most would accept hospice care but have not thought of it. The medical staff, too, value control of symptoms, home nursing, and psychological counseling, and want to continue to follow their patients through the dying process and hospice care. However, medical institutions give little support to psychological counseling for the dying.

Physicians working with the dying aged are the bearers of a professional tradition that orients them toward the cure of diseased individuals. Research into the care of the dying indicates that physicians continue to care for and about their patients when they are dying and that this loyalty is important to the patients. Physicians must collaborate with other caretakers — professional and informal — to deal effectively with a condition that is increasingly nonmedical. It is important that these preeminent authorities explain reality to the dying aged: Reality is much less frightening than fantasy, and the aged can guide this information process by asking for and accepting only what they can tolerate.

Physicians have difficulty dealing with dying patients. Research indicates that physicians fear death, and begin to fear death at an earlier age (6 to 12 years) than others. They are negative and blocked about the subject of death, reject the idea of their own deaths, personalize the deaths of others, and do not want to tell others about their incurable diseases. They use the profession of medicine to defend themselves against fears of death and to master it. When they are faced with death, their anxieties increase, and they distance themselves psychologically from it and focus on the physiological and technological aspects of medicine. This emotionally isolates incurable patients, thus hastening the emotional process of dying.

It is important that the dying aged maintain life that is useful and meaningful in their terms and that the prolongation of life not be confused with the prolongation of dying. The physician must learn, in this situation, to be a helper rather than a healer, to care rather than cure. When the physician's goal can change from that of curing patients to that of trying his best to help and to care for the patient, then success is much less related to whether the patient lives or dies. As White has pointed out: "The death of such a patient is no less a tragedy if cure is not your goal, but it makes the death of a patient less of a personal failure on your part."

## EMOTIONAL AND COGNITIVE ASPECTS OF PROFESSIONAL HEALTH CARE

### Health Care Professionals

The practices of health care professionals are determined not only by knowledge and skills but by attitudes, values, and ideologies (Gurland, 1985), which vary from discipline to discipline and from health care setting to health care setting. These variations may be influenced by professional education and socialization, and by the operating environments and cultures of health care institutions, but they also are powerfully determined by the personalities and personal experiences of the individuals invested with professional roles. People bring themselves to professional practice. Thus, it is problematic whether professionals can be taught to be interested in and empathize with the aged, to value goals of maintenance and restoration of function, and to share authority and respect with other disciplines, much less patients and families. Those who have the perspectives, values, and attitudes that make these professional functions possible may be taught to recognize, develop, and implement them more effectively. Perhaps those who do not have them should be recognized and directed to other professional practices.

Health care disciplines, too, have their own cultures and histories. These orient them to certain goals, technical practices, and territories of professional practice. For instance, nurses were first nurturing women who cared for the human needs and comforts of soldiers and other isolates. They continue to focus on the comprehensive care and education of patients through intensive contact with them, but nurses have assumed many of the technical and theoretical functions and perspectives of physicians. Their battles are to practice their "medicalized" roles without the direction of the physicians who have dominated this field. In contrast, psychologists were first researchers into mental processes. Clinical psychologists apply the testing and modification of mental processes to human mental illness and behavior. Their battles are to reserve psychological testing for themselves and to expand their treatment of mental illness, while practicing independently. These histories, goals, and practices affect the ways these disciplines perceive and act upon the emotions and cognitive function of the aged.

Oliver Wendell Holmes, Sr., noted that "medical knowledge and practice, which is thought to be rooted in objective research, is no less responsive to the current politics, religion, and fashion than the barometer is to the air pressure." The science of the day is an aspect of the social philosophy of the day, and both are manifestations of the sociological status of contemporary society.

Politicoeconomic factors affect the goals and practices of health professionals. The labor, time, and money available powerfully influence "what is practical" in caring for the aged. Health care institutional goals determine the goals of the program and the allocation of resources. The economic resources society finds available for health care and for the care of the aged set limits and directions for health care institutions and are ultimately a reflection of society's social priorities. At present the trend is toward reduction of human services in favor of production of goods and economic growth. At the same time, the numbers, needs, and political influence of the aged are growing. On balance, health-care professionals are supported in responding to the health needs of the aged but must do so according to short-term and acute-care models.

These factors have practical implications for the care of the emotional and cognitive aspects of the aged. It cannot be assumed that the same expertise and responsiveness will be forthcoming in any health care setting: the aged and emotional and cognitive issues will be perceived differently by different individuals, disciplines, and health care institutions. The aged, their advocates, and referring professionals must have some sophistication about the nature of the problems, the care that will be most effective, and the characters of the various health care resources available, and must make selective referrals. It also follows that it is necessary for the aged and their advocates to be active in the diagnostic and treatment process, since there is a component of values and ideology as well as professional expertise in the understanding of problems and appropriate treatment. This militates toward the collaborative model of health care, rather than the authoritative one. Finally, there is a need to provide consultation and education to professionals. One goal is to heighten their awareness of the part attitudes, values, and ideologies play in the perception and manifestation of emotional and cognitive issues both in the aged and in professional practice. Another is to sharpen their sensitivity and skill in dealing with these issues in non-psychiatric contexts, such as physical illness and the changes of normal ageing. Much of the frontline professional caretaking of emotional and cognitive problems is done by non-psychiatric disciplines, such as primary care physicians, nurses, and clergymen. Skills in evaluation, counseling, resource-finding, and coordination can be enhanced with training. And it is worth attempting to educate health care professionals to each other's expertise and practices, and to methods of collaborating efficiently and flexibly in some approximation of interdisciplinary practice.

### Health Care Institutions

There is a tendency for the aged in institutions to become patients or residents rather than independent citizens. This role necessarily involves diminution of individuality, and certainly loss of the social and physical environment that made this individuality possible. The tendency is to shape self-images and behaviors to fit institutional regimens, resources, physical environments, and goals. Often good patients or residents are those who accept that role, abide by rules, obey professional authorities, and do not present too many individual needs or behaviors. Thus a dependent, passive, and regimented role may be fostered.

- An 83-year-old widow had completed college and worked for many years as a technician and supervisor in a defense laboratory. After her husband's death she lived alone, and was competent, active, and strong-minded. Increasing forgetfulness, dangerous behavior, and panic calls to her daughter caused concern, and she was eventually (reluctantly) convinced to move into a nursing home. She expected to continue her independent activities, including walks in the neighborhood. She resented the company of old, mentally disabled people, and did not want to feel that she was like them. She also resented being scolded by the concerned but strict nursing director for taking unauthorized and unaccompanied walks, being restricted to the house in punishment, and having her daughter informed and scold her as well. On several occasions she became angry and intolerant of the nursing home, and decided to "take a powder": She waited until evening or early morning, when the staff was limited and busy, and fled the nursing home with the intention of walking back to her old home. The nursing home staff became fearful for her safety and for their responsibility if she were hurt. They insisted that her behavior be curbed by discipline and/or psychotropic medication, or she would be moved to another facility. Her daughter was torn between sympathy for her mother's violated independence and concern for her care and safety.

The loss of familiar surroundings, people, and activities may be more than unhappy. It may deprive the aged of the stimulation and orientation that make it possible for them to function with limited capacities. Those who are mildly demented may become disoriented and disorganized in new and unfamiliar surroundings. Those who have explosive tempers or mistrustful views of other people can no longer withdraw to their homes or refuse to associate with some (or most) people as defenses; they may then become troublesome or dangerous. The loss of control and information about their lives and care, which is usually left to professional caretakers, encourages disorientation, helplessness, and despair. It is an important contributor to the adjustment reactions and depression found in such high frequency among the institutionalized aged, as discussed earlier.

Health care institutions sensitive to the functional needs of the aged provide frequent and well-paced activities for social and physical stimulation. In institutions that attend only to food, shelter, clothing, and the safety skills of self-care, intellectual vigor and social interaction are not exercised and so these abilities atrophy. People may lose the capacity to concentrate on reading or a discussion, becoming quickly bored and in need of attention. They may forget to pay attention to others' needs and activities and become self-centered and irritable. They may forget how to button clothes or which article of clothing to put on first and thus become helplessly dependent on the care of others. Senility and being "old" in the dysfunctional sense becomes a self-fulfilling expectation.

These things can happen in acute-care hospitals as well as in long-term care institutions, because the aged tend to have longer stays than others because of multiple disabilities, longer recovery times, and vulnerability to complications. In fact, the patterns, equipment, and staffing at acute-care hospitals are less attuned to maintenance of function than those at long-term care facilities. It is important to look upon the institutionalized aged as rather finely tuned functioning systems that need careful preventive maintenance and exercise in order to preserve them in running order. What is not used may be lost, and once lost it may be difficult or impossible to recover because of the impairment of new learning and limited resources for more than current function.

Social isolation from family and acquaintances exacerbates the losses and further reduces the social network of the aged. Institutionalization may even tend to isolate them from other patients, when individual accommodation and attention from staff are the principles of care, rather than group activities and self-help. And relationships with staff may not be consistent, as staff rotate shifts, are absent on vacations, and turn over at a high rate. The result is not only grief for the loss of past relationships but a reluctance to make new ones in the expectation they will be superficial and temporary. The obvious corrective is to maintain former social relationships by means of liberal visiting policies, outings into the community, and the involvement of outside caring people in institutional caring roles. Within the institution, self-help, mutual help, and activity among the aged should be maximized, and staff should be assigned long-term to individual residents.

### Health Care-Produced Disabilities

It is well to be aware of the toxic effects and side effects of health care as a whole. People function best in the environment in which they have learned to function and which contains the resources they use in functioning. Intruding — even to help — is dangerous. A wise pathologist, Norman Bolker, offered the adage: "Never give a treatment unless the risk of *not* giving it is *even greater* than the risk of *giving* it."

Many of the risks have been mentioned previously:

- Exclusion from functioning society produces depression and loss of positive self-image, and contributes to paraphrenia and paranoid illness.
- Institutionalization brings the risk of loss of autonomy and loss of capacity for the activities of daily living and social skills.
- Medications may cause delirium, sedation, falls (and injury), pseudodementia, loss of self-care capacity, and impairment of various physical functions (muscular incoordination, constipation, intestinal obstruction, urinary retention, kidney failure, cardiac arrhythmias, etc.).
- Health testing may produce anxiety and hypochondria, as well as anemia from blood loss.
- Inactivity and bed rest create muscle atrophy, orthostatic hypotension, ataxia, pressure sores, infections (including pneumonia and urinary tract infections), osteoporosis, and constipation.
- Residence in institutions brings the risk of infections, both through close contact with groups and because the people contacted are very likely to be infected with pathogens. The infections are also more likely to be resistant to ordinary antibiotics, since they are due to microorganisms that are constantly exposed to antibiotics.

The response to the risks of health care–imposed disability is the recognition of and defense against them by both the aged and health care professionals. Again, the collaborative model of health care is indicated. The aged and their advocates must take active roles. Disabilities, the sick role, the passive status of being treated by experts, and the imposing organization, staffing, and physical environment of health care institutions make it difficult for people to maintain the perspective, confidence, and assertiveness required to be effective participants in the health care process. Advocates are needed. These may be family members or formal appointees, such as hospital ombudsmen and officials of city and state departments of elder affairs or public health. In addition, there is increasing regulation of the health care of the aged and increasing legal protection of their rights and safety. However, the ultimate guarantees of attentive and responsible health care are the active involvement of the aged and the sophistication and integrity of the health professionals.

*Society*

The influences of the society at large on clinical care must not be overlooked. They have very practical implications for the individual's life, health, and treatment. The chapters in Part III, Interpersonal and Societal Issues, speak to many of these concerns. Here we will only mention a few specifically.

Legal issues, addressed in Chapter 11, influence the emotional state of the aged, as when self-direction, as well as the self-esteem that it engenders, is affirmed and protected by civil rights statutes and elder-abuse protection policies. Conversely, self-esteem, trust, and the will to maintain effort and even life may be undermined when civil commitment, conservatorship, and guardianship affirm only the incompetence of the aged and consign them to dependent status. An impaired cognitive state may trigger legal interventions and bring helpful guidance and protection. Without these interventions, cognitive impairments may degrade self-care, prevent appropriate use of professional health care, and weaken family and social supports. Thus, legal intervention, like any other "helping intervention," must be used circumspectly, with due consideration for its positive and negative mental health effects.

Long-term health care, addressed in Chapter 12, likewise has positive and negative effects on emotional and cognitive health. Silverman (1989) has demonstrated the supportive effects of long-term care institutions on the maintenance of identity and self-esteem for the aged who rely on the structure and supports these institutions provide when they are truly "homes for the aged." When they are inhumane storage facilities, however neat and clean, they may crush the emotional and spiritual — and even physical — life out of their inmates, as Sarton (1973) has poignantly portrayed. Institutions can even degrade cognitive functions through demoralization and enforced passivity (see earlier discussion of the pseudodementia of depression). The lesson here is: "Use with caution."

Economics as facilitator of and obstacle to the health care of the aged is discussed in Chapter 13. We might note here only the fact that economics determines the availability of health care. On the societal/systems level, the supply and allocation of health care personnel, technology, and specific procedures are determined by politicoeconomic forces. Unmanaged systems may concentrate care on powerful and profitable segments of the population — often the urban and wealthy. The aged may not be attractive consumers. Managed systems have struggled with priority decisions. The aged have not come out high on the list by reason of their large consumption of health care, increasing its cost, or by reason of their low worth in society (as a result of their lack of valued contributions). On the personal health care level, the expertise of the health care practitioner available may be economically determined, that of the experienced going to the well-to-do, whereas aides treat the not-so-well-to-do. In the same way, the readiness of availability, access to high-technology procedures, and even the possibility of certain types of care may be controlled by personal payment, privately-purchased insurance, and government-financed services.

## EXAMINATION OF THE EMOTIONAL AND COGNITIVE STATUS OF THE AGED

Good health care of the aged is good health care for anyone. The principle concern is not to deviate from good practice just because the subjects of care are aged. However, some special precautions and emphases are necessary.

It is important to evaluate the vision and hearing of the aged, which are important to communication, as normal aging often impairs these special senses. Unrecognized impairments may lead at least to confusion and frustration on the part of both the aged and the examining professional and, at worst, to erroneous diagnosis and treatment, invoking the ever-present prejudice about senility. Simple questioning as to whether the aged can hear and see the examiners and situation clearly or require louder voice, brighter light, or retrieval of hearing aids or eyeglasses suffices in most cases. In some cases, specific testing of hearing and vision is needed to verify problems. It is probably wise to examine the aged in especially well-lighted rooms that are free of masking background noise. Aids such as a magnifying glass and an assisted hearing device that anyone can use to amplify sound may be useful.

We must remember that understanding, memory, and decision making are slowed with age even when there is no cognitive deficit. Responses that are not promptly forthcoming may be mistaken for the inability to respond. Therefore, examining professionals must schedule ample time to communicate as part of the examination, and give aged people enough time to absorb what is presented to them and respond to it. Timed tests are probably less valid than tests without arbitrary time limits.

The slowed absorption of communication with aging, as well as the higher prevalence of cognitive deficit, may make the aged less reliable historians and reporters. There is a human need to respond to requirements and to appear competent, so the aged may fill in the hiatuses in their knowledge with plausible fictions or agreement with examiners' suggestions. Therefore, the examining professional must be careful not to suggest answers or "lead the witness." Also, seek third-party historians for corroboration. These may be family members, neighbors, previous health care givers, or medical or other records.

The aged are vulnerable to current stresses and losses of resources, both as primary causes of emotional and cognitive problems and as aggravators of preexisting problems. They themselves are concerned about the state of their health and well-being and the changes in them. Therefore, it is important for examiners to carefully assess environmental stresses and resources as pathogenic agents. In addition, in planning treatment it is essential to determine what is possible in terms of the resources available.

The aged are much involved with their families and other social supports. Their disabilities require assistance from others, and their sense of vulnerability leads them to seek supportive relationships. In turn, those in key relationships with them have a sense of responsibility that makes them protective. Disability and health care often require that the aged have helpers. For all these reasons health professionals must plan to deal with families and others interested in the aged. They must leave time for them, include them in planning and reviewing conferences, and schedule communication with them. These helping people are not intruders or unwanted burdens, but essential parts of the lives of the aged and facilitators of health care.

Emotional and cognitive issues pervade the lives and health of the aged because feeling and thinking are essential parts of their beings. It is incumbent on health care professionals to know and be prepared to deal with these essential aspects of the aged and their care.

## REFERENCES

Blythe, R. (1979). *The view in winter: Reflections on old age.* New York: Harcourt Brace Jovanovich.
Estes, C. L., with Lee, P. R., Lenore, G., & Noble, M. (1979). *The Aging Enterprise.* San Francisco: Jossey-Bass.

Gonda, T. A., & Ruark, J. E. (1984). *Dying dignified: The health professional's guide to care.* Menlo Park, CA: Addison-Wesley.

Gurland, L. (1985). *Who you are is what you do: A study of the health care attitudes, values, and ideologies of clinicians who work with the elderly.* Unpublished doctoral dissertation, Massachusetts School of Professional Psychology, Boston, Massachusetts.

Johnson, C. J., & McGee, M. (1986). *Encounters with eternity: Religious views of death and life after death.* New York: Philosophical Library.

Lindemann, E. (1956). The meaning of crisis in individual and family living. *Teachers College Record, 57,* 310.

Mace, N. L., Rabins, P. V. (1981). *The thirty-six hour day: A family guide to caring for persons with Alzheimer's disease, related dementing illnesses, and memory loss in later life.* Baltimore, MD: Johns Hopkins University Press.

Miner, J. (1986). *Labor crowned with favor: The relationship of work to identity and self-esteem in old age.* Unpublished doctoral dissertation, Massachusetts School of Professional Psychology, Boston, Massachusetts.

Sarton, M. (1973). *As we are now.* New York: W. W. Norton.

Silverman, D. (1989). *A phenomenological study of self-identity in nursing home residents.* Unpublished doctoral dissertation, Massachusetts School of Professional Psychology, Boston, Massachusetts.

Sadavoy, J., Lazarus, L. W., & Jarvik, L. F. (1991). *Comprehensive review of geriatric psychiatry.* Washington, DC: American Psychiatric Press.

Townsend, P. (1957). *The family life of old people.* Glencoe, IL: The Free Press.

# 4

# Oral Health and Treatment of the Aged

Athena S. Papas
Maureen C. Rounds

Since the turn of the century there has been a ninefold increase in the aged population primarily because of an increase in life expectancy. According to the U.S. Bureau of the Census, when the "baby boomers" become elderly, the elderly will comprise 22% of the U.S. population, reaching 66 million in the year 2030. The growth of this group is paralleled by an increased need for dental care. Just as we see characteristic medical problems in the aged population, we see characteristic dental problems, such as root decay, recession of the gingiva (gums), periodontal disease, advanced alveolar bone resorption due to long-term denture use, xerostomia (dry mouth), and oral cancer.

Although most common oral diseases usually are not fatal, they can have critical effects on life and general health and well-being. A misjudgment in the oral care of a patient undergoing chemotherapy, bone marrow transplant, or head and neck radiation therapy, can be fatal. Oral factors also have been implicated in death from food asphyxiation, especially in people who have dentures.

Virtually all of the aged suffer from at least one chronic disease. Any disease, chronic or acute, can stress the body, depleting nutrient reserves and turning marginal nutritional status into overt deficiency. Furthermore, there are approximately 200 systemic diseases that have manifestations in the oral cavity and that can, in turn, affect nutrition. Poor oral health can also profoundly influence the desire and ability to eat, which may then lead to poor nutrition. Because compromised nutritional status can impair immune response, healing, and resistance to infection in the aged, it can, in turn, seriously affect oral health.

Appearance is an essential component of self-esteem, self-expression, and well-being. Without healthy teeth and oral tissues, the quality of life can be undermined from both emotional and social standpoints. The aged with ill-fitting dentures may be reluctant to talk for fear of "whistling," clicking, or even dropping dentures, thus withdrawing from social contacts. Others with missing teeth may refrain from smiling, always appearing serious or even dour. These behaviors, in some extreme cases, may lead friends to misinterpret expressions and withdraw and may lead to self-imposed isolation due to embarrassment. Without social interactions, a downward spiral of psychological and general health problems begins. Conversely, the aged who have regular oral care have a better self-image, may be more outgoing and active, and tend to adjust better to the aging process.

In our society at present, more individuals are retaining teeth longer than in the past. However, with this increase in dentate status comes an increase in other oral problems such as periodontal diseases and root caries. Both periodontal disease and root caries have multifactorial etiologies. Dietary and nutritional factors, heredity, age, sex, salivary gland function, oral treatment patterns, oral hygiene practices, exposure to fluoride, psychosocial history, economic status, disease and medication history, and tobacco and alcohol use, all play a role.

## THE HEALTHY MOUTH

As seen in Figure 4.1, in the adult mouth, teeth are set in two arches: the maxilla (upper) and the mandible (lower). The different teeth perform different functions: incisors cut, canines tear, and premolars and molars grind food. When the upper and lower teeth meet, they touch one another simultaneously. Since the upper arch is slightly larger, the outside surfaces of the upper teeth face slightly more toward the cheeks than do the lower teeth. There is some overlap of the upper teeth over the lower, particularly in the front.

The tooth consists of two parts, the crown and the root (see Figure 4.2). The crown is covered by enamel, which is the hardest tissue in the body. Once formed, it cannot regenerate itself. It relies on saliva to maintain its hardness since it no longer has access to blood supply. Enamel is milky white in color and translucent.

The root is covered by a thin yellow layer of cementum, which is similar to bone in structure and hardness. Unlike enamel, it is capable of regenerating itself, providing a

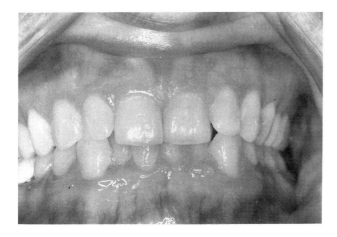

FIGURE 4.1 The healthy oral cavity.

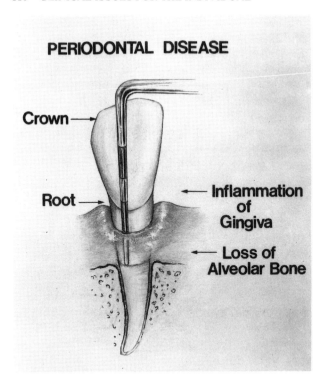

FIGURE 4.2 Tooth with root exposed after periodontal disease.

surface for the attachment of fiber bundles. The fiber anchors the tooth to bone, providing stability and resistance for the tooth and acting much like shock absorber.

The next layer of the tooth, found in both the crown and the root, is dentin. It is slightly harder than bone and since it is not as hard as enamel, it provides elasticity to the tooth. Dentin is yellowish in color and slightly translucent. Nutrients are supplied to the dentin by the blood vessels found in the pulp. Cells (odontoblasts), present in the pulp, form new dentin.

The pulp occupies the center of the tooth and is confined by the inner layer of dentin. It is comprised of blood vessels, nerves, and fibers, and provides both nutrition and sensation to the tooth. The nerves and blood vessels enter the tooth through the bottom of the root.

The tooth does not exist in the mouth in isolation, but is supported and held in place by the periodontium (*perio* means "to surround"; *dont* means "tooth"). As seen in Figure 4.3, it consists of gingiva (gums), alveolar bone, periodontal ligament, and cementum.

The individual tooth is set into a socket in the alveolar bone. Periodontal ligament fibers extend from the bone to the cementum covering the root of the tooth. These fibers attach the tooth to the bone and provide stability. They also act as shock absorbers to cushion the force of biting. The gingiva is soft tissue that is pink in Caucasians and pigmented in blacks or people from the Mediterranean area. It surrounds the tooth and alveolar bone. The upper portion of the gingiva is not attached to the tooth surface; conse-

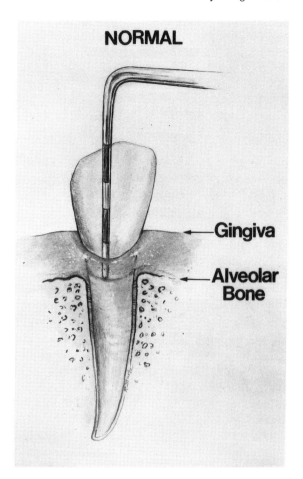

FIGURE 4.3 Normal tooth.

quently, there is a natural space, called the sulcus, between the outer layer of tooth and the inner layer of gingiva, like a cuff on a pant leg. Lining the oral cavity is a mucous membrane called the oral mucosa.

## ORAL DISEASES

### Caries

Dental caries is one of the most prevalent diseases in humans (see Figure 4.4). Several factors affect susceptibility or resistance to caries: bacteria adhering to and metabolizing on the tooth surface; the resistance of the person and tooth surface; the oral environment, composed of saliva, other microorganisms and their products, and food residues; and the duration of exposure of the tooth surface to organic acids resulting from foods.

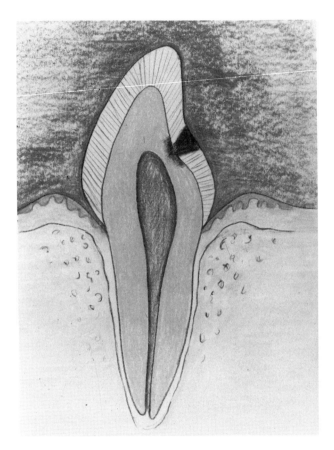

FIGURE 4.4 Caries pene-
trating into dentine.

The organisms associated with caries on top of the tooth (coronal caries) are *S. mutans*
and lactobacillus. Although the organisms involved in root caries have not been fully
identified, the major ones implicated are *S. mutans*, lactobacillus, diphtheroids, and fila-
mentous organisms, especially *Actinomyces viscous.*

### Gingival Disease

Microbial, environmental, and systemic factors influence periodontal disease as well.
Periodontal lesions (pockets) harbor a variety of mostly anaerobic, amino acid ferment-
ing organisms that require certain serum factors for growth (e.g., *B. melaninogenicus*
requires hemin and vitamin K). Some of the environmental factors are food impaction,
overhanging or irregular restorations, the degree of plaque and calculus (hardened
plaque) accumulation, and tobacco use. Systemic factors include nutrition, endocrine
conditions, and inherited characteristics. Subgingival plaque, unlike supragingival
plaque, is not affected by local dietary factors and saliva; instead, gingival fluid, host
cells, and the tooth itself supply the necessary nutrients. Some food extracts have been
shown to initiate the immune response directly. Thus, impacted food could lead directly
to the initiation of periodontal inflammation.

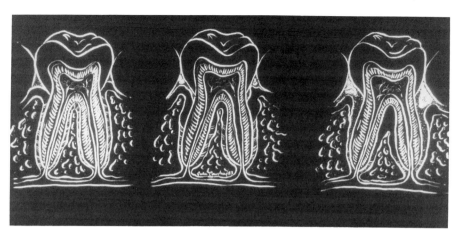

FIGURE 4.5  Progression of periodontal disease.

When the gingiva becomes irritated, inflammation occurs. Inflammation represents the body's defensive response to injury by the toxins produced by plaque. Gingival inflammation is characterized by swelling, redness, heat, pain, and loss of function. Bleeding is a sign of gum inflammation and should be considered a warning that an unhealthy condition exists. The inflammation may be localized or generalized, depending on how many areas have accumulated plaque.

Calculus below the gum line provides some physical irritation to the gums but, more importantly, additional plaque adheres to the outer surface of the calculus and produces its toxins. Bacterial plaque, which adheres to the rough surface of the calculus, is not as easily removed as that which attaches to the smoother tooth surface. Therefore, it is important to have calculus removed regularly by the dental hygienist or dentist.

As seen in Figure 4.5, left untreated, gingival inflammation will worsen: The amount of redness will increase, the triangular-shaped tissue between the teeth will appear swollen, and gums are likely to bleed when brushed. If this condition is allowed to persist, the redness and swelling eventually subside. However, this does not mean that the gum tissue is healthy. In fact, the texture of the gums changes: tissue that was once resilient becomes fibrotic and hard. Blood flow to the gums is reduced; consequently, the inflow of nutrients and outflow of the waste products of metabolism are diminished. The tissue becomes very pale. In this condition, gums heal slowly after injury or infection. The gums recede gradually, exposing the root of the tooth (hence the expression "long in the tooth" to indicate old age). The exposed root surfaces are susceptible to decay.

## Periodontal Disease

When periodontal disease develops, deep scaling or surgery may be necessary. Changes also occur within the sulcus (space around the tooth). If irritants are constantly present in the sulcus, a destructive process occurs in which the tissue that forms the bottom of the sulcus gradually moves further down the root away from the irritants. The result is a deeper space or "pocket" that is impossible to clean with normal methods (i.e., tooth brushing and flossing). A vicious cycle is set up: Bacteria in the deep pocket remain undisturbed and multiply rapidly. As more bacteria produce more toxins, the pocket deepens still more, and so on. As the destructive process moves gradually farther down the root, it involves not only soft gingival tissues but the ligament and bone as well. This is called periodontitis. As the ligaments and bone provide support and stability for the teeth, if these structures are gradually destroyed the tooth loosens and eventually will fall out if nothing is done to stop the destruction of the supporting tissues.

It is not uncommon for the teeth of an aged person to "spread" or "flare" when they have loosened. This is initially treated by deep scaling. If the periodontitis persists, surgery is recommended unless the person's medical status contraindicates this. Periodontal surgery consists of the removal of diseased soft tissue and the smoothing of the jagged surface of the bone left in the aftermath of bone destruction.

Secondary factors may predispose the individual to periodontal disease. Among these are:

1. Areas of decay, in which bacteria can reside
2. Smoking or chewing of tobacco
3. Brushing with a hard bristled brush or hard "scrubbing" of the teeth with a brush, which results in wearing away of the gums
4. Malnutrition, which lowers the body's resistance to the disease.

The recently completed National Dental Survey of Oral Health of United States Adults (1987) indicates that 42% of those attending senior centers are edentulous. The average number of teeth in those retaining natural teeth was only 17. Although these figures indicate an improvement since past national surveys, they are still not indicative of good oral health. The oral health of the inner-city poor who do not attend senior centers is likely to be even worse than this. Of the elderly who had retained some of their teeth, 22% exhibited signs of periodontal disease as defined by at least one periodontal pocket with the depth of at least 4 mm. Eighty-eight percent had gingival recession in at least one site, exposing roots to the oral environment. The mean number of decayed or filled teeth was 7.6. The prevalence of root caries is much higher in the elderly than among younger adults. Sixty-seven percent of the males and 61% of the females of the 1985 National Study of Senior Center Population, 83% of terminally ill institutionalized elderly patients, and 89% of patients suffering advanced periodontal disease had root caries. In contrast, such lesions were much less prevalent in younger populations (Banting, 1986).

Despite the high level of caries, only 37.5% of the seniors had received dental care within the past year — almost half the percentage found in younger adults.

LOSS OF TEETH

As noted earlier, forty-two percent of the aged have lost all of their teeth (U.S. Department of Health and Human Services, 1987). This has several effects:

1. The elder may experience a decline in chewing ability or in the desire to eat.
2. The elder may be embarrassed and become reclusive.
3. Infection and inflammation are possible.
4. Digestive ability may suffer.

However, none of these effects is universal, and the aged manage quite well with dentures or even without teeth or dentures. If dentures are so poorly fitted that they irritate gums, aged people may have difficulty chewing and may limit their food intake. Resultant nutritional deficiencies can further aggravate the condition. As a result of poorly fitting dentures or fears about their ability to eat with dentures, the aged may follow self-imposed diet restrictions, such as soft and liquid diets. Protein intake may be low because of a hesitancy to eat meats, which require chewing. Some of the aged may avoid fibrous foods, such as fruits and vegetables, because of the embarrassment of poorly functioning dentures. This may lead to bowel problems. Others may avoid foods that are hard, sticky, or irritating because they may become trapped in the sulcus.

Furthermore, when food is not chewed properly, digestion is less efficient since the rate of digestion is directly related to the surface area of the food exposed to intestinal enzymes.

## THE EFFECT OF DENTATE STATUS ON NUTRIENT QUALITY OF THE DIET

The relationship between dentate status and dietary quality was studied in 181 aged free-living volunteers enrolled in the Tufts Dental Pilot study, a substudy of the Nutritional Status Survey (NSS). The entire survey consisted of 691 individuals aged 60 to 98, who were surveyed by the epidemiology group of the United States Department of Agriculture's Human Nutrition Resource Center at Tufts University in the early 1980s. The survey has been described in detail by McGandy et al. (1986).

The data obtained include the following: blood chemistry, three-day food diary, modified physical examination, dental examination, anthropometric measure, current and past medical history, current and past medication use, subjects living, shopping and cooking arrangements, tobacco, alcohol or beverage consumption, age, sex, education, dental knowledge, attitudes, and behaviors.

The NSS population is characterized by a high educational level and is 98% Caucasian (despite the fact that an attempt was made to recruit a more diverse population). Dietary-intake data revealed low intakes of certain nutrients, Vitamin D, $B_6$ and $B_{12}$, as well as folic acid and the minerals zinc and calcium, in both sexes. Three lifestyle characteristics were associated with reduced food intake and dietary quality: low educational attainment, low median family income, and partial or full dentures.

Analysis of nutrient intakes including total calories revealed a statistically significant decrease of approximately 20% for 19 of the nutrients in the diets of those who had one or two full dentures compared to those who have teeth and no dentures, or partial dentures. Similar findings emerged on a subset of 75 subjects in the Dental Longitudinal Study population whose 3-day diaries were analyzed (Wayler & Chauncy, 1985). Many edentulous people are able to chew well with gums alone (which may become callused), maintaining an adequate diet.

The cariogenicity of a food is its relative potential to promote caries. Among the food-related factors that affect cariogenicity are the chemical composition of the food, the physical form in which it is eaten, the frequency with which it is eaten, the oral clearance time, and the concentration and the organoleptic effect of the food (Schachtele & Jensen, 1983;

Burt & Ismail, 1986). Only certain "fermentable" carbohydrates (e.g., mono- and disaccharides and possibly starch) can be decomposed by the caries promoting oral bacteria *S. mutans* and *L. acidophilus*, which in turn produces acid and subsequent decay. Acid conditions below *p*H 5.5 cause dissolution of calcium and phosphate from enamel; any combination of oral factors can cause demineralization (Rosen & Willett, 1985). The simple sugars, especially sucrose, are clearly important in causing coronal caries and appear to be significant in root caries development as well. Starch has a somewhat lesser effect on caries; however, preliminary data suggest that it is also important (Papas, 1992).

## Coronal Caries

It is important to measure total fermentable carbohydrates rather than sucrose alone, since other sugars and starches also contribute to the incidence of caries. The sucrose content of food is not directly related to acidogenic potential, nor is acid production necessarily related to the amount of enamel dissolved (Krasse, 1985). The Consensus Conference on Cariogenicity (1986) concluded that confirmatory results of any two studies (including animal studies, *in vitro* studies, and interproximal plaque *p*H studies) could be used to determine if a food is noncariogenic. Because one food is mixed with other foods prior to and during ingestion, the sequence of eating is important (e.g., if cheese or peanuts is eaten after a sugar exposure, the duration of the *p*H drop is reduced (Schachtele, Rosamond, & Harlander, 1985; Jensen, 1984; Dodds & Edgar, 1986). Changes in the form in which food is eaten, time of day, length of intervals between eating, rate of ingestion, and the presence of cariostatic factors can influence cariogenicity.

Sugar consumption rises again in older age groups: males and females in the 65- to 74-year-old group consume 53% and 47% more sugar-containing foods than young adults 19 to 24 years old (Schachtele et al., 1985). Therefore, it is important help the aged develop eating habits that are not cariogenic.

## Root Caries

Dietary factors have been shown to play a role in root caries: Studies of New Guineans and Aborigines (Schamschula, Keyes, & Hornabrook, 1972; Schamschula, Barnes, Keyes, & Guilbinat, 1974; Holloway, James, & Slack, 1963) and observations of ancient skulls (Hardwick, 1960) have shown that such populations who subsist on diets high in complex carbohydrates have a low prevalence of coronal caries but a high prevalence of root caries. Patients suffering from periodontal disease exhibit statistically significant correlations between their frequency and consumption of fermentable carbohydrates and root caries (Hix & O'Leary, 1976; Ravald, Hamp, & Birked, 1986). The Tufts Nutrition and Oral Health Study (NOHS) confirmed such observations (Papas et al., 1984; Papas, Palmer, McGandy, Hartz, & Russell, 1987; Papas et al., 1989). Preliminary data from subjects in the NOHS population and the Forsyth Root Caries Center show that both starch and sugar consumption correlate well with the prevalence of root caries (Papas et al., 1989). Where sugars were separated into categories based on form and retention, people who developed root caries consumed almost twice as much of sugary liquids and 25% more cakes and cookies (solid fermentable carbohydrates) as those who did not have root caries. Vekhalahti and Paunio (1988) found similar results. Additionally, the incidence of root and coronal caries in our population was similar to that found by Beck in a representative sample of 451 rural, aged, free-living Iowans (Hand, Hunt, & Beck, 1988).

Diets containing dairy products (especially cheese) exert a caries-protective effect. Many mechanisms of action have been hypothesized: Caseinates and other organic phosphates found in milk products have been found *in vitro* to help reduce demineralization by augmenting the action of the acquired pellicle-inhibiting adhesion of normal microbial flora (Reynolds, Riley, & Storey, 1982; Reynolds & Wong, 1983; Reynolds & del Rio, 1984; Reynolds, 1987; Harper, Osborn, Clayton, & Hefferren, 1987; Hayes & Hyatt, 1974; Vratsanos & Mandel, 1984; Bowen, 1974). Calcium-phosphate buffering systems and common ion effects present in dairy products can affect the critical *p*H through the diffusion of calcium and phosphate into plaque. They may also stimulate the salivary secretion rate and composition, and increase the rate of oral clearance (Tabak, 1988). Further, lipids derived from dairy products coat the tooth surface, although it has not been verified that fatty acids inhibit bacterial growth. In addition, calcium lactate, calcium propionate, and fluoride may have other cariostatic effects. Silva, Burgess, and Sandham (1987a, 1987b) have found that cheese extracts reduce acid demineralization *in vitro*. Supportive data include studies of *in vitro* dentin demineralization (Jenkins & Harper, 1983), *in vitro* and *in vivo* enamel demineralization studies (Silva et al., 1987a, 1987b), plaque *p*H studies (Schachtele & Jensen, 1982) on experimental animals (Reynolds & del Rio, 1984; Reynolds & Johnson, 1981; Edgar, Bowen, Amsbaugh, Monell-Torrens, & Brunell, 1982; Edgar, 1983; Krobicka, Bowen, Pearson, & Young, 1987; Harper et al., 1983; Harper, Osborn, Hefferren, & Clayton, 1986; Harper et al., 1987), seven-day intraoral cariogenicity tests (Silva et al., 1986), and epidemiological observations of human subjects (Rugg-Gunn et al., 1984). In preliminary studies at Tufts and Forsyth conducted by Papas et al. (1987), it was found that people who were free of root caries ate 50% more cheese and 25% more other dairy products than those who had root caries.

### Relationship between Diet, Nutrition, and Oral Disease

Systemic nutritional deficiencies may influence the ability of the periodontium to resist adverse microbiologic and environmental challenges or may modify the progression of existing periodontal disease (Alfano, 1976; Vogel & Alvares, 1985).

Systemic nutritional factors could indirectly influence an individual's susceptibility to caries by affecting preeruptive tooth composition, size, and morphology; saliva quantity, composition, and function; and, perhaps, immunological responses. Unfortunately, firm data from human studies are not available.

## CHANGES THAT OCCUR WITH AGE

The relative composition of the body changes with age. Mean body mass and water decrease, whereas fat increases.

### Muscle Changes

The loss in lean body mass (muscle) is due to a decrease in the total number of muscle cells and atrophy caused by lack of exercise. At age 80 only one half of the muscle cells once present in the body remain. Although body weight may be the same at age 75 as at age 35, the body composition may not be the same. If weight is maintained, it is due to accumulation of fat. Despite continued physical exercise, there is reduced muscle, which is replaced with fat and fibrous connective tissue (Wantz & Gay, 1981).

In the face, muscles may sag, making it difficult to adapt to a denture and keep it in place. Difficulty in chewing may result from weakened masticatory muscle. Muscle weakness of the tongue and throat may lead to swallowing problems, choking, and difficulty in breathing while asleep, as well as difficulty in closing the mouth completely.

### Skin Changes

The color and texture of the skin change. There may also be a reduction in the amount of subcutaneous fat and loss of elasticity of the skin, making it appear matte smooth. With these changes, the lining of the oral cavity (the oral mucosa and gingiva) is affected, and there may be delayed healing after trauma or treatment for periodontal disease. Proper nutrition through an adequate diet may help minimize these changes.

The decreased immunological competence of the aged makes them more susceptible to infection and slower healing. Nonetheless, they can respond to periodontal treatment when oral hygiene is good.

### Vascular Changes

Another condition frequently observed in older individuals is ischemia (diminished blood flow) in both the central and peripheral blood vessels. Among the consequences of ischemia are poor inflammatory response and delayed healing after periodontal surgery. The top surface of the tongue may become bald and salty, and sweet taste may diminish. Gingival recession may occur, exposing the roots of the teeth. Poor blood flow in combination with poor oral hygiene and an ill-fitting upper denture can cause a condition called papillary hyperplasia, an excess growth of gum tissue between the teeth that has the appearance of tiny rosebuds.

### Hard-Tissue Changes

OSTEOPOROSIS. Bone "remodeling" occurs throughout life through constant absorption of old bone and deposition of new bone. Sometime in the fifth decade, bone absorption becomes more rapid than deposition, resulting in net loss of bone. This is manifested by progressive thinning of bone walls and an overall decrease in skeletal mass. Severe bone loss of this type is referred to as osteoporosis.

Osteoporosis may be one of the most prevalent age-related health problems in the aged population. It is characterized by loss of bone density, which increases the risk of fracture. It has been estimated that 90% of all fractures in individuals past 60 are due to osteoporosis. In the United States osteoporosis accounts for 5.3% of all hospitalized patients over age 65. This increases to 10.2% after age 85. Osteoporosis probably has multiple etiologies, involving racial, genetic, hormonal, physical, and nutritional factors. The bone loss progresses twice as fast in women as in men, possibly because of a variety of factors:

1. Lack of physical activity and immobilization
2. Decline in renal function
3. Changes in endocrine controls affecting calcium metabolism
4. Abnormal calcium:phosphorus ratio

*Alveolar Bone.* Alveolar bone, which supports the teeth or dentures, is usually the first area affected by osteoporosis. This may cause periodontal problems and possible loss of healthy teeth. In denture wearers, premature loss of the bone that supports the dentures may result in ill-fitting dentures.

OSTEOMALACIA. Osteomalacia (adult rickets) is characterized by softening and weakening of bone due, in this case, to Vitamin D deficiency. Vitamin D is required for the absorption of calcium from the intestine. With a deficiency of Vitamin D, bones become soft because they fail to mineralize as they undergo remodeling. Vitamin D is synthesized in the presence of ultraviolet light from substances normally found in the skin and can also be obtained in the diet.

In this country, osteomalacia is usually a secondary result of defective intestinal absorption or renal abnormalities. It is also seen in women who stay inside away from sunlight and have diets that are low in dairy products.

ENAMEL. With age, the enamel layer of the tooth becomes thin as a result of mineral loss. This occurs because of wear or erosion of outer enamel layers, or loss of mineral with no replacement from saliva. This will result in exposure of underlying dentin, and the teeth will have a yellowish appearance. Long-term accumulation of metal ions from saliva can also cause teeth to look yellow.

PULP. As an individual ages, layers of dentin form on the inner surface of the dentin, making the pulp chamber smaller. This causes restriction of blood and nutrient flow to the dentin, making the tooth brittle and more easily fractured.

The infection of dental pulp in an older individual is more likely to be chronic, but the pain tends to be less severe than in younger individuals. Treatment is still necessary, however.

### Digestive Changes

Elders often complain of a variety of digestive disturbances and intolerances. Yet changes in the ability to digest food as a result of aging is controversial. Some authors report an increase, others a decrease, in digestive capability (Wantz & Gay, 1981). At least 25% of those over age 60 have achlorhydria (loss of gastric acidity as a result of gastric atrophy (Sandstead, 1987). This may result in a bacterial overgrowth and malabsorption of folic acid, while cations secretion of digestive juices decreases. The secretion of ptyalin, an enzyme that digests starch in the mouth, decreases by 20%. In the stomach, trypsin decreases by 30% and pepsin by 20%. There may be a decrease in the ability to digest protein, an increased requirement for iron and vitamin $B_{12}$, a decrease in fat absorption (resulting in the common complaint of abdominal discomfort), and a decrease in absorption of fat vitamins. There is a decrease in gastric emptying rate and an increase in the number of diverticula in the colon and intestinal tract, along with a thinning of muscle layers. Although there is a decrease in blood flow and the number of absorbing cells, all these do not affect absorption. The decreased digestive capacity that occurs with age may be a result of drug therapy, gastrointestinal surgery, or alimentary tract disease.

People who wear dentures frequently complain of dyspepsia. This is caused by the decreased masticatory function, which is 23% of that found in people with natural dentition (Manly & Vinton, 1951), leading to an increase in the size of the particles swallowed.

Inability to digest lactose (milk sugar) is common with the aged. Normally the enzyme lactose in the lining of the small intestine hydrolyzes, or digests, the milk sugar. However, in the lactose-intolerant individual, lactase secretion is insufficient and lactose passes through the intestinal tract where bacteria act on it and form gas. This causes the bloating and pain associated with lactose intolerance. Individuals who are lactose intolerant often have a deficiency in calcium and should supplement their diets with vitamins.

There is also a decrease in intestinal motility with age. Intestinal tone decreases and intestinal activity lessens. Constipation, abdominal discomfort, and abuse of laxatives are common. Certain drugs, among them codeine and morphine, and other narcotics are constipating, as are iron and calcium preparations.

The abuse of laxatives commonly leads to fluid and potassium depletion. In an effort to avoid the unpleasantness of constipation and other digestive discomfort, the elder may refuse or become afraid to eat.

Increasing dietary fiber may be helpful in improving regularity; however, the aged must be cautioned that too much fiber may lead to diarrhea and decreased absorption of essential minerals, especially calcium.

### Changes in Total Body Water

Water is essential to life. In fact, the cells and tissues of the body are comprised primarily of water. The human body can survive for weeks without proteins, carbohydrates, or fats, but lack of water for even a few days will lead to death.

Body water performs various functions. It lubricates joints, muscles, and tendons, to make them flexible so that they can move easily; and it transports nutrients and removes waste products; it maintains body heat by acting as a reservoir. Dehydration affects the body in many ways. The skin develops wrinkles when water is lost from the skin tissues. This is usually noticed first in the face, because it is the most visible part of the body and because facial skin is exposed to sun and weather. Muscle mass shrinks and sags and muscle strength diminishes. When this happens to the facial muscles, facial contours collapse. Body secretions diminish. A decrease in sweat and sebaceous secretions manifests itself in dry skin. The production of tears diminishes, resulting in dry eyes.

With a decrease in total body water, the effect of drugs is enhanced; therefore, doses should be adjusted. Temperature changes are felt more acutely because the body's water reservoir is diminished.

## Oral Changes

DRY MOUTH. The secretion of saliva and perception of moisture is dependent on several physiological, biochemical, and neurological factors. Salivary secretion is regulated by the autonomic nervous system. Neurotransmitters (NE, ACH, and peptide) initiate secretion but can be modulated by secondary factors, such as insulin, thyroid hormones, vitamin D, androgens, estrogen, and parahormone, among other body secretions (Fox, Van der Ven, Sonies, Wieffenbach, & Baum, 1985). Proper salivary gland function requires proper nerve supply, mucosal and glandular integrity, and higher cortical integrative functions.

Dry mouth, or xerostomia, could be caused by altered salivary fluid and electrolyte production by acinar cells, alteration of the salivary ducts, perturbed exocrine protein synthesis and release, and altered neurological or hormonal function, and altered cognitive function.

Xerostomia is commonly found in older individuals. Since adequate saliva flow is essential to the health of the oral structures as well as to digestion of food, it is important to understand the causes, consequences, symptoms, and treatment of this condition. It should be noted that xerostomia is not a direct consequence of the aging process, but may result from one or more etiologic factors affecting the salivary secretion.

Emotions, especially fear or anxiety; neuroses; organic brain disorders; and drug therapy have all been known to produce xerostomia. At least 400 drugs are known to produce dry mouth as a side effect. Some of the main groups are antihypertensives, anticonvulsants, anti-Parkinson drugs, antidepressants, and tranquilizers. In addition, salivary gland function may be diminished by obstruction of the duct with a stone, therapeutic radiation for treatment of head or neck cancer, and such infections as mumps. Also implicated are autoimmune disorders, such as Sjögren's syndrome, rheumatoid arthritis, systemic lupus erythematosus, primary biliary cirrhosis, polymyositis or dermatomyositis, graft versus host diseases, sarcoid, and autoimmune hemolytic anemia.

Since saliva lubricates the oral mucosa, the lack of saliva creates a dryness and often pain. In addition, saliva helps in cleaning food debris from the mouth. Without significant saliva flow, the debris remains in the mouth, where bacteria ferment it to cause decay and produce acids. With adequate saliva, acids are buffered and neutralized, as well as diluted. Saliva also aids in the remineralization of tooth structure because it contains calcium phosphates. Lack of saliva can affect nutrition in several ways:

1. Chewing ability may decline because saliva aids by moistening food.
2. The mouth may become sore and chewing painful.
3. Swallowing may be difficult because of the loss of saliva's lubricating effect and formation of food into an easily swallowed bolus.
4. Taste perception may change, resulting in a decreased interest in eating.

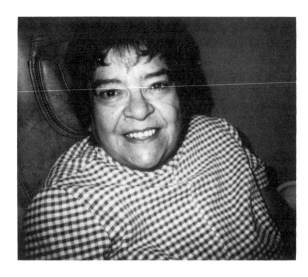

FIGURE 4.6  A patient with Sjögrens.

Patients suffering from Sjögrens syndrome (see Figure 4.6) have a number of problems. Along with xerostomia, Sjögrens syndrome may affect all the glands in the body, but the full-blown disease may not have shown itself except in the mouth. Chronic xerostomia often does not respond to treatment, if acinar cells are destroyed.

As a result of the absence of appropriate salivary enzymes, the patient may have digestive problems as well. Most important, without the minerals from saliva, the teeth will demineralize and eventually break off, and no amount of restorative dentistry can prevent this from happening. Mucositis related to xerostomia leads to constant discomfort, which affects the patient's quality of life.

In 1979 a comprehensive oral health management system for patients suffering from xerostomia was instituted at Tufts University School of Dental Medicine. The results over the years have been impressive in that most of the oral complications in these patients can be successfully prevented or markedly reduced in severity. In this program, intensive fluoride treatments are used over a 1-month period to raise the fluoride concentration of both the surface and underlying tissues to levels that give protection against caries. Supersaturated calcium/phosphate mouth rinses are also utilized to augment the physiological maintenance system and provide new nucleation sites for mineral growth. In order to stimulate salivary secretion, the patients are supplied with inert chewing gum. They are also given individual instruction on proper oral hygiene, as well as nutritional counseling.

EFFECT OF CHRONIC DISEASES ON DENTAL HEALTH
AND NUTRITIONAL STATUS

It is rare for an individual to be totally free from illness or disability throughout a lifetime. In the young and middle-aged, acute diseases prevail, whereas in the aged, disease tends to be chronic. It is estimated that 86% of all aged suffer from at least one chronic disease. Most people over the age of 65 have at least two medical problems, which are exacerbated by the medications required in the management of these problems.

### Cardiovascular Disease

Cardiovascular disease is the most prevalent of the chronic diseases. Of these, arteriosclerotic heart disease, characterized by thickening and hardening of the arterial walls, is one of the most common. Antihypertensive medications have mild to moderate xerostomia as a side effect (see the section on xerostomia for its management). Seniors with heart murmurs and valvular protheses require antibiotic prophylaxis prior to dental treatment. Any oral infection or trauma of the gingival tissues (gums) could lead to an infection of the heart valve (subacute bacterial endocarditis). Therefore, cardiac patients with a history of valvular heart disorders should take particular care with oral hygiene and have frequent cleanings to prevent gingival inflammation and periodontal disease. Coumadin therapy can lead to spontaneous gingival bleeding, especially in patients with poor oral hygiene.

### Stroke

The stroke patient may experience loss of motor function (especially in the cheek and tongue), resulting in loss of chewing ability or drooling. Because there is loss of muscular activity on one side, debris will accumulate on this side. More frequent and effective oral cleaning is required.

### Endocrine Disorders

DIABETES MELLITUS. Impaired glucose tolerance is common with aging. In most cases, the patient is not clinically diabetic and may not require special therapy or severe dietary restrictions. Causes of impaired glucose tolerance are obesity, decreased pancreatic function (Beta cells), altered intracellular glucose metabolism, reduced physical activity.

Decreased resistance to infection in combination with the circulatory problems seen in diabetes make the gingival tissues vulnerable. This results in increased gingival swelling, bleeding, and ultimately periodontal disease. Burning tongue is frequently a presenting symptom. Candidiasis and *Lichen planus* are more common in the diabetic patient. Effective oral home care is an important factor in preventing gingival infection.

CORTICOSTEROID DISORDERS. Increased levels of corticosteriods, either through drug therapy or an adrenal disorder (Cushing's syndrome), will lead to increased vulnerability to infection, hot flashes, "mooning" of the face, and profound bone loss. Increased home care is necessary to prevent oral infections. Loss of alveolar bone can lead to periodontal disease or loss of the alveolar ridge in edentulous patients.

### Diseases of the Nervous System

Many neurological diseases become more prevalent in the aging population, including vascular and degenerative diseases.

TRIGEMINAL NEURALGIA. Trigeminal neuralgia, or "tic douloureux," is characterized by excruciating pain of the lips, gums, or chin, which is usually one-side and triggered by contact with certain areas of the face, lips, tongue, or elsewhere. It is seen primarily in older populations and usually does not have an assignable cause, except occasionally it may be seen in patients with multiple sclerosis or herpes zoster. Other neuralgias may occur in the tongue, pharynx, and ear.

If a patient complains of this type of pain, he should be referred to an oral surgeon or physician for treatment. Trigeminal neuralgia responds to carbamazine (tegretol) or phenytoin, alcohol injection, or, if all else fails, surgery to sever the nerve.

MUSCULAR DYSTROPHY. Muscular weakness, followed by wasting of the muscular tissue, characterizes muscular dystrophy. Patients are unable to relax muscles after contracting them. Patients may have difficulty chewing, pursing the lips, and turning the head. Since the facial muscles may become involved, it is very important that the patients keep their natural teeth because severe problems in keeping dentures in position may occur in the patient without teeth. Mouth breathing, xerostomia, and edema of the oral mucous membranes because of medications (especially quinine) make oral health difficult. Additionally, enlargement of the tongue because of fatty deposits and weakness of facial muscles may cause teeth to flare out. Thus, effective oral hygiene and treatment of the concomitant xerostomia is necessary, especially if the patient has teeth.

MULTIPLE SCLEROSIS. In multiple sclerosis, multiple lesions due to demyelination of nerves in the brain and spinal cord may lead to paralysis of some parts of the body, or the part of the body below the spinal cord injury, sudden loss of vision, and muscle coordination. Trigeminal paraesthesia or anesthesia also may occur. Infection is common.

Weakness of the tongue may be the presenting symptom for multiple sclerosis. The patient may have difficulty wearing and caring for a denture. Effective home care is essential, especially in dentate individuals. Trigeminal neuralgia frequently is seen in patients with multiple sclerosis.

PARKINSON'S DISEASE. Parkinson's disease is a slow, progressive, degenerative process of the basal ganglion of the brain and is the major cause of chronic disability in individuals over the age of 50. With this disease, muscle tremors and rigidity occur, resulting in a masklike appearance of the face and eventual total loss of movement.

Loss of precision in lip and tongue movements manifests itself in monotonous speech, a weak and feeble voice, and difficulty in articulation. Tremor and rigidity of the mouth and tongue often develop, resulting in difficult swallowing and drooling. This may lead to angular cheilosis, or cracks or sores at the corners of the mouth. L-dopa therapy may cause purposeless chewing, grinding, or tongue thrusting.

Because of the moderate to severe xerostomic side effects of most anti-Parkinsonian medications, more frequent and effective oral home care, including fluoride and mineralizing rinses for teeth, become necessary. Application of Vaseline or some other emollient to the lips will help the patient's lips from cracking.

SEIZURE DISORDERS. Seizure disorders, or epilepsy, are due to intermittent, excessive, and disorderly discharge of cerebral neurons. This condition causes varying degrees and combinations of disturbances in sensation, consciousness, convulsive movements, and behavior. It can usually be controlled by anticonvulsant medications.

Patients who are treated with Dilantin for seizure disorders can develop enlarged gingival tissue as a side effect of the medication. There is no pain or bleeding; the gum tissue is pink and firm. Effective oral hygiene is important in controlling Dilantin hyperplasia.

## Oral Cancers

Depending on the type of tumor and its location, one or more of the following treatments will be given: radiation therapy, chemotherapy, or surgery. Radiation therapy to the head and neck causes xerostomia, a decrease in vascular supply, and nervous transmission. Special precautions in oral care are very important to prevent necrosis of the jaw bone. Many chemotherapies have oral side effects, among them mucositis, candidiasis, osteoradionecrosis, and loss of salivary flow, which can be minimized with a rigorous home care program. Home care can also help healing after surgery.

## Nutritional Implications

Well-nourished patients are better able to undergo and recover from surgery, illness, or infection and to withstand the stress of and higher doses of chemotherapy and radiation therapy. Radical surgery of the head and neck often leads to difficulties in chewing and swallowing, problems that may be further complicated by radiation therapy. Radiation therapy can result in mouth sores (stomatitis), dry mouth (xerostomia), loss of taste and reduced food acceptance, or an increased risk of osteoradionecrosis (necrosis of bone due to radiation). Chemotherapeutic drugs also cause a variety of symptoms that may discourage eating: stomatitis, sore throat, change in taste sensation, stomach cramping, feeling of fullness, nausea, vomiting, or diarrhea. Nutrition care is essential for the cancer patient since malnutrition is a common sequelae of the disease.

Recommendations include the following:
1. The treatment of xerostomia was discussed previously (see Dry Mouth).
2. For stomatitis, food textures should be modified by means of soft and liquid diets. The use of a straw will facilitate eating, and the head should be tilted back. Soft, cold foods should be encouraged; highly acidic foods, spices, salt, and alcohol avoided.
3. To maintain weight and counteract catabolism caloric intake and protein should be optimized. Increased calorie nutritional supplements may be useful for these patients.
4. For decreased appetite, the aged person should eat small amounts frequently; food textures should be modified to counteract anorexia and early satiety. Strong odors and hot and spice foods, which may decrease the appeal of food, should be avoided.

### Other Oral Pathologies Observed in the Aged

FISSURED TONGUE. With age, deep grooves can appear on the top side of the tongue. Food and debris may lodge in these furrows and lead to irritation. Tongue brushing is very important in individuals with fissured tongue.

GEOGRAPHIC TONGUE. Geographic tongue is characterized by red patchy areas seen on different days in various areas on the top surface of the tongue. The condition, which is produced by the loss of papillae on multiple areas of the tongue has been associated with stress, emotional problems, and the common cold, among other things.

HAIRY TONGUE. If the papillae have become elongated and do not slough off, the tongue looks hairy. The tongue surface may be white, especially as a result of saliva loss, dehydration, common cold, or poor oral hygiene. Tobacco, candy, coffee, or tea can make the tongue appear brown or black. Better oral hygiene and improved hydration, especially through ingestion of vegetable or chicken soups, should improve this condition.

FORDYCE GRANULES. Eighty percent of the population have small multiple yellow-white spots, which are misplaced sebaceous glands. These are harmless.

TORIS. Hard swellings protruding from the lower jaw or roof of the mouth are known as toris. They are excess normal bone.

ENAMEL EROSION. Severe vomiting over a prolonged period of time as a result of bulimia, constant consumption of beverages with phosphoric acid (e.g., carbonated beverages), or sucking on lemons, can destroy the enamel layer on teeth. This exposes the more vulnerable dentin layer, which is more easily attacked by decay-producing bacterial acid.

HYPOPLASIA AND HYPOCALCIFICATION. Any trauma to the teeth (e.g., high fever, malnutrition, or a blow to the mouth) while the tooth is forming will cause weakened white, chalky areas (the result of hypocalcification), or brown areas (the result of hypoplasia) on the tooth surface. Those areas are more vulnerable to decay and would benefit from fluoride treatment.

ABRASION. Habits such as chewing or holding a pipe, holding bobby pins with one's teeth, or biting one's nails, can wear away the enamel layer. Vigorous tooth brushing may cause similar damage.

ATTRITION. This is the normal wearing of teeth by chewing, clenching, and grinding one's teeth.

BRUXING. The side-to-side grinding of one tooth is referred to as bruxing. This often occurs at night, and the patient is frequently unaware of it. This will not only lead to wearing down of the teeth themselves but will also weaken the bone around the teeth.

TEMPOROMANDIBULAR JOINT DISEASE. The temporomandibular joint (TMJ), which allows one to open and close one's mouth, can be affected by arthritis, causing degeneration, dislocation, or muscular spasms. People may have severe pain, spasms of the muscles around the jaw, and trouble opening their mouths. Often an improper bite can trigger bruxing or clenching, which can in turn cause pain in the TMJ. Stress or physical or emotional problems may also be factors in causing bruxing and clenching. Pain in the TMJ may be caused by loss of teeth, which leads to a collapsed bite, arthritis, and congenital problems.

## *Pathologic Changes of Oral Soft Tissues*

ASPIRIN BURN. People sometimes place aspirin in their mouth and hold it in one spot, or keep aspirin-containing chewing gum in one area. The aspirin resting on the tissues causes burns.

CHEEK BITING. Frequently the cheeks will show a white fibrous area along the biting surfaces in patients with lower teeth that overlap the uppers or in people who have a habit of chewing the sides of their mouths. A thin white line is normal, but a pronounced area shows that trauma is occurring.

CANDIDIASIS. Candidiasis is an infection of oral tissues caused by a fungus. It appears as a white curdlike patch that can be wiped off. The area beneath the patch is usually red. Antibiotic therapy or any condition that disturbs the normal balance of organisms within the mouth (especially debilitating diseases such as cancer) allows the normally harmless candida to become infectious. Candidiasis should be treated by a dentist or physician. Good oral hygiene and frequent rinses are important in preventing and managing this condition.

LICHEN PLANUS. Often observed in postmenopausal references women, lichen planus affects the skin and the oral tissues. It appears in the mouth as a number of tiny white spots having a lacelike appearance. Lichen planus can be distinguished from candida in that these white spots cannot be scraped off. Sometimes the mucosa under the spots can erode and be painful. The area should be kept clean to prevent infection. The dentist or physician should reassure the patient that it is not cancer.

PEMPHIGUS. Pemphigus is another skin disorder that can affect the oral tissues. It can be dangerous because in a later stage, large blisters form that can rupture, leaving large denuded areas on the skin or oral mucosa through which loss of fluid occurs, as in a severe burn. In the early stages it produces oral lesions. Since pemphigus can be fatal, the patient should see a physician or dentist for treatment.

HERPES ZOSTER. Ten percent of the population develops primary herpes, small vesicles or blisters that rupture and form an ulcer with a red halo. These will last 10 to 14 days and disappear. The tongue and gums may also be inflamed. This condition is rare in a geriatric patient, but cold sores or fever blisters, a secondary herpes infection around the lips, are common.

### Other Viral Infections

HERPANGINA. Small vesicles usually seen in the back of the throat (Cox sakie infection) is the result of herpangina.

HERPES ZOSTER. Shingles is characterized by an eruption of vesicles or blisters that occurs only one side of the body in a linear pattern along nerve fibers. Severe pain sometimes accompanies this infection.

APHTHOUS ULCER. The aphthous ulcer is a small ulcer in the mouth usually brought on by stress, either physical or emotional. It will heal within 2 weeks. Any nonhealing oral ulcer should be evaluated by a dentist or physician.

TRAUMATIC ULCER. Traumatic ulcer is caused by burns from hot food or beverages, or cuts due to injury. It should heal within a 2-week period; if it does not, the patient should be referred to physician or dentist for biopsy.

## DENTAL HEALTH CARE AMONG THE AGED

Although the geriatric population utilizes the greatest proportion of health care dollars (29%), it has the lowest utilization rate of dental services (37.5%) at the time of life when the need for dental treatment is the greatest. Nursing-home residents use dental services the least because of the perception among them that they do not need dental care at their age. Since dental problems usually are not acute among the aged, they rarely present dental emergencies. Instead, they have chronic infections with possible low-grade "fevers" of unknown origin. Thus, if dental services are provided on a request basis rather than after dental screening, the aged may suffer from chronic infection and discomfort.

The issue of the effect of oral health on quality of life is also important. Many nursing-home residents expressed an immense enthusiasm for receiving dental care when presented with a treatment plan. In a study conducted by Tufts University, 75% of the residents required treatment. Even though 20% stated that they had their own dentists, most patients reported not having seen a dentist since their admission. The 1.7% who had seen a dentist reported that they generally received only emergency care without adequate follow-up. It was not uncommon for patients to report that they had received a new denture 1 or 2 years ago without a standard follow-up examination and any necessary adjustments. All too often a denture ends up sitting in its plastic container because the patient is unable to wear it. This could result in the patient's feeling abandoned.

Since many elders earn less than $10,000 annually, financial need could account for some of their failure to use dental services. In Massachusetts, the Branch Study found that elders who had had more formal education did not receive Medicaid and who reported maintaining good nutritional status were more likely to use dental services. Medicaid coverage was negatively associated with use of dental services. This phenomenon has been reported in other studies.

Both local and national attitudinal studies indicate that the major reason the aged do not seek dental treatment is the lack of awareness of a need for dental treatment. The best predictors of the use of dental services were found to be perceived importance of dental care and perceived need for treatment (Branch, Antczak, & Stason, 1986). Bomberg and Enst (1986) found that in old age people continue patterns of dental health that they established when they were younger but that these patterns can be modified by educational programs, which the elders themselves acknowledge as beneficial.

Clinical examinations of the aged have shown a discrepancy between actual dental need and dental need as perceived by the aged themselves. Branch et al. (1986) conducted a longitudinal study from 1974 to 1980 of 776 noninstitutionalized Massachusetts residents aged 65 and over and found that 70% needed services but only 37% perceived a need for dental care and only 41% had used dental services during the past year. The use of dental services was influenced more by the importance that the aged placed on dental care than by ability to pay for care or other barriers to access. Therefore, if the aged can be convinced of the need for dental care, they will seek it. Branch et al. (1986) reported that among the population aged 75+, the factors affecting the perception of need were dentate status, perception of dental health status, and the frequency with which they saw a dentist.

## DENTAL CARE FOR THE AGED

The aged whose oral cavities have been damaged by dental disease can benefit from recent advances in dental technology by which teeth may be restored or replaced by protheses and periodontal tissues (bone and gingiva or gums) restored to health. Dentists today use high-speed drills that no longer vibrate and can remove decay (dental caries) in a few minutes, thus reducing the discomfort associated with dental treatment.

Progress has also been made in the development and administration of local anesthetics. There are now many different anesthetics, with varying durations of action, that are safe compared to earlier procaine anesthetics, which carried with them the risk of anaphylaxis due to allergic reactions. Also, various methods of sedation have made extractions and surgery less frightening.

Dental implants have now been used successfully in some cases for 30 years (Bränemark, 1983). This can be the answer for someone who no longer can keep a lower denture in place. Two implants and a bar between them can anchor the denture and stop clicking and eating problems. Implant procedures are also used to replace missing teeth in a partially edentulous person.

We now know that dental caries in adults can be reduced through proper diet, removal of dental plaque through brushing and flossing, and fluoride. Dental caries can be prevented through the use of fluoride toothpaste, fluoride rinses, and fluoride in the drinking water. Even if caries have begun to form, they can be reversed in their early stages through remineralization. Caries formation is believed to involve the intermittent dissolution of enamel.

When carbohydrate is ingested, the $pH$ drops because of acid formation, and there is some demineralization. During the interval between meals, thère is a rise in the $pH$, which results in a certain amount of remineralization. The greater the concentration of fluoride released from the dissolved enamel or already present in the plaque, the more will remineralization be favored and the more will the carious process be slowed (Johansen, Papas, & Fong, 1987). In the presence of fluoride and saliva, the remineralizing enamel, cementum, and dentin are more resistant to subsequential acid attack.

Once the aged have acknowledged the need for care, dental professionals, making use of the new technology available to them, can provide comprehensive care that can restore the oral cavity to optimal health and provide the aged or their caretakers with the knowledge and skills necessary to maintain oral health.

No one is too old for dental treatment. With proper management, even a healthy 90-year-old can use dental implants as successfully as a 50-year-old, even when there is little or no remaining alveolar bone (which supports the teeth or denture).

When proper medical precautions are taken, comprehensive dental care is as possible for an older patient as it is for a younger patient. With appropriate treatment, such as root canal therapy, implants, crowns and bridges, and periodontal treatment, the aged can keep their teeth for a lifetime. If teeth have been lost, a dental prosthesis, such as a complete or partial denture, can be provided. Although a prosthesis is never as good as one's own teeth, an individual can learn to use it effectively and continue to function well.

Dentists are now able to provide comprehensive dental treatment to the homebound and nursing-home aged through the use of mobile equipment and mobile vans. But aside from bringing care to the aged, a major challenge facing health professionals who work with the aged will be to make them aware of the need for dental treatment and then inform them that dental professionals possess new procedures and materials with which optimal health and function can be restored. Finally, the perception that the elderly are too old for proper dental care must be attacked. Just as one would not remove a diseased limb and replace it with a prosthesis if one didn't have to, one should not remove teeth and replace them with dentures unless periodontal disease or caries are too advanced to save the teeth.

## REFERENCES

Alfano, M. C. (1976). Controversies, perspectives and clinical implications of nutrition in periodental disease. *Dental Clinics of North America, 20,* 519.

Banting, D. W. (1986). Epidemiology of root caries. *Gerontology 5*(1), 5–11.

Bomberg, T. J., & Enst, N. S. (1986). Improving utilization of dental care services by the elderly. *Gerodontics, 2,* 57–60.

Bowen, W. H. (1974). Effect of restricting oral intake to invert sugar or casein in the microbiology of plaque in *Macaca fascicularis* (IRUS). *Archives of Oral Biology, 19,* 231–239.

Branch, L. G., Antczak, A. A., & Stason, W. B. (1986). Toward understanding the use of dental services by the elderly. *Special Care in Dentistry, 5*(1), 38–41.

Bränemark, P. I. (1983). Osseointegration and its experimental background. *Journal of Prosthetic Dentistry, 50,* 399–410.

Burt, B. A., & Ismail, A. I. (1986). Diet, nutrition, and food cariogenicity. *Journal of Dental Research, 65* (Special Issue), 1475–1484.

Dodds, M. W., & Edgar, W. M. (1986). Effects of dietary sucrose levels on $pH$ fall and acid-anion profile in human dental plaque after a starch mouth rinse. *Archives of Oral Biology, 31*(8), 509–512.

Edgar, W. M., Bowen, W. H., Amsbaugh, S., Monell-Torrens, E., & Brunell, J. (1982). Effects of different eating patterns on dental caries in the rat. *Journal of Caries Research, 16,* 384–389.

Edgar, W. M. (1983). The role of sugar in the etiology of dental caries. III. The physio-chemical evidence. *Journal of Dental Research, 11*(3), 199–205.

Fox, P. C., Van der Ven, P. C., Sonies, B. C., Weiffenbach, T. M., & Baum, B. J. (1985). Xerostomia: Evaluation of a symptom with increasing significance. *Journal of the American Dental Association, 110,* 519–525.

Hand, J. S., Hunt, R. J., & Beck, J. D. (1988). Incidence of coronal and root caries in older adults. *Journal of Public Health Dentistry, 48*(1), 14–19.

Hardwick, J. L. (1960). The incidence and distribution of caries throughout the ages in relation to the Englishman's diet. *British Dental Journal, 108,* 9.

Harper, D. S., Osborn, J. C., & Clayton, R. (1983). Cariostatic potential of four cheeses evaluated in a programmed-fed rat model. *Journal of Dental Research, 62,* 283.

Harper, D. S., Osborn, J. C., Hefferren, J. J., & Clayton, R. (1986). Cariostatic evaluation of cheeses with diverse physical and compositional characteristics. *Caries Research, 20*(2), 123–130.

Harper, D. S., Osborn, J. C., Clayton, R., & Hefferren, J. J. (1987). Modification of food cariogenicity in rats by mineral-rich concentrates from milk. *Journal of Dental Research, 66,* 42–45.

Hayes, M. L., & Hyatt, A. T. (1974). The decarboxylation of amino acids by bacteria derived from human dental plaque. *Archives of Oral Biology, 19,* 361–369.

Hix, J. O., III, & O'Leary, T. J. (1976). The relationship between cemental caries, oral hygiene status and fermentable carbohydrate intake. *Journal of Periodontology, 47*(7), 398–404.

Holloway, P. J., James, P. M. C., & Slack, G. L. (1963). Dental diseases in Tristan da Cunha. *British Dental Journal, 115,* 19–25.

Jenkins, G. N., & Harper, D. S. (1983). Protective effects of different cheeses in an *in vitro* demineralization system (abstract). *Journal of Dental Research, 62,* 284.

Jensen, M. E. (1984). Diet, nutrition, and oral health. *Journal of the American Dental Association, 109,* 20–32.

Johansen, E., Papas, A., Fong, W. & Olsen, T.T. (1987). Remineralization of carious lesions in elderly patients. *Gerodontics, 3*(1), 47–50.

Krasse, B. (1985). The cariogenic potential of foods: A critical review of current methods. *International Dental Journal, 35,* 36–42.

Krobicka, A., Bowen, W. H., Pearson, S., & Young, D. A. (1987). The effects of cheese snacks on caries in desalivated rats. *Journal of Dental Research, 66*(6), 1116–1119.

Manly, R. S., & Vinton, P. (1951). A survey of chemical ability of denture wearers. *Journal of Dental Research, 30,* 314–321.

McGandy, R. B., Russell, R. M., Hartz, S. C., Jacob, R. A., Tannenbaum, S., Peters, H., Sahyoun, N., & Otradovec, C. L. (1986). Nutritional status survey of healthy noninstitutionalized elderly: Energy and nutrient intakes from 3-day diet records and nutrient supplements. *Nutrition Reviews, 6,* 785–798.

Oral health of U.S. adults: The national survey of oral health in U.S. employed adults and seniors (1985–1986, national findings). NIH Pub. No. 87–2868.

Papas, A., Herman, J., Palmer, C., Rounds, M., Feldman, R., Russell, R., McGandy, R., Hartz, S., & Jacob, R. (1984). Oral health status of the elderly with dietary and nutritional considerations. *Gerondontology, 3*(2), 147–155.

Papas, A., Palmer, C., McGandy, R., Hartz, S., & Russell, R. (1987). Dietary and nutritional factors in relation to dental caries in elderly subjects. *Gerodontics, 3,* 30–37.

Papas, A. S., Palmer, C. A., Rounds, M. C., Herman, J., McGrandy, R. B., Hartz, S. C., Russell, R. M., & DePaola, P. (1989). Longitudinal relationships between nutrition and oral health. *Annals of the New York Academy of Sciences, 561,* 124–142.

Papas, A. S. (1992). Oral Health. In S. C. Hartz, R. M. Russell, & I. H. Rosenberg (Eds.). *Nutrition and the Elderly: The Boston Nutritional Status Survey.* London: Smith-Gordon.

Proceedings: Scientific Consensus Conference on methods for assessment of the cariogenic potential of foods. *Journal of Dental Research, 65,* 1475–1543 (1986).

Ravald, R., Hamp, S.-E., Birked, D. (1986). Long-term evaluation of root surface caries in periodontally treated patients. *Journal of Clinical Periodontology, 13,* 758–767.

Reynolds, E. C., & Johnson, J. H. (1981). Effect of milk on caries incidence and bacterial composition of dental plaque in the rat. *Archives of Oral Biology, 26,* 445–451.

Reynolds, E. C., Riley, P. F., & Storey, E. (1982). Phosphoprotein inhibition of hydroxyapatite dissolution. *Calcified Tissue International, 34,* 552–556.

Reynolds, E. C., & Wong, A. (1983). Effect of adsorbed protein on hydroxyapatite zeta potential and *Streptococcus mutans* adherence. *Infection and Immunity, 39,* 1285–1290.

Reynolds, E. C., & del Rio, A. (1984). Effect of casein and whey protein solutions on caries experience and feeding patterns in the rat. *Archives of Oral Biology, 29,* 927–933.

Reynolds, E. C. (1987). The prevention of subsurface demineralization of bovine enamel and change in plaque composition by casein in an intraoral model. *Journal of Dental Research, 66,* 1120–1127.

Rosen, S., & Willett, N. P. (1985). Nutrient requirements, regulation, and interdependence of microbes in dental plaque. In R. L. Pollack & E. Kravitz (Eds.), *Nutrition in Oral Health and Disease.* (pp. 119–127). Philadelphia: Lea & Febiger.

Rugg-Gunn, A. J., Hackett, A. F., Appleton, D. R., Eastoe, J. E., & Jenkins, G. N. (1984). Correlations of dietary intakes of calcium, phosphorus, and Ca/P ratio with caries rates in children. *Caries Research, 18,* 149–152.

Sandstead, H. H. (1987). Nutrition in the elderly. *Gerodontics, 3,* 3–13.

Schachtele, C. F., & Jensen, M. E. (1983). The acidogenic potential of reference foods and snacks at interproximal sites in the human dentition. *Journal of Dental Research, 62*(8), 889–892.

Schachtele, C. F., & Jensen, M. E. (1982). Comparison of methods for mascatory changes in the $pH$ of human dental plaque. *Journal of Dental Research, 61*(10), 1117–1125.

Schachtele, C. F., Rosamond, W. D., & Harlander, S. K. (1985). Diet and aging: Current concerns related to oral health. *Gerodontics, 1*(3), 117–124.

Schamschula, R. G., Keyes, P. H., & Hornabrook, R. W. (1972). Root surface caries in Lufa, New Guinea. I. Clinical observations. *Journal of the American Dental Association, 85,* 603–608.

Schamschula, R. G., Barnes, D. E., Keyes, P. H., & Guilbinat, W. (1974). Prevalence and interrelationships of root surface caries in Lufa Papua, New Guinea. *Community Dentistry and Oral Epidemiology, 2,* 295–304.

Scientific Consensus Conference on methods for assessment of the cariogenic potential of food (1986). American Dental Association Health Foundation Research Institute. *Journal of the American Dental Association, 112*(4), 535.

Silva, M. F. deA., Jenkins, G. N., Burgess, R. C., & Sandham, H. J. (1986). Effects of cheese on experimental caries in human subjects. *Caries Research, 20*(3), 263–269.

Silva, M. F. deA., Burgess, R. C., & Sandham, H. J. (1987a). Effects of water-soluble components of cheese on experimental caries in humans. *Journal of Dental Research, 66*(1), 38–41.

Silva, M. F. deA., Burgess, R. C., & Sandham, H. J. (1987b). Effects of cheese extract and its fractions on enamel demineralization *in vitro* and *in vivo* in humans. *Journal of Dental Research, 66,*(10), 1527–1531.

Tabak, L. A. (1988). Roles of saliva (pellicle), diet, and nutrition on plaque formation. Paper presented at the 11th International Conference on Oral Biology, Hong Kong.

Vehkalahti, M. M., & Paunio, I. K. (1988). Occurrence of root caries in relation to dental health behavior. *Journal of Dental Research, 67*(6), 911–914.

Vogel, R. I., & Alvares, O. F. (1985). Nutrition and periodontal disease. In R. L. Pollack & E. Kravitz, (Eds.), Nutrition in Oral Health and Disease. (pp. 136–150). Philadelphia: Lea & Febiger.

Vratsanos, S. M., & Mandel, I. D. (1984). Plaque in caries: Resistant versus caries-susceptible adults. *Journal of Dental Research, 64,* 422–424.

Wantz, M. S., & Gay, J. E. (1981). *The aging process: A health perspective.* pp. 194–202. Cambridge, MA: Winthrop.

Wayler, A. H., & Chauncey, H. H. (1985). Longitudinal study of dentition stability and food selection patterns. Collected abstracts of the 13th International Congress of Gerontology: no. 130.

# Protocol for Head and Neck Inspection of Elderly Individuals

One of the best measures for early detection and treatment of disease in your patient is a brief but thorough head and neck inspection. This will take about 15 minutes and should be done as part of your routine evaluation of the patient. Since only 42% of the elderly have contact with dental health professionals, you — as a health-care provider — may be the only person in a position to detect pathology in the head and neck area. The importance of your inspection of these areas cannot be overemphasized. Such attention could result in two benefits to the patient in addition to early detection of pathology:

- It could increase your patient's awareness of his oral structures and their importance to his well-being.
- It could give you an opportunity to dispel some of the fears and myths your patient may have about dentistry.

Your objective in head and neck inspection is to look for the presence of any obvious or suspicious-looking areas and record them on the inspection record which appears in the Appendix. If your inspection produces positive findings, it is important that you personally refer the patient to a dentist or a physician.

Your steps for head and neck inspection are as follows (more complete instructions appear on the recording form that follows — which may be photocopied for use each time you perform an inspection):

*Note:* Wear disposable gloves.

Before beginning your inspection, ask the patient if he has noticed any changes in his mouth, head, or neck. Be specific: "Is there any area that is painful? Have you noticed any swelling?"

1. Look at the head and face for any asymmetry and/or lesion. Check behind the ears.
2. Standing behind the seated patient and using two hands, feel the cheeks and neck and under the chin for any swellings.
3. Retract the lips and look for swellings or red, white, or red-and-white lesions, blisters, or ulcers on the inner aspect of the lips and cheeks. Remember, in the middle of the cheek there is a white line which occurs where upper and lower teeth meet. This is normal.
4. Inspect the roof of the mouth.
5. Have the patient extend his tongue
   (a) Look at the front of the top surface.

(b) Take hold of the tongue with gauze, pull it out, and inspect the posterior of the top surface. Have the patient say "Aah" and inspect the throat area. If you are unable to see the throat, use a tongue depressor to depress the tongue.

(c) Pull the tongue to each side and inspect the sides for red, white, or red-and-white lesions, blisters, or ulcers, especially in the area of the lingual tonsil.

6. Instruct the patient to touch the roof of his mouth with the tip of his tongue. Now inspect the floor of the mouth and the under-surface of the tongue.

7. Inspect the tonsillar area and pharynx. Look for
   •Red or red-and-white area;
   •White area; or
   •Sores

8. Inspect the teeth and gums. Look for
   •Decayed or broken teeth;
   •Loose teeth;
   •Bleeding gums; or
   •Pus

9. Look for soft tissues which appear red and dry. Observe the saliva to see if it is thick and ropey. Ask the patient if his mouth is dry.

| Area | Action | Findings |
|------|--------|----------|
| FACE | Look | Bruises |
| | | Asymmetry |
| | | Red or discolored area |
| | | Sores |
| | | Swelling |
| | | Irritation under eyeglasses |
| | Feel | Lump |
| | (press inner & outer | Tender area |
| | surfaces of cheeks) | |
| NECK | Look | Swelling |
| | | Discolored area |
| | | Sores Swelling |
| | Feel | Lump |
| | (move fingers up & down | Tender area |
| | all sides of neck) | |
| LIPS | Look | Swelling |
| | | Cracks |
| | | Sores |
| | | Blister |
| | Feel | Lump |
| | (press inner & outer | Tender area |
| | surfaces) | |

| Area | Action | Findings |
|------|--------|----------|
| CHEEK (inside surface) | Look (retract w/fingers or tongue blade) | Sore<br>Red area<br>White area<br>Generalized redness of mucosa<br>Dry, shiny mucosa<br>Lump |
| ROOF OF MOUTH | Look (tilt head back & open wide, or use mouth mirror) | Red area<br>White area<br>Sores<br>Lump |
| | Feel | Lump<br>Tender area |
| TONGUE | Look (have patient extend tongue; wrap tip in gauze & move to either side) | *Top surface*<br>  Sores<br>  Swelling<br>  White coating<br>  Dark "hairy" appearance<br>  Smooth, red shiny surface<br><br>*Sides*<br>  Red area<br>  White area<br>  Blister<br>  Sores<br>  Lump |
| | Look (have patient touch tip of tongue to roof of mouth) | *Under surface*<br>  Red area<br>  White area<br>  Blister<br>  Sores<br>  Lump |
| FLOOR OF MOUTH | Look (have patient touch tip of tongue to roof of mouth) | Red area<br>White area<br>Blister<br>Sores<br>Swelling<br>*Blue areas may be varicose veins |
| | Feel (press inner surface & outer surface, under chin) | Lump<br>Tender area |
| TONSILAR AREA | Look (pull out tongue w/gauze) | Red area<br>White area<br>Sores |
| TEETH | Look | Broken teeth<br>Loose teeth<br>Decayed teeth<br>Missing fillings |

| Area | Action | Findings |
|------|--------|----------|
| GUMS | Look | Redness |
| | | Bleeding |
| | | Swelling |
| | | Blister |
| | | Sores |
| | | Pus |
| | | Dryness |
| SALIVA | Look | *Obvious lack of saliva |
| | | *Saliva is thick & stringy |
| | Look (dry inside of cheek w/gauze) | *No wetness appears on inside of cheek |

ADDITIONAL INSPECTION FOR DENTURE WEARER

*Directions*: Circle any findings.

| | Action | Findings |
|------|--------|----------|
| DENTURE IN MOUTH | Observe | Denture appears loose |
| | | Denture slips when elder speaks |
| | | Denture slips when elder chews |
| | | Denture appears too large for size of mouth |
| | Ask questions to elicit information | Denture feels comfortable |
| | | Problems in chewing with denture |
| | | Problems in speaking with denture |
| | | Wears denture always, except to clean it |
| | | Wears denture all day; leaves out overnight |
| | | Wears denture only when eating |
| | | Wears denture only when socializing |
| | | Wears denture seldom |
| | | Never wears denture |
| DENTURE OUT OF MOUTH | Inspect denture | Areas of food retention |
| | | Soft debris |
| | | Hard debris (calculus, tartar) |
| | | Stain |
| | | Denture is warped |
| | | Denture is chipped |
| | | Denture is cracked |
| | | Denture teeth missing |
| | | Broken clasp on partial denture |

# 5

# DRUG THERAPY
# IN THE AGED PATIENT

Joseph M. Scavone

The use of drugs in the aged patient continues to be an issue of considerable social and medical concern. Problems associated with the proper selection of drugs by the clinician, the patient's ability and desire to take medications as prescribed, the effects of aging on drug therapy, and the misunderstandings about the goal(s) of drug therapy have led to many discussions about the appropriateness of the use of drugs in aged patients. Whenever a patient's clinical status is evaluated, at some point the medications must be reviewed. This review usually raises many questions about how the drugs that the patient is taking may influence the patient's lifestyle and coexistent disease states. All health-care providers are concerned about how medications may help or aggravate the situation they are specifically evaluating, but often the questions that are raised and the concerns that are expressed go unanswered. Sometimes the absence of information translates to speculation that drug therapy may be hazardous and that aged patients are especially overmedicated. Prescription and over-the-counter drugs are often implicated in causing many problems in the aged patient. Many times the mention of medications for an aged patient conjures up negative thoughts for everyone involved in the patient's care, including the patient and their family. However, many health-care providers forget that there are specific reasons for the use of drugs in the medical management of a patient, and generally many patients tolerate their effects very well.

Monitoring drug therapy in the aged is sometimes difficult because both the frequency of drug therapy and the number of drugs taken progressively increases with age. It has been estimated that two thirds of all Americans over the age of 65 years take at least one prescription drug. At hospital discharge, 25% of the aged patients receive prescriptions for 6 or more drugs. In nursing homes it is not uncommon for some patients to be receiving 12 to 15 drugs. Obviously the job of monitoring the effects of all of these drugs has to be a cooperative effort between the physician, nurse, pharmacist, other health-care providers, and the patient.

In addition, aged patients commonly purchase over-the-counter medications. Almost 70% of aged people regularly use such medications, as compared to about 10% of the general adult population. Approximately 55% of the over-the-counter drugs used by the aged are analgesics. It is estimated that the over-the-counter preparations probably account for at least 40% of all drugs used by the aged. Since the incidence of adverse drug effects increases with age and number of medications used, it is not surprising that aged persons suffer adverse drug reactions 1½ to 3 times more than the younger and middle-aged adult population.

Compliance with prescribed drug regimens by aged patients is reported to be very low. It has been estimated that greater than 60% are noncompliant to their prescription drug regimens. Many patients either omit doses or take extra doses, as dictated by their symptoms. Furthermore, it is not uncommon for the aged to self-medicate with nonprescription drugs or to take the wrong medication for a particular symptom.

The purpose of this chapter is to present information about the use of drugs in the aged patient and to describe the elements of drug therapy that are affected by the aging process. To accomplish this goal it will be necessary to explain in detail the factors that govern drug disposition and response. This chapter will also discuss the physiologic aspects of drug therapy; the mechanisms of drug interactions and adverse effects; the patient's influence on and expectations of the therapeutic outcome; compliance; over-the-counter drug use; and the individual categories of pharmacologic agents.


DRUG THERAPY

To understand the differences in the way the aged react to medications compared to younger patients, it is necessary to understand some basic concepts about how the body responds to drugs. It is important that the patient receives "the right drug for the right disease," but it also has to be prescribed in the right dosage form, at a correct interval, and through an acceptable route of administration. When a certain drug is chosen for a patient, the pharmacologic action of the drug is always considered. The positive effect is referred to as its therapeutic effect and the unacceptable effects are known as toxic or adverse effects. Each drug has a certain mechanism of action that results in acceptable and often coexistent unacceptable result(s). A clinician has to weigh the positive and negative effects when selecting a certain drug therapy. Many drugs such as digoxin, theophylline, warfarin, phenytoin, lithium, antiarrhythmics, antibiotics, and others have to be dosed so that the resultant drug concentration in the patient's serum or plasma lies within a defined "therapeutic range." Some drugs correlate very well to a range that will offer the most benefit with the least toxic effects. Thus, drugs are categorized into two major groups: those with a "narrow" therapeutic range and those with a "wide" therapeutic range (Figure 5.1, Table 5.1). A wide therapeutic range suggests that large fluctuations in serum or plasma drug concentration can occur without resulting in toxicity. Therapeutic drug monitoring is useful in evaluating the effect of drugs with a narrow therapeutic margin, whereas its value is limited when monitoring drug therapy with those medications having a wide therapeutic range. As expected, drugs with a narrow therapeutic range can cause the most problems in the aged patient if drug therapy is not carefully monitored since pharmacologic and toxic effects closely parallel serum and plasma drug concentration.

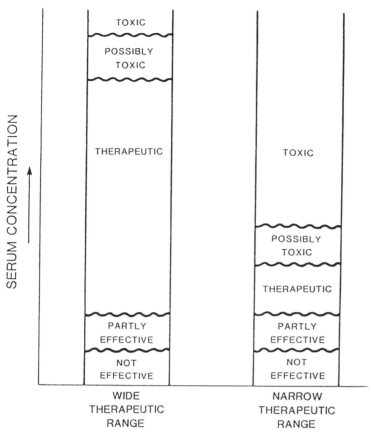

FIGURE 5.1. Based on serum or plasma drug concentrations, some drugs are associated with having wide or narrow therapeutic margins. Small fluctuations in plasma/ serum concentration are unlikely to be clinically important for drugs with a wide therapeutic margin, but for drugs with a narrow therapeutic margin, small fluctuations in concentration most likely will result in a change in clinical response.

TABLE 5.1  Therapeutic Ranges

| Examples of drugs with a narrow therapeutic range | | Examples of drugs with a wide therapeutic range | |
|---|---|---|---|
| Phenytoin | Vancomycin | Valium | Atenolol |
| Theophylline | Lithium | Librium | Ibuprofen |
| Digoxin | Quinidine | Lorazepam | Imipramine |
| Gentamicin | Procainamide | Oxazepam | Amitriptyline |
| Tobramycin | Lidocaine | Temazepam | Buspirone |
| Kanamycin | | Propranolol | |

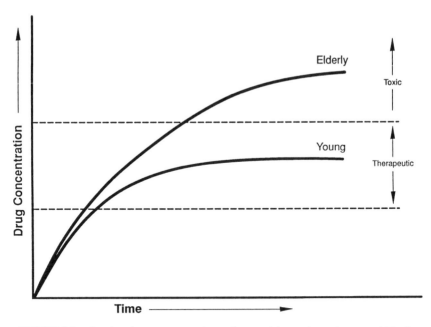

FIGURE 5.2.   Aged patients may experience drug toxicity at doses that are within the usual therapeutic range for younger adults.

## THE EFFECTS OF AGING ON DRUG THERAPY

In recent years drug use in the aged and its untoward effects have received much attention. It is well known that the aged may exhibit an exaggerated response to medications and that a significant portion of hospital-related morbidity and mortality is related to drug use. A therapeutic response may develop in aged patients at doses far below what is recommended for younger adults. In addition, aged patients may experience drug toxicity at doses that are within the usual therapeutic range (Figure 5.2).

Studies of drug response in the aged have suggested that at least two types of phenomena may explain these changes in sensitivity. The first is the possibility that the ability to biotransform (metabolize) or eliminate drugs from the body declines with age. If the total elimination (clearance) of a drug is reduced, then chronic therapy with any given dose will lead to higher steady-state (mean drug concentration following multiple dosage) blood concentrations, and the likelihood of toxicity is increased. The second explanation is pharmacodynamics; it is possible that receptor-site sensitivity to the pharmacologic action of drugs may increase with age. Thus, at any given drug concentration the presence of the drug at the receptor site may lead to a greater response. Such an increase in drug sensitivity may be evident clinically as a greater likelihood of excessive drug effect(s) or toxicity at what are usually regarded as safe therapeutic doses. It should be noted that reduced drug sensitivity in the aged can also occur but it has only been described in a few cases (Figure 5.3).

### Drug Sensitivity in the Elderly

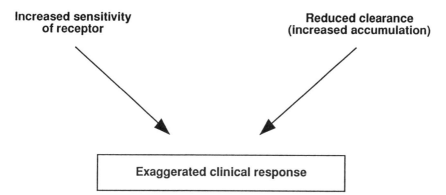

FIGURE 5.3.   Drug sensitivity in the elderly resulting in alterations in clinical response can be explained by the complex interaction of pharmacokinetics and pharmacodynamics.

### *Pharmacokinetics and Pharmacodynamics*

When studying the effects of drugs in the aged, one is quickly introduced to the many terms that are used to describe the consequences of drug therapy. The term *pharmacokinetics* is often encountered and usually causes a fair amount of apprehension to those who are not familiar with the basic concepts. Pharmacokinetics is the mathematical analysis of the time course of drug concentration in a body fluid or tissue. It describes the amount of drug in the body over time and includes factors that control the time course of drug absorption, distribution, biotransformation, and elimination. These parameters are also collectively referred to as drug disposition. The pharmacokinetic profile of a drug is based on several interrelated factors that include the relationship of plasma or serum drug concentrations to the size and frequency of dose, the free or unbound drug concentration to the amount that is bound to proteins or other blood components, the equilibrium of ionized and unionized bound and unbound drug with receptors and the dissipation of drug effects in relationship to the elimination of the drug from the receptor site (Ogilvie, 1983). Other factors that can influence the pharmacokinetics of drugs are listed in Table 5.2.

It is important to realize that absorption, distribution, biotransformation (often referred to as metabolism) and elimination (also called removal or excretion) occur simultaneously at rates that change over time. The process is complex, but the essentials of pharmacokinetics should be understood by all persons involved in prescribing and monitoring the effects of pharmacologic agents. Since the goal of drug therapy is to treat a patient in such a way that medications provide a therapeutic yet nontoxic way to manage various disease states, the understanding of and cautious application of pharmacokinetic principles can assist the clinician in making correct decisions when choosing or evaluating a patient's drug therapy (Greenblatt & Shader, 1985). They can also allow for more educated decisions about drug selection, dose, frequency of administration, route of adminis-

TABLE 5.2   Factors that can affect the pharmacokinetics of drugs

| Patient variables | Medical conditions |
| --- | --- |
| Age | Congestive heart |
| Gender | failure |
| Body composition | Kidney disease |
| Body weight | Cirrhosis |
| Drugs | Hepatitis |
| Nutritional status | Fever |
| Ethanol use | Sepsis |
| Cigarette smoking | Burns (severe) |
| | Anemia |

tration and monitoring therapeutic response, ineffectiveness or toxicity. The application of the principles of pharmacokinetics are extremely important for safe and effective drug therapy but should never replace careful clinical judgment. Pharmacokinetics provides the framework for understanding drug behavior, but it still oversimplifies the complicated physiologic events that govern drug disposition.

The other term that often appears in discussions about drug use in the aged is *pharmacodynamics*, which refers to the interaction of the drug molecule with its target receptor site. The interaction of drug and receptor is analogous to an enzyme-substrate or lock-and-key type of interaction (Figure 5.4). To fully understand how and why a drug causes a particular effect, its pharmacodynamics must be defined. The effects of aging on recep-

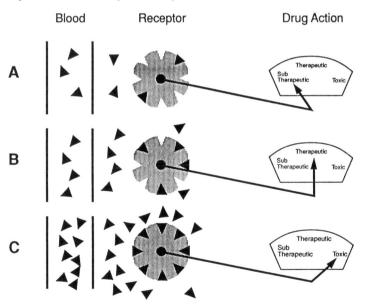

FIGURE 5.4.   For many drugs a relationship between plasma/serum drug concentration and the availability of drugs at the receptor site translates to clinical effect.

tor sensitivity, specificity, number, and affinity are now being studied. When the pharmacodynamic effects of aging are correlated with pharmacokinetic changes and other variables such as tissue sensitivity, altered homeostasis, co-existing disease states and drug interactions, it will enable the health-care provider to predict more accurately the effects of drugs in the aged patient.

## Absorption

In general, the safest, most convenient, and most economical delivery route for drugs intended to have systemic effect is by the oral route. When patients receive drugs orally, they must be absorbed from the gastrointestinal tract into systemic circulation so that they can distribute to the site of action. Numerous factors govern the absorption process. Most important is the intention of drug therapy. Drugs can be administered as a single dose for a specific time-limited situation or in multiple doses for chronic therapy. For example, if the patient is taking a medication as a single dose for the treatment of acute pain, as a sedative, or to assist in falling asleep, it is important that the drug be absorbed quickly and that it produce a high enough blood level for a long enough time to solve the patient's problem. However, if a patient needs to take a medication for a long period of time, it is more important that the drug provide an average or steady-state concentration in the blood. For single-dose drug therapy, the time to reach a desired concentration is very important. Thus, the time to produce an effective concentration and the amount of drug that gets absorbed in terms of rate and extent will affect the desired therapeutic outcome.

In discussions of drug absorption, three variables that describe the bioavailability (i.e., systemic availability) of a drug should be identified: time of peak plasma drug concentration ($T_{max}$), peak plasma drug concentration ($C_{max}$), and the area under the plasma drug concentration–time curve (AUC) (Figure 5.5). Knowledge of the bioavailability of a drug is important to the clinician because it can be used as a guide when choosing between a "brand name" and generic form of a drug, or when changing from one dosage form or product to another (Lamy, 1982). For example, solutions are absorbed faster and often more completely than either suspensions, capsules, or tablets. Likewise, suspensions are absorbed more quickly than capsules, which are absorbed more quickly than tablets. Soft gelatin liquid-filled capsules are more quickly absorbed than the hard gelatin dry powder–filled capsules (Figure 5.6). For example, except in the United States, the benzodiazepine hypnotic drug temazepam is available in a soft gelatin liquid-filled capsule. Following the ingestion of the capsule, temazepan dissolves rapidly, has a short time of onset of action, and is most useful for treating insomnia caused by the inability to fall asleep because of increased sleep onset or sleep latency. However, when temazepam was marketed in the United States it was manufactured as a hard gelatin dry powder–filled capsule. As a result of this change in dosage form, it took nearly 1 to 2 hours for the drug to become absorbed. Unfortunately, the drug was no longer useful in treating patients who had difficulty in falling asleep but was more appropriate for patients who have frequent nocturnal awakenings and/or early morning awakenings. Despite what is known about the result of the change in dosage form and its consequences, many clinicians still

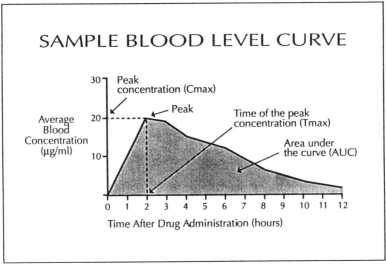

Adapted from Bioequivalence of Solid Oral Dosage Forms; PMA Presentation, September 1986

FIGURE 5.5.   Rate and extent of absorption is described using a graph of plasma concentration versus time after dose. $C_{max}$, $T_{max}$, AUC, absorption, distribution and elimination phases are described.

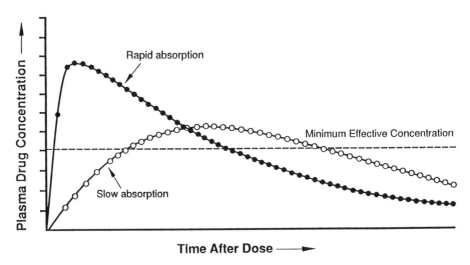

FIGURE 5.6.   The rate of absorption is an important determinant of the onset of clinical activity (e.g., analgesics, sedatives, hypnotics). Shown here is an example of a drug administered in the fasting state (rapid absorption) and the same drug co-administered with food (slow absorption).

prescribe temazepam for sleep latency. When patients complain about the drug not working, they usually increase the dose rather than choose a more appropriate drug.

After a tablet or capsule is swallowed, it must disintegrate before the active drug can dissolve in gut fluid and become absorbed into the bloodstream. If a drug does not get absorbed from the stomach, it will pass into the small intestine where actually most drugs are absorbed. Factors that govern the absorption of drugs from the gut include the amount of fluid that is coingested with the dosage form, pharmaceutical aspects of the dosage form such as tablet coatings, formulation and hardness, the presence of other substances (other drugs, antacids, food, ethanol) in the stomach, gastric emptying time, and intestinal transit time. All these variables influence the bioavailability profile of a drug. Other considerations include medications that can delay gastric emptying and gastrointestinal transit time (anticholinergics or opiates), drugs that accelerate gastric emptying (metoclopramide), and drugs that can bind other drugs (antihypercholesterolemic resins, kaopectate, psyllium-type laxatives).

Another concern is that some drugs such as nonsteroidal anti-inflammatory agents (including salicylates), potassium tablets and capsules, and iron supplements can be extremely irritating to the gut mucosa. Gastrointestinal bleeding, ulceration, and perforation have all been reported with the aforementioned drugs. A simple way around this problem is to require the patient to take these drugs with food or milk and/or at least 4 to 6 oz of fluid. This will essentially buffer the effects of the drug on the gastrointestinal mucosa and prevent the damaging effects of the drugs. It seems like such simple and intuitive instruction, but because of its simplicity, it is often forgotten. The presence of food or milk usually causes a delay in drug absorption, but it should not be a clinically important problem if the drugs are taken as chronic therapy. The risks of gastrointestinal ulcerations, bleeding, and perforation associated with nonsteroidal anti-inflammatory drug therapy, especially in aged and debilitated patients, are so great that the U.S. Food and Drug Administration required the manufacturers of these agents to include a highlighted warning about the occurrence of these problems in the package information inserts, which also appear in the Physician's Desk Reference.

Enteric coated tablets are specially coated to dissolve in the higher *p*H of the small intestine. This type of tablet is useful in preventing irritation by the drug of the gastric lining. Since the tablet is designed to dissolve in a higher *p*H, drugs which increase gastric *p*H such as antacids and histamine$_2$ antagonists (i.e., cimetidine, ranitidine, nizatidine, and famotidine) may cause the tablet to dissolve in the stomach. Therefore, these drugs should be taken separately or coadministered with meals. Sustained-release tablets that provide a slow release of medication either by dissolution over varying ranges of *p*H, by ion exchange, or by leaching the drug slowly out of a special matrix, may also be affected by changes in gastrointestinal *p*H transit time. Patients react differently to the effects of the gastrointestinal tract on drug absorption. Whether or not the aged patient reacts more frequently is not known at this time. It is suspected but there is no data from well-controlled studies to support this speculation.

Other routes of administration that involve drug absorption include the oral route in which a drug can be used sublingually, buccally, or as a perioral spray, the intramuscular route, subcutaneous route (including injection and implantation), intranasal route, ophthalmic route, and the transdermal route (Figure 5.7). There is not much information about the effects of aging on the absorption of drugs from the aforementioned routes, with the exception of oral ingestion. It is assumed that aging does not significantly affect the absorption of drugs from these routes either. However, there is a theoretical concern about sublingual or buccal absorption. Anecdotal information suggests that if an aging person has diminished salivary production and if they are taking an anticholinergic drug

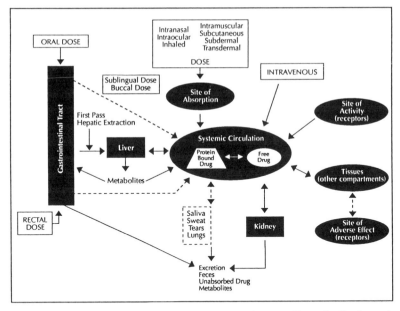

FIGURE 5.7.   Drugs can be administered by several routes. Drug distribution and clearance are determined by many factors which are interrelated.

such as an antihistamine, tricyclic antidepressant, or antipsychotic medication, this may sufficiently dry the mouth so that it will take longer for the tablet to dissolve. Although this has not yet been studied in a controlled fashion, it may explain why some aged patients have difficulty with sublingual dosage forms. The sublingual route of drug administration is becoming more popular because in some patients oral administration may be undesirable because of nausea, vomiting, or other situations when the use of the gastrointestinal tract needs to be avoided. Drugs such as triazolam, alprazolam, captopril, opiate analgesics, antiarrhythmics, nitroglycerin and other drugs are administered by this route (Scavone, Greenblatt, & Friedman, 1986; Scavone et al., 1992).

The coingestion of food and other drugs can significantly affect the bioavailability of a drug. Certain drugs such as propranolol, griseofulvin, and others actually have an increased bioavailability when taken with food, whereas the coingestion of food can delay absorption of analgesics, hypnotics, and other drugs so dramatically that the desired clinical effect following a single dose will not occur. Thus, it is important for the clinician to be familiar with the variable that can affect bioavailability.

When drugs are given in multiple doses as chronic therapy, the amount of drug absorbed (AUC) is more important than either $T_{max}$ or $C_{max}$. Since the object of drug therapy is to maintain an average blood level of the drug, the time course of absorption is less important than the actual amount of drug replacing that which has been cleared by the body.

Numerous studies performed on the effects of aging on the gastrointestinal tract suggest the possibility of altered drug absorption in the aged gut (Greenblatt, Sellers, & Shader, 1982; Ouslander, 1981). Reasons for this include increased gastric $pH$ because of a reduction in gastric parietal-cell function, resulting in decreased gastric acid output (Geokas & Haverback, 1969), decreased splanchnic blood flow resulting from a decrease in cardiac output (Stevenson, 1984); a reduction in gastric emptying time; and a decrease in gastrointestinal motility (Evans, Triggs, Cheung, Broe, & Creasey, 1981). In addition, altered active transport processes of some nutrients in the aged have suggested that drug absorption may be similarly impaired (Montgomery et al., 1978). However, for most drugs used in clinical practice, the rate and extent of absorption are determined by passive diffusion during contact with the surface of the proximal small intestine (Greenblatt, Sellers, & Shader, 1982). Despite speculation to the contrary, there is essentially no evidence that drug absorption is impaired in the aged (Kramer, Chapron, Benson, & Mercik, 1978; Ochs et al., 1979; Ochs, Otten, Greenblatt, & Dengler, 1982). Any changes, if they actually do occur, are often small and unlikely to be of any clinical importance, especially during chronic therapy (Stevenson, 1984). For example, well-controlled studies of acetaminophen (Divoll, Ameer, Abernethy, & Greenblatt 1982) and lorazepam (Greenblatt et al., 1979) suggest that the rate and extent of gastrointestinal absorption are not important in the aged. In summary, changes in drug absorption appear to be the least important of the age-related pharmacokinetic changes.

*Distribution*

Once in the body, a drug will distribute to various body fluids and tissues. Fat-soluble drugs such as digoxin, diazepam, and imipramine distribute readily and have relatively large distribution volumes, whereas water-soluble drugs such as cephalosporins, penicillins, and aminoglycosides are considered to have small volumes of distribution. Understanding drug distribution is sometimes difficult because the distribution volumes or compartments are actually derived from mathematics rather than anatomy and physiology. Thus, pharmacokinetic compartments are imaginary mathematical spaces and do not correspond to actual anatomic entities, even though the compartments are assigned numeric dimensions of volume (milliliters, liters) (Greenblatt & Shader, 1985).

After a drug reaches systemic circulation, its passage into body tissue and fluids depends on the drug's molecular size, degree of ionization, solubility, and ability to cross biological membranes. The goal is to have the drug reach the receptor at the intended site of activity and to cause the desired effect. If too much reaches the receptor site, toxicity could result and if not enough drug reaches the target, a subtherapeutic response can result. Furthermore, if the drug is available to reach other sites, adverse effects may occur. For example, an antihistamine may be prescribed for the treatment of an allergy but in addition to alleviating the allergic symptoms, it can act in the central nervous system (CNS), causing drowsiness and confusion; in the eyes, causing a mydriasis and a blurring of vision; in the gastrointestinal tract, causing a decrease in gut motility resulting in constipation; and many other areas resulting in urinary retention, diminished salivary flow, and various other effects. If the drug is able to penetrate many areas in the body, the range of adverse effects can be dramatic.

Certain drugs are specifically designed to have different lipid and water solubility characteristics so that the intended action is more predictable based on its distribution profile. For example, if a patient requires an antibiotic for the treatment of a bone infection, a drug with a relatively large volume of distribution is chosen because of its ability to permeate distant body compartments. On the other hand, if a patient requires an antibiotic for the treatment of an uncomplicated urinary tract infection, choosing a drug with a wide volume of distribution is not important because a drug that confines itself to body water, involving a smaller volume of distribution, may be more desirable. Since many drugs need to be present at the site of activity at a certain minimum effective concentration, a drug's distribution profile can be used clinically to actually plan on a desirable duration of effect. For example, the benzodiazepine midazolam is administered intravenously as a preanesthetic/induction agent for surgery. It is an extremely fat-soluble substance, so it readily distributes throughout the body following the administration of the dose. Because of its extensive distribution, the CNS concentrations diminish to a level at which the drug is not active any longer. Thus, the termination of clinical effect is governed by the distribution of drug throughout the body, causing a dilution of the amount available to the brain and not by the biotransformation or excretion of drug from the body (Figure 5.8).

If a lipid-soluble drug with a large volume of distribution is given chronically, as is often the case with diazepam, the compartments will sequester drug and the result will be the accumulation of drug in various tissues. This can lead to residual effects secondary to increased total body levels of drug. In other words, the level of response to a medication may increase over time independent of an increase in dose to the patient. Although this concept is extremely important, many clinicians forget that drug accumulation can occur. Some reasons for this include that the body maintains homeostasis through adaptive mechanisms at the receptor site. For example, when the body experiences a constant

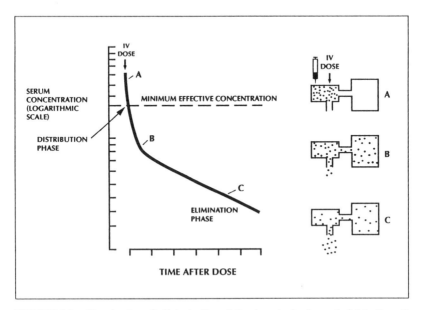

FIGURE 5.8.   Termination of clinical effect following single dose administration of lipophilic drugs is a function of distribution.

exposure to a given drug, receptors react to that particular agent and adapt by changing receptor number, sensitivity, concentration, and affinity and by the production or termination of endogenous agonist or antagonist substances that can modulate the effect of the drug. It is a rather complicated process, but the message is that despite the protective mechanisms, the body's defense can be overridden after a period of time because of changes in reserve capacity. This topic will be discussed in more detail later in the chapter, when age-related changes in pharmacodynamics are presented.

Several factors such as decreased cardiac output; increased peripheral vascular resistance; decreased blood flow to the liver and kidney blood flow; and increased fraction of cardiac output to cerebral, coronary, and skeletal muscle circulations, affect the distribution of drugs in the aged person (Ouslander, 1981; Bender, 1965). In addition, age-related changes in body habitus (composition) can affect drug distribution (Figure 5.9). The aged generally experience a decrease in body water, extracellular fluid, muscle, and lean body mass and a relative increase in the proportion of adipose tissue. For example, the fat content in the body of young adult males is approximately 18% and can increase to approximately 36% in aged males. The percentage of fat in young adult females is approximately 33% and can increase to approximately 48% in aged females (Greenblatt, Sellers, & Shader, 1982). These changes in body habitus can affect the volume of distribution of drugs depending on their fat and water solubility. Thus, it appears that there is a gender-related difference in the aged regarding the volume of distribution of drugs. Women will have a larger distribution of fat-soluble drugs and a smaller distribution volume for relatively water-soluble drugs (Greenblatt, Allen, Harmatz, & Shader, 1980; Divoll, Ameer, Abernethy, & Greenblatt, 1982; Allen, Greenblatt, Harmatz, & Shader, 1980; Greenblatt et al. 1981). Various fat-soluble drugs such as diazepam and lidocaine

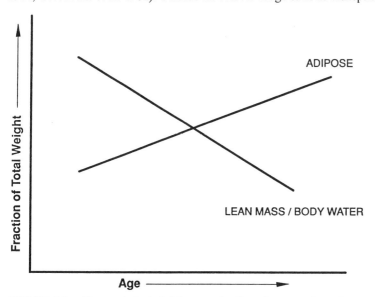

FIGURE 5.9. Changes in body habitus as a function of age are shown here. As one ages there tends to be a reduction in lean body mass and total body water and an increase in adipose tissue.

are more extensively distributed in the aged, whereas various relatively water-soluble drugs (i.e., less lipid-soluble) such as ethanol, antipyrine, and acetaminophen have a decreased volume of distribution in aged individuals (Greenblatt, Sellers, & Shader, 1982; Vestal et al., 1977; Nation, Triggs, & Selig, 1977; Maklon, Barton, James, & Rawlins, 1980; Klotz, Avant, Hoyumpa, Schenker, & Wilkinson, 1975).

After drugs enter the systemic circulation, they become bound to circulating plasma proteins. Albumin and alpha-one acid glycoprotein (AAG), an acute-phase reactant, are the two most important proteins to which drugs can bind. The attachment of drugs to a protein involves a reversible bonding of the ionic, hydrogen, or van der Vaal's type, which is relatively weak and loose (Richey & Bender, 1977). Acidic drugs preferentially bind to albumin (e.g., nonsteroidal anti-inflammatory agents, salicylates, benzodiazepines, warfarin, and phenytoin), whereas basic drugs (e.g., tricyclic antidepressants, beta-adrenergic antagonists, and lidocaine) bind to alpha-one acid glycoprotein. Not all drugs are equally bound and the actual binding of drugs is a dynamic process. In any given situation, an equilibrium is established between the amount of drug that is bound and the amount of drug that is unbound or free. The percentage of free drug is known as the free fraction and represents a ratio between the free-drug concentration and the total (free plus bound) drug concentration. The distribution of drug to plasma proteins contributes to the actual volume of distribution because only the unbound drug is available to leave the systemic circulation and travel to the receptor site. Additionally, it is the free drug that is available for elimination from the body and to other body tissues and fluids. Although some controversy exists, an age-related reduction in plasma albumin concentrations and age-related increases in alpha-one acid glycoprotein have been consistently reported (Dybaker, Lauritzen, & Krakaner, 1981; Greenblatt, 1979). Aged patients who are undernourished, severely debilitated or have advanced disease especially have a substantial decrease in plasma albumin concentrations (MacLennan, Martin, & Mason, 1977). Healthy, well-nourished aged persons have lower albumin concentrations than young persons even though they may not fall below the usual normal range (Greenblatt, Sellers, & Shader, 1982). Thus, the degree of drug binding to plasma proteins may be reduced in the aged because of the decrease in the amount of albumin. Even though it has been reported, no consistent or convincing evidence exists that the affinity of albumin for drugs is altered by the aging process (Ouslander, 1981; Richey & Bender, 1977) (Figure 5.10).

The clinical implications of protein binding have often been overestimated. Plasma protein binding, or changes in binding that may occur as a result of drug interactions or disease, seldom have any direct clinical importance. It is neither a benefit nor disadvantage for a drug to be extensively bound to plasma protein because the free-drug concentration is that which is pharmacologically active, as well as that which is available to the hepatocytes for biotransformation. The free concentration depends only on the drug dosing rate and the clearance of free drug, not on the actual extent of protein binding (Greenblatt & Scavone, 1986). Drugs that are considered highly protein bound are generally bound to an extent greater than 80% (Table 5.3). Changes in free fraction could be important for drugs that are 80% to 90% bound but much more important for those that are bound to an extent greater than 90%. When the free fraction is small, slight variations can have important consequences. Drugs that are less than 80% bound generally imply

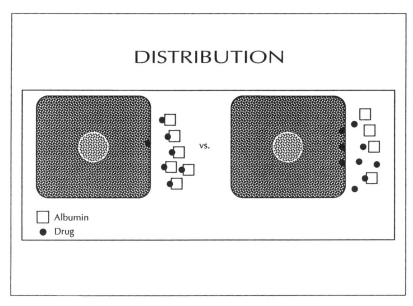

# DISTRIBUTION

Albumin
Drug

FIGURE 5.10. Drugs are bound to plasma proteins. This diagram describes the relationship between drug bound to albumin, unbound or free drug in the plasma, and drug at the receptor site, site of toxicity or site of biotransformation. The left side of the diagram represents a young adult and the right side represents the arrangement of drug and albumin in an aged adult. Note the reduction in the amount of albumin, the decrease in affinity of drug for albumin and the resultant increase in free fraction of drug in plasma and the amount of drug at the site of action, toxicity and/or biotransformation.

TABLE 5.3   Examples of protein-bound drugs

| Greater than 90% bound | 80% to 90% bound |
| --- | --- |
| Warfarin | Chlorpromazine* |
| Ibuprofen | Lorazepam |
| Phenylbutazone | Sulfisoxazole |
| Indomethacin | Salicylates |
| Diazepam | Phenytoin |
| Chlordiazepoxide | Oxazepam |
| Temazepam | Clofibrate |
| Oxazepam | Haloperidol* |
| Furosemide | Methadone* |
| Thiazide diuretics | Quinidine* |
| Oral hypoglycemics (first generation) | Tricyclic antidepres- |
| Propranolol* | sants* |

*Bound to alpha-one acid glycoprotein. Drugs without asterisk are bound to albumin.

that the consequences of protein binding are relatively unimportant (Greenblatt & Shader, 1985).

While protein binding does not influence clinical activity, alterations in binding can have an enormous effect on the interpretation of total serum or plasma drug concentrations. When drug levels in the serum, plasma, or whole blood are monitored, the laboratory reports the total (free plus bound) amount of drug even though it is only the free drug that is available to cross cell membranes and interact with the receptor. The reason for this is that the evaluation of the unbound drug concentration is technically more complex than the evaluation of the total amount. Luckily, the free concentration remains stable over the course of a patient's therapy, and the variability between and within patients is relatively small (Friedman & Greenblatt, 1986).

When more than one highly protein-bound drug is given to a patient, drug binding to serum protein may be substantially altered. A "new" drug added to a therapeutic regimen can displace the present drug(s) from their protein-binding site(s), resulting in a reduction in binding accompanied by an increase in free fraction (Koch-Weser & Sellers, 1976; Sellers, 1979). Such interactions have been misinterpreted as leading to immediate drug toxicity. In reality, these interactions are unlikely to be clinically important because the increased free concentrations will be transient because of the rapid equilibrium that occurs with other tissues and the availability of the unbound drug to be biotransformed and cleared from the body (Koch-Weser & Sellers, 1976; Sellers, 1979; Greenblatt, Sellers, & Shader, 1982; McElnay & D'Arcy, 1983). However, the total drug concentration will be reduced as a result of redistribution and may result in a lowering of the therapeutic and toxic ranges for the total serum or plasma drug level (Friedman & Greenblatt, 1986).

For example, if a patient who was taking phenytoin (Dilantin) for the treatment of a seizure disorder and routinely had steady-state plasma concentrations averaging about 15 µg/ml (micrograms per milliliter) and was well controlled (seizure and side effect free) received a prescription for aspirin, a drug interaction will most likely occur because of the displacement of phenytoin from protein-binding sites by the salicylate. Initially the free concentration of phenytoin would increase, but soon after the steady-state phenytoin plasma concentration would actually decrease because the more unbound drug is available for clearance by the liver. The resulting phenytoin plasma level could now be around 10 µg/ml and the patient would still be well controlled. However, the free fraction of phenytoin increased even though the free concentration remained the same. In other words, if the free fraction of phenytoin was 10% when the total plasma level was 15 µg/ml, the free concentration would be 1.5 µg/ml. If the salicylate caused the free fraction of phenytoin to increase to 15%, the resulting total plasma concentration is 10 µg/ml and the free concentration would still be 1.5 µg/ml. The fraction of unbound drug has increased, but the total concentration has decreased because more free drug is available for removal from the body. The result is no change in either the free concentration or the clinical status of the patient. This drug interaction would unlikely be of clinical importance with respect to toxicity, provided the clinician does not increase the phenytoin dosage to compensate for the lower than expected total phenytoin levels (Fraser, Ludden, Evens, & Sutherland, 1980).

As one can now appreciate, protein-binding interactions are complex yet transient, and the net result is usually harmless to the patient. The misinterpretation of what actually occurs is the main problem and could result in an inappropriate and potentially hazardous intervention. Since the aged take more medications, the frequency as well as the confusion of such interactions is much greater than in younger patients.

In summary, a change in drug binding to plasma proteins does not itself alter clinical drug effects. However, alterations in binding may influence the interpretation of plasma or serum drug concentrations (blood levels) used to monitor therapy (Greenblatt, Sellers, & Shader, 1982). For highly protein-bound drugs whose binding is decreased and resulting free fraction increased, clinicians should anticipate lower ranges of both toxic and therapeutic plasma or serum concentrations of total (free plus bound) drug. Regarding drug distribution, altered drug distribution itself in the aged will not alter steady-state plasma concentrations during chronic drug administration because the maintenance of steady-state plasma concentrations depends only on the dosing rate and the total clearance of the drug. The concept of clearance will be discussed in the next section.

## Clearance

To understand how the body eliminates drugs from the body, it is important to be familiar with terms such as *clearance* and *elimination* half-life. Understanding these concepts will enable the health-care provider to fully appreciate how aging affects the biotransformation and elimination of drugs.

The concept of total clearance is extremely important when evaluating the pharmacokinetic properties of all drugs. Clearance is expressed in units of volume divided by time (such as milliliters per minute, ml/min, or liters per hour, L/hr) and is the single most reliable index of an organism's capacity to biotransform (i.e., metabolize) or excrete a given drug (Greenblatt & Scavone, 1986). Clinicians are most familiar with the concept of clearance in the context of renal function, for which the clearance of creatinine is used as an index of kidney function. Creatinine clearance schematically represents the total volume of blood, plasma, or serum for which creatinine is completely removed per unit time. The clearance of drugs is conceptually similar. Most drugs are primarily cleared by either the liver or the kidney. A given drug's clearance numerically describes the capacity of a given individual to remove that drug from the body. A drug's clearance cannot exceed the rate of drug delivery or blood flow to the clearing organ. Thus, when drugs are biotransformed by the liver, their clearance cannot exceed hepatic blood flow. For drugs removed by the kidney, renal clearance likewise cannot exceed renal blood flow.

Clearance is important in clinical practice because it is a major determinant of steady-state plasma or serum concentration during multiple dosage. In fact, the total clearance of a drug will influence a patient's therapeutic outcome. When a medication has been administered as a multiple dose long enough for steady state to occur, the general equation describing the steady-state concentration in blood, plasma, or serum ($C_{ss}$) is as follows:

$$C_{ss} = \frac{\text{Dosing rate}}{\text{Clearance}}$$

It is important for the clinician to appreciate this equation, because dosing rate is the variable over which they have control; it is the rate of drug administration, expressed in units of amount of drug divided by time (such as milligrams per hour, mg/hr, or grams per day, g/d). By varying the size of each dose or the interval between doses (i.e., dosage schedule), the clinician can directly control the dosing rate and ultimately the steady-state concentration. Clearance appears in the denominator of this equation as the biologic variable describing the individual's capacity to remove the drug from the body. In general, for any given drug in an individual patient, the actual numerical value for clearance is usually unknown unless it has been specifically identified. However, in a medically stable patient, the clearance of a drug is assumed to be constant. Changes in hepatic or renal status secondary to aging or disease or the addition or deletion of drugs that affect liver function, such as cigarette smoking, ethanol ingestion, and drugs that are hepatic microsomal enzyme inducers or inhibitors, and kidney function, such as drugs that compete for renal tubular absorption or secretion, may dramatically change an individual's clearance rate. Thus, at any given dose rate, $C_{ss}$ will increase as clearance decreases (Greenblatt, Sellers, & Shader, 1982). If aging is associated with the reduction in total clearance of a given drug, $C_{ss}$ will increase accordingly. Knowing this, the clinician can either extend the dosing interval or give a lower maintenance dose to the aged patient for a desired steady-state concentration.

Knowledge of a drug's pathway of biotransformation and of factors that could influence its clearance can help clinicians to anticipate patient characteristics, drug interactions, or disease states that might alter clearance and signal the need to adjust the dosage or choose a more appropriate drug. Many drugs yield active metabolites upon biotransformation which contribute to the therapeutic or toxic effect of the parent compound. The ultimate goal of multiple-dose drug administration is to achieve a steady-state plasma concentration that lies within a "therapeutic" range and to avoid toxic or clinically ineffective blood levels (Greenblatt & Scavone, 1986).

### Elimination Half-Life

Elimination half-life is probably the most commonly discussed and most misinterpreted pharmacokinetic variable for drugs used in clinical practice. Most drugs are eliminated by a characteristic kinetic behavior known as a first-order process. In order for a drug to fit this first-order model, the rate of change of drug concentrations over time must vary continuously in relation to the concentration (Greenblatt & Shader, 1985). In other words, the drug concentrations in body fluids usually decline with time, and when the concentrations are high (i.e., following drug administration), the rate of decline is also high and when concentrations are low, the rate of decline is smaller (Figure 5.11). Since the rate of drug disappearance varies continuously as a function of time as the concentration changes, an exponential function is used to describe this behavior. Luckily, first-order exponential processes can be described using the concept of half-life. The elimination half-life of a drug is the time necessary for the drug concentration in blood, serum, plasma, or any other body fluid or tissue to fall by one half, or 50%. Each time an interval equal to a half-life elapses, the concentration falls to one half of the value at the beginning of that interval (Greenblatt & Shader, 1985). For example, if the initial drug concentration was 80 mg/ml and the elimination half-life of that drug was 2 hr, the concentration would fall to 40 mg/ml after 2 hr had elapsed (1 half-life), to 20 mg/ml after 4

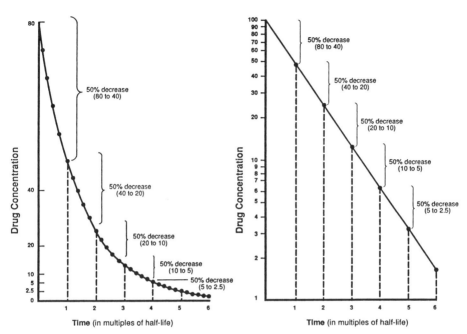

FIGURE 5.11.   Elimination half-life of a drug is represented in a linear-linear plot (left) and a log-linear (semi-logarithmic) plot (right). The x-axis represents time in multiples of elimination half-life and the y-axis represents plasma or serum concentration.

hr (2 half-lives), to 10 mg/ml after 6 hr (3 half-lives), to 5 mg/ml after 8 hr (4 half-lives) and to 2.5 mg/ml after 10 hr (5 half-lives) had elapsed. The amount of drug that has been eliminated from the system decreases with the passing of each half-life, but the percentage or ratio of change (50%) is always constant. The important facts (Greenblatt & Shader, 1985) to remember about the clinical use of half-lives is that:

1. All first-order processes are more than 90% complete after four half-life intervals have elapsed.
2. First-order processes are never 100% complete no matter how much time elapses.
3. It takes approximately 4 to 5 half-lives to elapse before a drug is considered to be in the steady-state condition.
4. It takes approximately 4 to 5 half-lives to elapse before a drug is considered to be virtually eliminated from the system even though first-order processes are considered to be essentially complete after approximately 8 half-life intervals.

It is also important that clinicians understand that the elimination half-life is a dependent biological variable related to a drug's volume of distribution (*Vd*) and inversely related to its total clearance as follows:

$$\text{Elimination half-life} = \frac{0.693 \times Vd}{\text{Clearance}}$$

If the volume of distribution is relatively constant, then the elimination half-life will be inversely related to total clearance. Therefore, when clearance is low, half-life is long, and conversely, when clearance is high, half-life is short. However, when the volume of distribution is not constant, changes in volume of distribution may influence elimination half-life without a change in clearance (Abernethy, Greenblatt, Divoll, & Harmatz, 1981). The potential pitfalls of elimination half-life must always be recognized.

Elimination half-life is a clinically important variable, because it is related to the rate and extent of drug accumulation during multiple dosage. When a drug is administered at dosing intervals that are shorter than its elimination half-life, a large fraction of each prior dose will remain in the body when the next dose is administered. This leads to drug accumulation, which continues until the steady-state condition is reached, at which point there is no further accumulation (Figure 5.12). Likewise, the time necessary to reach steady state following the start of multiple-dose therapy is also related to the drug's elimination half-life. This concept is used clinically in situations where a loading dose is administered to a patient in order to quickly initiate a therapeutic response.

Many categories of drugs contain representatives in their class that vary widely in their elimination half-life. This raises questions about which type of drug is more appropriate for a particular patient. There are benefits as well as disadvantages for both long elimination half-life and short elimination half-life compounds. Drugs with relatively short values of elimination half-life (such as ibuprofen, triazolam, temazepam, lorazepam, and alprazolam) are usually termed "nonaccumulating." For these drugs, the steady-state condition is reached rapidly after the start of therapy. This may provide some therapeutic benefit in terms of ease of dosage titration, because little delay occurs between initiation of treatment and the attainment of steady state. Short half-life compounds also have some potential disadvantages, since multiple daily doses are usually required to maintain adequate plasma levels throughout the day. Furthermore, when

## DRUG ACCUMULATION

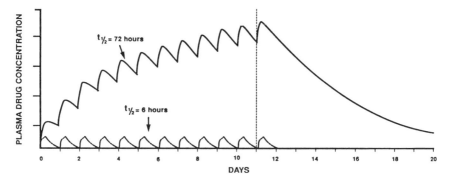

FIGURE 5.12.   Accumulation of a drug with a long elimination half-life versus no accumulation of a drug with a short elimination half-life following the administration of multiple doses. Note the time course of drug elimination in the drug with a long elimination half-life.

treatment is discontinued, or if doses are inadvertently or deliberately missed, serum concentrations will fall rapidly, which may lead to rapid recurrence of symptoms, withdrawal, or rebound effects. For long half-life compounds (such as piroxicam, oxaprozin digoxin, diazepam, chlordiazepoxide, and desmethyldiazepam), a theoretic disadvantage is that attainment of steady state may be delayed. There is also a delay in the achievement of a new steady-state condition if the dosage must be increased or decreased. Upon discontinuation of the drug there is also a long elimination (wash-out) phase that must be accounted for when a patient's treatment response is reevaluated after starting a different drug therapy. On the other hand, a potential advantage is that the number of doses that the patient takes per day is decreased, which could possibly translate into enhanced patient compliance. Furthermore, when treatment is discontinued, or when doses are missed, plasma levels will not fall promptly, thereby minimizing the likelihood of a rapid recurrence of symptoms.

Clinicians who are aware of the elimination half-life values of individual drugs will be in a better position to judge their potential benefits and disadvantages, and to choose a kinetic profile suitable for an individual patient (Greenblatt & Scavone, 1986).

## *Biotransformation*

Biotransformation, commonly referred to as drug metabolism, is a considerably complex process that primarily occurs in the liver. Liver cells carry out many biotransformation reactions that contribute to the removal of drugs from the body. Oxidation and conjugation are the two most important subdivisions of hepatic clearance. These reactions can be categorized into either Phase I, also referred to as preparative reactions, or Phase II, also known as synthetic reactions (Figure 5.13). Phase I biotransformation includes the oxidation reactions, such as hydroxylation, dealkylation, sulfoxidation, nitroreduction, and hydrolysis. These reactions generally constitute minor molecular modifications, usually resulting in a more water-soluble (polar) metabolite. The product of these reactions also retains part or all of the pharmacologic activity of the parent compound (Greenblatt,

## BIOTRANSFORMATION

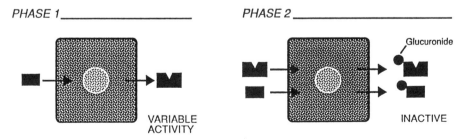

FIGURE 5.13.    Phase I (oxidation) versus Phase II (conjugation) biotransformation pathways are shown in this figure. Phase I reactions may yield the formation of active metabolites whereas Phase II reactions result in the inactivation of a drug.

Divoll, Abernethy, Harmatz, & Shader, 1982). Examples of drugs that undergo Phase I biotransformation reactions yielding active metabolites include (parent drug to active metabolite): diazepam to desmethyldiazepam, flurazepam to desalkylflurazepam, imipramine to desipramine, and amitriptyline to nortriptyline. Hepatic microsomal oxidation is often termed a "susceptible" metabolic pathway, in that its activity can be impaired by numerous factors, such as old age, hepatitis, cirrhosis, severe debilitation, or the coadministration of many agents known to impair oxidizing capacity (Williams, 1983; Gibaldi & Perrier, 1975). The hepatic microsomal enzymes that are responsible for Phase I reactions appear to be significantly impaired in the aged. The result is a reduction in total drug clearance, higher steady-state plasma drug concentrations during multiple dosage and an increase in elimination half-life. Phase II reactions involve the attachment or conjugation of the drug molecule to a glucuronide, sulfate, or acetate moiety. The resulting conjugates are generally pharmacologically inactive (except for some acetylated metabolites), are much more polar than the parent molecule, and are usually excreted in the urine (Greenblatt, Sellers, & Shader, 1982). Hepatic conjugation is considered to be a "nonsusceptible" pathway and is relatively uninfluenced by old age, disease states, or drug interactions (Greenblatt et al., 1981; Greenblatt & Scavone, 1986). Thus, a prior knowledge of a drug's major metabolic pathway (oxidation versus conjugation) may be of help to the clinician in predicting whether clearance is susceptible to change in a specific clinical situation (Tables 5.4 and 5.5). In addition, it can be helpful in drug selection for the aged patient. For example, the benzodiazepines diazepam, chlordiazepoxide, desalkylflurazepam, and desmethyldiazepam are all subject to oxidation reactions during the clearance from the body. Thus, the clearance of these drugs is

TABLE 5.4   Examples of drugs biotransformed by Phase I (preparative) reactions

| | |
|---|---|
| Alprazolam | Flurazepam |
| Amitriptyline | Glutethimide |
| Antipyrine | Ibuprofen |
| Barbiturates | Imipramine |
| Carbamazepine | Lidocaine |
| Chloramphenicol | Meperidine |
| Chlorpromazine | Methamphetamine |
| Clonazepam | Nortriptyline |
| Codeine | Midazolam |
| Desipramine | Phenacetin |
| Desmethyldiazepam | Phenylbutazone |
| Diazepam | Phenytoin |
| Dimenhydrinate | Prazepam |
| Doxylamine | |

TABLE 5.5   Examples of drugs biotransformed by Phase II (synthetic) reactions

| | |
|---|---|
| Acetaminophen | Nitrazepam |
| Acetylsalicylic acid | Oxazepam |
| (aspirin) | Phenelzine |
| Clonazepam | Procainamide |
| Hydralazine | Sulfanilamide |
| Lorazepam | Temazepam |

reduced in aged patients and the likelihood for increased accumulation is a concern in this patient population. Since the metabolism of the parent drug yields metabolites that are also clinically active, there is a concern about the accumulation of not only the parent drug but the active metabolites as well. The accumulation of metabolites could theoretically contribute to the development of adverse or increased effects. On the other hand, the benzodiazepines oxazepam, temazepam, and lorazepam undergo conjugation reactions, have no active metabolites, and are relatively unaffected by old age. Thus, drug selection for the aged patient can essentially make more sense if the prescribing clinician considers the drug's metabolic fate.

Hepatic blood flow can be more important for some drugs than microsomal enzyme activity as a major determinant of total drug clearance (Wilkinson & Shand, 1975). Partially as a result of an age-related reduction in cardiac output, liver blood flow declines an estimated 40% to 45% in aged persons as compared to young adults (Geokas & Haverback, 1969). Hepatic size, both in absolute terms and as a percentage of total body weight, decreases with age. One would expect that the clearance of high liver blood flow–dependent drugs would be uniformly affected, but the data are conflicting. For example, a reduction in the total clearance occurs for propranolol but not for lidocaine (Nation et al., 1977; Vestal, Wood, & Shand, 1979; Casteleden & George, 1979). Theoretically, the bioavailability of drugs that have a high first-pass hepatic extraction (following drug absorption from the gastrointestinal tract before reaching the general systemic circulation) may also be affected by aging, but there is no conclusive evidence available at this time.

It is difficult to predict the influence of age on biotransformation, since hepatic-drug metabolizing capacity may not be uniformly affected. Changes in total clearance of drug oxidation reactions mediated by hepatic microsomal enzymes can be impaired in an aged individual even though the patient has normal liver function tests. Thus, normal values on liver function tests do not imply normal drug metabolism. In addition, the effect of age on hepatic drug clearance depends on the metabolic pathway of the drug in addition to the influence of liver blood flow, size, and other co-ingested substances and drugs.

Various drugs can either induce or inhibit drug metabolism (Table 5.6). Stimulation of hepatic mixed-function oxidase enzymes is a slow process, which can take anywhere from a few days to a few weeks to become clinically evident (Greenblatt & Shader, 1985). Conversely, enzyme inhibitors impair metabolic function and exert their clinical

TABLE 5.6   Partial list of drugs that induce or inhibit hepatic microsomal mixed-function oxidase enzymes

| Enzyme inducers | Enzyme inhibitors | |
|---|---|---|
| Barbiturates | Chloramphenicol | Methylphenidate |
| Carbamazepine | Cimetidine | Propoxyphene |
| Ethyl alcohol (chronic) | Disulfiram | Quinolones |
| Glutethimide | Erythromycin | Tricyclic |
| Phenytoin | Estrogens | antidepressants |
| Rifampin | Ethyl alcohol (acute) | |
| | Isoniazid | |

effect rapidly. Drugs with a narrow therapeutic range that are biotransformed in the liver by microsomal enzymes represent the most clinically important drug interactions if enzyme inducers or inhibitors are added or deleted from a patient's drug regimen.

### Elimination (Renal Clearance)

In contrast with hepatic biotransformation, the effect of age on renal drug clearance is more straightforward and predictable. Glomerular filtration rate decreases by about 35% over a person's lifetime so that drugs excreted mainly by the kidney can be expected to have reduced total clearance (Ouslander, 1981; Greenblatt, Sellers, & Shader, 1982; Vestal, 1978; Rowe et al., 1976). To adequately predict the effect of the aging kidney on total drug clearance, it is necessary to know the status of a patient's level of renal function. This is usually accomplished by evaluating a serum creatinine level or estimating a glomerular filtration rate (GFR), using creatinine clearance as an indicator. Serum creatinine concentration depends on endogenous creatinine production as well as renal creatinine clearance. Evaluating renal function based on serum creatinine is oftentimes misleading because the age-related decrease in lean body (muscle) mass results in a decrease in daily endogenous creatinine production. As a result, in the aged person creatinine clearance must fall to a greater extent than in a younger person before the serum creatinine increases (Rowe et al., 1976). Thus, the use of serum creatinine concentration as the

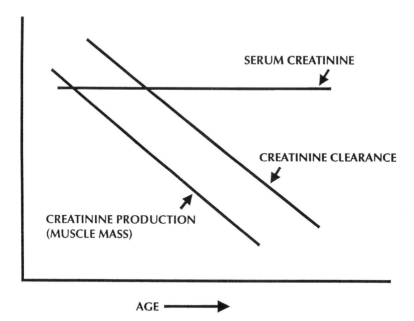

FIGURE 5.14.    Serum creatinine may overestimate renal function in the elderly. With less muscle mass, less creatinine is formed and is presented to a kidney with reduced function. Normal serum creatinine values usually result even when there is a significant decline in renal function.

TABLE 5.7   Examples of drugs excreted by the kidney

| | |
|---|---|
| Amantadine | Nitrofurantoin |
| Amikacin | Penicillins |
| Cephalosporins | Phenobarbital |
| Cimetidine | Procainamide |
| Digoxin | Quinidine |
| Erythromycin | Sulfonamides |
| Furosemide | Tetracycline |
| Gentamicin | Tobramycin |
| Lithium | Vancomycin |
| Methanamic acid | |

only indicator of renal function may actually overestimate renal function. In an aged patient, serum creatinine may be in the normal range, whereas renal function is substantially reduced (Ouslander, 1981; Greenblatt, Sellers, & Shader, 1982) (Figure 5.14). Ideally, creatinine clearance determinations based on 24-hr urinary excretion should be used along with serum creatinine to evaluate renal function. In reality this is not always feasible, so the clinician must rely only on serum creatinine concentrations. However, there are various nomograms and formulas available to estimate creatinine clearance from serum creatinine. One formula (Cockroft & Gault, 1976) that is considered useful (Ouslander, 1981) is the following:

$$\text{Creatinine clearance in males} = \frac{(140 - \text{age}) \times \text{body weight (kg)}}{72 \times \text{serum creatinine level}}$$

$$\text{Creatinine clearance in females} = 0.85 \times \text{above value}$$

where creatinine clearance is in milliliters per minute (ml/min), serum creatinine is in milligrams per deciliter (mg/dl), age is in years, and weight is in kilograms (kg).

In general, the dosage of a drug that is excreted principally by the kidney must be reduced to prevent excessive accumulation of the drug (Table 5.7). Following reduction in the initial doses of drugs excreted by the kidney, the clinical status of the patient can be reviewed, along with a serum or plasma drug concentration, and the dose can be subsequently titrated to the desired level.

### *Pharmacodynamics: The Effects of Aging on Drug Sensitivity*

It is generally regarded that the aged are more sensitive to drug effects than the young and consequentially experience more adverse reactions (Ouslander, 1981; Greenblatt, Divoll, Abernethy, Harmatz, & Shader, 1982). These observations have stimulated much speculation about the cause of these clinical impressions, but conclusive evidence is still lacking about the reasons and mechanisms for altered responsiveness. Since it is not possible in many cases to measure in humans the true *in vivo* receptor sensitivity, many of these questions will go unanswered (Stevenson, 1984). Data from experiments using animal models, tissue, and/or cell cultures and studies in humans correlating serum, plasma, or tissue level to a resulting pharmacodynamic response are the basis for evaluating the effects of aging on drug response.

There are conflicting data and considerable debate about the mechanisms underlying the altered sensitivity to drugs in aged humans. There are basically two interrelated hypotheses which are used to explain the differences. The pharmacodynamic hypothesis suggests that receptors change in their sensitivity to certain drugs in such a way that a given drug concentration at the receptor site leads to a greater effect in an aged individual than in a young individual. The age-related changes appear to occur at the level of either the affinity of the receptor for a drug, the number of functioning receptors, the concentration or density of receptors in a given area, the sensitivity of the receptor, the presence or absence of second or subsequent messengers, or the cellular responsiveness to these messengers (Ouslander, 1981). The second possible mechanism for altered drug sensitivity is a pharmacokinetic one. Previously in this chapter age-related changes in pharmacokinetics were discussed. Information about a decrease in total metabolic clearance and changes in volume of distribution raised the issue that at any given dosing rate, steady-state concentrations will be higher in the aged than in young individuals. Since the effects of many drugs parallel receptor occupancy, the more drug available to the receptor at a given dose results in increased pharmacodynamic (therapeutic or toxic) activity.

Studies in humans documenting a change in pharmacodynamic sensitivity to drugs among the aged are less numerous than those describing pharmacokinetic changes. This is because it is often difficult to isolate aging from confounding variables such as coexistent medical or psychiatric disease, drug therapy, and altered nutritional status and body habitus. No consistent generalizations can be made about drug effects in the aged because intrinsic changes in drug sensitivity are difficult to quantitate in well-controlled studies (Greenblatt, 1989). Drug responses in the aged may be increased, decreased, or unchanged depending on the nature of the study population and the particular variable evaluated. Thus, the interpretation of altered drug sensitivity in the aged has to be described for each drug category.


DRUG SELECTION

Generally, the fewest drugs the aged patient takes the better. There are no specific rules about which drugs should only be used in the aged patient because many factors contribute to drug and dose selection. Some variables include a patient's medical status, other drugs the patient is taking and specific pharmacokinetic and pharmacodynamic aspects of individual drugs and combinations. From the information presented earlier in this chapter some helpful guidelines can be suggested about how certain drugs are selected over others.

The design of a dosage form (tablet, capsule, or liquid), such as the size and taste of the medication can be used to guide drug selection. The choice of a sustained-release drug product instead of a single-release dosage form may make more sense in certain patients because they do not have to take the drug as frequently. However, if the patient has had a prior history of problems with sustained-release products, e.g., dose dumping or short duration of clinical effect, avoidance of time-release drug formulations makes sense. If a patient is already in the habit of taking other prescription medications at certain times, the choice of a drug with an overlapping administration schedule makes the most sense.

Another important selection variable is the elimination half-life of a drug. In general, the shorter the half-life the less likelihood that the drug will cause problems secondary to accumulation. Likewise, if an adverse reaction or side effect occurs, abatement of the problem occurs sooner for a drug with a short elimination half-life versus a long half-life. Classes of drugs that are assumed to be therapeutically equivalent can be categorized based on elimination half-lives. Depending on the treatment objective, drugs with a shorter half-life should be tried first for the aged patient (e.g., triazolam versus temazepam versus flurazepam).

The clearance route of a drug can also be used to guide drug selection. For drugs that are predominantly cleared by the liver, a drug that undergoes conjugation (Phase II biotransformation) is more desirable than one that is metabolized via oxidation (Phase I) pathways. If the choice is between drugs that are oxidized, the drug with the least number of active metabolites should be chosen. In this situation, further assessment of the lipophilicity and elimination half-life of the metabolites will help to select the most appropriate agent. An example would be the choice of alprazolam, lorazepam, or oxazepam over diazepam, clorazepate, or chlordiazepoxide.

The volume of distribution of a drug should also be considered when selecting or reevaluating a patient's medications. The relative fat versus water solubility of a drug may predict or explain the clinical effects of a medication. For example, if a beta-adrenergic antagonist, that is, propranolol (lipophilic), is prescribed for a hypertensive patient and the patient complains of nightmares and/or daytime somnolence but is otherwise experiencing an acceptable therapeutic response, the clinician can simply switch to atenolol (hydrophilic). Atenolol is a less fat-soluble beta-blocker that has fewer CNS effects than propranolol. Alternatively, if a beta-blocker is being prescribed for the management of physical symptoms of anxiety, that is, palpitations, nervousness, and tremor, a more lipophilic version may be more desirable than a hydrophilic one. Volume of distribution concerns related to body habitus and accumulation are important determinants in drug selection in the aged.

The route of excretion is also a factor that must be considered. For drugs that are primarily excreted through the kidney, an appropriate evaluation of renal function is essential. In a patient who has compromised renal function, adjustments in dose and/or dosing interval will have to be made. However, if an alternative drug that is biotransformed by the liver rather than excreted by the kidney exists, selection of this agent would be prudent. Likewise, if a patient's liver function is compromised or if the patient is taking drugs that may affect hepatic microsomal mixed-function oxidase enzymes, it would make more sense to select a drug that is excreted by the kidney.

The drug interaction profile of a drug can also guide the selection process. Potential drug-drug, drug-disease state, and drug-food/nutrition interactions should be considered before a certain drug is used in a patient. The adverse effect (side effect) profile can also be used as selection criteria. Avoidance of drugs with overlapping side-effect profiles, that is, anticholinergics, CNS depressants, gastrointestinal tract irritation, and others, should be avoided if possible because of synergistic or additive effects. Likewise, if patients are experiencing side effects from their medications, an assessment of all the prescription and nonprescription medications in terms of their adverse-effect profile should be performed. Simply changing one or more of the medications may be all that is necessary.

The cost of medications is another important factor. Various therapeutic alternatives can be more or less expensive for the patient. Certain generic forms of drugs may be available and consideration of less expensive alternatives may be more reasonable for aged patients on fixed incomes. For example, it is less expensive for the patient if ampicillin or a sulfa drug is chosen instead of a cephalosporin for the treatment of an uncomplicated urinary tract infection. Aspirin could be used before more expensive nonsteroidal anti-inflammatory drugs for the management of rheumatoid arthritis. However, all generic versions may not be therapeutically equivalent. Therefore, the person prescribing the drug should know the criteria that pharmacists use in selecting the generic drugs that they dispense.

There are many variables that can contribute to the appropriate selection of drugs for the aged patient. Factors such as the clinical pharmacology of a drug and socioeconomic and psychosocial factors all have to be balanced in order to ensure that the patient is receiving optimal therapy.

In the following section, selected drug and therapeutic categories will be discussed in relation to the effects of aging on drug therapy.

## SLEEP DISORDERS AND THE USE OF HYPNOTICS

Sleep disorders are extremely common in the aged. Each year, approximately 10 million Americans consult a physician about their sleep problems and about half of these receive prescriptions for hypnotic medications (Dement, Miles, & Carskadon, 1982). Insomnia is the second most common indication requiring drug therapy. More than 50 million prescriptions are dispensed annually for hypnotic drugs and countless more over-the-counter hypnotics are sold (Lasagna, 1972).

Insomnia is the major complaint among aged patients seeking help for a sleep disorder. Insomnia is sometimes used as a catch-all term for different types of sleep disturbances. Therefore, it is necessary for the clinician who is evaluating the patient to obtain a thorough history and description of the condition causing the complaint. Sleep disturbances are often clinical manifestations of other diseases or problems, such as psychiatric illness, incontinence, cardiac conditions, pain, and others. Thus, the complaint of insomnia may be secondary to a problem that can be readily treated. If a patient with a sleep problem, which is secondary to another condition, is treated with a hypnotic agent, aggravation of the preexisting condition and/or worsening of the primary disorder could ensue. The presence of other disturbances that may be associated with symptoms of sleep disturbance must be ruled out before hypnotics are prescribed for the patient.

The complaint of insomnia may be further clarified into either one or a combination of the following: difficulty in falling asleep (increased sleep latency), frequent nocturnal awakenings, and/or early morning awakenings with the inability to fall back to sleep. Each problem may have to be treated differently because of the characteristics of the available drug therapies.

### Hypnotic Drug Therapy

Hypnotic drugs are among the most widely used in clinical medicine. Recent surveys have reported that insomnia is the second most common indication requiring drug therapy. Prescription hypnotic agents are widely used by both hospitalized and nonhospitalized patients and account for more than 50 million prescriptions yearly. When the large number of over-the-counter sleep medications is also considered, the overall use of drugs to assist in sleep is staggering. Since there are so many agents available for the treatment of sleep disorders, it is important that health-care providers be familiar with the positive and negative aspects of the various available drug therapies (Scavone, 1987).

### Chloral Hydrate

Chloral hydrate was introduced in 1832 and is one of the oldest sedative/hypnotic agents. It continues to be a useful drug for the short-term treatment of insomnia. Chloral hydrate is metabolized to its active ingredient trichloroethanol by alcohol dehydrogenase. The major route of elimination for trichloroethanol is through conjunction with glucuronic acid in the liver and subsequent excretion of trichloroethanol glucuronide (urochloralic acid) by the kidney. Some of the trichloroethanol is biotransformed in the liver to trichloroacetic acid by means of oxidative pathways. Trichloroacetic acid has been reported to be capable of competing with other drugs such as coumadin and coumadin-related drugs for binding sites on plasma proteins. The clinical importance of this observation is controversial but if chloral hydrate and coumadin are used concomitantly, close monitoring of prothrombin times is necessary.

Chloral hydrate in usual doses (0.5–1.0 g) produces drowsiness and sleep within an hour and is more effective in inducing sleep than in prolonging it. Since chloral hydrate is irritating to mucosal membranes, it is probably not an appropriate choice for patients with gastritis or peptic ulcer disease. It can also produce nausea and vomiting if taken on an empty stomach, so patients should be advised to take this drug with either a glass of milk or a little food if they are experiencing any gastrointestinal discomfort after taking the dose. Tolerance to chloral hydrate is well known and occurs frequently following repeated dosage. Therefore, in order for patients to regain therapeutic benefit, the dosage will have to be increased.

Chronic use of chloral hydrate at higher than therapeutic doses may result in hypotension, skin eruptions, or physical dependence. Death has occurred with as little as 6 g, but some patients have survived as much as 38 g. Chloral hydrate poisoning is similar to that of barbiturate poisoning and resembles the overall "toxic-to-therapeutic ratio" of barbiturates. Also, reports of the development of serious cardiac arrhythmias following overdose with chloral hydrate have led to the speculation that it may cause cardiac depression. This drug is also contraindicated in patients with significant impairment of liver and kidney function because of the potential for accumulation. It has also been suggested that chloral hydrate may induce hepatic microsomal enzymes, but the evidence for this is unclear. It is advisable that patients do not take this drug with alcohol because of its synergistic effect. Hangover effects with chloral hydrate do occur but are minimal when compared to other hypnotic agents.

In summary, chloral hydrate in doses of 0.5 to 1.0 g administered occasionally appears to be well tolerated in the aged patient. This agent has been proved effective and does not appear to suppress rapid-eye movement (REM) sleep at usual therapeutic doses.

## Barbiturates

The first barbiturate, barbituric acid, was synthesized in 1864 by Adolf von Baeyer. Approximately 50 derivatives of barbituric acid have been marketed as hypnotics over the past 80 years. Barbiturates are rapidly absorbed from the gastrointestinal tract, distributed throughout the body, and have a profound depressant effect upon the central nervous system. To a lesser extent, they affect skeletal, smooth, and cardiac muscle. Their onset and duration of action is determined by their lipid solubility. The ultra short-acting barbiturates are extremely lipophilic and are used as anesthetic agents. The long-acting barbiturates are used in the treatment of seizure disorders and the short to intermediate action barbiturates are used as sedative/hypnotic agents. The efficacy of barbiturates as hypnotics is unquestioned, but other aspects of their pharmacology are such that oral therapy with barbiturates is rarely indicated other than for the treatment of seizure disorders.

The neurophysiology of barbiturate-induced sleep differs considerably from that of natural sleep. Many studies have shown that the time spent in the REM stage of sleep is reduced following barbiturate treatment. The extended use of REM-suppressing drugs leads to "REM rebound" when the drug is withdrawn. "REM rebound" is associated with significantly increased dreaming time, nightmares, daytime confusion, and resultant insomnia, which could contribute to the continued use of the drug. Paradoxical reactions, especially in the aged, are also associated with barbiturates. Patients may become confused, incoherent, restless, excited, agitated, or delirious after taking a barbiturate. Barbiturates induce hepatic microsomal enzymes. Most clinicians feel that this class of drugs is contraindicated in the aged patient.

Barbiturates are also very addicting and their "toxic-to-therapeutic" dose ratio is among the least favorable of the hypnotics available. In fact, they are a very popular and effective means of suicide. Many patients may be maintained on the same or escalating doses of barbiturates for several years. As a result, they may experience psychologic dependency and/or physical dependence. Some patients may gradually increase their barbiturate dose over time and the development of tolerance is usually proportional to the total dose and duration of barbiturate use. Caution must be exercised when these drugs are discontinued, because abrupt withdrawal of barbiturates in chronic users may result in seizures. Barbiturates also show a synergistic effect with ethanol and the concurrent use of these two agents should be discouraged.

In summary, barbiturates are extremely efficacious in producing sleep. Unfortunately, their toxicity, addiction potential, drug interaction capabilities, adverse-effect profile (especially in the aged), and adverse effect on REM sleep, support the impracticality of using these drugs for the treatment of sleep disorders.

## Glutethimide

Glutethimide, introduced in 1951, is a derivative of piperidinedione and is structurally related to phenobarbitone. It is administered as a hypnotic in doses of 0.5 to 1.0 g and is an inhibitor of REM sleep. Initially it gained popularity because it was first thought to have a greater therapeutic margin for safety and less addictive liability than the barbiturates. Glutethimide has a potential for producing tolerance and dependence at least as great as the short-acting barbiturates. Overdosage with this drug was and still is a significant and serious problem. It is highly lipid soluble, poorly dialyzable, and a potential cardiac depressant. Relatively small doses may produce deep coma and death. Glutethimide also stimulates the production of hepatic microsomal enzymes and affects the metabolism of other drugs. At present, the popularity of glutethimide has waned because of the availability of benzodiazepines.

In summary, glutethimide is rapidly absorbed and is undoubtedly effective. However, there are biases against its use because of its toxicity. The use of glutethimide in outpatients cannot be justified and since there are no specific clinical indications for the use of this drug, many clinicians feel that this agent should be removed from the market.

## Ethchlorvynol

Ethchlorvynol, introduced in 1955, is a halogenated non-cyclic tertiary alcohol whose sedative/hypnotic properties have received little attention from sleep researchers. In doses of 0.5 to 1.0 g, it is a potent short-acting hypnotic. It induces sleep within 30 min, is metabolized rapidly by the liver and as a result, is not detectable in the blood after 3 hr. Common side effects are hypotension, nausea, vomiting, unpleasant aftertastes, dizziness, and facial numbness. Hangover and confusion have also been reported. It appears that ethchlorvynol may interfere clinically with oral anticoagulants. However, the mechanism of the interaction is unknown. Physical dependence has developed in patients taking 1.5 g daily, and seizures and psychotic behavior have followed abrupt withdrawal. Although its effect on REM sleep has not yet been evaluated, ethchlorvynol provides no special benefit in terms of efficacy or safety.

## Antihistamines and Anticholinergics

The antihistamines diphenhydramine hydrochloride, doxylamine succinate, phenyltoloxamine citrate, and pyrilamine maleate are available in over-the-counter products that are marketed as sleep-inducing agents. Antihistamines are classified into different groups according to chemical structure. Diphenhydramine, doxylamine, and phenyltoloxamine are ethanolamines and have the highest sedative effect and the lowest incidence of gastrointestinal side effect. The effect of aging on the pharmacokinetics of doxylamine have been studied, and it appears that clearance is reduced in aged males but not in aged females (Friedman et al., 1989). Pyrilamine is classified as an ethanolamine diamine and produces relatively less sedation and drowsiness. It is also associated with a higher incidence of gastrointestinal side effects than the ethanolamine derivatives. Methylpyrilamine, also a member of the ethanolamine diamine group, was withdrawn from the U.S. market because of its potential carcinogenicity. Other antihistamines such as chlorpheniramine, an alkylamine, chlorcyclizine, a piperazine, and promethazine, a phenylthiazine derivative, are not suitable for use in the treatment of insomnia. Scopolamine has also been available in some over-the-counter sleeping medications.

The sedative effects of antihistamines may vary between individuals and some patients may feel that these products are ineffective. Aged patients are particularly sensitive to the anticholinergic side effects that are produced by these drugs and that have been associated with many problems. Confusion, dizziness, blurred vision, drying of mucous membranes, decreased gut motility resulting in constipation, and urinary retention (which may cause problems, especially in aged males with prostatic hypertrophy) may occur. If a patient suffers from occasional difficulty in falling asleep, antihistamines may be used safely if they are not taken on a chronic basis. There are many drugs and clinical conditions that could possibly interact with these types of medications, and anticholinergic agents can be clearly contraindicated in numerous situations. If patients feel the need to rely on antihistamines for longer than a 3-week period in order to fall asleep or to maintain sleep, they should be referred to a physician or other appropriate clinical practitioner for evaluation of their sleep disorder.

## L-tryptophan

L-tryptophan is an amino acid used to treat insomnia. It is not currently approved by the U.S. Food and Drug Administration as a hypnotic agent but is readily available as a nutritional supplement. Doses ranging from 1.0 to 10.0 mg have been effective in decreasing sleep latency and increasing total sleep time. There is also evidence suggesting that L-tryptophan may suppress REM sleep. L-tryptophan offers an alternative to some of the classical hypnotic agents, especially in alcoholics, but more clinical trials are needed to determine the clinical utility of this substance. The association of L-tryptophan (or a contaminant) with a potentially fatal disorder called eosinophilia-myalgia syndrome has resulted in its withdrawal from the U.S. market.

## Benzodiazepines

Data on the efficacy and toxicity of benzodiazepine hypnotics following single dosage and during chronic use are available from sleep laboratory studies and from controlled clinical trials. Results from these two research settings do not always agree, but some generalizations have been made. The clinical efficacy of benzodiazepines used in the short-term or intermediate-term treatment of insomnia that is unrelated to identifiable medical or psychiatric disease is well known. The use of hypnotic agents to treat insomnia constitutes only one management option in the overall clinical approach to patients with insomnia. Individualized clinical judgment must be used when deciding which patients are candidates for hypnotic medications. Most patients with insomnia do not require long-term treatment, and the hazards of well-monitored therapy of limited duration with hypnotic drugs appear to be small. Currently there are four benzodiazepine derivatives that are indicated specifically for the treatment of sleep disorders in the United States. A number of other benzodiazepines are equally useful as hypnotics, although they do not carry specific labeling for the insomnia indication (Greenblatt et al., 1983). It would be incorrect to state that hypnotic benzodiazepines have important neuropharmacologic differences from anxiolytic benzodiazepines. In fact, all of these drugs act as antianxiety agents at low doses and as sedative/hypnotics at higher doses. The primary approved therapeutic indication reflects a combination of research direction taken during clinical development and testing, together with specific pharmacokinetic properties that might make a particular drug suitable as a hypnotic. The information in this section will focus on pharmacokinetic similarities and differences among benzodiazepine hypnotics, and on a potential relationship of these properties to their use in clinical practice.

A clear relationship between plasma benzodiazepine concentrations and clinical sedative and/or anxiolytic effects has not yet been demonstrated. Therefore, it cannot be stated with certainty that the pharmacokinetic profile of a particular benzodiazepine derivative explains its clinical properties. Observations during clinical and sleep laboratory studies of the various benzodiazepine hypnotics are highly consistent with the pharmacokinetic properties of these drugs.

The principal determinant of the onset of action of hypnotic drugs is the rate of absorption. The faster the rate of absorption, the quicker and more intense is the onset of action.

The duration of clinical effect following a single dose is governed mainly by distribution and not by the elimination half-life. However, for a drug with an extremely short elimination half-life such as triazolam, elimination does contribute to the termination of action.

Multiple-dose effects are a combination of the effect of any given dose together with residual effects from prior doses (Greenblatt et al., 1983). Elimination is a major determinant of accumulation. Accumulation of compounds with long elimination half-lives increases the likelihood of continued efficacy during repeated dosage and minimizes the probability that rebound insomnia will occur upon discontinuation of the drug. The chance of the occurrence of residual effects such as daytime drowsiness and impairment of performance is also increased, but is partly offset by adaptation and/or tolerance. Nonaccumulating hypnotics with short elimination half-lives have a reduced likelihood of adverse daytime sequelae. Although previously disputed, evidence now indicates that there is an increased probability of transient rebound insomnia following the discontinuation of hypnotics with short elimination half-lives.

The relevance of these pharmacokinetic principles becomes evident when the properties of the benzodiazepine hypnotics are considered individually.

### Flurazepam

Flurazepam hydrochloride was the first benzodiazepine to become available in the United States for specific use as a hypnotic agent. Flurazepam has been extensively used since its introduction in 1970. As a result, most other hypnotic agents are compared to flurazepam in clinical trials.

The pharmacokinetic profile of flurazepam in humans is extremely complex. Flurazepam appears to act as a mixture of short- and long-acting hypnotics. When the blood or serum from a patient taking flurazepam is evaluated, a number of active substances are found to be present. Flurazepam has at least three metabolites that are pharmacologically active. Hydroxyethyl flurazepam and flurazepam aldehyde appear and disappear rapidly, so they are termed "short-acting substances." These two metabolites are likely to contribute to the induction of sleep. Desalkylflurazepam, the principal metabolite, both appears and is eliminated slowly. Flurazepam is a complicated compound with respect to what is actually inducing sleep, what is maintaining sleep, what is causing residual effects, and what is accumulating following multiple dosage.

The metabolic pathway of desalkylflurazepam involves hepatic hydroxylation, which is an oxidative reaction. It is influenced by aging (especially in males), liver disease, and microsomal enzyme inducers and inhibitors. The elimination half-life of desalkylflurazepam in healthy, normal adults ranges from 40 to 200 hr and may be as long as 300 hr in the aged. Accumulation of desalkylflurazepam during multiple dosage with flurazepam occurs and is directly related to its long elimination half-life and clearance.

Aged males accumulate desalkylflurazepam to a greater degree than do young males. However, values for aged females are no different than those for young females (Greenblatt, Divoll, Abernethy, & Shader, 1982).

Clinical ratings of sleep patterns and daytime sedation have also been correlated with pharmacokinetic data. Results indicate an increase over time in daytime sedation in addition to improvement in sleep parameters, which are generally consistent with the profile of desalkylflurazepam accumulation. The changes over time in clinical effects did not occur in parallel with the increases in desalkylflurazepam plasma concentration, probably because of the capacity of benzodiazepines to produce clinical tolerance and adaptation to their effect.

As a result of the long elimination half-life of desalkylflurazepam in the aged because of a reduction in clearance, many clinicians avoid its use in patients over 60 years old. Short-term occasional doses of flurazepam (15 mg) have been shown clinically to be "safe" for the aged. Issues dealing with carryover, residual, or hangover effects compared with tolerance and adaptation are still unclear at this time, so definitive recommendations cannot be made. Flurazepam at a dosage of 15 mg appears to be safe in most patients younger than 60 years old, but caution must be emphasized with its use in aged patients who may receive chronic therapy.

### Quazepam

Quazepam is available as a product named Doral (formerly Dormalin). Claims that quazepam is selective for the BZ-1 receptor that affects the neural pathways involved in the generation of natural sleep remain to be proved. Quazepam is a precursor of desalkylflurazepam and as such can be expected to be an accumulating hypnotic agent, especially in the aged. The same cautions for flurazepam apply to quazepam.

### Temazepam

Temazepam was introduced as a hypnotic agent in 1981. It is a 3-hydroxybenzodiazepine derivative, which is biotransformed in the liver by conjugation rather than oxidation. The major metabolite is glucuronide conjugate. Temazepam glucuronide has no pharmacologic activity and is excreted in the urine. Smaller amounts of temazepam are metabolized by N-demethylation to yield oxazepam, which then appears in the urine as oxazepam glucuronide.

Following administration of the hard-gelatin capsule preparation of temazepam that is currently available in the United States, the appearance rate of temazepam in plasma is slow. Peak concentrations are reached in an average of 2.5 hr after administration (Ochs, Greenblatt, & Heur, 1984). Part of this slow rate of appearance is the result of the formulation of the hard-gelatin capsule and part is due to temazepam's intrinsic physicochemical properties. Clearly, temazepam is not ideal for patients with insomnia characterized primarily by difficulty in falling asleep (increased sleep latency), particularly when the drug is taken directly at bedtime. This is consistent with clinical studies showing its minimal efficacy in sleep latency insomnia (Greenblatt, Divoll, Abernethy, & Shader, 1982). The slow absorption of temazepam may be partly offset by ingestion of the dose 1 to 2 hr before bedtime rather than immediately at the time of retiring. However, if the dose is co-ingested with food, there may be a further delay in the time to reach peak plasma concentrations and the onset of clinical effect.

It must be emphasized that clinical studies of temazepam performed in the United Kingdom and Europe are not applicable to the use of temazepam in the United States. The soft-gelatin capsule preparation of temazepam that is available in Europe provides a much more rapid rate of absorption than does the hard-gelatin capsule. Thus, it is impossible to extrapolate or compare clinical trials using one or the other preparation. Since the patient on temazepam has expired, a number of companies are currently performing clinical trials with a reformulated soft-gelatin-capsule dosage form. This will possibly lead to the reevaluation of temazepam as an appropriate agent for patients who complain of difficulty of falling asleep.

The mean elimination half-life of temazepam is approximately 13 to 14 hr, with a range of 10 to 20 hr. In some individuals it can be longer than 30 hr. Therefore, temazepam is characterized as having an intermediate rather than a short half-life. As a result, an intermediate degree of accumulation will occur, with the accumulation profile falling between the extremes of benzodiazepines with long as opposed to short elimination half-life values (Ochs et. al, 1984). The clinical consequence of the temazepam accumulation profile is not clearly established.

Because temazepam is biotransformed by conjugation rather than oxidation, its metabolic pathway is less likely to be influenced by factors such as aging. It is speculated that despite its absorption problems, temazepam may be more appropriate for the treatment of frequent nocturnal awakenings and/or early morning awakenings, especially in the aged.

In summary, temazepam is an intermediate-acting benzodiazepine with no long-acting metabolites. Doses of 15 to 30 mg increase total sleep time and decrease the frequency of duration of nocturnal awakenings in insomniac patients. Temazepam does not appear to decrease the latency to sleep onset and therefore would not be appropriate for a patient whose only complaint is difficulty in falling asleep. In the aged, a dose of 15 mg daily should be used initially and the patient should be reevaluated before it is increased to 30 mg.

### Triazolam

Triazolam (Halcion) is a triazolobenzodiazepine hypnotic with a short elimination half-life. In the majority of individuals, the elimination half-life falls between 1.5 and 5 hr. A typical dose is almost completely eliminated 12 to 15 hr after ingestion. Therefore, triazolam is an essentially nonaccumulating hypnotic. This lack of accumulation probably minimizes the likelihood of residual daytime effects.

The absorption rate of triazolam is in the intermediate range, with peak concentrations occurring between 1 and 2 hr after dosage. Triazolam can also be administered sublingually. Following sublingual administration, there is approximately a 28% increase in bioavailability, presumably due to avoidance in first-pass hepatic extraction (Scavone et al., 1986). Triazolam is metabolized principally by hepatic microsomal oxidation. The effects of age, liver disease, or metabolic inhibitors or enhancers on its pharmacokinetic profile cannot yet be generalized. Factors influencing the pharmacokinetic profile of triazolam may differ from those of other oxidized benzodiazepines (Greenblatt, Divoll, Abernethy, & Shader, 1982).

The current recommended initial starting dose of triazolam in adults is 0.25 mg unless the patient is unresponsive. In the aged, dosages greater than 0.25 mg are not recommended. Aged patients should initially be started at a dose of 0.125 mg. If this appears to be too much, then one half of a 0.125 mg tablet (0.0625 mg) can be given. The use of triazolam for several consecutive nights may lead to a transient period of rebound insomnia, which usually lasts for one to two nights following the abrupt discontinuation of the drug. This effect should be anticipated and can be minimized by tapering treatment over time.

Triazolam, in addition to other benzodiazepines, can also cause "anterograde amnesia." The intensity and duration of this effect appears to increase with dosage. It is not clearly established at this time if the amnestic effects are any more frequent or severe than those that occur during treatment with other benzodiazepine derivatives. Various psychologic disturbances have been anecdotally associated with triazolam but controlled clinical trials suggest this is not a substantial concern (Greenblatt et al., 1982c).

In summary, triazolam is a short-acting benzodiazepine. In doses of 0.125 to 0.25 mg it increases sleep duration and decreases nocturnal awakening in latency to sleep onset. Triazolam alters the distribution of REM sleep during the night, but has little if any effect on the total amount of REM sleep. Triazolam also appears to have no effect on delta sleep, which distinguishes it from chlordiazepoxide, diazepam, flurazepam, and temazepam. In comparative studies, triazolam is subjectively judged to be equal to or better than flurazepam, diazepam, or oxazepam (Greenblatt et al., 1983). Clearly this appears to be the benzodiazepine hypnotic of choice in an aged patient who has trouble falling asleep.

### Other Benzodiazepines

Other benzodiazepines may also serve as hypnotics. The lack of a Food and Drug Administration–approved specific indication for sleep disorders by no means precludes the use of a benzodiazepine as a hypnotic agent. Many benzodiazepines indicated primarily for anxiety can serve equally well as sleep-inducing agents, provided the clinical approach is adapted for this objective and the drug's kinetic properties are well understood. Both diazepam and clorazepate are rapidly absorbed from the gastrointestinal tract and can be very useful in the treatment of sleep disorders characterized by difficulty in falling asleep. Furthermore, their extensive volume of distribution tends to minimize residual hangover effects. However, the cumulative profile of desmethyldiazepam during multiple dosage closely resembles that of flurazepam, with the associated risks and benefits. Lorazepam and oxazepam may also be used as hypnotics. The rate of lorazepam and oxazepam absorption and elimination half-life is intermediate. Therefore, it is best taken approximately an hour before bedtime if it is used in patients with increased sleep latency. During multiple dosage, an intermediate degree of accumulation can be anticipated.

Benzodiazepines are clearly superior to other classes of hypnotic agents in safety and possibly in efficacy. Clinically meaningful differences among the various benzodiazepines are often subtle but could result in a significant alteration in clinical response. Therefore, understanding the pharmacokinetic similarities and differences among the various benzodiazepine sedative-hypnotics is extremely important and should help the health-care practitioner to make a more informed judgment as to the appropriateness of a choice of a particular agent for a patient.

### Choosing the Correct Therapy for the Patient

The key for choosing the correct therapy for a patient who is suffering from insomnia begins with proper diagnosis of the problem. Secondary causes of insomnia must be ruled out before a prescription for a hypnotic agent is written. In addition, a thorough history concerning the onset, duration, disease profile, other drug therapies, and social habits is needed from the patient. Certain situations may contribute to the existence of stress and anxiety and these may have to be dealt with accordingly. Certain disease states and drug therapies may result in situations causing the sleep problem. Social habits such as caffeine intake, ethanol use, exercise, heavy eating, late-night snacks, daytime napping, and smoking tobacco may all contribute to the person's inability to sleep. These factors all have to be addressed before drug therapy is initiated.

When it is decided to choose a drug for a patient or evaluate a preexisting therapy, certain properties of the drug have to be considered. The ideal hypnotic must provide a reliable and predictable form of treatment. It should be safe and effective and not cause any residual or hangover effects or produce drug dependence. It should not accumulate, and its clinical effect should be sufficient to cover the patient throughout the night but not affect daytime performance. The benzodiazepine hypnotics are the closest to the ideal hypnotic agent that is currently available. Hypnotic agents, if used correctly and are properly chosen, provide many beneficial effects to the insomniac.

In summary, there is much that goes into treating the patient with a sleep disorder. Once the diagnosis is properly made, an appropriate agent must be chosen. Knowledge of the pharmacokinetic properties of the drug and the clinical manifestation of the type of problem that the patient has must be correlated with the other medications the patient is receiving, as well as with any coexistent disease states. With proper selection and monitoring, drug therapy can offer many benefits to the patient suffering from a sleep disorder.

### Antianxiety Agents

Benzodiazepines are the most frequently prescribed anxiolytic agents. They are usually recommended for the short-term relief of anxiety, whereas psychotherapy or counseling is chosen for long-term management (Thompson, Moran, & Nies, 1983). The effects of aging on some benzodiazepines have already been discussed in the section on hypnotics. In general, the aging process does not result in any change in the absorption rate of benzodiazepines. Age-related changes in body habitus can result in accumulation of the more lipophilic and so-called long-acting benzodiazepines (i.e., diazepam, desmethyldiazepam, flurazepam, desalkylflurazepam, quazepam, prazepam, clorazepate, and chlordiazepoxide) and their metabolites because of a larger volume of distribution. These long-acting benzodiazepines are cleared via the hepatic microsomal mixed-function oxidase system and will be metabolized at a slower rate in the aged. Age-related changes in clearance and volume of distribution result in a prolongation in the elimination half-life. These pharmacokinetic changes coupled with increased sensitivity in pharmacodynamic effects in the aged explain why this group experiences a more profound drug effect at any given dose (Thompson et al., 1983; Pomara et al., 1985; Greenblatt et al., 1989). The benzodiazepines lorazepam and oxazepam are less lipid soluble than the others and undergo conjugation in the liver as their means of clearance. This biotransformation pathway is relatively unaffected by aging, so these drugs are better choices for the aged. Alprazolam is comparatively an intermediate-acting drug, which is primarily cleared by Phase I biotransformation. However, it does not yield any clinically important metabolites. In lower doses it is also a reasonable choice for the aged.

All benzodiazepines can produce lethargy, sedation, cognitive impairment, and CNS depression, which can lead to ataxia and motor incoordination (Lamy & Love, 1988; Greenblatt et al., 1983; Jenike, 1982a). They can also interact synergistically or additively with other CNS depressants. They are contraindicated in patients with sleep apnea and respiratory depression because of their respiratory depressant effects.

In summary, for the aged patient short- to intermediate-acting benzodiazepines (i.e., those with short to intermediate elimination half-life) are preferred to long-acting agents (i.e., those with long elimination half-life) and hydrophilic alternatives that are metabolized by means of conjugation reactions are preferred to those that are oxidized and yield active metabolites. Drug interactions with benzodiazepines and the potential aggravation of underlying medical or psychiatric conditions must be considered before these drugs are prescribed for the aged.

Buspirone is a nonbenzodiazepine anxiolytic that is classified as an azapirone. Its exact mechanism of action is not known, but it appears to involve complex interactions among CNS neurotransmitters, especially serotonin (Goa & Ward, 1986; Eison & Temple, 1986; Kastenholz & Crimson, 1984). Buspirone is metabolized to active and inactive metabolites, but aging does not appear to affect its clearance. It is an appealing drug for treating the aged because of its lack of serious side effects. Buspirone lacks the sedative, muscle-relaxant, and anticonvulsant effects of benzodiazepines (Kastenholz & Crimson, 1984). The most common adverse effects are dizziness, nervousness, and headaches, which are dose-related. Buspirone does not cause cognitive or psychomotor impairment, does not interact with alcohol or other CNS depressants, and does not decrease respiratory function or impair driving skills (Goa & Ward, 1986; Kastenholz & Crimson, 1984). It has also been shown to be as effective as other benzodiazepines in the treatment of anxiety (Rickels et al., 1982). The major drawback with buspirone is the lag time of approximately 1 to 2 weeks before its anxiolytic effect occurs. This should not preclude its use, but patients should be counseled about therapeutic expectations. It also seems to work better in benzodiazepine-naïve patients because many patients who have taken benzodiazepines miss the characteristic "buzz," which does not occur following the ingestion of buspirone. In summary, buspirone is a reasonable drug for use in the aged because of its safety and efficacy profile.

Antihistamines, beta-adrenergic blockers, antidepressants, and neuroleptics are also used to treat anxiety. Beta-blockers are useful when patients have somatic components to anxiety such as palpitations, diaphoresis, tremulousness, urinary frequency, and tachycardia (Jenike, 1982a). Antihistamines may be useful in patients with depressed respiratory function, such as those with chronic obstructive pulmonary disease. Neuroleptics are useful in patients who suffer from severe anxiety and agitation, and antidepressants are useful in anxious patients with coexisting depression. These drugs are discussed elsewhere in this chapter.

## Antidepressants

Antidepressants can be safely prescribed for the aged if underlying medical conditions and concurrent drug therapy are carefully evaluated. It is important to consider the many drugs that a patient is taking that cause or contribute to depression (Table 5.8). Various medical conditions may also aggravate or contribute to depression, and other medical conditions could be adversely affected by drug therapy. The choice of which antidepressant is most appropriate for a given patient is determined largely by its adverse-effect profile (i.e., sedative, cardiovascular, and anticholinergic), the patient's ability to tolerate its side effects, prior patient response to the drug or other antidepressants, the patient's medical and psychiatric status, and age-related changes in the pharmacokinetics of a drug and its metabolites (Peabody, Whiteford, & Hollister, 1986; Baldessarini, 1989; Lamy & Love, 1988; Blazer, 1989). Generally, antidepressant drug doses for the aged should be 30% to 50% of those used in younger patients and the dosage should be gradually increased until the desired therapeutic effect is achieved or until intolerable or potentially dangerous adverse effects develop. If side effects occur, the drug should be substituted for another, usually from the same class, with a lower incidence of the adverse effect that occurred (Thompson et al., 1983). The aged patient must be closely monitored for both side effects and response. Antidepressants should be continued for a minimum of 4 weeks before a decision is made that they are not

TABLE 5.8   Some drugs that cause or contribute
to depression

| | |
|---|---|
| Benzodiazepines | Methyldopa |
| Carbamazepine | Reserpine |
| Cimetidine | Hypnotics |
| Clonidine | Nonsteroidal anti-inflam- |
| Corticosteroids | matory agents |
| Digoxin | Beta-adrenergic blockers |
| Estrogen | Ethanol |
| Levodopa | Opiates |

effective (Peabody et al., 1986). The aged may take longer to respond to therapy than do younger patients (Lazarus, Davis, & Dysken, 1985). It should be noted that electro-convulsive therapy and psychotherapy are safe and effective treatments for depression in the aged but they will not be addressed in this chapter.

Tricyclic antidepressants are considered the drugs of choice in treating depression in the aged (Jenike, 1985; Blazer, 1989; Peabody et al., 1986). The mechanisms of action of tricyclic antidepressants include inhibition of the reuptake of biogenic amines, especially norepinephrine and serotonin; muscarinic acetylcholine receptor antagonism; and histamine ($H_1$ and $H_2$) receptor antagonism (Peabody et al., 1986). The tricyclics differ from one other by their relative anticholinergic and sedative effects (Hollister, 1978). The aged are especially sensitive to the anticholinergic effects of tricyclics, which include blurred vision, urinary retention, tachycardia, dry mouth, mild memory loss, orientation difficulties, confusional reactions, constipation, and precipitation of narrow angle glaucoma. Aged patients may not differ from younger patients in the likelihood of becoming hypotensive on tricyclics, but they are more likely to experience serious complications after falls (Peabody et al., 1986). Of these agents, amitriptyline and doxepin are the most sedative, protriptyline is the least sedative, amitriptyline, trimipramine, doxepin and pro-triptyline have the highest anticholinergic activity, desipramine has the weakest anti-cholinergic effects, and nortriptyline may cause less orthostatic hypotension than the other tricyclics (Lamy & Love, 1988; Peabody et al., 1986).

Tricyclics can also be categorized by chemical structure and biotransformation. The tertiary amines (amitriptyline, doxepin, imipramine and trimipramine) are metabolized in the liver by demethylation to yield active metabolites, which are secondary amines. The age-related decrease in the rate of hepatic biotransformation has been previously discussed. Thus, there tends to be a higher ratio of tertiary to secondary amines. Generally, the tertiary amines produce greater anticholinergic, hypotensive, and cardiac effects than the secondary amines so it appears to be more reasonable that the secondary amines (desipramine, nortriptyline and protriptyline) are used initially in the aged patient (Lamy & Love, 1988).

In summary, the tricyclic antidepressants are especially useful and effective in the aged patient. When the patient is properly diagnosed and coexisting medications, medical, and psychiatric problems are evaluated in terms of their effect on depression and how they might be affected by tricyclic antidepressants, appropriate drug and dose selection will often result in safe and effective therapy.

*Monoamine Oxidase Inhibitors*

Monoamine oxidase (MAO) inhibitors are not used as much as the tricyclics in the aged. Reasons for this include severe orthostatic hypotension and interactions with tyramine-containing foods and sympathomimetic drugs resulting in hypertensive crisis (Rabkin et al., 1985; Peabody et al., 1986; Scavone & Marx, 1983). MAO inhibitors still need to be further evaluated in the aged because monoamine oxidase increases with age, whereas the synthesis of biogenic amines decreases (Robinson, 1971), they do not produce cardiac arrhythmias, have few anticholinergic effects and do not adversely affect cognitive function (Peabody et al., 1986).

## Other Drugs

Trazodone is a phenylpiperazine derivative that selectively inhibits the uptake of serotonin (Riblet & Taylor, 1981). The major side effect of trazodone is sedation, which is less pronounced with chronic dosing than acute dosing. The drug most likely does not impair psychomotor function or memory in aged patients; it has few anticholinergic effects and a low incidence of cardiovascular toxicity; and its safety profile in overdosage is good. Dry mouth and constipation do occur, but they are thought to be a result of alpha-adrenergic blocking activity. Major cardiovascular side effects include a mild reduction of heart rate, blood pressure, and some recent reports of the exacerbation of preexisting arrhythmias (Peabody et al., 1986). The worst adverse effect is priapism. Trazodone offers many advantages over tricyclic antidepressants and MAO inhibitors in the management of depression in the aged.

Maprotiline is a tetracyclic antidepressant that blocks the reuptake of norepinephrine and has antihistaminic and peripheral anticholinergic effects (Richelson, 1984). Unfortunately, maprotiline is associated with a high incidence of seizures at therapeutic levels, has cardiovascular side effects similar to those of the tricyclics, and is considered to be extremely toxic in overdosage. Its use is not favored in any age group (Gruter & Poldinger, 1982; Burckhardt et al., 1978).

Amoxapine is a demethylated metabolite of loxapine, a neuroleptic, and belongs to the dibenzoxapine class of tricyclics. It is a dopamine antagonist and a potent inhibitor of norepinephrine uptake. It has a relatively benign cardiac toxicity profile, but it has been associated with atrial arrhythmias and conduction abnormalities at therapeutic doses in the aged (Peabody et al., 1986).

Amoxapine can also cause tardive dyskinesia, dystonias, parkinsonism, akinesias, and neuroleptic malignant syndrome, which effects make it a poor choice for aged patients (Steele, 1982).

Bupropion is a phenylaminoketone that has dopaminergic properties but no significant effect on norepinephrine or serotonin (Dufresne, Weber, & Becker, 1984). It has no cardiovascular effects, minimal anticholinergic effects, a mild anxiolytic effect, and no sedative effects. Dry mouth is the major side effect. Dose-related seizures have been reported, but its implication to aged patients is not known at this time (Peabody et al., 1986).

Fluoxetine is a bicyclic antidepressant that inhibits the presynaptic reuptake of serotonin with an apparent impressive side-effect profile. It is biotransformed in the liver to its demethylated metabolite norfluoxetine. One study evaluating the effect of aging on the pharmacokinetics of fluoxetine found no difference between young and aged subjects (Bergstrom, 1983). The frequency of side effects is low and dose-related, with the most common being nausea, anxiety, insomnia, anorexia, diarrhea, and nervousness (Sommi, Crimson, & Bowden, 1987). Fluoxetine is still considered a new drug at this writing, so more experience with using fluoxetine in the aged is necessary in order to support or refute its safety profile. To date, there have been no deaths reported following intentional overdose with fluoxetine (Sommi et al., 1987).

## Antipsychotic Agents

Antipsychotic drugs or neuroleptics are used for treating chronic schizophrenia, psychotic paranoid states, bipolar disorders, agitated depression, and agitation and confusion of delirium and dementia (Thompson et al., 1983). Chlorpromazine, thioridazine, thiothixene, haloperidol, perphenazine, trifluoperazine, and fluphenazine are of equal therapeutic efficacy if prescribed in equipotent dosages. Haloperidol and fluphenazine are considered to be high-potency antipsychotics and have the greatest incidence of extrapyramidal effects, pseudo- parkinsonism, akathesias, and dystonias (Thompson et al., 1983). However, they are associated with a lower incidence of sedation, hypotension, and anticholinergic effects. Because of age-related changes in the central nervous system, the aged are more likely to have side effects of the pseudo-parkinsonian type and tardive dyskinesia but less likely to have dystonias than younger patients (Hamilton, 1966). Chlorpromazine and thioridazine are classified as low-potency drugs. They are associated with a higher incidence of sedation and anticholinergic effects. Side effects related to alpha-adrenergic antagonism, such as orthostatic hypotension, myocardial infarction, cerebrovascular accidents, and hypersensitivity reactions, are more common with chlorpromazine and thioridazine (Thompson et al., 1983; Lamy & Love, 1988). Higher plasma levels of chlorpromazine occur in the aged following similar doses to younger patients (Rivera-Calimlim et al., 1977). In summary, age-related increases in sensitivity to antipsychotic drugs appear to be explained by a combination of pharmacokinetic changes involving decreased clearance and pharmacodynamic alterations related to changes in receptor sites (i.e., number and density) and receptor sensitivity. It is presumed that aged patients require reduced doses of antipsychotic drugs, but interpatient variability is high. As with most other drugs, antipsychotic drug doses should start out low and be gradually increased until the desired clinical response is reached with minimal side effects.

### Lithium

Lithium is primarily excreted via the kidneys. Since renal function declines secondary to aging, a predictable decrease in lithium clearance occurs. Therefore, serum lithium levels should be closely monitored in aged patients. Many drugs can also affect lithium clearance. Diuretics may cause sodium depletion, resulting in lithium retention, and methyldopa and nonsteroidal anti-inflammatory drugs can decrease the renal clearance of lithium (Thompson et al., 1983). It has been suggested that red-blood-cell lithium binding decreases in the aged, but this is unconfirmed. The major age-related change in lithium disposition is related to decreased renal function.

## ANTIHYPERTENSIVE AGENTS

Most aged people are hypertensive (both combined diastolic and systolic, >140/90 mmHg; or isolated systolic >160 mmHg) and, if diagnosed, are receiving antihypertensive therapy (Havlick et al., 1989). Epidemiologic studies have demonstrated the increased risk of cardiovascular morbidity and mortality associated with untreated hypertension in the aged (Tjoa & Kaplan, 1990; Kannel, 1989). Nonpharmacologic therapies such as weight reduction in the obese, moderated sodium restriction (2 g of sodium or 5 g of sodium chloride), moderation of alcohol, and exercise are just as effective in the aged as they are in younger patients and usually result in decreases of about 9 mmHg for both diastolic and systolic pressures (Stuart et al., 1989). If drug therapy is chosen, equal hypotensive effect can be expected in both younger and aged patients. In general, there are no risk-free or universally effective drugs and no single drug or combination of drugs is regarded as the best for the aged (Tjoa & Kaplan, 1990). As with younger patients, blacks respond less well to angiotensin-converting enzyme inhibitors and beta-adrenergic antagonists. Similar to other drugs, specific therapy should be tailored to each patient. It is wiser to initiate antihypertensive drug therapy with a reduced dose (approximately one half of the normal) and to titrate slowly and gradually.

## Diuretics

Diuretics are commonly used as monotherapy in the aged. When given at reduced dosage (12.5 mg/day of hydrochlorothiazide or its equivalent), diuretics are well tolerated (Tjoa & Kaplan, 1990; Hulley et al., 1985; Goldstein et al., 1990). Adverse effects are dose related, and doses greater than 25 to 50 mg daily of hydrochlorothiazide are of little therapeutic benefit (Materson et al., 1990). Advantages of diuretics over other antihypertensives include usefulness in patients with heart failure, peripheral edema, proven efficacy, low cost, and convenient dosing (Tjoa & Kaplan, 1990). Adverse effects include hypokalemia, hyponatremia, hyperuricemia, hyperglycemia, azotemia, and hypercholesterolemia. Furosemide and metolazone are useful in patients with renal insufficiency.

## Beta-Adrenergic Reception Antagonists

Beta-blockers are effective antihypertensive agents in the aged despite theoretical concerns about the aged having decreased beta-receptor response and low renin state. They are especially useful in patients with angina pectoris and tachyarrhythmias. Both hydrophilic and lipophilic beta-blockers cause CNS effects such as depression, sleep disturbance, and lethargy, but, anecdotally, many aged patients tolerate the water-soluble drugs better than the lipophilic versions. Adverse effects to beta-blockers include atrioventricular conduction delay or block, increased peripheral vascular resistance, negative inotropy, hypertriglyceridemia, lowered high density lipoprotein cholesterol, bradycardia, and bronchospasm in asthmatics.

## Angiotensin-Converting Enzyme Inhibitors

Angiotensin-converting enzyme (ACE) inhibitors act as peripheral vasodilators by blocking the effect of the renin-angiotensin-aldosterone system. They appear to work equally well in younger and aged patients (Tjoa & Kaplan, 1990). The advantages of ACE inhibitors are their ability to reverse left ventricular hypertrophy, their usefulness in the treatment of congestive heart failure, and their lack of peripheral vascular symptoms, orthostatic hypotension and CNS effects. However, ACE inhibitors can worsen renal function in patients with congestive heart failure. Other adverse effects include a nonproductive cough and hyperkalemia, especially in patients taking potassium supplements or potassium-sparing diuretics.

### Calcium Channel Antagonists

Calcium channel blockers may be slightly more effective in aged than younger individuals (Kaplan, 1989). As a class of drugs, calcium channel blockers do not affect electrolyte, lipid, or hormonal levels, have few contraindications, and rarely cause orthostatic hypotension, or CNS side effects (Tjoa & Kaplan, 1990). The most common problems associated with calcium channel blockers are abdominal discomfort and constipation, but these problems are managed with the use of smaller doses and by increasing the patient's intake of dietary fiber.

Age-related decreases in clearance resulting in increased plasma concentrations have been shown for verapamil and sustained-release nifedipine (Abernethy, Schwartz, Todd, Luchi, & Snow, 1986; Chase, 1989). No differences in the clearance and elimination half-life of diltiazem were found following the administration of a single intravenous dose and chronic oral doses to aged and young hypertensive patients (Abernethy & Montamat, 1987).

### Alpha₁ Antagonists

Prazosin and terazosin are selective $alpha_1$ antagonists that reduce blood pressure by decreasing peripheral resistance. These drugs can cause orthostatic hypotension, which is enhanced in the aged patient secondary to impaired baroreceptor reflex (Tjoa & Kaplan, 1990). Orthostasis is usually avoided if an initial dose of not greater than 1 mg is taken at bedtime following abstinence of diuretics for 2 to 3 days. Little reflex tachycardia or tachyphylaxis and no compromise in cerebral blood flow has been observed in the aged (Ram et al., 1987; Tjoa & Kaplan, 1990).

### Centrally Acting Alpha₂ Agonists and Direct-Acting Vasodilators

Clonidine, guanabenz, guanfacine and methyldopa reduce blood pressure by decreasing central sympathetic outflow. They are associated with many CNS side effects, such as dry mouth, sedation, and orthostatic hypotension. Although effective, they are not used in the aged because of their adverse effects and the availability of safer agents (Tjoa & Kaplan, 1990).

Hydralazine, a direct-acting vasodilator, is generally well tolerated and does not cause orthostasis. In the aged it may reduce blood pressure and cause less reflex tachycardia than in younger patients so that concomitant beta-adrenergic blockers or other sympatholytic agents may not be necessary (Tjoa & Kaplan, 1990). However, hydralazine is not used frequently because of its inability to cause a regression in left ventricular hypertrophy and its association with increased adverse effects in blacks and patients with renal insufficiency.

In summary, diuretics, beta-adrenergic blockers, calcium channel blockers, and ACE inhibitors are all useful in treating the aged hypertensive patient. Calcium channel blockers and ACE inhibitors are appealing because of the relatively low incidence of hemodynamic, electrolyte, CNS, and metabolic adverse effects. As with the treatment of many disease states, low doses, careful titration, and the use of nondrug therapies, result in safe and effective management of hypertension in the aged.

## DIGOXIN

The extensive use of digoxin in the aged may not be clinically justified because the chance of digitalis toxicity may outweigh the therapeutic benefit (Stults, 1982). Digoxin is used in the treatment of left ventricular failure, of chronic atrial fibrillation with a rapid ventricular response rate, and for the prevention of some atrial tachyarrhythmias. The peak age of onset of chronic atrial fibrillation is between 65 and 70 years of age (Morris & Hurst, 1980).

Digoxin is a drug with a narrow therapeutic margin. Age-related changes in digoxin disposition do occur. As a result, steady-state serum digoxin concentrations resulting from a given maintenance dose are on the average twice the level in patients older than 80 years of age (average elimination half-life is 70 hr) than in patients between the ages of 30 and 50 (average elimination half-life is 30 to 40 hours) (Cusack et al., 1979; Ewy et al., 1969; Stults, 1982).

Digoxin, approximately 75% of it, is primarily eliminated from the body by the kidney. Thus, the age-related decline in glomerular filtration rate results in accumulation of digoxin. In addition, digoxin is distributed primarily to lean body mass, which diminishes in the aged. These changes result in higher serum digoxin concentrations for any given dose. In the aged population, the range in magnitude of the changes in digoxin pharmacokinetics is variable and unpredictable. Therefore, digoxin dosage must be carefully tailored to the individual patient, using a combination of clinical judgment, estimates of renal function (calculated creatinine clearance), and serum digoxin concentrations (Stults, 1982). Adverse effects resulting from digoxin toxicity include anorexia, nausea, vomiting, bradycardia, bigeminy, delirium, delusions, confusional states, visual and auditory hallucinations, and disturbances in color vision and visual acuity. Potassium depletion secondary to diuretic therapy can predispose patients to digoxin toxicity.

In summary, digoxin use in the aged is a controversial subject. However, it appears to be safe when close patient monitoring accompanies its use. Digoxin doses should be calculated for aged patients based on creatinine clearance, lean body weight, and steady-state serum concentrations.

## ANTIARRHYTHMICS

In the aged, the incidence of lidocaine toxicity was found to be twice that of younger patients (Pfeiffer, Greenblatt, & Koch-Weser, 1976). The volume of distribution of lidocaine is also greater in the aged, which may account for a significant increase in elimination half-life without a change in plasma clearance in aged patients compared to young patients (Nation et al., 1977; Cusack et al., 1980). Additionally, variables such as congestive heart failure, hepatic disease, and decreased hepatic blood flow are associated with increased lidocaine toxicity (Thomson et al., 1973).

Steady-state serum concentrations of procainamide and its active metabolite n-acetylprocainamide have been found to increase in the aged (Reidenberg, Comacho, Kluger, & Drayer, 1980). This change is associated with the age-related decrease in renal function and a decrease in renal tubular secretion. Both the hepatic and renal clearance of quinidine decrease with age and therefore lower initial doses and gradual increases should be used in the aged (Ochs, Greenblatt, & Woo, 1977; Ochs, Greenblatt, & Woo, 1978; Drayer, Hughes, Lorenzo, & Reidenberg, 1980). Disopyramide has potent anticholinergic effects, which account for a majority of side effects in the aged. It is especially not tolerated well by males with benign prostatic hypertrophy and urinary retention (Baines, Davies, Kellett, & Munt, 1976). The effects of aging on beta-adrenergic blockers and calcium-ion antagonists have already been addressed in this chapter. In summary, the effects of aging on antiarrhythmics mostly result in an increase in elimination half-life, leading to higher steady-state blood levels. Dosage reduction and careful monitoring of serum or plasma drug concentrations are necessary when these drugs are used in aged patients.

## ANTICOAGULANTS

Anticoagulant use in the aged is associated with higher risks of complications. Although the pharmacokinetic parameters of heparin are poorly understood, patients greater than 60 years (particularly females) experience an increased incidence of bleeding (Garnett & Barr, 1984; Jick, Slone, Borda, & Shapiro, 1968; Vieweg, Piscatelli, Houser, & Proulx, 1970).

Warfarin is highly plasma protein bound. Since aging is associated with a decrease in plasma albumin concentrations, the aged have less circulating albumin, which results in a decrease in bound warfarin and an increase in free (unbound) warfarin (Garnett & Barr, 1984). Thus at any given dose, aged patients effectively have a higher free warfarin concentration, are at an increased risk for dose-related complications, are more likely to experience bleeding, and are less likely to achieve a desired therapeutic outcome. When the pharmacokinetics of warfarin were evaluated in young versus aged patients, no differences were found in elimination half-life, volume of distribution, or clearance (Hayes, Langman, & Short, 1975a; Hewick, 1975).

Other factors that may contribute to the development of problems associated with anticoagulant therapy in the aged include a decrease in hematostatic response resulting from a 33% to 50% decrease in the synthesis of clotting factors in the aged versus the young; the increased potential for drug interactions with warfarin; age-related reductions in receptor sensitivity to vitamin K; increased clearance of vitamin K; and age-related increases in the active metabolite of warfarin, vitamin K oxide, in the aged (Garnett & Barr, 1984). Thus, when aged patients receive anticoagulant therapy, they should be very closely monitored for signs of bleeding. When warfarin is used, a dose reduction for aged patients is in order and cautious titration of dose should be accompanied with frequent monitoring of prothrombin times and/or INRs.

## GASTROINTESTINAL DRUGS

Drugs used to treat peptic ulcer disease are frequently prescribed for the aged. Options for treatment include the use of histamine$_2$ (H$_2$) receptor antagonists, sucralfate, antacids, omeprazole, and misoprostil; pirenzepine, colloidal bismuth, carbenoxolone, and antibiotics are still under investigation at this time. Of these, $H_2$ antagonists and sucralfate are considered to be the safest and most efficient choices for the treatment of peptic ulcer disease. Four $H_2$ antagonists are approved in the United States: cimetidine, ranitidine, famotidine, and nizatidine. The major difference between these drugs is their advance effect and drug interaction profiles. Cimetidine, the first available $H_2$ antagonist, is associated with the most problems. Cimetidine binds to hepatic cytochrome P-450 microsomal mixed-function oxidase enzymes and inhibits their function. As a result, clinically important decreases in clearance resulting in an increase in elimination half-life of drugs such as phenytoin, warfarin, theophylline, and others can occur (Somogyi & Muirhead, 1987; Gerber, Tejwani, Gerber, & Bianchine, 1985; McInnes & Brodie, 1988; Griffin, May, & DiPiro, 1984). Since aged patients may take many medications, alterations in the clearance of drugs, especially those with a narrow therapeutic margin, can result in increased adverse effects and/or toxicity. In addition to drug interactions, cimetidine use is associated with mental confusion, elevations of creatinine, increased values for liver function tests, and antiandrogenic effects (Gordon, 1981; Brier et al., 1980; Jenike, 1982b). Ranitidine, nizatidine, and famotidine are not associated with clinically significant changes in drug clearance (Mitchard, Harris, & Mullinger, 1987; Krishna & Klotz, 1988). Thus, it is reasonable to recommend that if $H_2$ receptor antagonists are to be used in aged patients who are taking other drugs that are hepatically metabolized by oxidative biotransformation, ranitidine, famotidine, or nizatidine should be used instead of cimetidine.

Sucralfate is an interesting alternative to the $H_2$ antagonists. It is not absorbed systemically and has few side effects. If patients experience problems with the $H_2$ antagonists or if systemic therapy is not desired, sucralfate can be used. The only clinically important problems associated with the use of sucralfate are constipation, the potential for sucralfate to bind to other drugs and interfere with their absorption, and the tablet's being so large that some patients have trouble swallowing it.

Antacids can be useful in some situations, but because they taste bad, patient compliance is the biggest problem. Aluminum-containing antacids can cause constipation, and magnesium- and calcium-containing products can cause diarrhea. The sugar content of antacid products is especially important for diabetic patients (Lamy, 1982).

Other gastrointestinal drugs such as hypocholesterolemics, prokinetics (e.g., metoclopramide), anti-inflammatory, antibacterial, and antidiarrheal drugs have not been sufficiently studied in the aged so that recommendations about their use in this population cannot be made. The use of laxatives in the aged should be avoided if possible. Nonpharmacologic measures such as increasing fluid intake, exercise, and dietary fiber should be used before drugs are prescribed. Evaluation of the drugs a patient is taking such as anticholinergics and iron salts should be performed and alternative agents should be substituted if possible. Stool softeners such as dioctyl sodium sulfosuccinate or dioctyl calcium sulfosuccinate should be considered if diet and exercise are ineffective.

ANTIBACTERIAL AGENTS

A review of the effects of aging on antibiotics reveals that for most agents, the age-related decrease in renal clearance results in predictable prolongation in elimination half-life (Meyers & Wilkinson, 1989). Therefore, dose reductions for most antibacterial agents are indicated for the aged patient. The reduction of dose should be carefully managed so that the blood level or tissue concentration necessary for bacteriocidal or bacteriostatic activity is achieved. Beta-lactam drugs such as the penicillins and cephalosporins, tetracyclines, and sulfonamides have an extremely good safety profile in the aged. Aminoglycosides, quinolones, vancomycin, and beta-lactams, all excreted by the kidney, may require dose adjustments based on creatinine clearance. The toxicity of aminoglycosides (ototoxicity and renal toxicity) cannot be overstated and dose reductions for aged patients are almost always required.

Antibacterials that are primarily cleared by the liver may also require dosage reduction. These drugs include isoniazid, metronidazole, quinolones, rifampin, and the macrolides (i.e., erythromycin). Thus, when antibacterial agents are used in the aged patient, the clinician should anticipate decreased clearance and an increase in elimination half-life.

Most of the agents are inherently safe so that changes in pharmacokinetics could present as an increased likelihood of adverse effects. On the other hand, aminoglycosides and vancomycin should be monitored and used with extreme caution since their toxicities are dose related and usually avoidable.

MISCELLANEOUS DRUGS

Studies evaluating the effects of aging on the pharmacokinetics and pharmacodynamics of other drugs exist, but often the studies raise more questions about the clinical relevance of their results than they answer. Reasons for this include the study of drugs in normal healthy (disease free) aged volunteers, the study of pharmacokinetics without pharmacodynamic evaluation, and likewise the evaluation of clinical response or toxicity in the absence of pharmacokinetic determinations. Other problems include the study of patients with concomitant disease states who may be taking other medications. Predictable age-related changes in clearance, plasma protein binding, and volume of distribution occur for many drugs, and we cannot overemphasize the necessity for starting therapy in aged patients with smaller doses than those used in younger adults and for adjusting therapy gradually.

The anticonvulsant phenytoin has been reported to be susceptible to age-related changes in protein binding and clearance. However, studies have shown that plasma phenytoin level may either increase or decrease as a function of aging (Patterson, Heazelwood, Smithhurst, & Eadie, 1982; Hayes, Langman, & Short, 1975b; Houghton, Richens, & Leighton, 1975). However, reports of the increased incidence of neurologic and hematologic toxicity in elderly patients is often dose related so if patients are maintained at lower steady-state plasma phenytoin concentrations, these complications can be avoided.

Narcotic analgesic use in the aged is often associated with increased incidence of adverse effects such as nausea, hypotension, and excess respiratory depression. In addition, increased pain relief from normal adult doses occurs in aged patients. The pharmacokinetic and pharmacodynamic reasons for these effects are not completely understood, but lower initial doses and cautious titration are usually adequate to solve these problems. However, care must be taken to avoid the undertreatment of pain (Wallace & Watanabe, 1977). No significant age-related effects have been reported for either aspirin or acetaminophen.

There is no evidence that the aged respond any differently to theophylline than the young. However, theophylline is mainly biotransformed in the liver, and the clearance may be decreased in the aged. Monitoring serum theophylline concentrations will adequately protect patients from overdosage.

The delivery of insulin to systemic circulation, the metabolic clearance, and the sensitivity of insulin do not change with age (Garnett & Barr, 1984; Barbagallo-Sangiorgi, 1970). The clearance and volume of distribution of oral hypoglycemic agents may be affected by aging, but lower doses and monitoring of serum glucose levels result in the selection of appropriate doses for the patient.

In summary, it is difficult to predict how aged patients will respond to various medications. With knowledge of how a drug is distributed and cleared from the body, reasonable assumptions can be made, especially if the therapeutic outcome is determined before treatment is initiated and if some endpoint or serum drug concentration can be evaluated.

## MEDICATION COMPLIANCE

Taking medications properly is something that is difficult for many patients to do. Too often patients forget to take their medications as prescribed, stop taking a medicine without informing their health-care provider, take their medications only when they think they need them, or take more medication than prescribed. These situations are all referred to as noncompliance. Actually, they can be subdivided into undercompliance, overcompliance, or erratic use. It appears that this classification (e.g., compliance) places the responsibility of following directions on the patient. The appropriate term should be "cooperation" instead of "compliance." If patients are adequately informed about what the medication is for, how it works, how it will help them, how long they should expect to take it, what will happen if they do not take it as prescribed, and what adverse or side effects may occur, they will be more likely to understand the importance of taking the medication properly and assuming an active role in their treatment plan.

The prevalence of noncompliance is a serious problem. The errors in medication use can be summarized as follows: 40% of patients miss drug doses or take medication "holidays" for three or more days; 50% of all patients make mistakes in the timing of doses; approximately 10% of patients take too high a dose of their medication; and approximately 100 million prescriptions per year go unfilled or unrefilled due to decisions not to take a medication. In a study of cardiovascular and respiratory medications, approximately 33% of patients changed the dose and dosage regimen themselves without consulting with or informing the prescriber. In a public opinion poll 75% of respondents who were noncompliant did not take their medication because they "felt better," 63% stated that they "just forgot," and more than 80% said that they were likely to take a little less medication or take it less frequently than what was prescribed (Mara, 1989).

The many problems that contribute to noncompliance patients being "forgetful," lack of knowledge of treatment goals, embarrassment about being labeled "noncompliant," lack of finances, asymptomatic illness, cultural biases about drug-taking behaviors, adverse effects, lack of access to a pharmacy, inability to open child-resistant containers, and frequency of administration. Factors that have been identified as high-risk character-istics of patients for drug noncompliance include a previous history of noncompliance, the use of multiple medications, the number of health-care providers, patients who live alone, decreased mentation, the high cost of medications, visual problems, and hearing impairment (Tideiksaar, 1984).

Factors related to the patient, clinician, illness, and drug regimen can also affect drug compliance. Illness-related items include severity of disease, severity of disability, and duration of treatment. Patient-related variables include the level of satisfaction with the clinician; the relationship of the clinician-patient interaction; the level of understanding of the disease and treatment and various personality traits of the patient, such as level of anxiety, level of responsibility, fear of the disease, fear of taking drugs, and the patient's unwillingness to participate in the treatment. Clinician-related variables include duration of office visit (i.e., long office waiting times negatively influence compliance), adequacy of the explanation of disease and treatment, the duration of time spent with the patient, willingness to negotiate a treatment plan, and the level of follow-up. Items related to the drug regimen include the number of drugs, cost of medication, frequency of dosing, route of administration, adverse effects, and the type of pill dispenser (Tideiksaar, 1984).

Evaluating noncompliance is often very difficult. Methods for measuring compliance include pill counts, prescription refill counts, measurement of blood and urine drug and metabolite levels, observation of therapeutic effect, and the actual patient interview.

Solutions to medication noncompliance have been offered but generalizations are dif-ficult. Patients may benefit from one or a combination of any of the following memory aids: medication calenders; drug reminder charts; color-keyed systems; pill organizers that have daily, weekly, and/or hourly compartments; blister packages; unit-dose packag-ing; computerized bottle caps; an alarm clock or watch; individual envelopes; and egg cartons. However, it is generally recognized that if patients know something about what they are being treated for, why they should take the medication as prescribed and what, if any, alternatives exist, they are more likely to accept the therapy and participate in their treatment plan.

If a clinician suspects that there is a compliance problem with a patient, it should be addressed in such a manner that the patient does not become defensive. If the problem can be identified and the appropriate solution instituted, the patient's therapeutic out-come will be improved as a result of cooperation with the treatment plan.

SUMMARY

The information presented in this chapter offers a comprehensive review of clinical phar-macology and the effects of aging on drug therapy. Absorption processes do not appear to be altered by the aging process but distribution, biotransformation, and renal elimina-tion may be affected so that the results are clinically important. When choosing dosages for aged patients, a smaller dose (i.e., one third to one half those recommended for young adults) should be tried initially, and depending on the desired clinical effect, subsequent doses should be gradually adjusted. For actual drug selection, drugs that will not interact with a patient's other drug therapies or disease states should be chosen. In pharmacokinetic terms, drugs that alter gut motility could affect the absorption or toxicity profile of other medications. Drugs that may compete for protein binding could affect the disposition of other drugs.

Accumulation can also occur, depending on a drug's route of clearance or metabolite profile. Care should be taken in noting which drugs the patient is currently using that could alter the metabolism of the drug being selected, or whether the new therapy could affect the clearance of a patient's coexisting drug therapy. Optimally, a drug with the least number of active metabolites should be selected. Additionally, drugs that undergo conjugation rather than oxidation as their primary route of biotransformation should be chosen first. Likewise, a drug that has a shorter elimination half-life should be selected over one with a long half-life. If drugs that are primarily excreted intact by the kidney are selected, care must be used in evaluating the patient's renal function so that the appropriate dose is selected. Other factors such as dosage form, cost, and the frequency of drug administration should be considered when drug selection is made.

A complete review of a patient's medications is extremely important. This review should include a listing of all current medications, both over-the-counter and prescription. A complete drug history should also include questions about prior drug sensitivities, adverse drug reactions, and allergies.

Whenever a prescription is written, it should be properly explained to the patient. Information should be provided as to what the generic and brand names are; what the drug is for; how it should be taken in relation to other medications, meals, and alcoholic beverages; how long it should be taken; what the patient should expect in terms of therapeutic effects and side effects; and what the patient should do if he or she experiences any problems. All of this information should be provided by the person prescribing the medication and should be explained in an understandable way and in sufficient detail so that the patient understands the medications they are taking. Ideally this information should be reinforced by the patient's pharmacist and nurse. Patients should also be instructed about whom they should contact if they have any problems or questions. This may also positively influence compliance since a patient is more likely to trust his or her drug therapy if it is understood.

If possible, the clinician should also try to choose drugs that can be taken in a dosing pattern similar to that of the rest of the patient's medications. This will help to ensure that the patient takes the drug on a familiar schedule.

There are many factors that govern appropriate drug therapy in the aged patient. With the number of new drugs introduced each year, the increasing numbers of elderly patients and the sophistication of medical care, choosing drugs for a patient can be extremely difficult. Often a patient's clinical condition is delicately balanced, and care must be taken not to upset homeostatic compensatory mechanisms. Knowledge of clinical pharmacology, pharmacokinetics, pharmacodynamics, and the effects of aging on all these parameters will help the members of the health-care team to provide the most appropriate care to their patient.

## REFERENCES

Abernethy, D. R., Greenblatt, D. J., Divoll, M., & Harmatz, J. S. (1981). Alterations in drug distribution and clearance due to obesity. *Journal of Pharmacology and Experimental Therapeutics, 217,* 681–685.

Abernethy, D. R., & Montamat, S. C. (1987). Acute and chronic studies of diltiazem in elderly versus young hypertensive patients. *American Journal of Cardiology, 60* (Suppl I), 116I–120I.

Abernethy, D. R., Schwartz, J. B., Todd, E. L., Luchi, R., & Snow, E. (1986). Verapamil pharmacodynamics and disposition in young and elderly hypertensive patients. *Annals of Internal Medicine, 105,* 329–336.

Adler, A. G., McElwain, G. E., Merli, G. J., & Martin, J. H. (1982). Systemic effects of eyedrops. *Archives of Internal Medicine, 142,* 2293–2294.

Allen, M. D., Greenblatt, D. J., Harmatz, J. S., & Shader, R. I. (1980). Desmethyldiazepam kinetics in the elderly after oral prazepam. *Clinical Pharmacology and Therapeutics, 28,* 196–202.

Baines, M. W., Davies, J. E., Kellett, D. N., & Munt, P. L. (1976). Some pharmacologic effects of disopyramide and a metabolite. *Journal of International Medical Research, 4* (Suppl 1), 5–7.

Baldessarini, R. J. (1989). Current status of antidepressants: clinical pharmacology and therapy. *Journal of Clinical Psychiatry, 50,* 117–126.

Barbagallo-Sangiorgi, G. (1970). The pancreatic beta cell response to intravenous administration of glucose in elderly subjects. *Journal of the American Geriatrics Society, 18,* 529–538.

Bender, A. D. (1965). The effect of increasing age on the disturbances of peripheral blood flow in man. *Journal of the American Geriatrics Society, 13,* 192–198.

Bergstrom, R. F. (1983). The pharmacokinetics of fluoxetine in elderly subjects. Abstracts of the Second World Conference on Clinical Pharmacology and Therapeutics. Washington, DC. *2,* 120.

Blazer, D. (1989). Depression in the elderly. *New England Journal of Medicine, 320,* 164–166.

Brier, K. L., Dasta, J. F., Kidwell, G. A., & Shonfeld, S. A., & Couri, D. (1980). Cimetidine and mental confusion. *Critical Care Medicine, 8* (12), 760–761.

Burckhardt, D., Rueder, E., Müller, V., Imhoff, P., & Neubauer, H. (1978). Cardiovascular effects of tricyclic and tetracyclic antidepressants. *JAMA, 239,* 213–216.

Casteleden, C. M., & George, C. F. (1979). The effect of age on the hepatic clearance of propranolol. *British Journal of Clinical Pharmacology, 7,* 49–54.

Chase, S. L. (Ed.) (1989). Calcium antagonists and cardiovascular diseases of the elderly. *Phil Col Pharm Sci, 1,* 1–31.

Cockroft, D. W., & Gault, M. H. (1976). Prediction of creatinine clearance from serum creatinine. *Nephron, 16,* 31–41.

Cusack, B., Kelly, J. G., Lavan, J., Noel, J., & O'Malley, K. (1980). Pharmacokinetics of lignocaine in the elderly. *British Journal of Clinical Pharmacology, 9,* 293–294.

Cusack, B., Kelly, J., O'Malley, K., Noel, J., Lavan, J., & Horgan, J. (1979). Digoxin in the elderly: pharmacokinetic consequences of old age. *Clinical Pharmacology and Therapeutics, 25,* 772–776.

Dement, W. C., Miles, L. E., & Carskadon, M. A. (1982). "White Paper" on sleep and aging. *Journal of the American Geriatrics Society, 30,* 25–35.

Divoll, M., Abernethy, D. R., Ameer, B., & Greenblatt, D. J. (1982). Acetaminophen kinetics in the elderly. *Clinical Pharmacology and Therapeutics, 31,* 151–156.

Divoll, M., Ameer, B., Abernethy, D. R., & Greenblatt, D. J. (1982). Age does not alter acetaminophen absorption. *Journal of the American Geriatrics Society, 30,* 240–244.

Drayer, D. E., Hughes, M., Lorenzo, B., & Reidenberg, M. M. (1980). Prevalence of high (3S)-3-hydroxyquinidine/quinidine ratios in serum, and clearance of quinidine in cardiac patients with age. *Clinical Pharmacology and Therapeutics, 27,* 72–75.

Dufresne, R. L., Weber, S. S., & Becker, R. E. (1984). Bupropion hydrochloride. *Drug Intelligence and Clinical Pharmacy, 18,* 957–964.

Dybaker, R., Lauritzen, M., & Krakauer, R. (1981). Relative reference values for clinical chemical and haematological quantities in 'healthy' elderly people. *Acta Medica Scandinavica, 209,* 1–9.

Eison, A. S., & Temple, D. L. (1986). Buspirone: Review of its pharmacology and current perspectives on its mechanism of action. *American Journal of Medicine, 80* (Suppl 3B), 1–9.

Evans, M. A., Triggs, E. J., Cheung, M., Broe, G. A. & Creasey, H. (1981). Gastric emptying rate in the elderly: implications for drug therapy. *Journal of the American Geriatrics Society, 29,* 201–205.

Ewy, G. A., Kapadin, G. G., Yao, L., Lullin, M., & Marcus, F. I. (1969). Digoxin metabolism in the elderly. *Circulation, 39,* 449–453.

Fraser, D. G., Ludden, T. M., Evens, R. P., & Sutherland, E. W. (1980). Displacement of phenytoin from plasma binding sites by salicylate. *Clinical Pharmacology and Therapeutics, 27,* 165–169.

Friedman, H., & Greenblatt, D. J. (1986). Rational therapeutic drug monitoring. *JAMA, 256,* 2227–2233.

Friedman, H., Greenblatt, D. J., Scavone, J. M., Burstein, E. S., Ochs, H. R., Harmatz, J. S., & Shader, R. I. (1989). Clearance of the antihistamine doxylamine reduced in elderly men but not elderly women. *Clinical Pharmacokinetics, 16,* 312–316.

Garnett, W. R., & Barr, W. H. (1984). *Geriatric pharmacokinetics* (pp. 1–27). Kalamazoo, MI: The Upjohn Company.

Geokas, M. C., & Haverback, B. J. (1969). The aging gastrointestinal tract. *American Journal of Surgery, 117,* 881–892.

Gerber, M. C., Tejwani, G. A., Gerber, N., & Bianchine, J. R. (1985). Drug interactions with cimetidine: An update. *Pharmacology and Therapeutics, 27,* 353–370.

Gibaldi, M., & Perrier, D. (1975). Clinical pharmacokinetics. New England Journal of Medicine, 293, 702–705, 964–970.

Goa, K. C., & Ward, A. (1986). Buspirone: A preliminary review of its pharmacological properties and therapeutic efficacy as an anxiolytic. *Drugs, 32,* 114–129.

Goldstein, G., Materson, B. J., Cushman, W. C., Reda, D. J., Freis, E. D., Ramirez, E. A., Talmers, F. N., White, T. J., Nunns, S., Chapman, R. H., Khatri, I., Schnaper, H., Thomas, J. R., Henderson, W. G., & Fye, C. (1990). Treatment of hypertension in the elderly: II. Cognitive and behavioral function: Results of a Department of Veterans Affairs cooperative study. *Hypertension, 15,* 361–369.

Gordon, C. (1981). Differential diagnosis of cimetidine-induced delirium. *Psychosomatics, 22* (3), 251–252.

Greenblatt, D. J. (1979). Reduced serum albumin concentration in the elderly: A report from the Boston Collaborative Drug Surveillance Program. *Journal of the American Geriatrics Society, 27,* 20–22.

Greenblatt, D. J. (1989). Disposition of cardiovascular drugs in the elderly. *Medical Clinics of North America, 73,* 487–494.

Greenblatt, D. J., Abernethy, D. R., Divoll, M., Harmatz, J. S., & Shader, R. I. (1983). Pharmacokinetic properties of benzodiazepine hypnotics. *Journal of Clinical Psychopharmacology, 3,* 129–132.

Greenblatt, D. J., Allen, M. D., Harmatz, J. S., & Shader, R. I. (1980). Diazepam disposition determinants. *Clinical Pharmacology and Therapeutics, 27,* 301–312.

Greenblatt, D. J., Divoll, M., Abernethy, D. R., Harmatz, J. S., & Shader, R. I. (1982). Antipyrine kinetics in the elderly: Prediction of age-related changes in benzodiazepine oxidizing capacity. *Journal of Pharmacology and Experimental Therapeutics, 220,* 120–126.

Greenblatt, D. J., Divoll, M., Abernethy, D. R., & Shader, R. I. (1982). Benzodiazepine hypnotics: Kinetic and therapeutic options. *Sleep, 5,* S18–S27.

Greenblatt, D. J., Divoll, M., Puri, S. K., Ho, I., Zinny, M. A., & Shader, R. I. (1981). Clobazam kinetics in the elderly. *British Journal of Clinical Pharmacology, 12,* 631–636.

Greenblatt, D. J., Ehrenberg, B. L., Gunderman, J., Scavone, J. M., Tai, N. T., Harmatz, J. S., & Shader, R. I. (1989). Kinetic and dynamic study of intravenous lorazepam: Comparison with intravenous diazepam. *Journal of Pharmacology and Experimental Therapeutics, 250,* 134–140.

Greenblatt, D. J., & Scavone, J. M. (1986). Pharmacokinetics of oxaprozin and other nonsteroidal antiinflammatory agents. *Seminars in Arthritis and Rheumatism, 15* (Suppl. 2), 18–26.

Greenblatt, D. J., Sellers, E. M., & Shader, R. I. (1982). Drug disposition in old age. *New England Journal of Medicine, 306,* 1081–1088.

Greenblatt, D. J., & Shader, R. I. (1985). Pharmacokinetics in clinical practice. Philadelphia: W. B. Saunders.

Greenblatt, D. J., Shader, R. I., Franke, K., MacLaughlin, D. S., Harmatz, J. S., Allen, M. D., Werner, A., & Woo, E. (1979). Pharmacokinetics and bioavailability of intravenous, intramuscular, and oral lorazepam in humans. *Journal of Pharmaceutical Sciences, 68,* 57–63.

Griffin, J. W., May, J. R., & DiPiro, J. T. (1984). Drug interactions: Theory versus practice. *American Journal of Medicine, 77* (Suppl. 5B), 85–89.

Gruter, W., & Poldinger, W. (1982). Maprotiline. *Modern Problems of Pharmacopsychiatry, 18,* 17–48.

Hamilton, L. D. (1966). Aged brain and the phenothiazines. *Geriatrics, 21,* 131–138.

Havlik, R. J., LaCroix, A. Z., Kleinman, J. C., Ingram, D. D., Harris, T., & Cornoni-Huntley, J. (1989). Antihypertensive drug therapy and survival by treatment status in a national survey. *Hypertension, 13* (Suppl. 1), I28–I32.

Hayes, M. J., Langman, M. J., & Short, A. H. (1975a). Changes in drug metabolism with increasing age: I. Warfarin binding and plasma proteins. *British Journal of Clinical Pharmacology, 2,* 69–72.

Hayes, M. J., Langman, M. J. S., & Short, A. H. (1975b). Changes in drug metabolism with increasing age: II. Phenytoin clearance and protein binding. *British Journal of Clinical Pharmacology, 2,* 73–79.

Hewick, D. D. S. (1975). The effect of age on the sensitivity to warfarin sodium. *British Journal of Clinical Pharmacology, 2,* 189P–190P.

Hollister, L. E. (1978). Tricyclic antidepressants. *New England Journal of Medicine, 2,* 1106–1109.

Houghton, G. W., Richens, A., & Leighton, M. (1975). Effect of age, height, weight and sex on serum phenytoin concentration in epileptic patients. *British Journal of Clinical Pharmacology, 2,* 251–256.

Hulley, S. B., Furberg, C. D., Gurland, B., MacDonald, R., Perry, H. M., Schnaper, H. W., Schoenberger, J. A., Smith, W. M., & Vogt, T. M. (1985). Systolic Hypertension in the Elderly Program (SHEP): Antihypertensive efficacy of chlorthalidone. *American Journal of Cardiology, 56,* 913–920.

Jenike, M. A. (Ed.). (1982a). Treatment of anxiety in elderly patients. Topics in *Geriatrics, 1,* 9–12.

Jenike, M. A. (1982b). Cimetidine in elderly patients: Review of uses and risks. *Journal of the American Geriatrics Society, 30,* 170–173.

Jenike, M. A. (1985). Handbook of geriatric psychopharmacology. Littleton, MA: PSG Publishing.

Jick, H. D., Slone, D., Borda, I. T., & Shapiro, S. (1968). Efficacy and toxicity of heparin in relation to age and sex. *New England Journal of Medicine, 279,* 284–286.

Kannel, W. B. (1989). Risk factors in hypertension. *Journal of cardiovascular pharmacology, 13* (Suppl. 1), 504–510.

Kaplan, N. M. (1989). Calcium entry blockers in the treatment of hypertension: current status and future prospects. *JAMA, 262,* 817–823.

Kastenholz, K. V., & Crimson, M. L. (1984). Buspirone, a novel nonbenzodiazepine anxiolytic. *Clinical Pharmacology, 3,* 600–607.

Klotz, U., Avant, G. R., Hoyumpa, A., Schenker, S., & Wilkinson, G. R. (1975). The effects of age and liver disease on the disposition and elimination of diazepam in adult man. *Journal of Clinical Investigation, 55,* 347–359.

Koch-Weser, J., & Sellers, E. M. (1976). Binding of drugs to serum albumin. *New England Journal of Medicine, 294,* 311–316, 526–531.

Kramer, P. A., Chapron, D. J., Benson, J., & Mercik, S. A. (1978). Tetracycline absorption in elderly patients with achlorhydria. *Clinical Pharmacology and Therapeutics, 23,* 467–472.

Krishna, D. R., & Klotz, U. (1988). Newer H$_2$-receptor antagonists: Clinical pharmacokinetics and drug interaction potential. *Clinical Pharmacokinetics, 15,* 205–215.

Lamy, P. P. (1982). Over-the-counter medication: The drug interactions we overlook. *Journal of the American Geriatrics Society, 30* (Suppl), S69–S75.

Lamy, P. P., & Love, R. C. (1988). Psychotropic agents. *Elder Care News, 4,* 9–15.

Lasagna, L. (1972). Hypnotic drugs. *New England Journal of Medicine, 287,* 1182–1184.

Lazarus, L. W., Davis, J. M., & Dysken, M. W. (1985). Geriatric depression: A guide to successful therapy. *Geriatrics, 40,* 43–53.

MacLennan, W. J., W. J., Martin, P., & Mason, B. J. (1977). Protein intake and serum albumin levels in the elderly. *Gerontology, 23,* 360–367.

Maklon, A. F., Barton, M., James, O., & Rawlins, M. D. (1980). The effect of age on the pharmacokinetics of diazepam. *Clinical Science, 59,* 479–483.

Mara, J. (Ed.). (1989). Medicine use errors: Where families need help. National Council on Patient Information and Education (*NCPIE*), *1,* 1–12.

Materson, B. J., Cushman, W. C., Goldstein, G., Reda, D. J., Freis, E. D., Ramirez, E. A., Talmers, F. N., White, T. J., Nunn, S., Chapman, R. H., Khatri, I., Schnaper, H., Thomas, J. R., Henderson, W. G., & Fye, C. (1990). Treatment of hypertension in the elderly: I. Blood pressure and clinical changes: Results of a Department of Veterans Affairs cooperative study. *Hypertension, 15,* 348–360.

McElnay, J. C., & D'Arcy, P. F. (1983). Protein binding displacement interactions and their clinical importance. *Drugs, 25,* 495–513.

McInnes, G. T., & Brodie, M. J. (1988). Drug interactions that matter: A critical re-appraisal. *Drugs, 36,* 83–110.

Meyers, B. R., & Wilkinson, P. (1989). Clinical pharmacokinetics of antibacterial drugs in the elderly: Implications for selection and dosage. *Clinical Pharmacokinetics, 17,* 385–395.

Mitchard, M., Harris, A., & Mullinger, B. M. (1987). Ranitidine drug interactions – A literature review. *Pharmacology and Therapeutics, 32,* 293–325.

Montgomery, R., Haeney, M. R., Ross, I. N., Sammons, H. G., Barford, A. V., Balakrishnan, S., Mayer, P. P., Culank, L. S., Field, J., & Gosling, P. (1978). The ageing gut: A study of intestinal absorption in relation to nutrition in the elderly. *Quarterly Journal of Medicine, 47,* 197–211.

Morris, D. C., & Hurst, J. W. (1980). Atrial fibrillation. *Current Problems in Cardiology, 5,* 1–12.

Nation, R. L., Triggs, E. J., & Selig, M. (1977). Lignocaine kinetics in cardiac patients and aged subjects. *British Journal of Clinical Pharmacology, 4,* 439–448.

Nolan, L., & O'Malley, K. (1988). Prescribing for the elderly: Sensitivity of the elderly to adverse drug reactions. *Journal of the American Geriatrics Society, 36,* 142–149.

Ochs, H. R., Greenblatt, D. J., Allen, M. D., Harmatz, J. S., Shader, R. I., & Bodem, G. (1979). Effect of age and Billroth gastrectomy on absorption of desmethyldiazepam from clorazepate. *Clinical Pharmacology and Therapeutics, 26,* 449–456.

Ochs, H. R., Greenblatt, D. J., & Heur, H. (1984). Is temazepam an accumulation hypnotic? *Journal of Clinical Pharmacology, 24,* 58–64.

Ochs, H. R., Greenblatt, D. J., & Woo, E. (1977). Reduced clearance of quinidine in elderly humans. *Clinical Research, 25,* 513A.

Ochs, H. R., Greenblatt, D. J., & Woo, E. (1978). Reduced quinidine clearance in elderly persons. *American Journal of Cardiology, 42,* 481–485.

Ochs, H. R., Otten, H., Greenblatt, D. J., & Dengler, H. J. (1982). Diazepam absorption: Effects of age, sex, and Billroth gastrectomy. *Digestive Diseases and Sciences, 27,* 225–230.

Ogilvie, R. I. (1983). An introduction to pharmacokinetics. *Journal of Chronic Diseases, 36,* 121–127.

Ouslander, J. G. (1981). Drug therapy in the elderly. *Annals of Internal Medicine, 95,* 711–722.

Patterson, M., Heazelwood, R., Smithhurst, B., & Eadie, M. J. (1982). Plasma protein binding of phenytoin in the aged: In vivo. *British Journal of Clinical Pharmacology, 13,* 423–425.

Peabody, C. A., Whiteford, H. A., & Hollister, L. E. (1986). Antidepressants and the elderly. *Journal of the American Geriatrics Society, 34,* 869–874.

Pfeifer, H. J., Greenblatt, D. J., & Koch-Weser, J. (1976). Clinical use and toxicity of intravenous lidocaine. *American Heart Journal, 92,* 168–173.

Pomara, N., Stanley, B., Block, R., Berchou, R. C., Stanley, M., Greenblatt, D. J., Newton, R. E., & Gershon, S. (1985). Increased sensitivity of the elderly to the central depressant effects of diazepam. *Journal Clinical Psychiatry, 46,* 185–187.

Rabkin, J. G., Quitkin, F. M., McGrath, P., Harrison, W., & Tricamo, E. (1985). Adverse reactions to monoamine oxidase inhibitors: Part II. Treatment correlates with clinical management. *Journal of Clinical Psychopharmacology, 5,* 2–9.

Ram, C. V. S., Meese, R., Kaplan, N. M., Devous, M. D., Bonte, F. J., Forland, S. C., & Cutler, R. E. (1987). Antihypertensive therapy in the elderly: Effects on blood pressure and cerebral blood flow. *American Journal of Medicine, 82* (Suppl. 1A), 53–57.

Reidenberg, M. M., Comacho, M. C., Kluger, J., & Drayer, D. E. (1980). Aging and renal clearance of procainamide and acetylprocainamide. *Clinical Pharmacology and Therapeutics, 28,* 732–735.

Riblet, L. A., & Taylor, D. P. (1981). Pharmacology and neurochemistry of trazodone. *Journal of Clinical Psychopharmacology, 1* (Suppl. 1), 17S–22S.

Richelson, E. (1984). The newer antidepressants: Structures, pharmacokinetics and proposed mechanisms of action. *Psychopharmacology Bulletin, 20,* 213–223.

Richey, D. P., & Bender, A. D. (1977). Pharmacokinetic consequences of aging. *Annual Review of Pharmacology and Toxicology, 17,* 49–65.

Rickels, K., Weisman, K., Norstad, N., Singer, M. M., Stoltz, D., Brown, A., & Danton, J. (1982). Buspirone and diazepam in anxiety. *Journal of Clinical Psychiatry, 43,* 81–86.

Rivera-Calimlim, L., Nasrallah, H., Gift, T., Kerzner, B., Griesbach, P. H., & Wyatt, R. J. (1977). Plasma levels of chlorpromazine: Effect of age, chronicity of disease, and duration of treatment. *Clinical Pharmacology and Therapeutics, 21,* 115–116.

Robinson, D. S. (1971). Relation of sex and aging to monoamine oxidase activity of human brain, plasma, and platelets. *Archives of General Psychiatry, 24,* 536–539.

Rowe, J. W., Andres, R., Tobin, J. D., Norris, A. H., & Shock, N. W. (1976). The effect of age on creatinine clearance in man: A cross-sectional and longitudinal study. *Journal of Gerontology, 31,* 155–163.

Scavone, J. M. (1987). Treatment of sleep disorders. *Pharmatherapeutica, 13* (3), 1–10.

Scavone, J. M., Greenblatt, D. J., & Friedman, H. (1986). Enhanced bioavailability of triazolam following sublingual versus oral administration. *Journal of Clinical Pharmacology, 26,* 208–210.

Scavone, J. M., Greenblatt, D. J., Goddard, J. E., Friedman, H., Harmatz, J. S., & Shader, R. I. (1992). The pharmacokinetics and pharmacodynamics of sublingual and oral alprazolam in the post-prandial state. *European Journal of Clinical Pharmacology, 42,* 439–443.

Scavone, J. M., & Marx, C. M. (1983). Drug-food and drug nutrition interactions. *NARD* (National Association of Retail Druggists) *Journal, 5,* 55–59.

Sellers, E. M. (1979). Plasma protein displacement interactions are rarely of clinical significance. *Pharmacology, 18,* 225–227.

Sommi, R. W., Crimson, M. L., & Bowden, C. L. (1987). Fluoxetine: A serotonin-specific, second generation antidepressant. *Pharmacotherapy, 7,* 1–15.

Somogyi, A., & Muirhead, M. (1987). Pharmacokinetic interactions of cimetidine. *Clinical Pharmacokinetics, 12,* 321–366.

Steele, T. E. (1982). Adverse reactions suggesting amoxapine induced dopamine blockade. *American Journal of Psychiatry, 139,* 1500–1501.

Stevenson, I. H. (1984). Drugs for the elderly. In L. Lemberger & M. M. Reidenberg (Eds.), Proceedings of the Second World Conference on Clinical Pharmacology and Therapeutics (pp. 64–73). Bethesda, MD: American Society of Pharmacology and Experimental Therapeutics.

Stuart, E. M., Deckro, J. P., Mamish, M. E., Friedman, R., & Benson, H. (1989). Non-pharmacologic treatment of the elderly hypertensive patient. *Circulation, 80* (Suppl. II), 189–190.

Stults, B. M. (1982). Digoxin use in the elderly. *Journal of the American Geriatrics Society, 30,* 158–164.

Thompson, T. L., Moran, M. G., & Nies, A. S. (1983). Psychotropic drug use in the elderly. *New England Journal of Medicine, 308,* 134–138, 194–199.

Thomson, T. L., Melmon, K. L., Richardson, J. A., Cohn, K., Steinbrunn, W., Cudihee, R., & Rowland, M. (1973). Lidocaine pharmacokinetics in advanced heart failure, liver disease, and renal failure in humans. *Annals of Internal Medicine, 78,* 499–508.

Tideiksaar, R. (1984). Drug noncompliance in the elderly. *Hospital Physician, 20,* 92–101.

Tjoa, H. I., & Kaplan, N. M. (1990). Treatment of hypertension in the elderly. *JAMA, 264,* 1015–1018.

Vestal, R., Wood, A. J. J., & Shand, D. G. (1979). Reduced beta-adrenoceptor sensitivity in the elderly. *Clinical Pharmacology and Therapeutics, 26,* 181–186.

Vestal, R. E. (1978). Drug use in the elderly. *Clinical Pharmacokinetics, 1,* 280–296.

Vestal, R. E., McGuire, E. A., Tobin, J. D., Andres, R., Norris, A. H., & Mezey, E. (1977). Aging and ethanol metabolism. *Clinical Pharmacology and Therapeutics, 21,* 343–354.

Vieweg, W. V. R., Piscatelli, R. L., Houser, J. J., & Proulx, R. A. (1970). Complication of intravenous administration of heparin in elderly women. *JAMA, 213,* 1303–1306.

Wallace, D. E., & Watanabe, A. S. (1977). Drug effects in geriatric patients. *Drug Intelligence and Clinical Pharmacology, 11,* 597–603.

Wilkinson, G. R., & Shand, D. G. (1975). A physiological approach to hepatic drug clearance. *Clinical Pharmacology and Therapeutics, 18,* 377–390.

Williams, R. L. (1983). Drug administration in hepatic disease. *New England Journal of Medicine, 309,* 1616–1622.

# 6

# Nutritional Concerns and Problems of the Aged

Johanna T. Dwyer

Health and quality of life have not been enjoyed by most of the elderly in our society in the 1980s. By 1990, however, the Surgeon General of the United States hoped to reduce the average annual number of days of restricted activity because of acute and chronic conditions by 20%, that is, to fewer than 30 days per year (Surgeon General of the United States, 1979). Similar goals were formulated for the year 2000 (U.S. Public Health Service, 1989). The goals of maintaining the vitality and independence of older people include increasing average life expectancy (years of healthy life expected) at age 65 to at least 14 years for men and 16 years for women.

How will such a goal be implemented? Its optimism assumes that it is not age itself but rather functional impairments that limit activity and detract from quality of life among the aged. If we hope to achieve the goal, we must increase the number of adults who can function independently. This can be done by decreasing the disease-related social and psychological factors that cause dependency. Moreover, premature deaths of older persons from curable conditions such as influenza and pneumonia need attention. And finally, we must ensure quality of life as much as we can by ensuring functional independence, by enhancing living conditions for the elderly, and by ensuring their emotional and social well-being.

## NUTRITIONAL CONCERNS OF THE AGED

Concerns about dependency, disease, and death cause much anxiety among the aged today. Increasing dependency is a reality of aging. The average 68-year-old man living in this country today has a life expectancy of 13 years; self-care suffices for 9 years, followed by 4 years of progressive incapacity. A 68-year-old woman in the circumstances can look forward to 20 more years of life, 11 of which are likely to consist of independent living with self-care, followed by 9 years in more sheltered settings for coping with progressive disability and increasing dependence.

One way of allowing the aged some measure of independence is to educate them about nutrition and the ways they can influence health.

Brillat-Savarin, the famous 19th-century gastronomist, claimed that the pleasures of the table outlasted those of all the other senses and indeed this seems to be the case. Thus, food shopping and preparation as well as sitting down to the table and eating should be encouraged as long as possible in the elderly. For many, the psychological and social gratifications surrounding eating continue to be high points of their daily lives. It is a source of solace as other sensory pleasures begin to wane.

## WHY THE AGED ARE NUTRITIONALLY VULNERABLE

The prevalence of nutritional deficiencies because of low dietary intakes appears to be quite high among the aged. In recent national population and community-based surveys, those over 65 years of age, especially the poor among them, were deficient in calcium, thiamine, vitamin D, folic acid, vitamin $B_6$, zinc, and overall caloric intake (O'Hanlon & Kohrs, 1978).

The aged are particularly at high risk of developing nutritional problems because of various social, psychological, and physical factors (Coe & Miller, 1984). Age, living alone (especially if this is due to recent bereavement or to a significant negative life event), lack of an effective family or neighbor support network, and low income, all contribute to poor nutrition. Psychological factors such as depression, mental deterioration, and impaired self-concept also increase nutritional risk. Physical factors such as functional dependence, sensory impairment, and limited mobility, especially when they are associated with a severe chronic degenerative disease, take a tremendous toll. Indices of nutritional risk using these factors are proving useful in identifying the aged more at risk for malnutrition and hospitalizations than their peers (Wolinsky, Coe, Miller, & Prendergast, 1984). These are summarized in recent publications (Dwyer, 1991; Nutrition Screening Initiative, 1992).

Aside from the particular needs of individuals suffering from debilitating disease, normal aging is accompanied by decrements in physiological function and inability to restore homeostasis once it is disrupted, increasing vulnerability to nutritional insults (Shephard, 1986). Chapter 2, Physical Health Problems and Treatment of the Aged, discusses these issues in greater depth. Also, the prevalence of many chronic degenerative diseases rises with advancing age. Atherosclerosis, diabetes mellitus, hypertension, cancer, renal disease, and dental disease may have synergistic negative effects on individuals whose physiological function is already compromised because of the aging process. Indeed, in most surveys the lowest nutrient intakes and the preponderance of frank malnutrition occur among those who are housebound because of chronic illness or disability, especially among those over age 75 years (Coe & Miller, 1986). That is, malnutrition appears to be the consequence not solely of age, but rather of a combination of age, disease, and poverty.

Many of these conditions have dietary implications, altering needs for nutrients, the physical form in which nutrients are delivered, and the activities of daily living relating to food and eating. Some of these conditions and the nutritional problems they give rise to are summarized in Table 6.1. Modifications in the type or amount of calories, the calorie-providing nutrients, vitamins, and minerals may all be called for to provide nutritional support or to control disease. Dietotherapy for the aged suffering from these conditions is beyond the scope of this chapter, but the reader is referred to recent reviews of the topic by Flynn (1984) and the American Dietetic Association (1992).

The aged are also especially vulnerable to malnutrition because there is little direct experimental evidence available on appropriate standards for their nutritional status or for dietary intake, especially among those age 85 years or over. The general problem of lack of nutrient standards for the aged has recently been reviewed by Lowenstein (1986). Specific examples of the difficulties in estimating protein needs among the aged are also available (Young, 1984).

The quality of diet required by the aged is high, which is another factor increasing nutritional vulnerability. Calorie needs are low (owing to reduced basal metabolic rates and lower physical activity), whereas their needs for protein, vitamins, and minerals stay more or less constant. Thus, the nutrient density (i.e., nutrients per calorie) necessary to fulfill recommended dietary allowances is higher for the aged than it is for younger adults.

The high use of pharmacologic agents also increases the vulnerability of the aged to malnutrition. Diet-drug interactions occur at all ages, but because so many of the aged take prescription and over-the-counter drugs on a regular basis, they are probably more common in this group. (See Chapter 5 for further discussion of these problems.) Also, age-related changes in gastrointestinal function, body composition, and liver and renal function alter both drug and nutrient metabolism. Coexisting disease, undernutrition, and malnutrition may further complicate these interactions in some cases (Roe, 1985; Bidlack , Kirsch, & Meskin, 1986; see also Chapter 2).

The simplest means by which drugs may affect nutritional status is through their effect on appetite. More commonly, absorption, metabolism, and excretion of dietary constituents are altered by various drugs. Dietary factors such as water consumption, amount of food consumed, timing of meals in relation to drug intake, and the constituents consumed may affect absorption and oxidative drug metabolism (Roe, 1982; Roe, 1985).

## PREVENTIVE NUTRITIONAL MEASURES FOR THE AGED

Preventive nutritional strategies for the aged differ somewhat from those that are most effective earlier in life (Branch & Jette, 1984). For example, diet-drug interactions rarely cause malnutrition in younger persons but, in the elderly, these side effects are much more common and may be partly preventable. Several measures can help keep diet-drug interactions to a minimum among the aged (Roe, 1982).

1. Reviewing medication schedules and over-the-counter drug use) and eliminating harmful drug-drug or drug-diet combinations.
2. Making certain that the patient is not abusing antacids, drugs, or alcohol.
3. Monitoring the nutritional status of all patients on drugs carefully.
4. Avoiding drugs with unwanted nutritional effects whenever possible, especially among the aged who are already malnourished due to disease.

Many other nutritional measures involving health promotion also act at the level of primary prevention and deserve greater attention (Surgeon General of the United States, 1979).

TABLE 6.1 Nutritional Problems in the Elderly

| Disease or Condition | Related Problems in Diet and Eating |
|---|---|
| Alzheimer's disease, senile dementia, organic brain syndrome | Cachexia and emaciation because of poor selfcare and poor eating habits. |
| Celiac sprue | Malabsorption, diarrhea, steatorrhea, weight loss, and malabsorption with secondary vitamin deficiencies, often corrected by gluten-free diet and vitamin-mineral supplements. |
| Chronic mesenteric ischemia (abdominal angina) | Abdominal pain after food ingestion, weight loss, malabsorption. |
| Diabetes mellitus | For adult-onset diabetes, it is necessary to limit energy intake in the obese. For insulin-dependent diabetes, it is necessary to control alcohol, simple sugars, time of eating, and energy intake. |
| Diverticular disease | Gastrointestinal pain and bowel discomfort. With diverticulitis, bleeding and infection may occur. Also, inappropriate dietary restrictions or lack of appetite may lead to loss of weight. |
| Emphysema | Dyspnea due to compromised lung function, which leads to lack of appetite and difficulty in eating. |
| Frequent constipation | Prolonged transit time of food from mouth to anus which is especially marked in bedridden, immobile elderly people. Constipation may be due to low intakes of dietary fiber; low intake of water and other fluids; small amounts of food consumed; or decreased colonic motility due to increased elasticity of the rectal wall, or secondary to drugs and disease. Among the elderly, the urge to defecate may be more frequent because maximal tolerable fecal volume in the rectum is reduced. Straining at stool is increased because higher rectal pressures are necessary at the same rectal volume for defecation among the aged. Fecal impaction may result if constipation is not prevented. Laxative use is also common in the elderly and may lead to laxative abuse and overdependence on laxatives to the point where normal defecation is no longer possible. |
| Gallbladder disease | Gallstones increase with age. Acute cholecystitis or acute pancreatitis due to common bile duct stones may ensue. Certain foods may be restricted and others may be repugnant, so undernutrition may ensue. |
| Gastrointestinal disorders (chronic) of lower gastrointestinal tract | Diverticular disease of the colon and colonic and rectal cancer all increase with age, and each may have nutritional implications. Increased intakes of dietary fiber may decrease symptoms of diverticular disease. Colon cancers, if untreated, may cause malabsorption. If treated by surgery, chemotherapy, or radiation, dietary alterations may be necessary in some instances to compensate for altered function and malabsorption due to resection of colon, radiation enteritis or chemotherapy. |
| Gastritis and duodenitis | Gastric secretion decreases, and gastric atrophy and atrophic gastritis rise with age, increasing risk of malabsorption of vitamin $B_{12}$ and iron with subsequent deficiencies. Certain foods may be restricted and others repugnant, so undernutrition may ensue. |
| Hiatal hernia | Increases with advancing age, as does gastroesophageal reflux (regurgitation) due to incompetent lower esophageal sphincter. Heartburn and dysphagia are common. |

196

| Disease or Condition | Related Problems in Diet and Eating |
|---|---|
| Liver disorders | Certain foods may be repugnant, others may be restricted (such as protein), and medication dose levels may change. Aside from specific disease, drug metabolizing systems of the liver operate more slowly. |
| Obesity | Calorie restriction is usually necessary, but energy intakes may already be very low, and it is important not to compromise intake of other essential nutrients. |
| Osteoarthritis | Difficulties in food getting and cooking, increased symptomatology with excess weight. |
| Osteoporosis | Difficulties in food getting and cooking, with very severe osteoporosis dyspnea if vertebral collapse causes distortion of rib cage and lungs which often causes lack of appetite, difficulty in eating, and decreased food intake. |
| Peptic ulcer | Gastric ulcer incidence increases with age, and complications such as obstruction, bleeding, and perforation are more common. Dysphagia, dyspepsia, and retrosternal discomfort are common. Antacid overuse may occur. Certain foods may be restricted and others may be repugnant, with undernutrition resulting. |
| Pernicious anemia | Incidence increases with age and causes vitamin $B_{12}$ deficiency and, if undiscovered, subacute combined degeneration of the spinal cord with dementia. |
| Renal disease | Limited ability to handle dietary protein, sodium, potassium, and water. |
| Severe coronary atherosclerosis | Dyspnea due to low cardiac output; if drugs used, leads to lack of appetite and constipation. |
| Stroke | Suppressed cough reflex resulting from stroke or extreme inanition, which may increase risk of choking; dysphagia. |

It is also important to consider secondary prevention, with early detection and nutrition-related support and treatment for various chronic degenerative diseases. The development of sensory deficits, eating and drinking problems related to mental health disturbances, diet-drug interactions, and failures of the social support system for the aged exacerbate and complicate their treatment (Stults, 1984). Special risk factors that involve nutritional problems include severe chronic illnesses, especially if the aged person is housebound or confined to an institution; social isolation, depression, and other mental disability; severe dental and periodontal disease; and low socioeconomic status (Kennie, 1984; Berkman, 1983).

Finally, nutritional support is an important part of tertiary prevention, or rehabilitation. Since most of the aged suffer from one or more chronic degenerative diseases, this type of prevention is especially important.

### Kidney Disease

Renal insufficiency is common in old age. Glomerular filtration rates, renal blood flow, and renal tubular function all decline, beginning in middle age. Atrophy of renal mass is usual and especially pronounced in the cortex, with decline in the number of nephrons, and hypertrophy and sclerosis in nephrons that remain, increasing the likelihood of renal insufficiency. In addition, chronic degenerative diseases, including hypertension, diabetes mellitus, and kidney disease, also often give rise to kidney damage. In end-stage renal disease, therapeutic diets are often prescribed to decrease the symptomatology and blood biochemistry disturbances. These include limitation of protein, sodium, and phosphorus (Cali, 1984; Walser, 1988). Although chronic renal insufficiency usually progresses so that additional measures, such as dialysis, may eventually be necessary, these dietary measures may offer symptomatic relief and decrease the frequency with which dialysis occurs.

The possibility that age-related deterioration in kidney function is not inevitable but that it results in part from chronic protein overnutrition earlier in life is now receiving attention (Brenner, Meyer, & Hostetter, 1982; Mitch, 1988; Rudman, 1988). The theory that protein restriction and meticulous control of blood pressure can decrease progression of chronic renal insufficiency is also being tested. Confirmation of this would alleviate much of the present suffering of the elderly.

### Congestive Heart Failure and Atherosclerosis

Therapy for congestive heart failure in the aged involves correction of sodium and water retention. Sodium-restricted diets are helpful, but the advent of effective diuretics has meant that extreme sodium restriction (e.g., to levels under 500–1,000 mg sodium per day) is no longer necessary. Because such extreme low-sodium diets are limited in palatability, this is a boon to the aged person's enjoyment of food (Kleiger, 1983; Hoy & Ponte, 1984).

Current recommendations for the aged are that modification of dietary fat (with respect to type and amount of fat) and cholesterol are in order, especially for those who have serum cholesterols over 250 mg/dl or above, since this is a major risk factor for coronary artery disease (National Cholesterol Education Program, 1988). At the same time, however, it is recognized that other therapeutic considerations are also important and that all of these must be integrated.

## STANDARDS FOR NUTRITION IN THE AGED

### Recommended Dietary Allowances

The most commonly used standards for adequacy of nutrient intakes in populations living in the United States are the recommended dietary allowances (RDAs), which are published periodically by the National Academy of Sciences (Committee on Dietary Allowances, 1989). They provide estimates of the amounts of essential nutrients that are adequate to meet the needs of virtually all healthy persons (95%) in different age and sex groups. While they are not intended for individual use, in clinical practice the RDAs are often used as a rough estimate of dietary adequacy: An individual who consumes the RDA is assumed to have adequate dietary intake. Difficulties in interpretation arise when failure to consume the RDA for a nutrient on a single occasion is equated with the presence of dietary inadequacy. It is more realistic to assume that, although the risk of dietary

TABLE 6.2   Recommended Dietary Allowances for Adults Ages 51 and Older

| Kilocalories | Males | Females |
|---|---|---|
| 51–75 years | 2,400 | 1,800 |
| 76+ years | 2,050 | 1,600 |
| | | |
| Protein, gm | 63 | 50 |
| Vitamin A, μg RE | 1,000 | 800 |
| Vitamin D, μg | 5 | 5 |
| Vitamin E, mg TE | 10 | 8 |
| Vitamin C, mg | 60 | 60 |
| Thiamine, mg | 1.2 | 1 |
| Riboflavin, mg | 1.4 | 1.2 |
| Niacin, mg mg | 1.5 | 1.3 |
| Vitamin B-6, mg | 1.2 | 2 |
| Folacin, micrograms | 200 | 180 |
| Vitamin B-12, μg | 2 | 2 |
| Calcium, mg | 800 | 800 |
| Phosphorus, mg | 800 | 800 |
| Magnesium, mg | 350 | 300 |
| Iron, mg | 10 | 10 |
| Zinc, mg | 15 | 15 |
| Iodine, μ | 150 | 150 |

*Source:* Committee on Dietary Allowances (1989), *Recommended Dietary Allowances*, 10th ed. Food and Nutrition Board, National Academy of Sciences.

inadequacy increases with intakes that chronically fail to meet the RDA, such a diagnosis can only be confirmed in the presence of positive anthropometric, clinical, or biochemical findings of malnutrition.

Recommendations for nutrient intakes based on RDAs are provided in Table 6.2. Data are lacking to permit breakdowns by decade according to age groups over 51 years. The special needs of the aged have not been given the attention they deserve. It is hoped that sufficient experimental evidence will be amassed to permit more specific recommendations in the future, and progress is being made in that direction (Young, 1982).

It is clear that energy needs are reduced, especially in the very old and frail. Differences in protein needs between the aged and younger populations are relatively slight, and recommendations for other vitamins and minerals vary because of altered absorption, metabolism, tissue stores, and excretion in the aged (Matcovik et al., 1979).

### *Dietary Guidelines for Americans*

First formulated in 1980 by the USDA and the US Department of Health and Human Services, the Dietary Guidelines for Americans provide additional advice for health promotion and risk reduction, especially for primary prevention of diet-related chronic degenerative diseases. The recommendations, which apply to the aged as well as to other groups, are to eat a variety of foods; maintain desirable body weight; increase intakes of starches and fiber; avoid too much fat, saturated fat, and cholesterol in the diet; avoid too much sugar; avoid too much sodium; and reduce to moderate intake the amount of alcoholic beverages consumed or avoid them altogether.

### Functional Assessment of Nutritional State

In the past few years, increasing attention has been paid to the importance of maintaining essential activities of daily living among the aged. To assess functional status simple questionnaires have been developed that appear to be closely associated with nutritional risk (Wolinsky et al., 1986). This type of assessment tool is important in evaluating overall nutrition-related functioning, since, even with the same diagnosis, individuals vary widely in their functional status. The instrument has been validated, and although correlations with clinical status and nutrition are rather low, the instrument is nonetheless useful (Wolinsky et al., 1985; Wolinsky et al., 1983; Wolinsky et al., 1984; Wolinsky et al., 1986).

Regardless of their relationship to nutritional status, functional assessments, such as those based on the activities of daily living and instrumental activities of daily living, provide critical insights into the well-being of the aged and their needs for assistance in eating, bathing, and so forth (Fillenbaum, 1980). Such information is now collected and reported on routinely (National Center for Health Statistics, 1987). These assessments deserve greater attention in clinical practice.

## NUTRIENTS OF SPECIAL IMPORTANCE TO THE AGED

Needs for the 44 essential nutrients remain qualitatively similar over the human life span; however, quantitative changes do occur for some nutrients. When diet-related disease is present, additional alterations in nutrients, other dietary constituents, the physical form of food, and the route for feeding (e.g., by mouth, by tube, or by vein) may also be called for.

When mean population intakes of a nutrient are below a standard such as the RDA, nutritionists regard it as a "problem" nutrient. Surveys of the aged reveal that mean intakes of calories and calcium are low and often problematic and that although mean intakes of protein are adequate, at least a third of those surveyed have intakes below the standard, suggesting low intakes in population subgroups (O'Hanlon & Kohrs, 1978; Kohrs & Czajka-Narins, 1986). Other vitamins and minerals present special problems for certain groups of the aged, and we will discuss some of these in detail. However, it is important to remember that any nutrient may be insufficient or in excess in certain individuals, groups, or situations, and can thereby constitute a problem nutrient.

### Calories

The RDA, which consists of just enough kilocalories to maintain energy balance, usually declines with age.

The recommended intake of calories from 51 to 75 years of age is 2,400 kilocalories (kcal) for men, and 1,800 kcal for women, with a range of from 2,000 to 2,800 kcal, and 1,200 to 2,000 kcal, respectively. For age 76 and older, the recommendation is for 2,050 kcal (a range of 1,650 to 2,450) for men, and 1,600 kcal (a range of 1,200 to 2,000) for women (Food and Nutrition Board, 1989).

CAUSES OF CURRENT DECLINES IN ENERGY INTAKES. Four major factors influence energy needs: resting energy expenditure, physical activity, growth, and thermogenesis (heat production secondary to food consumption, exercise, or cold stress), in that order. Resting energy expenditure and physical activity both decline with age, and thus energy needs are lower among the aged than among younger persons, all other things being equal. Linear growth does not occur in the aged organism, although during recovery and rehabilitation from wasting illnesses, lean body mass and fat may be laid down, requiring energy. Thermogenesis, a relatively minor contributor to energy needs at any age, is not known to differ between aged and younger persons.

Resting metabolic rate differs with age chiefly because lean body mass, which is the metabolically active tissue of the body, decreases by about 3 kg per decade after age 50. Cellular metabolic rate also decreases with aging, a factor of lesser importance since this decline is small. It is currently assumed that energy allowances should decrease by 6% from ages 51 to 75 years, and by another 6% after age 76, to account for reductions in resting metabolism.

Energy output in the form of physical activity declines with age because, after retirement, energy outputs from nondiscretionary physical activity often decline. Also, optional household tasks and discretionary physical activity often decline (Sidney & Shepherd, 1979). Currently, a decrease of 300 kcal in males and 200 in females is recommended for ages 51 to 75 years, with an additional 500 kcal (males) and 400 kcal (females) subtracted after age 76 years to account for reduced activity (Food and Nutrition Board, 1989) after the younger adult years.

ENERGY INTAKES AND BODY WEIGHT IN THE AGED. All national and most local surveys report that energy intakes among the aged are so low as to be inadequate for a significant proportion of the population. For example, in two recent population-based nutrition surveys conducted by the U.S. Department of Health and Human Services, the National Health and Nutrition Examination Survey I; (NHANES I); conducted from 1971 to 1974, and the NHANES II, conducted from 1976 to 1980, nearly half of the aged reported energy intake less than 67% of the RDA (Carroll, Abraham, & Dresser, 1983; Abraham, 1977). Most local surveys report similar findings (Kohrs & Czajka-Narins, 1986; Posner, 1979). One might conclude that in view of such low intakes, a larger proportion of the aged are extremely lean, if not emaciated. However, median weights at age 76 are 5 kg higher in males and 7 kg higher in females than among young adults (Abraham, 1979); these median weights are heavier by 9 kg for males and 7 kg for females than the desirable weights for height associated with lowest mortality in the actuarial statistics collected on younger persons. Certainly this argues against widespread starvation among the aged. One explanation for this discrepancy is that the energy intake standards are too high for actual energy outputs. Some evidence suggests that, in healthy individuals of desirable weight levels, energy intake recommendations and outputs agree closely (Calloway & Zanni, 1980). Many of the aged are ill, and with increasing age and illness interindividual differences in energy requirements and body weight become more pronounced (Widdowson, 1983). Limitations on physical activity caused by chronic disease such as arthritis, hip fractures, emphysema, osteoporosis, congestive heart failure, stroke, peripheral vascular insufficiency, and other degenerative conditions of the bones and joints probably limit physical activity and, consequently, reduce energy needs in at least a 10th of the population over 65 years of age. Among the very old, especially those who are in nursing homes, energy needs are often often slightly above basal levels. Thus, energy balance is apparently achieved at lower levels of energy output than recommended.

Although energy need is very low for some of the aged, it is extremely high for others. When neuromuscular coordination declines, with reduced mechanical efficiency of the limbs and increased difficulties in balance control, the energy cost of movement is also greatly increased. This is also true in cases of amputations or other handicapping conditions requiring prostheses or crutches.

Unfortunately, the aged with high energy needs are not necessarily those who have high intakes, nor is the converse the case. Thus both obesity and emaciation are observed.

In summary, a small but nevertheless significant proportion of the aged are undernourished and starved. This holds especially for those who are not only aged but also ill and poor and living at home. However, widespread undernutrition is uncommon. In interpreting data on energy intakes among the aged, methodological considerations must be kept in mind if valid and reliable measures are to be obtained. When 24-hour recalls of energy intakes are used, as is the case in many surveys, a large number of very low energy intakes result on any given day owing to intraindividual variation in eating patterns. These are not habitual and thus are not indicative of undernutrition or starvation. Also, underreporting is common, especially among the aged, when dietary survey methods rely on memory.

CLINICAL IMPLICATIONS

*Increasing Physical Activity Among the Aged.* The optimal level of physical activity varies among the aged because of differences in lifestyle; disabilities, if any; and disease. Evidence is rapidly accumulating that marked declines in physical activity among the aged are undesirable from a health standpoint. Reasonable levels of physical activity improve physical conditioning, may improve some aspects of endocrine function, contribute positively to bone health, increase cerebral oxygenation and alertness, and prevent muscle atrophy. Yet a substantial decrease in physical activity is common, particularly among those in institutions (Shepherd, 1987). Exercise can improve work capacity and cardiovascular function when it is undertaken with sufficient frequency, intensity, and duration. It also contributes to psychological and social health. This is discussed at greater length in Chapter 9. With exercising, body fat decreases, lean body mass increases, and endurance increases on aerobic training programs, with improvement in oxygen delivery and utilization (Barry et al., 1966; Sidney, Shepherd, & Harrison, 1977). Thus, individualized programs that emphasize physical activity as well as exercise are now recommended.

*Desirable Weights for the Aged.* The desirable weights for height associated with lowest mortality were derived from insured people aged 25 to 59. Median weights for the height of both males and females 65 to 74 years of age and older are higher by 10 to 15 lb than these weights, even though weight for height among the aged is decreased compared to middle age (Russell, 1983). Based on data collected in a longitudinal study on aging, Andres (1980) has argued that mortality among the aged is lower at weights that are higher than the desirable weights for height derived from younger populations. However, other studies suggest that, in fact, older individuals (e.g., 65 to 94 years) do have mean weights close to or even lower than desirable weights (Masters & Lasser, 1960). Therefore, at present, desirable weight tables are appropriate. At 90 years or older, weights 90% of desirable are closest to those exhibited in cross-sectional data of long-lived individuals. Those at all ages who are 20% below or above desirable weight levels for height should receive remedial attention, especially when diminished lean body mass or fat stores are indicated by midarm muscle circumferences 20% below the standard and triceps skinfolds 40% below. Obesity is signaled by a triceps skinfold 190% or more of the recently published HANES standard (Frisancho, 1981).

*Weight Reduction in the Aged.* Reducing diets are difficult to plan for the aged. Many of the aged are so sedentary that the usual 1,200 kcal diet produces only a very slight caloric deficit. Very low energy intake brings more rapid weight loss, but such a diet is usually low in iron, copper, and vitamin $B_6$, so that a multi-vitamin-mineral supplement at the RDA level may be necessary. Moreover, at very low levels of intake, resting metabolism and voluntary physical activity fall. Thus, whenever possible, moderately low-calorie diets (e.g., 1,200 kcal or more) should be coupled with increased physical activity.

## Protein

The current RDA for protein is 0.8 gm/kg of high-quality protein per day. This amounts to 56 gm for males and 44 gm for females of high-quality mixed protein per day for individuals who conform to RDA guidelines. Experimental studies of the aged have been limited, but most conclude their needs are at least this high and perhaps higher if long-term nitrogen balance is to be achieved (Lowenstein, 1986). The elderly are more likely to be affected by stresses such as disease, which may increase dietary protein requirements by two or more times (Young, 1984). The reduced contribution of muscle to body protein metabolism in the aged may decrease the ability of the organism to adapt during periods of restricted dietary energy or protein intake, when protein synthesis in vital organs is maintained by mobilization of amino acids from peripheral limbs (Cahill, 1970; Young, 1970). The reduction in energy intake is likely to increase protein needs because the efficiency of protein utilization depends somewhat on energy balance. And economic or social constraints, which limit the intake of high-quality protein, further increase need. Thus, protein need per unit of total body protein or lean body mass may be elevated. An allowance of 12% to 14% of total energy needs of the aged should probably come from protein (Young, 1984).

At present, the major clinical implication is to ensure that protein intakes are maintained at levels at least as high as those for younger people.

## Fat

At present, there is no RDA for dietary fat. However, the Dietary Guidelines for Americans recommend reductions in saturated fat and cholesterol from current levels. Recent recommendations of the American Heart Association and other groups suggest reductions in total fat, saturated fat, and cholesterol (American Heart Association, 1978; Committee on Diet and Health, 1989; National Cholesterol Education Program, 1990). The rationale is that the type and amount of dietary fat and cholesterol are risk factors for coronary artery disease, at least among middle-aged persons. Modifications in diet and other aspects of lifestyle have been found to decrease risks of coronary artery disease among young and middle-aged persons (McGill, 1986). Rigorous clinical trials of the effectiveness of such dietary changes are lacking for the aged since relevant studies involving this age group have not been carried out. However, it is known that total serum cholesterol, low-density lipoprotein cholesterol (LDL-C), triglyceride levels, and coronary artery disease rates all rise more rapidly with age among Americans and other populations consuming diets high in total fat, saturated fat, and cholesterol (Heiss et al., 1980; Connor et al., 1978) than they do in populations consuming lower intakes of these substances. Most of this age-related increase is in LDL-C and VLDL-C (very-low-density lipoprotein cholesterol) rather than HDL-C (high-density lipoprotein cholesterol). Although the association between plasma cholesterol and coronary heart disease is highest in early middle age, even among the aged the association is significant. However, LDL-HDL cholesterol ratios become better predictors of coronary artery disease risk over 70 years of age (Castelli et al., 1977). The alterations in lipoprotein structure and metabolism brought about by aging are unknown, although it is thought that cellular repair processes may be impaired, and that arterial lesions accumulate with age. Why LDL cholesterol levels rise with age is unknown, but it is theorized that they do so because of age-related changes in the body's ability to metabolize cholesterol, coupled with a diet that is high in saturated fat and cholesterol (Schoenfeld, 1984).

CLINICAL IMPLICATIONS

*Atherosclerosis.* Opinion is divided on whether diet modifications should be urged for the aged who have serum cholesterols over 250 mg/dl or high LDL-HDL cholesterol ratios. The limited evidence available on the effects of dietary alterations in the aged indicate that, although coronary artery disease mortality decreases, overall mortality may not decline (Dayton et al., 1969). Other arguments center on whether alterations in dietary fat and cholesterol should be given priority over other lifestyle-related risk factors (Flynn, 1984). As LDL-HDL cholesterol ratios rise in the aged, so do risks of coronary artery disease, and they are increased at higher blood-pressures.

On balance and extrapolating from studies of middle-aged persons, it seems wise to urge those over 65 years of age to adopt a fat-modified diet if they have not done so already. It is clear that LDL cholesterol levels can be changed by dietary measures, and such changes may reduce risk for coronary artery disease. Even among the aged, control over cardiovascular risk factors such as hypertension, serum cholesterol, impaired glucose tolerance, cigarette smoking, and weight control can decrease cardiovascular events (Kannel, 1986; National Cholesterol Education Program, 1988; Committee on Diet and Health, 1989). All of the atherogenic lipids (LDL cholesterol and triglycerides) rise with age up to age 60 and then decline. The decline is faster in men than in women, so that, at advanced aged, women have higher levels than men. Diastolic blood pressures rise until the 60s, while systolic pressures continue to rise into advanced age. These rises are associated with overweight, alcohol use, high serum lipids, high hematocrits, and low glucose tolerance levels. They are also associated with dietary factors, such as calories, fat, salt, and possibly lack of potassium, calcium, and magnesium.

The suggested guidelines for lowering cardiovascular disease risk in the elderly include dietary modifications to restrict saturated fat and cholesterol so as to lower LDL cholesterol. Ideally the diet should be approximately 30% fat with 8% to 10% of calories coming from saturated fat, and cholesterol kept well below 300 mg/day (Kannel, 1986). Weight reduction, exercise to raise HDL cholesterol, cessation of smoking, blood pressure control, control over diabetes if it is present, and moderation in alcohol use are also important. However, therapeutic priorities of other sorts must also be taken into account.

## Carbohydrates

Aside from an admonition that at least 100 gm of carbohydrate are needed per day to prevent ketosis, there is no RDA for carbohydrate, nor are there any specific recommendations for the aged. However, the Dietary Guidelines for Americans suggest that intake of complex carbohydrates and fiber should be increased and that of simple sugars decreased. Also, recent statements of the American Diabetes Association (1979, 1984) and the National Academy of Sciences (Committee on Diet and Health, 1989) recommend diets higher in complex carbohydrates and fiber and lower in simple sugars than most Americans probably currently consume, since serum lipids and blood glucose control appear to be improved on such regimens. The American Dental Association recommends diets low in retentive fermentable carbohydrates (i.e., carbohydrates that are retained in the mouth and that can be fermented by the bacteria in the mouth) to decrease risks of crown and root caries.

CLINICAL IMPLICATIONS

*Dental Health.* Both starches and sugars retained in the mouth can serve as substrates for the bacteria that are active in causing both crown and root caries (the latter type of caries being of particular concern in aged populations). However, good oral hygiene, which includes brushing, swishing, and flossing after meals, can minimize risks of periodontal disease and caries, even when fermentable carbohydrate intakes are high.

*Diabetes Mellitus.* Should the aged be advised to consume diets higher in complex carbohydrates and fiber than they currently do? At present, authoritative opinion favors some increase in carbohydrate (especially complex carbohydrate) in all individuals (Committee on Diet and Health, 1989). Modest reduction, but not total elimination, of simple sugars is suggested among diabetics. The rationale is that the effects of these constituents on blood glucose rise after eating (American Diabetes Association, 1984). Furthermore, increased calories from carbohydrates permit reduction in dietary fat, which may be advisable to reduce cardiovascular disease risk and to control energy intake. Slightly increased carbohydrate intake among all the aged is probably advantageous. Present evidence does not warrant dogmatic insistence solely on very high complex carbohydrate diets or avoidance of refined carbohydrates to control blood sugar for individuals of any age, be they diabetic or not. Instead, maintaining or achieving desirable weight and adoption of appropriate levels of physical activity deserve attention in controlling diabetes mellitus.

The carbohydrate-related concerns of the aged arise in large part from their own or their health advisers' outdated views about the causes of and dietary measures to control diabetes mellitus. Glucose intolerance usually increases with age, probably because of a combination of factors. These include poor dietary preparation prior to testing, inadequate diet with generalized undernutrition, physical inactivity, decreased lean body mass with consequent diminished capacity for metabolizing carbohydrate, decrease insulin secretion, and increased insulin resistance (perhaps because of increased adiposity) (Davidson, 1979). The relative strength of these factors probably varies from one individual to another.

The clinical importance of increased glucose intolerance among the aged is a matter of debate. Some experts claim that it is a normal accompaniment of aging; others believe that it indicates a pathological change requiring treatment. The present standards for diagnosing diabetes mellitus in aged adults are those of the National Diabetes Data Group (1979). Diabetes is considered to be present if fasting glucose concentrations exceed 140 mg/dl on more than one occasion; if the results of a standard oral glucose tolerance test with a 75 gm glucose dose reveal blood glucoses of 200 mg/dl or above at 2 hr and in one other sample during the test; or if plasma glucose is grossly and unequivocally elevated in the presence of classic signs and symptoms of diabetes, such as polyuria, polydipsia, ketonuria, or rapid weight loss. These standards are based on their value in predicting clinical outcomes. Those who have diabetes as defined above have increased risks of later health problems associated with the disease. These include diabetic symptoms (polydypsia, polyuria, and polyphagia), retinopathy, nephropathy, and disease of the large and small blood vessels. While the data on risk of lower complications is strongest for young and middle-aged persons, some studies are available on the aged. There is no clear evidence that mortality is affected. The evidence attesting to the adverse effect on morbidity is mixed, but it does appear to be elevated in most studies (Haavisto et al., 1983; Panzram & Zabel Langhennig, 1981; Tattersall, 1984). Therefore, it makes sense to control diabetes when it is present, including in the aged. Also, in view of the association between impaired glucose tolerance and increased incidence of large-vessel disease in the aged (even though microvascular disease and overt symptomatic diabetes is lower), those with oral glucose-tolerance test values in excess of 140 mg/dl at 2 hr should be considered for risk reduction by dietary and other means.

Before embarking on treatment, it is important to ensure that the glucose tolerance test used for diagnosis is valid. Undernourished individuals; those who have starved themselves for several days prior to the test; and those who have failed to eat the recommended high-carbohydrate diet prior to the test, consuming instead their usual diets, often give falsely high blood glucose values (Seltzer, 1983). Fasting blood sugars are not as sensitive to dietary influences.

The control of diabetes mellitus among the aged depends not only on diet but on weight control, physical activity, other lifestyle changes and, in some cases, on insulin or oral hypoglycemic agents. The basic principles are to keep blood glucose levels as normoglycemic as possible without substantial risks of hypoglycemia or unacceptably rigid restriction on lifestyle. Clinicians vary in the degree of hyperglycemia they are willing to accept, some settling simply for the control of polyuria and nocturnia, others requiring much stricter control because they believe it minimizes risks of infection, cataract formation, neuropathy, and thromboembolism (Horwitz, 1986).

The aged who have been newly diagnosed with diabetes should have a stepwise approach to dietary modification which gradually changes eating habits and lifestyle to bring about symptomatic and biochemical changes. More than 80% of aged diabetics suffer from Type II (non-insulin-dependent) diabetes mellitus with obesity. The major goal in Type II diabetes is to achieve and maintain desirable weight, since doing so reduces hyperglycemia, hyperlipidemia, and elevated blood pressure, often to the point where glucose intolerance normalizes sufficiently so that medications can be dispensed with. A strict "diabetic diet" with rigorous control over the type, amount, and timing of food portions as specified in diabetic exchange lists is neither necessary nor desirable for most aged patients, since they seldom suffer from insulin-dependent diabetes even if they are receiving insulin. In any event, attempts to make radical changes in eating patterns and habits are unlikely to succeed, since by old age those are well established. Horwitz (1982, 1986) provides sensible guidance for treating the aged diabetic. The principles he emphasizes are to make the fewest possible changes in diet (beginning with control of obesity if it is present); introducing changes gradually and with a good deal of professional assistance, especially if the person is living alone. The emphasis is on a balanced diet with calorie reduction if needed; regular mealtimes if the patient is insulin dependent and ketosis prone; modest restrictions in dietary saturated fat and cholesterol; and increased dietary fiber. A physical activity program should also be considered. For ketosis-prone individuals, more vigorous control may be necessary. Special attention needs to be paid to diet during illness among all diabetics.

Fewer aged diabetics have Type I (insulin-dependent) diabetes. For them, in addition to keeping body weight at desirable levels, consistency in the amount, type, and timing of food intake is important to balance blood sugar and insulin doses. This is best achieved by a diet which consists of 50% to 60% carbohydrate, 38% fat, and 12% to 20% protein.

Insulin dosage is related more to energy intake than to any other factor, so it is important to keep energy intake constant. High levels of carbohydrate in the diet improve glucose tolerance in diabetics by enhancing tissue sensitivity to insulin action, and for this reason high intakes of complex carbohydrates are called for, since these are absorbed more slowly than simple sugars. Low levels of dietary fat, especially saturated fat, decrease rates of atherosclerosis and gangrene in diabetic populations (West, 1980). Refined carbohydrates, which are rapidly absorbed, produce transient increases in glycemia and glycosuria, and make control of blood sugar difficult. Very high intakes of dietary fiber are recommended by some experts because of the serum cholesterol–lowering effects of high amounts of soluble fibers and the favorable effects of high amounts of insoluble fibers on normalizing blood glucose levels, but in general gradual and moderate increases in fiber obtained from natural foods are most appropriate for the aged.

Aged diabetics are particularly good candidates for secondary-prevention measures. They are especially prone to hypoglycemic reactions after taking insulin or oral hypoglycemic agents and often develop hyperosmolar nonketotic coma (Podolsky & El Behari, 1984). Many aged diabetics are also receiving long-term therapy with potassium-wasting thiazide diuretics and are at risk of hypoglycemia. If they become potassium depleted, their hyperglycemia can worsen. Therefore, either alternative medications that do not waste potassium should be used or at least 40 mEq per day of potassium from sources like oranges, apricots, bananas, supplements such as artificially sweetened potassium chloride, or waxy matrix potassium chloride tablets should be provided to the aged diabetic (Podolsky & El Behari, 1984). For the aged who do not like or cannot tolerate fruits, potassium supplements are mandatory.

## Alcohol

Alcohol is both a drug and a food and provides substantial amounts of energy. It is widely abused by individuals of all ages today. Among the aged its abuse is especially easy, the risks of intoxication from a given dose of alcohol being elevated because lean body mass and total body water decrease with age. The consequence is that the total volume of distribution of alcohol is smaller and peak blood alcohol levels are higher than in younger individuals (Vestal et al., 1975).

CLINICAL IMPLICATIONS

*Alcohol Abuse.* Greater physiological sensitivity to the effects of alcohol and greater psychological vulnerability to alcohol abuse because of depression, loneliness, and lack of meaningful social roles, combine to raise the risk of alcohol abuse among the aged. Alcohol use should be avoided entirely among the aged who have known organic brain disease, any disease that requires medication with psychoactive drugs, or a previous history of alcohol abuse, or who suffer from chronic and extreme depression, loneliness, or despair.

Moderate alcohol use (e.g., one or two drinks a day) is pleasant and often helpful as a socializing influence among the aged. Alcohol in moderation is an appetite stimulant, enhancing the taste of food. It may increase HDL cholesterol levels, thereby lowering the risk of atherosclerosis. Also, among the aged, moderate alcohol intake is associated with lowered rates of congestive heart failure (Alderman & Coltart, 1982). However, consumption of more than two drinks a day may increase high blood pressure. Since their energy intakes are already low, however, care must be taken to ensure that calories from alcohol do not displace other items in the diet that provide not only energy but protein, vitamins, and minerals. For this reason, and to minimize potential for abuse, one drink (approximately 100–200 cal) per day is probably a wise limit.

## Fiber

There is no RDA for dietary fiber. However, the Dietary Guidelines for Americans and several other sets of recommendations such as those published by the National Cancer Institute and the Diet, Nutrition and Cancer Committee of the National Academy of Sciences, suggest substantial increases in fiber intake to 20 or 30 gm per day or more. The rationale is that, in addition to sure benefits with respect to laxation, risks for certain forms of cancer, such as colon cancer, may be reduced by high-fiber diets.

CLINICAL IMPLICATIONS

*Laxation.* Two problems of the aged that can be alleviated in part by increased dietary fiber intake are atonic constipation and diverticular disease of the colon. The dietary fiber intake of the aged is often quite low. Some aged people avoid raw vegetables and whole grain breads and cereals, which are rich sources of fiber, because they have difficulty chewing; others live in nursing homes where these may not be served. Gradual increases in dietary fiber intakes to 25 to 40 g/day, coupled with liberal fluid intakes, often bring relief from constipation and may also decrease the frequency of flare-ups of diverticular disease. The mechanism for these effects is thought to operate by prevention of spasms in the muscles of the colon, which can give rise to both disorders. Such dietary alterations may be especially helpful in the aged who are housebound, institutionalized, and immobile. Otherwise, constipation problems may be severe and lead to an unnecessary dependence on laxatives, and it is clear that laxatives are too frequently used by the aged (Fanelli & Kaufman, 1985). In addition to their expense and disruption of normal bowel function, they may interact with other medications the aged must take, causing adverse drug reactions.

Increasing intakes of dietary fiber can be achieved by the use of more whole grain breads and cereals, potatoes, and raw fruits and vegetables. Dietary fiber supplements such as bran may also be advisable for patients who dislike vegetables and fruits. However, they should be accompanied by plenty of water or other fluids.

Those who suffer from hiatus hernia or irritable bowel syndrome need to have their tolerance to dietary fiber carefully monitored.

*Colon-Rectal Cancers and Other Diseases.* Evidence from cross-country studies and some clinical epidemiology studies suggests that dietary fiber may lessen symptomatology in diverticular disease of the colon in some individuals and perhaps also decrease colon cancer rates. These leads deserve to be tested (Committee on Diet and Health, 1989). As yet, they are not proven. Also of interest are recent observations that water-soluble dietary fibers lower serum cholesterol by approximately 3 to 5% (National Cholesterol Education Program, 1989).

## *Iron*

The current RDA for iron is 10 mg/day for individuals 51 years and older. Iron is a mineral for which needs decline with age among females, since after menopause iron is no longer lost through menstrual bleeding and childbearing. Now that postmenopausal estrogen replacement therapy is common, some bleeding with artificially induced menses does ensue, but this is much lower than among healthy menstruating women.

Although the aged require less iron, there is some evidence that the efficiency of iron absorption may decrease with age. This results from the presence of atrophic gastritis, with less hydrochloric acid available to reduce nonheme iron (i.e., iron present in the oxidized or ferric form) to an absorbable (ferrous) form (Freiman & Johnston, 1963). Decreased iron absorption among the aged is also due to the frequent use of antacids, calcium supplements, and tea, all of which form complexes with iron in the gut and make absorption more difficult. Some aged people decrease their intakes of red meat and other animal-flesh foods rich in highly bioavailable heme iron because of dental difficulties or limited incomes. Instead, they rely on plant foods, which are generally lower in bioavailable iron. Since the absorption of heme iron is close to 20%, while that of nonheme iron rarely rises above 5%, such dietary changes have the net effect of decreasing bioavailability. Some aged people also decrease their intakes of foods rich in ascorbic acid, thereby decreasing intakes of ascorbic acid and amino acids, two enhancers of iron absorption. Finally, some elderly people simply have very low dietary intakes of iron.

CLINICAL IMPLICATIONS

*Anemia.* Concerns about iron in the aged usually focus on its role in the blood and the part it plays in causing anemia. Evidence that iron deficiency or other anemias are normal outcomes of the aging process is weak. Experimental animal models do not show that aging is accompanied by anemia, although hematopoeitic reserve capacity, or the time it takes for hematocrit (volume of packed red blood cells) to recover after a stress such as phlebotomy (blood drawing) is increased (Lipschitz, Udupa, Milton, & Thompson, 1984). However, in human beings reductions in hematocrit that are not associated with dietary deficiency, chronic disease, or blood loss but rather with an abnormality in cellular proliferation, sometimes exist (Lipschitz et al., 1984). Anemias due to other causes are also common. Indeed, in contrast to popular belief, iron deficiency anemia is not the sole nor even the major cause of anemia in the aged. In addition to iron deficiency, nutritional anemias also result from deficiencies in ascorbic acid, vitamin $B_6$, vitamin $B_{12}$, folic acid, and protein-calorie malnutrition (Lipschitz & Mitchell, 1982). Hemolytic anemias and those due to chronic infection are the most common.

In spite of decreased losses of iron in the aged, many other factors increase risks of anemia in both sexes. Most groups in the United States meet the recommended iron intakes, except low-income black women, who have low intakes. However, because the aged eat less meat and no more ascorbic acid than younger individuals, the bioavailability of iron in their diets may be lower and is certainly not higher than in younger populations. Also, achlorhydria, malabsorption, and partial or total gastrectomy may decrease iron absorption. Blood losses may also be elevated through alcohol abuse, frequent use of aspirin, infection, ulcers, neoplasms, and renal and other diseases. Thus, any instance of anemia has a cause that should be explored; it should not be considered normal in aging (Garry, Goodwin, & Hunt, 1983).

Iron deficiency anemia is not epidemic among the aged, although some individuals are clearly at increased risk. In recent national population–based surveys, the prevalence of iron deficiency anemia, as measured by transferrin saturation levels below 16, was below 10% in all age groups, except for black women aged 65 to 74 years, who had levels of nearly 10% in NHANES I and 15% in NHANES II as well as the lowest dietary intakes of iron (Singer et al., 1982; Fulwood et al., 1982). Moreover, in both men and women, a smaller proportion of those over 65 were anemic compared with younger adults.

In addition to microcytic hypochromic anemias associated with iron deficiency, blood loss, and infection, there is evidence of megaloblastic anemias, which are occasionally apparent in certain high-risk groups because of folic acid deficiency. Included in this high-risk group are low-income people who rarely eat raw green leafy vegetables, alcoholics, and those who suffer from malabsorption (Young, 1983). Dietary intakes of folic acid often fall below the RDA of 400 µg, but biochemical evidence of folic acid deficiency is relatively rare.

## Calcium

The current RDA for calcium is 800 mg/day for those 51 years of age and older. However, a recent consensus conference suggests much higher needs on the basis of possible positive effects on bone health: 1,000 mg/day for premenopausal and postmenopausal women who are on estrogen replacement therapy, and 1,500 mg/day for those who are not (Consensus Conference, 1984).

Several factors militate against adequate calcium nutrition in the aged. Intake of calcium among the aged is low and frequently does not meet the RDA (Abraham, 1977; Carroll et al., 1983). Absorption of dietary calcium in the gut is poor (Bullamore, Gallagher, Wilkinson, & Nordin, 1970), and the ability to adapt to a low-calcium diet after a high-calcium diet decreases with age (Ireland & Fordtran, 1973). There are several possible explanations. Decreased sensitivity to parathyroid hormone decreases renal production of $1,25(OH)_2D_3$, which decreases serum $1,25(OH)_2D_3$ levels, ultimately decreasing calcium absorption from the gut (Armbrecht, 1984). Since passive absorption accounts for only half of the calcium absorbed by the gut, and the active transport process of calcium absorption requires $1,25(OH)_2D_3$ (calcitrol), decreases in this vitamin reduce absorption by 25% to 35% in early adulthood and by 20% to 30% in middle age (Heaney, 1986). Thus, dietary calcium absorbed by the gut contributes less to the maintenance of serum calcium, and bone is resorbed to maintain serum calcium. A final factor that increases the risk of poor calcium nutrition is the presence of protein in large amounts in the diet, which increases urinary calcium losses (Johnson, Alcantara, & Linksweiler, 1970), and the presence of high levels of phosphorus, which increases calcium fecal losses (Draper, Sie, & Bergen, 1974).

### CLINICAL IMPLICATIONS

*Osteoporosis, Bone Health, and Hypertension.* From what we know today, the most important influences on the amount of bone individuals possess are genetic and mechanical factors, not nutritional and hormonal influences.

Blacks have heavier skeletons throughout life than do whites and adapt better to lower calcium intakes. Individuals who engage in heavy mechanical work or rigorous athletics also have heavier bones. These appear to be due to more efficient calcium absorption and lower urinary calcium losses.

Although genetics and mechanical factors are the most potent determinants of bone mass, one can do little to change these factors. Diet and hormonal influences, however, are easier to manipulate, so they are currently receiving a great deal of attention.

Dietary calcium is thought to affect bone mass in two ways. Calcium intake during childhood and early adulthood influences whether the genetically determined amount of peak bone mass (reached at about 25 years of age) is achieved. Intakes thereafter minimize age-related decreases in bone mass. Since women have smaller skeletal mass to begin with, and their rate of bone loss with age is more rapid than men, they are more likely to exhibit age-related bone loss (Avioli, 1977).

Nutrients other than calcium also affect calcium utilization. Protein has profound effects on urinary calcium levels and on calcium nutrition, a doubling of dietary protein increasing urinary calcium by 50%. Since the kidney filters as much as 10 gm of calcium per day, these differences may be of great consequence in calcium metabolism (Heaney & Recker, 1982). Protein increases the obligatory renal loss of calcium — its sulphur-containing amino acids are oxidized to sulfate during metabolism, and the sulfates are eliminated by a compensatory decrease in the tubular reabsorption of calcium. Moreover, on high-protein intakes, the filtered load of calcium increases. Even in the presence of large amounts of phosphorus in the diet, its well-known effect of decreasing urinary calcium is not enough to prevent protein's negative effect, since high dietary phosphorus also increases calcium loss through digestive secretions (Heaney & Recker, 1982; Heaney, 1986). Therefore, the aged who eat high-protein diets have higher calcium requirements.

Sodium also increases urinary calcium loss at the tubular level (Heaney, 1986), and very high levels of dietary fiber in the diet may affect the absorption of calcium. However, 20 to 30 gm of dietary fiber per day has little effect. Both dietary fiber itself and the phytic acid (which is often associated with the bran portion of cereals) decrease calcium absorption. Oxalic acid in rhubarb and spinach also decreases calcium absorption.

Caffeine increases both the amount of calcium secreted in digestive juice and renal calcium losses — a cup of coffee probably increases it by about 8 mg, which would require a 25 to 30 mg increase in calcium intake to compensate for it. Alcohol increases urinary calcium losses as well. At very high levels, alcohol may have an adverse effect on bone cell metabolism.

Commonly used drugs that increase the need for calcium include aluminum-containing antacids, which in turn decrease phosphorus absorption, thus lowering plasma phosphorus; lower plasma phosphorus ultimately increases calcium excretion (Spencer & Lender, 1979). On the other hand, thiazide diuretics decrease calcium needs by decreasing urinary calcium losses and may have a positive effect on bone mass (Wasnich, Benfante, Yanok Heilbrun, & Vogel, 1983).

Diseases that damage kidney or endocrine function can profoundly affect calcium nutrition, since 10 gm or more of calcium per day are filtered by the glomerulus, the filtering unit of the kidney. In good health, most of this is reabsorbed in the renal tubules under the influence of parathyroid hormone. Gastrointestinal diseases that inhibit the reabsorption of this 150 mg or more of endogenous calcium (which enters the gut via sloughed cells and digestive-juice secretions as well as dietary calcium) can cause a net loss of calcium from the body.

One significant hormonal event that influences calcium nutrition is the menopause. Estrogens increase calcium absorption and decrease renal losses, so that on the same calcium intake, the estrogen-replete female utilizes dietary calcium better. Postmenopausal estrogen replacement therapy is helpful in preventing negative calcium balance and osteoporosis. Growth hormones and hormonal events such as pregnancy also increase absorption and decrease renal losses.

Populations consuming less than the RDA of calcium have slightly lower bone masses than do those on high intakes, but studies vary, and, in most cases, the differences are rather small (Garn, Solomon, & Freidl, 1981; Matkovic et al., 1979; Smith & Frame,

1965). If dietary calcium intakes are increased, greater net amounts of calcium are absorbed, even in the aged (Spencer, 1984). Increased calcium intake may also decrease bone resorption (Nordin, Morsman, & Gallagher, 1975).

Median intakes of calcium are much lower than the RDA for women at most ages after 12, although intakes approach reference standards for men (Abraham, 1977; Carroll et al., 1983). After age 50, women's daily median intake hovers around 500 mg, as opposed to the RDA of 800 mg. At these intakes, most middle-aged and aged women will be chronically deficient in calcium and in danger of losing bone (Heaney et al., 1978).

Recent studies of calcium needs among aging women indicate that mean requirements for calcium balance range from about 800 to 1,200 mg or more per day, levels much above the existing RDA (Heaney, 1982). Moreover, previous studies of calcium balance among the middle-aged and aged may have underestimated needs. In most studies, after changing the calcium intakes of subjects, insufficient time was allowed to elapse for bone remodeling rates to reach a new equilibrium. Since bone remodeling rates change slowly, it takes 3 to 6 months or more to observe the true effects of alterations in calcium intake on bone remodeling and ultimately bone mass. Calcium supplements temporarily change bone remodeling rates, and calcium balances transiently seem to be less negative or even positive simply as a result of the increased intake and decreased loss. At present, we do not know what this long-term steady state is because the long-term results of calcium supplementation have not been studied (Heaney, 1986).

The rationale for increasing calcium intakes among menopausal women and those who are within a few years of the menopause is that most but not all intervention studies have shown that intakes of 750 to 1,000 mg/day decrease the rates of cortical, long-bone loss among women who are 5 to 20 years postmenopausal (Freudenheim, Johnson, & Smith, 1986; Santora, 1987; Dawson-Hughes, 1986; Schaafsma et al., 1987; Riggs & Melton, 1986). In contrast, the rate of loss of trabecular bone (woven bone found in the central skeleton) and overall bone density do not appear to be affected by increased calcium intakes, especially in the early stages of menopause (Ruis et al., 1987; Ettinger et al., 1987). It is also important to ensure that vitamin D intakes are adequate.

However, the optimal amount of calcium needed to reduce bone loss is not yet known with certitude. The NIH's Consensus (1984) recommendations represent expert judgment. It is increasingly apparent that people differ in the amount of calcium they need to maintain bone mass, and that factors other than diet are also involved. For example, in early postmenopausal women, when a high-calcium intake (e.g., 1,500 mg) is combined with estrogen therapy, the estrogen required to prevent bone loss may be reduced (Ettinger, Genant, & Cann, 1987). Yet, estrogen therapy is more effective than calcium in preventing the accelerated loss of cortical bone (Riis, Thomsen, & Christiansen, 1987). Therefore, increased intake of calcium should be combined with, rather than substituted for, estrogen. The concerns some women have about estrogen causing increased risk of endometrial or breast cancer are legitimate. Use of estrogen-progesterone combinations appears to lower risks of endometrial cancers. As yet, the possibility that use of these estrogens is associated with increased breast cancers is being debated.

In addition to being a useful prophylaxis for some types of age-related bone loss, large doses of calcium in combination with vitamin D, fluoride, and hormones (Recker, Saville, & Heaney, 1977; Nordin et al., 1980) are being tested for their utility in treating symptomatic osteoporosis. The rationale is that large doses of calcium suppress parathyroid hormone, and thus bone remodeling rates slow down. Also, it is thought that the carbonate or phosphate anions accompanying the calcium may themselves have a positive effect upon bone metabolism (Heaney, 1986). The problem is that, when parathyroid hormone levels fall, the percentage of calcium absorbed in the gut also falls precipitously. Thus, very large (e.g., 2,000–8,000 mg) doses of calcium may be required.

It is clear that it is difficult to replace bone tissue once it is lost. Therapeutic regimens designed to do so involve very large doses of vitamin D, calcium, and other treatments that require careful medical supervision and should not be undertaken on one's own. The failure of dose levels of 1,500 mg of calcium to reduce the spurt of bone loss at menopause (Nilas et al., 1984) or among individuals who are immobilized in bed (Hantman et al., 1973) may be due to a true lack of effect or to insufficient dose. Possibly, there are many different forms of osteoporosis, only some of which respond to calcium treatment. Indeed, results to date suggest that the "senile osteoporosis" of old age, which is thought to be due to an intrinsic or possibly acquired defect in calcium absorption, is more amenable to calcium prophylaxis than in postmenopausal osteoporosis, which responds better to combination therapies including estrogen as well as calcium.

There is no cure for symptomatic osteoporosis, but partial relief can be had by taking several measures. First, a comprehensive general rehabilitation program that includes greater physical activity, spine stretching, and abdominal-strengthening exercises is employed in the hope that, by raising mechanical stress on bones, resorption rates will decrease. Increased muscle tone maximizes function and minimizes postural changes. Second, the use of various combinations of calcium, estrogen, vitamin D, and sodium fluoride may help in halting bone loss but cannot increase bone mass, unless they are begun within 3 to 6 years after the menopause (Aloia et al., 1982; Briancon & Meunier, 1981; Gallagher & Riggs, 1978). Both estrogen and calcium seem to be most effective in the early years after the menopause, whereas doses 6 or more years later have relatively little effect (Riggs et al., 1982). Usual dose levels are conjugated equine estrogen (0.625 mg/day) or ethinyl estradiol (20 mg/day).

Although calcium supplementation and estrogen replacement are currently suggested for postmenopausal women, the increased risk of endometrial cancer associated with estrogen use make ongoing gynecological monitoring mandatory (Shapiro et al., 1985; Hammond et al., 1979). The use of progestational agents, such as Premarin 0.685 mg/day for 1 to 25 days and Provera 70 mg/day on days 15 and 25, decrease this risk.

A relatively high intake of calcium (e.g., 1,000–1,500 mg/day) may also be helpful in decreasing blood pressures in hypertension (Karanja and McCarron, 1986; Villar, Repke, and Belizan, 1986). It is theorized this is either through its effect on phosphate metabolism or a sodium dependent effect on the cell membranes of vascular smooth muscle. Hypertensive patients who have low plasma renin activity, low serum ionized calcium levels, and a sodium sensitive hypertension may be especially helped by calcium supplements (Resnick, 1985). Intervention studies using calcium intakes of 1,000–1,500 mg/day are generally but not uniformly positive, with small but significant effects seen on systolic blood pressure especially in men and in hypertensives after several months of increased calcium intake (McCarron & Morris, 1985; Strazzullo et al., 1986).

Still speculative but intriguing is the influence of calcium in relatively large doses on colonic cell proliferation, which may be of significance in colon cancer risk.

In summary, there are several reasons for assuming that intake of calcium larger than the RDA may be beneficial for many of the aged, especially women. Increased calcium intake to at least 1,000 to 1,500 mg/day (depending on estrogen status), increased physical exercise involving the weight-bearing bones (such as walking or jogging), and not smoking are all advisable. Although several studies show some promise for the treatment of osteoporosis, results are not yet consistent enough for any one treatment regimen to be regarded as definitive (Recker et al., 1977; Nordin et al., 1980).

## Sodium

The Estimated Safe and Adequate Allowances for sodium encompasses a range of 1,100 to 3,300 mg/day, and this is not thought to vary with age. However, the sodium intake of most Americans greatly exceeds this, and the Dietary Guidelines for Americans suggest a reduction in dietary sodium intake, mainly because excessive intake is unnecessary and some individuals respond with increased blood pressure. Fortunately, most of the aged are able to maintain serum sodium levels within normal limits over a wide range of intake (e.g., 1–8 gm of salt per day) and neither hypernatremia nor hyponatremia often ensues. Hypernatremia manifests itself among the aged with net water loss because they are bedfast and unable to drink when thirsty or are denied water, or because sensation of thirst is decreased by impaired CNS function. Hyponatremia frequently is due to inappropriately prescribed or consumed diuretics (Fichman et al., 1971); dilutional hyponatremia (with water retention exceeding sodium retention) in edematous states such as congestive heart failure, hepatic cirrhosis, and renal disease; a syndrome of inappropriate secretion of antidiuretic hormone as is seen in malignancies, congestive heart failure, cirrhosis, nephrotic syndrome, renal failure, and pulmonary disease; and the ingestion of certain drugs such as sulfonylureas, thiazides, and antitumor agents (Lindeman, 1986).

### CLINICAL IMPLICATIONS

*Hypertension.* Diastolic blood pressure declines and systolic pressure increases with age, probably because of reduced blood vessel compliance and changes in pulse waves. With aging, the arterial system becomes less elastic and distensible so that systolic blood pressures rise. The arteriolar bed, especially the small arteries and arterioles, becomes thickened with hyaline deposits, and peripheral vascular resistance rises. Decreased baroreceptor sensitivity makes compensations in blood pressure more difficult. The prevalence of mild or definite hypertension in individuals 65 to 74 years of age is 59% in males and 75% in females. Much of this is isolated systolic hypertension (140 mmHg or more). The reason for concern is that elevated blood pressure increases cardiovascular disease by two- to threefold. Thus 30% to 60% of all cardiovascular disease among the aged is due to hypertension, and it often leads to target organ damage, especially stroke (Harris et al., 1985; Shea et al., 1985).

Systolic blood pressure is the best predictor of later cardiovascular events among the aged, and interventions to control it are currently being tested. Data are already available that show that control of diastolic hypertension and combined systolic and diastolic hypertension in the aged can reduce cardiovascular complications and stroke dramatically (Veterans Administration Cooperative Study Group on Antihypertensive Agents, 1972; National Heart Foundation of Australia, 1981; Hypertension Detection, 1979).

Several diet-related steps are recommended. Reduction of overweight can be helpful. Even relatively small losses reduce cardiac output and plasma norephinephrine values, with a consequent lowering in blood pressure (Havlik et al., 1983). Moderate sodium restriction to 75 to 100 mmol per day may also help individuals who have high blood pressures and low renin values (Kannel, 1986). Exercise can also be encouraged among those without significant atherosclerotic disease who are suffering from mild hypertension without end-organ damage. For those with severe hypertension and significant atherosclerotic disease, drug therapy is in order. Because many of the aged react poorly to antihypertensive drugs and may already be taking many other medications, drug choice and dosage schedules should be individualized. The use of "step care" with various graduated combinations of diet and drugs, starting with the most benign, may help to maximize the lowering of blood pressure while minimizing side effects, vascular insufficiency, and side effects altering the quality of life, such as dizziness, exhaustion, and impotence (Chobanian, 1983; National Heart, Lung and Blood Institute, 1981; National High Blood Pressure Education Program, 1982).

Dietary measures that appear to be the most helpful in reducing blood pressures among the elderly are weight reduction and sodium restriction. Other dietary measures, such as potassium supplementation to decrease sodium-to-potassium ratios, increased calcium or magnesium intake, decreased fat intake, and increased polyunsaturated fat intake have also been suggested to decrease blood pressure, but the effects are not as large or as consistent as the modifications in weight and sodium intake.

### Vitamin D

Vitamin D deficiency is defined biochemically as levels of calcitrol (25 (OH)D$_3$) below 3.8 $\mu$g/ml. Among the institutionalized and housebound aged in the British Isles who do not take vitamin D supplements, this biochemical indicator of vitamin D deficiency is relatively prevalent (McKenna et al., 1985; Vir & Love, 1979). In northern climates in the United States, low intakes of vitamin D may also be a problem in winter.

CLINICAL IMPLICATIONS

*Osteomalacia.* In this country osteomalacia, or undermineralized bone, sometimes contributes to the increased incidence of fractures among the aged (Jenkins et al., 1973; Slovik et al., 1981). However, because several foods are fortified with vitamin D in the United States, intakes of the vitamin are higher and deficiencies somewhat rarer than in the United Kingdom, where such foods are not widely available (Jenkins et al., 1973; Baker, Peacock, & Nordin, 1980). Nevertheless, they do exist. The causes of osteomalacia include vitamin D disturbances because of inadequate exposure to sunlight, use of sunblocks or sunscreen lotions, dietary deficiency, and altered absorption or metabolism of the vitamin resulting from disease. Also, kidney disease, familial inborn errors of hypophosphatemia, and tumors may be involved. A daily dose of 600 to 800 IU (15–20 $\mu$g) to the institutionalized aged can prevent osteomalacia due to vitamin D deficiency.

The housebound and those with malabsorption syndromes need special surveillance and treatment with supplements.

## Other Nutrients

Nutrient recommendations for the aged are listed in Table 6.2. Frank clinical deficiencies of nutrients in the United States are rare. When they do exist, they cluster among individuals who eat very little, who are suffering simultaneously from a disease, or who are extremely eccentric in their choice of foods. In most surveys, inadequate intakes of vitamins and minerals are associated with limited food consumption, sometimes caused by poverty, but probably more frequently by physical inactivity and associated very low energy intakes, disease, or depression with anorexia (Bidlack, Kirsch, & Meskin, 1986). Energy intakes for ages 51 to 75 are usually only 90% of those recommended for younger adults, and for ages over 75 only 75% to 80%. Yet recommended intakes of vitamins and minerals do not decline with age. Thus, in order to meet the recommended levels the diet must be higher in nutrient density (i.e., vitamins and minerals per calorie).

Many studies of the vitamin and mineral nutrition of the aged have revealed that mean or median dietary intake is below the RDA (Bidlack, et al., 1986). Whether these shortfalls in dietary intakes and altered biochemical indices are of functional significance, or whether supplementation is helpful, is not clear. From the clinical perspective, it is reasonable to recommend a multivitamin-multimineral supplement that provides RDA levels of nutrients if the individual is at risk.

## SOURCES OF NUTRIENTS IN DIETS OF THE AGED

### Food Sources of Nutrients

In planning to meet the nutrition needs of the aged, all of the following factors must be considered (Institute of Food Technologists, 1986):

- Nutrient profiles must be tailored to meet needs of the aged. The diet is lower in calories, especially in fat, and higher in nutrient density. Nutrients should be in forms that are highly bioavailable, and sufficient fluid must be included in the diet to permit normal laxation.

- The food must meet energy needs of the aged and maintain desirable weight.

- Therapeutic adjustments must be incorporated. For example, any adjustment necessary for therapeutic purposes need to be included, such as decreased sodium or increased fiber.

- Supplementation, if necessary, should be appropriate and not excessive. Unless prescribed by a physician, supplementation should not exceed the U.S. RDA. Aged women may require calcium supplements of 1,000 to 1,500 mg/day. Homebound aged who rarely go outdoors, who avoid milk products, or who use sunscreens on their skin may need 400 IU of a vitamin D supplement.

- Foods should appeal to the senses as well. Color, texture, odor, and taste need to be enhanced, since visual and gustatory acuity are decreased in the aged.

- Convenience should also be considered. Reading labels, storage, opening, preparation, and cleanup all become difficult tasks for the aged. Packaging in small quantities permits the aged person to avoid wasting food and, by allowing for greater variety in food servings, prevents dietary monotony. Toaster ovens, microwave ovens, and timers may be helpful devices for the elderly.

- The cost of food must be low enough to be affordable by those on limited budgets.

### Fluids

Fluids as well as solid foods are essential. Approximately 1.5 qt of water or other fluid of any type other than alcohol per day is a reasonable goal to strive for in the aged.

### Vitamin-Mineral Supplements

Because energy intakes decrease greatly among the aged, if recommended levels of vitamins and minerals are to be met, dietary quality needs to be higher in the elderly than it is at younger ages. A vitamin-mineral supplement providing 100% of the U.S. RDA can be helpful. Use of supplements is currently high among the aged, although those who use them are not necessarily those with the lowest dietary intakes (Hartz & Blumberg, 1986).

CALCIUM SUPPLEMENTS. It is difficult for most postmenopausal women to obtain 1,000 to 1,500 mg of calcium daily from food sources. This is especially true for the aged, given their low energy intake. Therefore, for most individuals a combination of food sources and a calcium supplement are helpful.

The richest food sources of calcium are milk and milk products. Recently, some of these products have been fortified with additional calcium. This mineral has also been added to a variety of other foods that do not normally contain it, such as orange juice, some cereals, and soft drinks, or that naturally contain only very low amounts. The bioavailability of the calcium in these products varies, but they are usually costly.

A very large number of calcium supplements are now sold over the counter in drugstores and supermarkets, but the safety of some of these products is questionable. Specifically, dolomite, bone meal, and calcium supplements taken in conjunction with megadoses of vitamin D (e.g., 10,000 IU per day are of dubious nutritional benefit. A mineral formed naturally in the earth, dolomite contains significant amounts of calcium carbonate (about 22% by weight) but also a variable mixture of other minerals such as magnesium, lead, uranium, arsenic, and cadmium. Some of these may have adverse effects upon health, and in any event no rationale for consuming them has been established. In addition, dolomite preparations are often expensive and also are not recommended for this reason. Bone meal consists of ground bone from animals, often elderly animals whose bones contain varying but frequently significant amounts of calcium phosphate (usually about 17% by weight). Bone meal also contains environmental contaminants, including heavy metals, such as lead and arsenic. Because bone meal products are not standardized, pure products, they too should be avoided.

Some physicians and many laypersons have become confused by reports of cures of osteomalacia among the aged living in northerly countries, and of experimental treatments of symptomatic osteoporosis that use very large doses of vitamin D. As a result, in addition to taking calcium supplements, some persons take separate vitamin D supplements in very large doses (e.g., 50,000 or more IU of vitamin D per week) or increase their dosage of vitamin D–containing calcium supplements to reach such levels. Neither of these procedures is advisable. Vitamin D toxicity can occur at intake levels of 10,000 IU per week. Very large amounts of calcium also pose problems, both in decreasing the absorption of other minerals and in increasing the risk of kidney stones among those predisposed to that condition. The aged who are suspect of suffering from vitamin D deficiency need evaluation (Parfitt et al., 1982). Prophylactic use of megadose supplements of vitamin D should be avoided. Calcium supplements with modest amounts of vitamin D (e.g., 400–800 IU per day) are probably safe, but unless the individual receives little or no vitamin D from sunlight or other food sources, the vitamin D is unlikely to provide any additional benefits over a calcium supplement alone.

An optimal calcium supplement is not contaminated, even if natural; dissolves quickly so as to facilitate absorption in the gut; is inexpensive; has a relatively high percentage of calcium by weight to minimize the amount that must be taken; is palatable; and is easy to ingest (Heaney, 1986). Examples of acceptable calcium supplements include calcium carbonate or phosphate salts, calcium salts of hexose carboxylic acids, calcium lactate complexes and chelates, effervescent tablets to be dissolved in water before ingestion, calcium gluconate, and calcium supplements in syrup for those who have difficulty swallowing pills.

Calcium preparations containing other anions generally provide less calcium by weight than does calcium carbonate. They range from 9% to 29% calcium. Although some persons may find these preparations more palatable because of their calcium density, they must be taken in considerable quantity, and this may adversely affect compliance.

The least expensive preparations are calcium carbonate in the form of generic oyster-shell calcium, chalk, or calcium-containing antacids. They all provide about 40% calcium by weight. Brand-name products are generally higher in price, although they are no different from the other calcium carbonate products from a chemical or physiological standpoint.

Persons at high risk of renal calculus should be cautioned against using high doses of calcium. Also, individuals who suffer from achlorhydria may absorb calcium poorly and require higher dose levels.

VITAMIN D SUPPLEMENTS. A multivitamin containing 400 IU of vitamin D per day or, if the individual is housebound, perhaps as much as 800 IU will prevent osteomalacia due to vitamin D deficiency. Vitamin D supplements as high as 10,000 IU per day have been used for treating osteomalacia after it has been identified by bone biopsy, but this treatment should never be undertaken by individuals on their own, and recent evidence suggests it is inefficacious.

## *Federal Food Assistance Programs*

Excellent information is now available on the effect of community nutrition services on the aged (Smiciklas-Wright & Fosmire, 1985; Fanelli & Kaufman, 1985). Both group-care and health-care facilities provide food and nutrition services for the aged.

MEALS FOR THE AGED. Under the auspices of the Older Americans Act, the federal government's Administration on Aging provides congregate and home-delivered meals to over 2.5 million Americans 65 years of age and older. Among those who participate in the "Meals on Wheels" program for the homebound aged, many are also poor and have multiple diseases, and suffer from a relatively high prevalence of nutritional deficiencies that could be corrected by provision of adequate food and nutritional supplements (Lipschitz et al., 1984).

At a minimum, the meals provide a third of the RDA, and in this sense are helpful in sustaining the nutrition of the aged. In addition, the regular visits to deliver meals to the homebound elderly provide an opportunity for social interaction, and may increase food intakes as well as improve the quality of life. The elderly who attend congregate meals tend to be healthier than those receiving home-delivered services. Besides furnishing substantial amounts of daily nutrient intakes, congregate meals permit the elderly to socialize, and they can be screened at the location of the meals for referral to other services (see Chapter 9, Work, Productivity, and Worth in Old Age).

FOOD STAMPS. The federal food stamp program is available for the aged poor. Only about 30% of the aged now participate. Although the program benefits amount to only about $60 per month, in the form of coupons to increase food purchasing power, this extra food money can be of great help in increasing diet quality. At present, many eligible, aged people fail to apply for or use this program (Villers Foundation, 1986). These issues are discussed in greater depth in Chapter 13, The Economics of the Health-Care System: Financing Health Care for the Aged Person.

FOOD AND NUTRITION SERVICES FOR THE AGED IN GROUP CARE AND HEALTH-CARE FACILITIES. The aged who reside in group-care or health-care facilities are in especially fragile health and often have special nutritional needs or feeding requirements. To participate in Medicare and Medicaid, institutions must maintain certain standards with respect to food and nutrition services to obtain certification and licensure. While ensuring that these standards are met, dietary and institutional consultants can plan and implement more extensive nutrition services as necessary, including formulation of appropriate menus that meet the RDA and therapeutic diet needs, extension of dining-room facilities, feeding assistance, and implementatation of food safety regulations (Fanelli & Kaufman, 1985).

## SPECIAL FEEDING

### *Tube Feeding*

Long-term tube feeding is indicated for aged patients with no irreversible, life-threatening problems, who have an acceptable quality of life, and when the family (or the patient, if capable) wants such feedings (Lo & Dorenbrand, 1986). From the nutritional stand-point, feeding by nasogastric tube, gastrostomy, or jejunostomy is technically feasible, and patients can be kept in excellent nutritional status. The formulas that are fed usually consist of milk- or soy-based mixtures, with vitamins, minerals, and dietary fiber added. Many different formulations are available, depending on energy intake, protein require-ments, and other patient needs. Special feeding routes are often needed because of surgery or other conditions that preclude feeding by mouth. For a full discussion of the many ethical issues involved in tube feeding, see Chapter 11, Legal Issues in the Care of the Aged.

### *Hyperalimentation*

Parenteral routes of alimentation are usually employed for short-term, acute health prob-lems in the elderly. Both central and peripheral veins can be utilized, and good nutri-tional status can be maintained. However, the procedure is stressful and expensive and should only be undertaken after consultation with experts in clinical nutrition. The con-tent of these feedings consists of the simplest form of nutrients, one similar to that of nutrients in usual diets after digestion and absorption.

The economic costs of these feeding methods are substantial, and the methods are not pleasant for the patient. The legal and ethical implications of withholding special enteral or parenteral alimentation once it has been started are also considerable (see Chapter 10, Ethical Issues at the End of Life).

## CONCLUSION

Greater attention must be paid to the promotion of health, prevention of disease, and maintenance of quality of life and independent functioning in the elderly by nutritional and other means. Table 6.3 outlines specific goals in these areas for the year 2000, all of which will be advanced by good nutrition.

TABLE 6.3  Summary Table of Objectives to Maintain
the Vitality and Independence of Older People

By the year 2000 . . .

*Health Status Improvement*

1.  Increase average life expectancy (years of healthy life expected) at age 65 to at least 14 years for men and 16 years for women. (Baseline: An estimated 12 years for men and 13.7 years for women at age 65 in 1986)
2.  Reduce the proportion of noninstitutionalized people age 65 or older who report needing assistance in two or more personal-care activities to no more than 30 per 1,000. (Baseline: 40.6 per 1,000 in 1984)
Special Population Target:
Among people age 85 and older: 120 per 1,000. (Baseline: 140.2 per 1,000 in 1984)
3.  Reduce the incidence of adverse drug reactions among people age 65 and older to no more than 8.5 per 100,000. (Baseline: An estimated 17 per 100,000 in 1986)
4.  Reduce suicide deaths among men age 65 and older to no more than 41 per 100,000. (Baseline: 46 per 100,000 in 1986)
5.  Reduce hip fractures among people age 65 and older to no more than 650 per 100,000 people. (Base-line: 748 per 100,000 in 1986)

Special Population Target:

Among white women age 85 and older: 2,380 per 100,000. (Baseline: 2,850 per 100,000 in 1986)

6.   Reduce influenza-associated deaths among people age 65 and older to no more than 40 per 100,000 people. (Baseline: 70 per 100,000 in 1987)

7.   Reduce pneumonia-related days of restricted activity among people age 65 and older to no more than 38 days per 100 people. (Baseline: 48 days per 100 people in 1987)

8.   Reduce certified heat-related deaths to no more than 150. (Baseline: 373 in 1986)

*Risk Reduction*

9.   Increase to at least 75% the proportion of people age 65 and older with urinary incontinence who seek diagnosis and treatment from a health-care professional. (Baseline: An estimated 50% in 1988)

10.   Increase to at least 40% the proportion of people age 65 and older who participate in moderate physical activities 3 or more days per week for 20 min or more per occasion. (Baseline: 31 percent in 1985)

11.   Increase to at least 20% the proportion of people age 65 and older who participate in vigorous physical activities that promote the development and maintenance of cardiorespiratory fitness 3 or more days per week for 20 minutes or more per occasion. (Baseline: 15% in 1985)

12.   Increase to at least 60% the proportion of women age 50 and older who receive a clinical breast examination and a mammogram within the preceding year. (Baseline: 19% in 1987)

13.   Increase to at least 85% the proportion of women age 70 and older with an intact uterine cervix who have received a Pap smear and to 85% the proportion who received a Pap smear within the preceding year. (Baseline: 69% "ever" and 38% "in preceding year" in 1987)

*Public Awareness Enhancement*

14.   Increase to at least 50% the proportion of older smokers ages 65 through 74 who know that quitting smoking even late in life is one of the most important actions a person can take to preserve his or her health. (Baseline data unavailable)

15.   Increase to at least 75% the proportion of people at high risk for glaucoma who know they should receive regular, comprehensive eye examination. (Baseline data unavailable)

*Professional Education and Awareness*

16.   Increase to at least 50% the proportion of primary-care providers and mental health professionals who have ever received specific training in geriatrics. (Baseline data unavailable)

17.   Increase to at least 75% the proportion of primary-care providers who are able to identify risk factors for suicide — bereavement, loneliness, and low self-esteem — in older people and know how to respond appropriately. (Baseline data unavailable)

18.   Increase to at least 75% the proportion of primary-care providers who are able to recognize the early signs and symptoms of dementia in older people and determine if the dementia is potentially reversible, such as those dementias caused by drug toxicity, metabolic disorders, depression, and hypothyroidism. (Baseline data unavailable)

*Services and Protection*

19.   Increase to at least 90% the proportion of postmenopausal women at high risk for osteoporosis who have been counseled about the benefits and risks of estrogen replacement therapy (combined with progestin, when appropriate). (Baseline data unavailable)

20.   Increase to at least 30 the number of states that have design standards for signs, signals, markings, lighting, and other charactristics of the roadway environment to improve the visual stimuli and protect the safety of older drivers and pedestrians. (Baseline data unavailable)

21.   Increase to 25% the proportion of work sites with 100 or more employees that have a formal policy for family leave, allowing caregivers the flexibility to meet health needs of children and aging parents. (Baseline data unavailable)

22.   Delay by 2 years from the time of disease onset the institutionalization of people with Alzheimer's disease. (Baseline data unavailable)

# REFERENCES

Abraham, S. (1977). Dietary intake findings, United States 1971–1974. In *National Health Survey, Vital and Health Statistics, Series II, No. 202* (HRA 77-1647). Washington, DC: U.S. Department of Health, Education and Welfare, Public Health Service.

Abraham, S. (1979). Height and weight of adults (DHEW Publication No. PHS 79-1659). Washington, DC: U.S. Government Printing Office.

Abraham, S., Lowenstein, F. W., & Johnson, C. L. (1974). *Preliminary findings of the first Health and Nutrition Examination Survey, United States 1971–72: Dietary intake and biochemical findings* (DHEW Publication No. (HRA) 74-1219-1). Washington, DC: U.S. Government Printing Office.

Alderman, E., & Coltart, D. (1982). Alcohol and the heart. *British Medical Bulletin, 38,* 77.

Aloia, J. F., Zanzi, I., Vaswani, A., Ellis, K., & Cohn, S. H. (1982). Combination therapy for osteoporosis with estrogen, fluoride and calcium. *Journal of the American Geriatrics Society, 30,* 13–17.

American Diabetes Association. (1984). Glycemic effects of carbohydrates. *Diabetes Care, 7,* 607–608.

American Diabetes Association. (1979). Principles of nutrition and dietary recommendations for individuals with diabetes mellitus. *Diabetes, 28,* 1027–1030.

American Dietetic Association. (1992). *Manual of clinical dietetics.* Chicago: Author.

American Heart Association. (1978). Diet and coronary heart disease. *Circulation, 58,* 762A–766A.

Andres, R. (1980). Influence of obesity on longevity in the aged. *Advances in Pathobiology, 7,* 238.

Armbrecht, H. J. (1984). Changes in calcium and vitamin D metabolism with age. In H. J. Armbrecht, J. M. Pendergast, & R. M. Coe (Eds.), *Nutritional intervention in the aging process* (pp. 69–86). New York: Springer Verlag.

Avioli, L. V. (1977). Osteoporosis pathogenesis and therapy. In L. V. Avioli, & S. M. Krane (Eds.), *Metabolic bone disease* (Vol. 1; pp. 307–370). New York: Academic Press.

Avioli, L. V. (1984). Calcium supplementation and osteoporosis. In H. J. Armbrecht, J. M. Prendergast, & R. M. Coe (Eds.), *Nutritional intervention in the aging process* (pp. 183–190). New York: Springer Verlag.

Baker, M. R., Peacock, R., & Nordin, B. E. C. (1980). The decline in vitamin D status with age. *Age and Aging, 9,* 249.

Barry, A. J., Daly, J. W., Pruett, E. D., Steinmetz, J. R., Page, H. F., Birkhead, N. C., & Rodahl, K. (1966). The effects of physical conditioning on older individuals: 1. Work capacity, circulatory respiratory function and work electrocardiogram. *Journal of Gerontology, 21,* 182–191.

Berkman, L. F. (1983). The assessment of social networks and social support in the elderly. *Journal of the American Geriatrics Society, 31,* 743–749.

Bidlack, W. R., Kirsch, A., & Meskin, M. S. (1986). Nutritional requirements of the elderly. *Food Technology, 40,* 61–70.

Branch, L. G., & Jette, A. M. (1984). Personal health practices and mortality among the elderly. *American Journal of Public Health, 74,* 1126–1129.

Brenner, B. M., Meyer, T. W., & Hostetter, T. H. (1982). Dietary protein intake and the progressive nature of kidney disease. *New England Journal of Medicine, 307,* 652–659.

Briancon, D., & Meunier, P. J. (1981). Treatment of osteoporosis with fluoride, calcium and vitamin D. *Orthopedic Clinics of North America, 12,* 629–648.

Bullamore, J. R., Gallagher, J. C., Wilkinson, R., & Nordin, B. E. C. (1970). Effect of age on calcium absorption. *Lancet, II,* 535–537.

Buset, M., Lipkin, M., Winower, S., Swaroop, S., & Friedman, E. (1986). Inhibition of human colonic epithelial cell proliferation in vivo and in vitro by calcium. *Cancer Research, 46,* 5426–5430.

Cahill, G. F. (1970). Starvation in man. *New England Journal of Medicine, 282,* 668–675.

Cali, T. J. (1984). Renal disease. In T. R. Covington, & J. I. Walker (Eds.), *Current geriatric therapy* (pp. 366–384). Philadelphia: W. B. Saunders.

Calloway, D. H., & Zanni, E. (1980). Energy requirements and energy expenditure of elderly men. *American Journal of Clinical Nutrition, 33,* 2088–2092.

Carroll, M. D., Abraham, S., & Dresser, C. M. (1983). *Dietary intake source data: United States 1976–1980 data from the National Health Survey Series II, No. 231* (DHHS Publication No. (PHS) 83-1681). Washington, DC: U.S. Government Printing Office.

Castelli, W. P., Doyle, J., Hames, C. G., Hjortland, M. C., Hulley, S. B., Kagan, A., & Zukel, W. J. (1977). HDL cholesterol and other lipids in coronary artery disease: The cooperative lipoprotein phenotyping study. *Circulation, 55,* 767–772.

Chobanian, A. V. (1983). Pathophysiological considerations in the treatment of elderly hypertensives. *American Journal of Cardiology, 52,* 49D–53D.

Coe, R. M., & Miller, D. K. (1984). Sociologic factors that influence nutritional status in the elderly. In H.

Armbrecht, J. M. Prendergast, & R. M. Coe (Eds.), *Nutritional intervention in the aging process* (pp. 3–12). New York: Springer Verlag.

Committee on Diet and Health. (1989). *Diet and Health: Implications for chronic disease risk.* Washington, DC: National Academy Press.

Committee on Dietary Allowances. (1989). *Recommended dietary allowances* (10th ed.). Washington, DC: Food and Nutrition Board, National Academy Press.

Connor, W. E., Cerquiera, M. T., Connor, R. W., Wallace, R. B., Malinow, M. R., & Casdorph, H. R. (1978). The plasma lipids, lipoproteins and diet of the Tarahumara Indians of Mexico. *American Journal of Clinical Nutrition, 31,* 1131–1142.

Consensus Conference. (1984). Osteoporosis. *Journal of the American Medical Association, 252,* 799–802.

Davidson, M. D. (1979). The effect of aging on carbohydrate metabolism: A review of the English literature and a practical approach to the diagnosis of diabetes mellitus in the elderly. *Metabolism, 28,* 688–805.

Dawson-Hughs, B. (1986). Osteoporosis and aging: Gastrointestinal aspects. *Journal of the American College of Nutrition, 5,* 393–398.

Dayton, S., Pearce, M. L., Hashimoto, S., Dixon, W. J., & Tomiyasu, U. (1969). A controlled clinical trial of a diet high in unsaturated fat on preventing complications of atherosclerosis. *Circulation, 40,* II1–II63.

Draper, H. H., Sie, T. L., & Bergen, J. G. (1974). Osteoporosis in aging rats induced by high phosphorus diet. *Journal of Nutrition, 102,* 1113–1142.

Dwyer, J. T. (1991). *Older Americans' nutritional health: Current practices and future possibilities.* Washington, DC: Nutrition Screening Initiative.

Ettinger, G., Genant, H. K., & Cann, C. E. (1987). Postmenopausal bone loss is prevented by treatment with low-dosage estrogen with calcium. *Annals of Internal Medicine, 106,* 40–45.

Fanelli, M. T., & Kaufman, M. (1985). Nutrition and older adults. In H. T. Phillips, & S. A. Gaylord (Eds.), *Aging and public health* (pp. 76–100). New York: Springer.

Fichman, M. P., Vorheer, H., Kleeman, C. R., & Telfern, W. (1971). Diuretic-induced hyponatremia. *Annals of Internal Medicine, 75,* 853–863.

Fillenbaum, G. G. (1980). *The well-being of the elderly: Approaches to multidimensional assessment* (WHO Offset Publication No. 84). Geneva: World Health Organization.

Flynn, M. A. (1984). Problems in the nutritional management of the elderly. In H. J. Armbrecht, M. Prendergast, & R. M. Coe (Eds.), *Nutritional intervention in the aging process* (pp. 307–314). New York: Springer Verlag.

Folds, C. C. (1983). Practical aspects of nutritional management of the elderly. *Clinical Nutrition, 2,* 15–18.

Frisancho, A. R. (1981). New norms of upper limb fat and muscle areas for assessment of nutritional status. *American Journal of Clinical Nutrition, 34,* 2540–2545.

Freiman, R., & Johnston, F. A. (1963). Iron absorption in the healthy aged. *Geriatrics, 18,* 716–720.

Freudenheim, J. L., Johnson, N. E., & Smith, E. L. (1986). Relationships between usual nutrient intake and bone-mineral content of women 35–65 years of age: Longitudinal and cross-sectional analysis. *American Journal of Clinical Nutrition, 44,* 863–876.

Fulwood, R., Johnson, C. L., Bryner, J. D., Gunter, E. W., & McGrath, C. R. (1982). *Hematological and nutritional biochemistry reference data for persons 6 months–74 years of age: United States, 1976–1980.* Hyattsville, MD: U.S. Department of Health and Human Services, Public Health Service, National Center for Health Statistics.

Gallagher, J. C., & Riggs, B. L. (1978). Current concepts in nutrition: Nutrition and bone disease. *New England Journal of Medicine, 298,* 193–195.

Garn, S., Solomon, M. A., & Freidl, J. (1981). Calcium intake and bone quality in the elderly. *Ecology of Food Nutrition, 10,* 131–133.

Garry, P. J., Goodwin, J. S., & Hunt, W. C. (1983). Iron status and anemia in the elderly: New findings and a review of previous studies. *Journal of the American Geriatrics Society, 31,* 389–398.

Haavisto, M., Mattila, K., & Rajala, S. (1983). Blood glucose and diabetes mellitus in subjects aged 85 years or more. *Acta Medica Scandinavica, 214,* 239–244.

Hammond, C. B., Jelsovek, F. R., Lee, K. L., Creasman, W. T., & Parker, R. T. (1979). Effects of long-term estrogen replacement therapy: II. Neoplasia. *American Journal of Obstetric Gynecology, 133,* 525–547.

Hantman, D., Vogel, J., Donaldson, C., Friedman, R., Goldsmith, R., & Julley, S. (1973). Attempts to prevent disuse osteoporosis by treatment with calcitonin, longitudinal compression, and supplementary calcium and phosphate. *Journal of Clinical Endocrinology and Metabolism, 36,* 845–858.

Harris, T. B., Cook, E. F., Kannel, W. B., Schatzkin, A., & Goldman, L. (1985). Blood pressure experience and risk of cardiovascular disease in the elderly. *Hypertension, 7,* 118–124.

Hartz, S. C., & Blumberg, J. (1986). Use of vitamin and mineral supplements by the elderly. *Clinical Nutrition, 5,* 130–136.

Havlik, R. J., Hubert, H. B., Fabitz, R. R., & Feinleib, M. (1983). Weight and hypertension. *Annals of Internal Medicine, 98,* 855–859.

Heaney, R. (1986). Calcium intake, bone health, and aging. In E. A. Young (Ed.), *Nutrition, aging and health* (pp. 165–186). New York: Alan R. Liss.

Heaney, R. P., & Recker, R. R. (1982). Effects of nitrogen, phosphorus and caffeine on calcium balance in women. *Journal of Laboratory and Clinical Medicine, 99,* 46–55.

Heaney, R. P., Recker, R. R., & Saville, P. D. (1978). Menopausal changes in calcium balance performance. *Journal of Laboratory and Clinical Medicine, 92,* 953–963.

Heiss, G., Tamir, I., Davis, C. E., Tyroler, H. A., Rifkind, B. M., Schonfeld, G., Jacobs, D., & Frantz, I. D. (1980). Lipoprotein-cholesterol distributions in selected North American populations: The Lipid Research Clinics Program Prevalence Study. *Circulation, 61,* 302–315.

Horwitz, D. L. (1986). Nutrition, aging and diabetes. In E. A. Young (Ed.), *Nutrition, aging and health* (pp. 145–163). New York: Alan R. Liss.

Horwitz, D. L. (1982). Diabetes and aging. *American Journal of Clinical Nutrition, 36,* 803–808.

Hoy, R. H., & Ponte, C. D. (1984). Cardiovascular disorders. In T. R. Covington, & J. I. Walker (Eds.), *Current geriatric therapy* (pp. 140–177). Philadelphia: W. B. Saunders.

Hypertension Detection and Follow-up Program Cooperative Group. (1979). Five-year findings of the Hypertension Detection and Follow-up Program 2: Mortality by race, sex and age. *JAMA, 242,* 2572–2577.

Institute of Food Technologists Expert Panel on Food Safety and Nutrition. (1986). Nutrition and the elderly. *Food Technology, 40,* 81–88.

Ireland, P., & Fordtran, J. S. (1973). Effect of dietary calcium and age on jejunal calcium absorption in humans studied by intestinal perfusion. *Journal of Clinical Investigation, 52,* 2672–2681.

Jenkins, D. H. R., Roberts, J. G., Webster, D., & Williams, E. O. (1973). Osteomalacia in elderly patients with fracture of the femoral neck. A clinical pathologic study. *Journal of Bone Joint Surgery, 5513,* 575–580.

Johnson, N. E., Alcantara, E. N., & Linksweiler, H. N. (1970). Effect of level of protein intake on urinary and fecal calcium retention of young adults. *Journal of Nutrition, 100,* 1425–1430.

Kannel, W. B. (1986). Hypertensive disease in the elderly: A consequence of arteriosclerosis or blood pressure? In H. Grobecker, A. Philippu, & S. Klaus (Eds). *New aspects of the role of adrenoceptors in the cardiovascular system* (pp. 31–50). New York: Springer Verlag.

Kannel, W. B. (1986). Nutritional contributors to cardiovascular disease in the elderly. *Journal of American Geriatrics Society, 34,* 27–36.

Karanja, N., & McCarron, D. A. (1986). Calcium and hypertension. *Annual Review of Nutrition, 6,* 475–494.

Kennie, D. C. (1984). Health maintenance in the elderly. *Journal of the American Geriatrics Society, 32,* 316–323.

Kleiger, R. E. (1983). Cardiovascular disorders. In F. U. Steinberg (Ed.), *Care of the Geriatric Patient* (6th ed.; pp. 92–104). St. Louis, MO: C. V. Mosby.

Kohrs, M. B. (1982). A rational diet for the elderly. *American Journal of Clinical Nutrition, 36,* 796–802.

Kohrs, M. B., & Czajka-Narins, D. (1986). Assessing nutrition of the elderly. In E. A. Young (Ed.), *Nutrition, aging and health* (pp. 25–59). New York: Alan R. Liss.

Langer, E., & Rodin, J. (1976). The effects of choice and enhanced personal responsibility for the aged: A field experiment in an institutional setting. *Journal of Personality and Social Psychology, 34,* 191–198.

Leaf, A. (1984). Dehydration in the elderly. *New England Journal of Medicine, 311,* 791–792.

Lindeman, R. D. (1986). Mineral metabolism, aging and the aged. In E. A. Young (Ed.), *Nutrition, aging and health* (pp. 187–210). New York: Alan R. Liss.

Lipschitz, D. A., & Mitchell, C. O. (1982). The correctability of the nutritional, immune and haematopoietic manifestations of protein-calorie malnutrition in the elderly. *Journal of the American College of Nutrition, 1,* 17–25.

Lipschitz, D. A., Mitchell, C. O., Steele, R. W., & Milton, K. Y. (1985). Nutritional evaluation and supplementation of elderly subjects participating in a "Meals on Wheels" program. *Journal of Parenteral and Enteral Nutrition, 9,* 343–347.

Lipschitz, D. A., Mitchell, C. O., & Thompson, C. (1981). The anemia of senescence. *American Journal of Hematology, 11,* 47–54.

Lipschitz, D. A., Udupa, K. B., Milton, K. Y., & Thompson, C. (1984). The effect of age on hematopoiesis in man. *Blood, 63,* 502–509.

Lo, B., & Dorenbrand, L. (1986). Guiding the hand that feeds. *New England Journal of Medicine, 311,* 402–404.

Lowenstein, F. W. (1986). Nutritional requirements of the elderly. In E. A. Young, (Ed.), *Nutrition, aging and health,* (pp. 61–89). New York: Alan R. Liss.

Lynch, S. R., Finch, C. A., Monsen, E. F., & Cook, J. D. (1982). Iron status of elderly Americans. *American Journal of Clinical Nutrition, 36,* 1032–1045.

Masters, A. M., & Lasser, R. P. (1960). Tables of average weight and height of Americans aged 65 to 95 years: Relationships of weight and height to survival. *JAMA, 172,* 658–662.

Matcovik, V., Kostial, K., Simonovic, I., Buzina, R., Brodarec, A., & Nordin, B. E. C. (1979). Bone status and fracture rates in two regions of Yugoslavia. *American Journal of Clinical Nutrition, 32,* 540–549.

McCarron, D. A., & Morris, C. D. (1985). Blood pressure response to oral calcium in persons with mild to moderate hypertension. *Annals of Internal Medicine, 103,* 825–831.

McGill, H. C. (1986). Nutrition, aging and atherosclerosis. In E. A. Young (Ed.), *Nutrition, aging and health* (pp. 211–228). New York: Alan R. Liss.

McKenna, M. J., Freaney, R., Meade, A., & Muldowney, F. P. (1985). Hypovitaminosis D and elevated serum alkaline phosphatase in elderly Irish people. *American Journal of Clinical Nutrition, 41,* 101–109.

Minkler, M. (1984). Health promotion in long-term care: A contradiction in terms. *Health Education Quarterly, 11,* 77–89.

Mitch, W. E. (1988). In W. E. Mitch & S. Klahr (Eds.), *Nutrition and the kidney* (pp. 154–179). Boston: Little, Brown.

Munro, H. N., Suter, P. M., & Russell, R. M. (1987). Nutritional requirements of the elderly. *Annual Review of Nutrition, 7,* 23–49.

National Center for Health Statistics. (1987, June). Analytic and Epidemiological Studies, Lin, B. M., Kovar, M. G. et al., Health Statistics on Older People. United States 1986, Vital and Health Statistics, Series 3, No. 25, DHHS Publ. No. (PHS) 87-1409, Public Health Service. Washington, DC: U.S. Government Printing Office.

National Cholesterol Education Program. (1990). Report on the National Cholesterol Education Program Expert Panel on Population Based Programs. Bethesda, MD: National Institutes of Health.

National Cholesterol Education Program. (1988). Report of the National Cholesterol Education Program Expert Panel on Detection, Evaluation and Treatment of High Blood Pressure in Adults. *Archives of Internal Medicine, 148,* 36–69.

National Diabetes Data Group. (1979). Classification and diagnosis of diabetes mellitus and other categories of glucose intolerance. *Diabetes, 28,* 1039–1057.

National Heart Foundation of Australia. (1981). Treatment of mild hypertension in the elderly: Report by the management committee. *Medical Journal of Australia, 2,* 398–402.

National Heart, Lung and Blood Institute, National High Blood Pressure Education Program. (1981, December). *1980 report of the Joint National Committee on the detection, evaluation and treatment of high blood pressure* (NIH Publication No. 82-1088). Washington, DC: U.S. Department of Health and Human Services, National Institutes of Health.

National High Blood Pressure Education Program Coordinating Committee (1982). *Statement of hypertension in the elderly, U.S. Dept. of Health and Human Services.* Washington, DC: U.S. Government Printing Office.

Nilas, L., Christiansen, C., & Rodbro, P. (1984). Calcium supplementation and postmenopausal bone loss. *British Medical Journal, 289,* 1103–1106.

Nordin, B. E. C., Horsman, A., Crilly, R. G., Marshall, D. H., & Simpson, M. (1980). Treatment of spinal osteoporosis in postmenopausal women. *British Medical Journal, xx,* 451–454.

Nordin, B. E. C., Horsman, A., Gallagher, J. C. (1975). Effect of various therapies on bone loss in women. In F. Kuhlencordt, & H. Kruse (Eds.), *Calcium metabolism, bone, and metabolic disease* (pp. 233–242). Berlin: Springer Verlag.

Norton, L., & Wozny, M. C. (1984). Residential location and nutritional adequacy among elderly adults. *Journal of Gerontology, 39,* 592–595.

Nutrition Screening Initiative. (1992). *Nutrition screening manual for older Americans.* Washington, DC: Author.

O'Hanlon, P., & Kohrs, M. B. (1978). Dietary studies of older Americans. *American Journal of Clinical Nutrition, 31,* 1257–1269.

Panzram, G., & Zabel Langhennig, R. (1981). Prognosis of diabetes mellitus in a geographically defined population. *Diabetologia, 20,* 587–591.

Parfitt, M. B., Gallagher, J. C., Heaney, R. P., Johnston, C. C., Weer, R., & Whedon, G. D. (1982). Vitamin D and bone health in the elderly. *American Journal of Clinical Nutrition, 36,* 1014–1031.

Podolsky, S., & El Behari, B. (1984). Nutrition and the elderly diabetic. In J. M. Ordy, D. Harman, & R. Alfin-Slater (Eds.), *Nutrition in gerontology* (pp. 167–187). New York: Raven Press.

Posner, B. M. (1979). *Nutrition and the elderly* (pp. 15–26). Lexington, MA: Lexington Books.

Recker, R. R., Saville, P. D., & Heaney, R. P. (1977). Effect of estrogens and calcium carbonate on bone loss in postmenopausal women. *Annals of Internal Medicine, 87,* 649–655.

Resnick, L. M. (1985). Calcium and hypertension: The emerging connection. *Annals of Internal Medicine, 103,* 944–946.

Riggs, B. L., & Melton, L. S. (1986). Involutional osteoporosis. *New England Journal of Medicine, 314,* 1676–86.

Riggs, B. L., Seeman, E., Hodgson, S. F., Traves, D. R., & O'Fallon, W. M. (1982). Effect of the fluoride/calcium regimen on vertebral fracture occurrence in postmenopausal osteoporosis: Comparison with conventional therapy. *New England Journal of Medicine, 306,* 446–450.

Riis, B., Thomsen, K., & Christiansen, C. (1987). Does calcium supplementation prevent postmenopausal bone loss? *New England Journal of Medicine, 316,* 173–177.

Roe, D. A. (1985). Therapeutic effects of drug-nutrient interactions in the elderly. *Journal of the American Dietetic Association,, 85,* 174–178.

Roe, D. A. (1982). Dietary control in human studies related to aging and drug disposition or response. *Journal of the American College of Nutrition, 1,* 199–205.

Rudman, D. (1988). Kidney senescence: A model for aging. *Nutrition Reviews, 46,* 209–214.

Russell, R. (1983). Evaluating nutritional status in the elderly. *Clinical Nutrition, 2,* 4–8.

Santora, A. C. (1987). Role of nutrition and exercise in osteoporosis. *American Journal of Medicine, 82*(Suppl. 1B), 73–79.

Schaafsma, G., Van Beresteyn, E. C. H., Raymakers, J. A., & Duursma, S. A. (1987). Nutritional aspects of osteoporosis. *World Review of Nutrition and Dietetics, 49,* 121–159.

Schoenfeld, G. (1984). Atherosclerosis and plasma lipid transport with aging. In H. J. Armbrecht, J. M. Prendergast, & R. M. Coe (Eds.), *Nutritional intervention in the aging process* (pp. 49–68). New York: Springer Verlag.

Seltzer, H. S. (1983). Diagnosis of diabetes. In M. Ellenberg & A. Rifkin (Eds.), *Diabetes mellitus: Theory and practice* (3rd ed.; pp. 415–420). New Hyde Park, NY: Medical Examination Publishing Co.

Shapiro, S., Kelly, J. P., Rosenberg, L., Kaufman, D. W., Helmrich, S. P., Rosenshein, N. B., Lewis, J. L., Knapp, R. C., Stolley, P. D., & Schottenfeld, D. (1985). Risk of localized and widespread endometrial cancer in relation to recent and discontinued use of conjugated estrogens. *New England Journal of Medicine, 313,* 969–972.

Shea, S., Cook, E. F., Kannel, W. B., & Goldman, L. (1985). Treatment of hypertension and its effect on cardiovascular risk factors: Data from the Framingham Heart Study. *Circulation, 71,* 22–30.

Shepherd, R. (1986). Nutrition and the physiology of aging. In E. A. Young (Ed.), *Nutrition, aging and health* (pp. 1–23). New York: Alan R. Liss.

Shepherd, R. J. (1987). *Physical activity and aging.* Rockville, MD: Aspen.

Sidney, K. H., & Shepherd, R. J. (1979). Activity patterns of elderly men and women. *Journal of Gerontology, 32,* 25–32.

Sidney, K. H., Shepherd, R. J., & Harrison, J. E. (1977). Endurance training and body composition of the elderly. *American Journal of Clinical Nutrition, 30,* 326–333.

Silverberg, A. B. (1984). Carbohydrate metabolism and diabetes in the aged. In H. J. Armbrecht, J. M. Prendergast, & R. M. Coe (Eds.), *Nutrition intervention in the aging process* (pp. 191–208). New York: Springer Verlag.

Singer, J. D., Granahan, P., Goodrich, N., Meyers, L. D., & Johnson, C. L. (1982). *Diet and iron status: A study of relationships, United States 1971–1974.* Hyattsville, MD: U.S. Department of Health and Human Services, Public Health Service, National Center for Health Statistics.

Slovik, D. M., Adams, J. S., Weer, R. M., Holick, M. R., & Potts, J. T. (1981). Deficient production of 1, 25 dihydroxyvitamin D in elderly osteoporotic patients. *New England Journal of Medicine, 305,* 372–374.

Smiciklas-Wright, H., & Fosmire, G. J. (1985). Government nutrition programs for the aged. In R. R. Watson (Ed.), *CRC handbook of nutrition in the aged* (pp. 323–334). Boca Raton, FL: CRC Press.

Smith, C. H., & Bidlack, W. R. (1984). Dietary concerns associated with the use of medications. *Journal of the American Dietetics Association, 84,* 901–914.

Smith, R. W., & Frame, B. (1965). Concurrent axial and appendicular osteoporosis: Its relation to calcium consumption. *New England Journal of Medicine, 273,* 72–78.

Spencer, H., Kramer, L., Lesniak, M., DeBartolo, M., Clemontain, N., & Osis, D. (1984). Calcium requirements in humans. *Clinical Orthopaedics and Related Research, 184,* 270–280.

Spencer, H., & Lender, M. (1979). Adverse effects of aluminum-containing antacids on mineral metabolism. *Gastroenterology, 76,* 603–606.

Strazzulo, P., Siani, A., Guglieloni, S., DiCarlo, A., Galletti, F., Cirillo, M., & Mancini, M. (1986). Controlled trial of long-term oral calcium supplementation in essential hypertension. *Hypertension, 8,* 1084–1088.

Stultz, B. M. (1984). Preventive health care for the elderly. *Western Journal of Medicine, 141,* 832–845.

Surgeon General of the United States. (1979). Healthy older adults. In *Healthy people: The Surgeon General's report on health promotion and disease prevention* (pp. 71–80). Office of the Assistant Secretary for Health and Surgeon General, U.S. Public Health Service (DHEW (PHS) Publication 7955071). Washington, DC: U.S. Government Printing Office.

Tattersall, R. B. (1984). Diabetes in the elderly: A neglected area. *Diabetologia, 27,* 167–173.

U.S. Department of Health and Human Services, U.S. Department of Agriculture. (1986, December). *Assessment of the existing scientific literature and research on dietary calcium and its importance in human health and nutrition: A report to Congress pursuant to the Food Security Act of 1985* (PL 99-198, Subtitle 13, Section 1453). Washington, DC: Author.

U.S. Public Health Service. (1989). *Promoting health, preventing disease: Year 2000 objectives for the Nation* (Draft for public review, pp. 7-1-7, 11). Washington, DC: U.S. Department of Health and Human Services.

Vestal, R. E., Norris, A. H., Tobin, J. D., Cohen, B. H., Shock, N. W., & Andres, R. (1975). Antipyrin metabolism in man: Influence of age, alcohol, caffeine and smoking. *Clinical Pharmacology and Therapeutics, 18,* 425–432.

Veterans Administration Cooperative Study Group on Antihypertensive Agents. (1972). Effects of treatment on morbidity on hypertension: III. Influences of age, diastolic pressure, and prior cardiovascular disease — further analysis of side effects. *Circulation, 45,* 991–1004.

Villar, J., Repke, J., & Belizan, J. M. (1986). Calcium and blood pressure. *Clinical Nutrition, 5,* 153–160.

Villers Foundation. (1986). On the other side of Easy Street: Myths and facts about the economics of old age. Washington, DC: Villers Foundation.

Vir, S. C., & Love, A. H. G. (1979). Nutritional status of institutionalized and noninstitutionalized aged in Belfast, Northern Ireland. *American Journal of Clinical Nutrition, 32,* 1934–1947.

Walser, M. (1988). Renal system. In D. M. Paige (Ed.), *Clinical nutrition* (2nd ed.; pp. 227–241). St. Louis, MO: C. V. Mosby.

Wasnich, R., Benfante, R., Yanok Heilbrun, L., & Vogel, J. (1983). Thiazide effect on the mineral content of bone. *New England Journal of Medicine, 309,* 344–347.

West, K. M. (1980). Recent trends in dietary management. In S. Podolsky (Ed.), *Clinical diabetes: Modern management* (pp. 67–89). New York: Appleton Century Croft.

Widdowson, E. M. (1983). How much food does man require? An evaluation of human energy needs. *Experientia, 44* (Suppl. 11), 25.

Wolinsky, F. D., Coe, R. M., Miller, D. K., & Prendergast, J. M. (1984). Measurement of global and functional dimensions of health status in the elderly. *Journal of Gerontology, 39,* 88–92.

Wolinsky, F. D., Coe, R. M., Chavez, M. N., Prendergast, J. M., & Miller, J. (1986). Further assessment of the reliability and validity of a nutritional risk index: Analysis of a three wave panel to study elderly adults. *Health Services Research, 20,* 977–990.

Wolinsky, F. D., Prendergast, J. M., Coe, R. M., & Chavez, N. M. (1985). Preliminary validation of a nutritional risk index. *American Journal of Preventive Medicine, 1,* 53–59.

Wolinsky, F. D., Coe, R. M., Miller, D. K., Prendergast, J. M., Creel, M. J., & Chavez, M. N. (1983). Health services utilization among the non-institutionalized elderly. *Journal of Health and Social Behavior, 24,* 325–337.

Young, E. A. (1983). Nutrition, aging and the aged. *Medical Clinic of North America, 67,* 295–313.

Young, E. A. (1982). Evidence relating selected vitamins and minerals to health and disease in the elderly population of the United States: Introduction. *American Journal of Clinical Nutrition, 36,* 979–985.

Young, V. R. (1970). The role of skeletal and cardiac muscle in the regulation of protein metabolism. In H. N. Munro (Ed.), *Mammalian protein metabolism* (pp. 585–674). New York: Academic Press.

Young, V. R. (1984). Impact of aging on protein metabolism. In H. J. Armbrecht, J. M. Prendergast, & R. M. Coe (Eds.), *Nutritional intervention in the aging process* (pp. 27–48). New York: Springer Verlag.

# 7

# Principles and Practice in Geriatric Rehabilitation

Jennifer M. Bottomley

Normal aging is not necessarily burdened with disability; however, almost all conditions that cause disability are more frequently seen in the older population. As a result, the aged are more likely to require assessment for rehabilitative services. The mutual exclusion of geriatrics and rehabilitation is unjustified, and functional assessment for needed rehabilitative services should be an essential part of the routine evaluations required by all the health-care disciplines working with the aged population. Geriatrics teaches as its fundamental objective that maximum functional capabilities be attained; thus, it can be argued that rehabilitation is the foundation of geriatric care. The purpose of this chapter is to supply health-care professionals with the knowledge they need of the principles and practices of geriatric rehabilitation to apply appropriate interventions and provide high-quality care to their aged patients.

The basic goal of geriatric rehabilitation is to assist the disabled aged in recovering lost physical, psychological, or social skills so that they may become more independent, live in personally satisfying environments, and maintain meaningful social interactions. This may be done in any number of settings, including acute- and subacute-care settings, rehabilitation centers, home and office settings, or in long-term care facilities such as nursing homes.

Because of the complexity of the interventions needed in dealing with the aged, an interdisciplinary team approach is required. The rehabilitation process also requires education of patients and their families. Finally, rehabilitation is more than a medical intervention: It is a philosophical approach that recognizes that diagnoses and chronological age are poor predictors of functional abilities, that interventions directed at enhancing function are important, and that the health-care team should always include the patients and their families.

## DISABILITY: A DEFINITION

The meaning of *disability* provides a key to understanding rehabilitation. When referring to alterations in people's function, three terms are often used interchangeably: impair-

230

ment, disability, and handicap. A distinct understanding of these concepts is useful in geriatric rehabilitation, in particular, within the context of a "systems approach." In this context, a problem at the organ level (e.g., an infarct in the right hemisphere) must be viewed not only in terms of its effects on the brain, but also in terms of its effects on the person, the family, the society, and, ultimately, the nation. It goes beyond the pure "medical model," in which only the current medical problem is assessed to determine the rehabilitative goals. From such a perspective, "impairment" refers to a loss of physical or physiologic function at the organ level. This could include alterations in heart function, nerve conduction velocity, or muscle strength. Impairments usually do not affect the ability to function. However, if an impairment is so severe that it inhibits the ability to function "normally," then it becomes a "disability." Rehabilitation interventions are most often oriented toward adaptation to or recovery from disabilities. Given the proper training or adaptive equipment, people with disabilities can pursue independent lives. However, obstructions in the pursuit of independence can arise when people with disabilities confront inaccessible buildings, or situations that limit rehabilitation interventions, such as low toilet seats, buttons on an elevator that are too high, or signs that are not readable. In these cases a disability becomes a "handicap." The social environment creates the handicap.

In this chapter we will be primarily concerned with the rehabilitative approaches employed to reduce disabilities.

## DEMOGRAPHICS OF DISABILITY IN THE AGED

The aged are disproportionately affected by disabling conditions when compared to younger cohorts. According to Wedgewood (1985), the "old-old" age group (85 years of age or older) comprises the highest percentage of disabled persons; indeed, 40% of all disabled persons are over the age of 65. Three fourths of all cerebrovascular accidents occur in persons over the age of 65 (Warshaw, 1982); the highest incidence of amputations have been reported in the aged (Clark, 1985); and hip fractures between the ages of 70 to 78, on the average (Kumar & Redford, 1984). The Federal Council on Aging (1981) has reported that, of all persons studied over the age of 65, 86% have at least one chronic condition, and 52% have limitations in their activities of daily living. It is the impact of these disabilities on the level of independence that needs to be considered, rather than the presence of an impairment or disability.

Disabilities in old age are associated with a higher mortality rate, a decreased life span, greater chronic health problems (cardiovascular, musculoskeletal, neurological, and so forth), and increased expenditures for health care. Disabilities resulting in an inability to ambulate, feed oneself or manage the basic activities of daily living like toileting or self-hygiene (e.g., bathing) are very strong predictors of loss of functional independence and an increased burden on caregivers (Enright & Friss, 1987). The greater the disability, the greater the risk of institutionalization. Rehabilitative measures can be cost effective by enhancing functional ability and attaining greater levels of independence. Higher functional capabilities and greater levels of independence have been associated with fewer hospitalizations and a lower mortality rate among the aged (Lehman et al., 1975; Rubenstein, Josephson, & Gurland 1984).

Geriatric rehabilitation includes both institutional and noninstitutional services for the aged with chronic medical conditions that are marked by deviation from the "normal" state of health and manifested in physical impairment. Unless treated, these conditions have the potential for causing substantial and frequently cumulative disability. Aged persons with disabilities need assistance with such daily functions as bathing, dressing, and walking. This increased need for help is often compounded when there is no spouse, nearby family, or able friends. With this social isolation, common in the aged, continuing professional medical care is required to ward off the debilitating affects of inactivity and depression.

## FUNCTIONAL ASSESSMENT OF THE AGED

The assessment of functional capabilities is the cornerstone of geriatric rehabilitation. The ability to walk, transfer from bed to chair, or chair to toilet, for example, and manage the basic activities of daily living independently often determines whether hospitalized aged patients will be discharged to their home or to an extended-care facility. Functional assessment tools, which are practical, reliable, and valid, are necessary to assist all interdisciplinary team members in determining the need for rehabilitation or long-term care services. In the home-care setting, precise assessment of patients' functioning can detect early deterioration and allow for immediate intervention.

In response to the growing importance of chronic diseases and the need for long-term care, the Commission on Chronic Illness was established in 1949 (Commission on Chronic Illness, 1957). The commission highlighted the importance of function and disability, and concluded that there was a need for a means of classifying the functional activities of daily living (Trussel & Elinson, 1959). Since that time functional assessment tools have gone through many evolutional stages. Early in this evolution, scales included variables such as locomotion and traveling, dressing, toileting, eating, and hand activities such as managing coins or knitting (Dinken, 1951). Some assessment tools addressed bowel and bladder function (Heather, 1960), whereas others had measures for muscle strength, overall functional capacity, communication, and behavior. From these early efforts, a series of more sophisticated methodologic scales were developed under the direction and sponsorship of the National Institute on Aging, the Administration on Aging, and the National Center for Health Services Research. These studies were concerned with the reliability, validity, and usefulness of the various tools proposed. Among those who helped to clarify the theoretical framework for functional assessment, Lawton proposed a behavioral model in which functioning is viewed within a hierarchy of domains (Rusk, 1958). Each domain includes a set of functions that can be ordered along a continuum from simple to complex activities. For example, following the simple task of picking up the telephone receiver is the more complex task of picking up the telephone receiver and dialing a number. This model outlined the activities of daily living in relation to different categories of self-maintainance functions and to broader, or more comprehensive, sets of functions. For instance, Lawton included mobility and ambulation (or locomotion) as basic self-maintainance functions that enabled aged individuals to adjust and adapt within their environment; the ability to ambulate one block and ascend and descend four steps would enable the aged person to walk to the bus stop and board a bus.

Lawton's conception of functional capacity defined three levels of activities of daily living: (1) the basic activities of daily living (ADL), including such self-care activities as bathing, dressing, toileting, continence, and feeding; (2) the instrumental activities of daily living (IADL), such as using the telephone, driving, shopping, housekeeping, cooking, laundry, managing money, and managing medications; and (3) mobility, described as a more complicated combination of the IADL, such as leaving one's residence and moving from one location to another by using public transportation. IADL and mobility are more complex and are concerned with people's ability to cope with their environments. This classification according to ADL, IADL, and mobility, has become standard in most functional assessment tools.

As a clinical tool, functional assessment scales are invaluable. Initial assessment identifies areas of functional deficit and can assist clinicians in developing treatment regimes that address specific needs. Subsequent assessments measure progress toward rehabilitation goals. On a broader scale, functional assessment can assist public policy-makers in the provision of health-care services by determining the levels of need in a population. Demographically, it is apparent that Americans are living longer; the question is, are these added years of life years of vigor and independence or years of frailty and dependence?

By design, functional assessment scales are meant to determine specific outcomes. Outcomes of interest to those working with the aged include mortality, hospitalization, institutionalization, special interventions, and declining physical function, to name a few. Numerous functional assessment tools are available to determine physical, emotional, cognitive, and social functioning in various care settings. Table 7.1 summarizes a number of ADL and IADL scales and indexes, including, but not limited to, those summarized by Branch & Meyers (1987). Though this table of functional assessment tools is not exhaustive, it represents a relatively comprehensive reference list of currently used scales. In reviewing this list, the reader will notice that some tools include only basic ADL skills, which tools are more useful in the institutional setting, whereas others are comprehensive and include all three levels of functioning defined by Lawton; these tools are more useful in discharge planning and the home-care setting.

## FUNCTIONAL ABILITIES OF THE CAREGIVER

Aged patients, given a choice, would prefer to stay at home rather than recuperate and rehabilitate in a institutional setting. The aged have strong ties to their homes, and the help of their spouses, other relatives, and friends is a crucial component in making rehabilitation in their homes possible. Home care, by professionals, can protect the health of informal caregivers and maximize patients' ability to perform the basic activities of daily living by including a systematic assessment of the living environment as a key part of care planning. Provision of such assistance openly acknowledges that caregivers (often

TABLE 7.1    Functional Assessment Scales and Indexes

| Scale Index | Domain | Assessor | Mode | Reliability | Validity | Reference |
|---|---|---|---|---|---|---|
| Katz ADL | Eating<br>Bathing<br>Dressing<br>Transfer<br>Continence<br>Toileting | Professional | Performance<br>Self-report | X | X | Katz et al., 1963;<br>Kane & Kane, 1981 |
| Modified<br>ADL Scale | Eating<br>Ambulation<br>Bathing<br>Dressing<br>Transfer<br>Personal<br>grooming<br>Continence<br>Toileting | Lay | Performance<br>Self-report<br>Proxy | X | X | Katz et al., 1963;<br>Branch et al., 1984;<br>Kane & Kane, 1981 |
| Pulses | Physical<br>condition<br>Upper limbs<br>Lower limbs<br>Sensory<br>Excretory<br>Social Function | Lay | Performance | | X | Moscowitz &<br>McCann, 1957;<br>Granger & Greer,<br>1976;<br>Kane & Kane, 1981 |
| Kenny<br>Self-care | Bed activities<br>Transfers<br>Locomotion<br>Continence<br>Dressing<br>Feeding | Professional | Performance | | X | Schoening & Iverson,<br>1968;<br>Kane & Kane, 1981 |
| Barthel<br>Index | Feeding<br>Grooming<br>Transfer<br>Toileting<br>Bathing<br>Walking<br>Continence | Professional | Performance | X | X | Sherwood et al.,<br>1977;<br>Kane & Kane, 1981 |
| Rapid<br>Disability<br>Rating | Eating/Diet<br>Medication<br>Speech<br>Hearing<br>Sight<br>Ambulation<br>Bathing<br>Dressing<br>Continence<br>Shaving<br>Safety<br>Bedfastness<br>Confusion<br>Cooperation<br>Depression | Professional | Performance | X | X | Linn, 1967;<br>Kane & Kane, 1981 |
| Range of<br>Motion | Motions:<br>Shoulders | Professional | Performance | X | X | Granger, 1974;<br>Eberl et al., 1976; |

234

| Scale Index | Domain | Assessor | Mode | Reliability | Validity | Reference |
|---|---|---|---|---|---|---|
| Range of motion (cont'd) | Elbows Wrists Hips Knees Ankles | | | | | Kane & Kane, 1981 |
| Patient Classification | Mobility Transfers Walking Wheeling Stairs Bathing Dressing Eating Toileting Bowel function Bladder function Communication Orientation Behavior Impairments Medical problems Sociodemographics | Both | Performance | X | X | Jones et al., 1974; US DHEW, 1978b; Kane & Kane, 1981 |
| Pace II | 7 ADL 17 Range of Motion 8 Strength Balance Coordination | Both | Performance Self-report Proxy | | | US DHEW 1978b; Kane & Kane, 1981 |
| Oars | Eating Dressing Grooming Walking Transfer Bathing Continence Toileting | Both | Self-report Proxy | X | | Duke University, 1978; Kane & Kane, 1981 |
| Functional Health of Institution-alized Elders | Transfer Eating Walking Bathing Dressing Toileting | Professional | Performance Self-report | X | X | Mossey & Tisdale, 1979; Kane & Kane, 1981 |
| Performance Activities of Daily Living (PADL) | Shave Wipe nose Drink from cup Comb hair File nails Eat with spoon Turn faucet Switch lights Button on and off Slippers on and off Brush teeth | Professional | Performance | X | X | Kuriansky & Guland, 1976; Kane & Kane, 1981 |

(continued)

Table 7.1 *(cont'd)*

| Scale Index | Domain | Assessor | Mode | Reliability | Validity | Reference |
|---|---|---|---|---|---|---|
| (PADL) *(cont'd)* | Telephone<br>Sign name<br>Turn key<br>Tell time<br>Stand and sit | | | | | |
| Philadelphia Geriatric Center | Toileting<br>Feeding<br>Dressing<br>Grooming<br>Ambulation<br>Bathing | Lay | Self-report<br>Proxy | X | X | Lawton & Brody, 1969;<br>Lawton, 1972 |
| Philadelphia Geriatric Center Scale II (PGCII) | Telephone<br>Shopping<br>Food Preparation<br>Housekeeping<br>Laundry<br>Public<br> Transportation<br>Medications<br>Finances | Both | Self-report<br>Proxy | X | X | Lawton & Brody, 1969;<br>Lawton, 1972;<br>Kane & Kane, 1981 |
| Functional Health Scale | Heavy Work<br>Current illness<br>Limitations in<br> activity<br>Walk 1/2 mi<br>Climb stairs<br>Socialize | Lay | Self-report<br>Proxy | | | Roscow & Breslau, 1966 |
| Pace II | Telephone<br>Finances<br>Shopping<br>Housekeeping<br>Meal preparation | Both | Self-report<br>Proxy | | | US DHEW, 1978a;<br>Kane & Kane, 1981 |
| Oars II Shopping | Telephone<br><br>Transportation<br>Meal preparation<br>Medication<br>Finance | Both | Self-report | X | 1978; | Duke University,<br><br>Kane & Kane, 1981 |
| Functioning for Independent Living | Vision<br>Hearing<br>Speech<br>Continence<br>Behavior<br>Orientation<br>Communication<br>Wandering | Professional | Performance<br>Self-report<br>Proxy | | X | Gross & Zimmer, 1978;<br>Kane, 1981 |

aged themselves) have some decreased physical ability whose effect on caring for disabled relatives needs to be considered. It has been demonstrated that more than 90% of persons 75 to 84 years of age can manage without help to perform such tasks as grooming, bathing, dressing, eating, and so forth. (Branch & Jette, 1981). In the performance of the more complicated skills of transferring and ambulation, more than 50% of persons aged 75 to 84 years of age require some assistance. These activities require greater assistance skills on the part of the caregiver.

Thus, assessment of the home environment must take into account the abilities (or disabilities) of the individual(s) providing care. Adaptive equipment such as a sliding board for transfers or a rolling walker for ambulation, can be made available to assist caregivers in caring for their spouse, relative, or friend. Attention to the abilities of the caregiver can facilitate care and decrease the burden placed on the caregiver.

## PRINCIPLES OF GERIATRIC REHABILITATION

Three major principles underly geriatric rehabilitation. First, variability in the capabilities of the aged must be considered. Functional variability is much more pronounced within an aged group than within younger cohorts. What one 80-year-old can do physically, cognitively, or motivationally, another may not be able to accomplish. Second, activity is essential. Much functional diminishment that occurs over time is attributable to disuse. Third, optimum health is directly related to optimum functional ability. In acute situations rehabilitation must be directed toward (1) stabilizing the primary problem(s); (2) preventing secondary complications, such as bed sores, pneumonias, and contractures; and (3) restoring lost functions. In chronic situations rehabilitation is directed primarily toward restoring lost functions. This can best be accomplished by promoting maximum health so that the aged can fully adapt to their care environment and to their disabilities. These principles of functional variability, activity, and optimum health will be discussed in greater detail in the following sections.

### *Functional Variability*

Unlike any other age group, the aged are more variable in their level of functional capabilities. In the clinic, we often see 65-year-old individuals who are severely physically disabled, yet, sitting right along side of them is a 65-year-old who is still building houses and felling trees. Even in the extremely elderly, the variability in physical and cognitive functioning is remarkable. A far cry from the frail bedridden 87-year-old persons in nursing homes who are not responsive to their environment, John Kelly at the age of 87 is still running the Boston Marathon. Cognitively as well, the spectrum spans from the demented institutionalized aged to those aged who are presidents and supreme court justices. Chronological age is a poor indicator of physical or cognitive function.

Awareness of the aged population's heterogeneity helps to combat the myths and stereotypes of aging and presents a foundation for developing creative rehabilitation programs. Given that older persons tend to be more different from themselves (as a collective group) than other segments of the population, interdisciplinary team members, policymakers, and planners in rehabilitation settings need to be prepared to design a wide range of services and treatment interventions. This becomes more difficult as the number of aged increase and budgets decrease. However, creating new and innovative rehabilitation programs could ultimately improve the functional capabilities and the resulting quality of life for many aged individuals.

EXAMPLES OF FUNCTIONAL VARIABILITY IN THE AGED. Reaction time is an important functional variable among the aged. Generally, reaction time tends to slow with age (Woollacott, 1990). This is not necessarily due to a decline in functioning of the nervous system, which would require reduction in the amount and intensity of exercise and rehabilitative measures. Recent research indicates that the aged who are more physically active are capable of performing as well as, and in some cases better than, younger subjects on reaction-time performance tasks (Woollacott, 1988). Reaction time itself is a complex variable and may be affected by disease or social stigma. For example, aged individuals with arthritis may react more flowly as a result of stiff and painful joints. Their discomfort may lead to a sense of physical instability and inadequate physical adaptability and result in a fear of falling. Evaluation of functional capabilities requires detection of underlying pathology or social parameters (i.e., fear or discomfort) that may have an impact on a person's functioning. Recognizing the variability of reaction-time response may help us determine causes for functional declines in other areas.

There is a marked range of visual capabilities in the aged that also affect reaction time and the ability to function safely in a given environment. Several changes normally occur within the aging eye. The lens begins to thicken and becomes yellowed, and the muscles that control dilation of the pupil weaken. The older eye needs three times the amount of light to function adequately. The thickening of the lens and delayed pupil dilation means that the glare and reflections often encountered in the environment cannot be tolerated (Andreasen, 1985). The older person has difficulty with depth perception and color differentiation, which can interfere with ambulation, the activities of daily living, and driving an automobile. The combination of these changes creates many obstacles for the aged person, whose overall functioning may ultimately be impaired by a decline in visual acuity. Even when errors of refraction are corrected, a loss of visual rceptors in the aging retina or macula will result in a decrease of acuity. Fortunately, with modern technology, the majority of older people are able to maintain a high degree of visual functioning and independence. Indeed recent research indicates that visual capabilities do not normally decline as part of aging. Instead, like so many other systems, the eyes are affected by nutritional deficits and environmental hazards such as intense sunlight, poor lighting, and air-borne contaminants, all of which are preventable causes of visual loss (Boyer, 1989; Kasper, 1988).

Physical strength is another variable that directly affects the ability of aged individuals to function at their maximum capability. Strength measures in a group aged 70 and older compared to a group of 40- to 50-year-olds (both male and female subjects) showed a greater range in strength values in the older group (Fitts, 1980). Part of the variability was due to factors that exist apart from age-dependent muscle changes but that also influence muscle strength, such as physical activity, disease, cardiovascular condition, and hormonal and neural influences. The younger group displayed fewer non-age-dependent factors. This variability in strength among the aged will be discussed further in the next section, Activity versus Inactivity.

Mental ability is another area that varies greatly within an aged population and directly affects the rehabilitation potential of an aged individual. The presence of pathology, such as Alzheimer's disease, can severely influence aged individuals' ability to function safely within their environment. In the absence of pathology, however, an individual's cognitive abilities have been shown to undergo little or no change (Schaie, 1984). What happens to intelligence and cognition with age? The answers are many, complex, and controversial. Some researchers say that cognition enters a process of irreversible decline in the adult years, because the brain becomes less and less efficient, just as the heart and lungs and other physical organs do (Wechsler, 1972). Other investigators say that intelligence and cognition are relatively stable throughout the adult years, with the brain providing more than enough capacity for anything we would want to comtemplate until serious disease sets in late in life (Siegler, 1983). Yet, other researchers indicate that cognition declines in some respects (e.g., in mental quickness) and increases in others (e.g., in knowledge about life) (Botwinick, 1978).

The decline of intelligence and cognition over the age of 65 or 70 is variable and subject to several interpretations. In addition to inevitable biological decrement, intellectual and cognitive decline can be attributed to social isolation, decreasing motivation to perform irrelevant tasks, disease, or a combination of such factors. All in all, many researchers have begun to believe that the search for a definition of "normal" deterioration in mental abilities is a fruitless task (Baltes & Schaie, 1986), finding that there is too much variability in age trends to postulate one of these as normal or basic. Some people decline in intellectual ability, others increase. Some abilities seem to increase with each new generation, others decrease. An environmental event—the development of television, for example—can change age trends for some people and have little effect on others. Thus the search goes on, but focusing more now on the determinants of change or stability and much less on inevitable and irreversible decrements. Application of the principle of variability in geriatric rehabilitation is essential in providing therapeutic interventions that address the range of mental capabilities. Though cognitive decline is bound to occur in the rehabilitative setting, it is also possible that healthy aged individuals who maintain an active intellectual life will show little or no loss of intellectual abilities even into their 80s and beyond.

## Activity versus Inactivity

The most common reason for losses in functional capabilities in the aged is inactivity or immobility. There are numerous reasons for immobilizing the aged. "Acute" immobilization is often considered to be "accidental," resulting from acute catastrophic illnesses, including severe blood loss, trauma, head injury, cerebral vascular accidents, burns, and hip fracture, to name only a few. Until acute illnesses become medically stable, the activity level of the patient is often severely curtailed. Chronic immobilization may result from long-standing problems that are undertreated or left untreated, such as cerebral vascular accidents (strokes), amputations, arthritis, Parkinson's disease, cardiac disease, pulmonary disease, and low back pain. A major cause of "accidental immobilization" in both the acute- and chronic-care settings, environmental barriers include bedrails; the height of the bed; physical restraints; an inappropriate chair; no physical assistance available; fall precautions imposed by medical staff; no clinical prescription for mobilization; social isolation; and obstacles such as stairs or doorway thresholds. Cognitive impairments; disorders of the central nervous system, disorders such as cerebral vascular accidents, Parkinson's disease, and multiple sclerosis; peripheral neuropathies resulting from diabetes; and pain with movement, can also severely reduce mobility. Affective disorders such as depression, anxiety, or fear of falling may also lead to accidental immobilization. In addition, sensory changes, terminal illnesses such as cancer or cirrhosis of the liver, acute episodes of illness like pneumonia or cellulitis, or an attitude of "I'm too sick to get up," can negatively affect mobility.

The process of deconditioning involves changes in multiple organ systems, including the neurological, cardiovascular, and musculoskeletal systems, in varying degrees. Deconditioning is probably best defined as the multiple changes in organ-system physiology that are induced by inactivity and reversed by activity (i.e., exercise) (Siebens, 1990). The degree of deconditioning depends on the degree of superimposed inactivity and the prior level of physical fitness. The term *hypokinetics* has been coined to describe the physiology of inactivity (Lewis, 1985). Deconditioning can occur at many levels of inactivity, the two major categories of which are (1) the acute hypokinetic effects of bedrest and (2) the chronic inactivity induced by a sedentary lifestyle (chronic-disease-induced hypokinetics).

Looking at the aging process with one eye on the adverse affects of bed rest or hypo-kinetics as a possible concommitant of deconditioning and disability has lead health professionals to explore the potential use of exercise as a primary rehabilitation modality. The phrase "use it or lose it" is a concept with tremendous ramifications for aging, especially in geriatric rehabilitation. However, exercise has not been viewed as an important factor in health until recently. Until the 1950s the rate-of-living theory was promoted. According to this theory, the body would be worn out faster and life shortened by expending energy through exercise (Holloszy, 1983). Conversely, studies in the past decade have shown that regular exercise does not shorten life span and may in fact increase it (Schneider & Reed, 1985). Exercise is becoming increasingly viewed as beneficial for both the primary and secondary prevention of disease (Astrand, 1987).

There are several challenges to understanding the interaction between inactivity and health in older persons. The first is that the process of aging itself causes changes that parallel those produced by inactivity. Several studies have provided strong evidence that the causes of such changes can be delineated (Bruce, 1984; Buskirk, 1985; Shephard, 1978; Shephard, 1987). It has been found that aged individuals *can* improve their flexibility, strength, and aerobic capacity to the same extent as younger individuals. It is obvious that some effects of "aging" can be directly related to inactivity. The second challenge in studying inactivity is to separate the effects of inactivity from those of disease (Bortz, 1982). Many aged individuals who are deconditioned may also suffer from an acute or chronic disease. Recent studies on younger subjects have helped to clarify some of the effects of inactivity alone (i.e., the effects of bed rest on physiological changes and funtional performance). The third challenge is to understand the relationship between physiologic decline and functional loss. Is the inability to climb stairs in an 85-year-old primarily due to cardiovascular deconditioning, muscle weakness, or impaired balance secondary to sensory losses or a sedentary lifestyle? Is there a new disease process beginning? Is this normal aging? An important concept in geriatric rehabilitation is that "threshold" values of physiologic functioning may exist (Young, 1986). Below these thresholds an aged person may suddenly lose an essential functional skill.

EFFECTS ON THE NERVOUS SYSTEM. Inactivity's effect on the nervous system has not been studied as intensely as for other organ systems. Perhaps this is because of the complexity of the nervous system and the lack of assessment techniques. In younger individuals changes in the nervous system that are brought about by inactivity are minimal. In the aged, however, especially those individuals with concurrent acute or chronic illnesses, the consequences of inactivity on the nervous system may be particularly severe (Miller, 1975).

Bed rest has been compared to the experience of sensory deprivation. In a study of prolonged immobilization (i.e., immobilization during the day followed by bed rest at night) Zubek & Wilgosh (1963) showed that occipital lobe frequencies on electroencephalograms (EEGs) were substantially decreased in awake subjects. Exercise prevented some of these changes (Zubek, 1963). In addition to physical changes, performance deteriorated on several intellectual tests, including verbal-fluency, color-discrimination, and reversible-figures tests. In another study of sensory deprivation, young subjects were put on bed rest and periodically stimulated by audiotapes of disjointed conversations (Downs, 1974). Within a 3-hour test period, the subjects' perception of time intervals became distorted and several subjects described hallucinatory experiences. Social isolation was also very disconcerting to the subjects and made them feel uncomfortable. Frequent complaints included feelings of loneliness and longing for some sign of recognition from the investigator. In young subjects, other emotions occur during prolonged bed rest, such as anxiety, irritability, and a depressed mood (Ryback, Lewis, & Lessard, 1971). Reactions were more intense in subjects who were not allowed to exercise than in those allowed to exercise three times a day (Ryback et al., 1971).

It has been found that bed rest also affects the EEG pattern of sleep. A longer period of time is spent in the deep stages of sleep, stages 3 and 4, in subjects on bed rest (Ryback, Lewis, & Lessard, 1971). This was even more pronounced in individuals who were not allowed to perform light supine exercise. Sleep periods involving rapid eye movement (REM) also increased in subjects on bed rest. In addition, there was a noted increase in mental lethargy observed during waking hours. In conditioned subjects, the onset of stage 3 sleep was sooner and the time spent in this deep slow-wave sleep was longer than in subjects who were deconditioned (Griffin & Trinder, 1978). These findings may have significant clinical implications in the aged person, especially one who is hypokinetic. Less time spent in deep sleep can lead to a feeling of tiredness, depression, and lack of motivation. All of these sequelae could have a significant impact on an aged individual's level of functioning and rehabilitation potential.

Thermoregulation is also altered by bed rest (Greenleaf & Reese, 1980). Both oral and skin temperatures show a decline. This may have important clinical implications for the aged individual who already has decreased thermoregulatory responses.

With inactivity, several neurological changes occur that affect motor performance. Balance decrements are significant after 2 to 3 weeks of bed rest (Haines, 1974). Muscle-strengthening exercises during bed rest did not reverse this deterioration. Recovery of the balance losses was accomplished within 3 to 5 days following cessation of bed rest. Testing included assessment with the eyes shut and with the eyes open. Allowing visual cues greatly improved the relearning rate and overall performance scores. Coordination was also found to decline with bed rest (Taylor, Henschel, & Keys, 1949). Pattern-tracing skill tests were used to test coordination. Performance of these activities decreased in accuracy by 10% after 3 weeks of bed rest and resolved within 4 days of the resumption of activity. Each of these changes has significant clinical implications for aged individuals on acute or chronic bed rest or whose level of activity has been severely restricted.

The neuropsychological consequences of a chronic level of inactivity, as in a sedentary lifestyle, are not easy to determine. Shepard (1987) found that a moderate level of physical activity makes a person feel better, leading to better intellectual and psychomotor development. The underlying mechanism may include increased arousal, improved self-esteem and body image, and a decreased level of anxiety, stress, and depression.

Chronic inactivity also negatively affects balance. Postural sway is known to increase with aging. Inactivity may contribute to the progression of this decline. Research indicates that balance is better in active compared to inactive older women (Rikli & Busch, 1986). Results were similar for different types of exercise, (for example, golf, walking, and range-of-motion (ROM) exercise). In a study by Emes, balance in standing on one foot was improved following a 12-week exercise program (Emes, 1979).

A sedentary lifestyle is also associated with prolonged reaction times (Buskirk, 1985; Rikli & Busch, 1986). A comparison between young versus older persons revealed an 8% decline in reaction and movement times when age was considered alone. A 22% decrement was present when nonactive young and old groups were compared. Spiraduso has proposed that "exercise prevents the cycle in which disuse increases brain metabolism leading to decreased blood flow and neuronal loss" (Spiraduso, 1980).

In conclusion, the effects of inactivity on the nervous system is of utmost significance in geriatric rehabilitation. Acute bed rest induces a number of cognitive changes, including distortion of time perception and decrements in some intellectual tests. Mood changes occur as well. The consequences of chronic inactivity on cognitive and emotional functioning may include a diminished sense of well-being. Prolonged reaction times are associated with chronic inactivity, and balance is impaired after both acute and chronic inactivity. Realizing how the effects of inactivity can superimpose themselves on the "normal" changes of aging, the rehabilitation team must seek to maintain activity and maximum functional capabilities in the aged person.

EFFECTS ON THE CARDIOVASCULAR SYSTEM. Changes in the cardiovascular system have been studied the most in relation to inactivity versus activity. An aged individual in good physical condition responds to submaximal exercise (exercise below maximal levels) without significant increases in heart rate or blood pressure. In contrast, a deconditioned person encountering minimal to moderate activity experiences a marked increase in these vital signs. Maximum workloads elicit similar increases in heart rate and blood pressure in both deconditioned and conditioned individuals; however, the recovery rate (i.e., the return to vital-sign values at rest) is slower in deconditioned individuals.

Within the first week of bed rest there is a noted increase in resting heart rate (Dietrick, Whedon, & Shorr, 1948; Saltin et al., 1968; Shepard, 1987). In other words, the work of the heart is increased inspite of the fact that the body remains at rest. In very early studies on the effects of bed rest on cardiovascular function, it was found that by the end of the third week of bed rest the morning heart rate increased by as much as 21% and the evening heart rate by 33%. This is an average increase in resting heart rate of approximately 1 beat for every 2 days of bed rest (Taylor, Henschel & Keys, 1949). Other investigations showed approximately a 4-beat increase, documenting lesser increases in resting heart rate over a 1-week period (Saltin et al., 1968). In each of these studies, 6 weeks of submaximal exercise was necessary before the resting heart rate returned to its baseline value.

Total blood volume has been found to decrease after several weeks of bed rest (Miller, Johnson, & Lamb, 1964). These findings were based on studies of astronauts in the areospace program, a presumably healthy group of individuals. It was determined that decrements in plasma volume were greater than those in red blood cell mass. Such a change could have a significant impact on older persons. There is a strong possibility that a decrease in total blood volume is correlated with orthostatic hypotension in the aged, though this has not been studied in an elderly population to date.

Orthostatic hypotension occurs within the first week of inactivity in young subjects. This, and other cardiovascular signs of deconditioning, occur even with arm-chair rest (Lamb, Stevens, & Johnson, 1965). Orthostasis resolves very slowly, even when the recovery period includes maximum exercise levels.

In addition to the deterioration of the cardiovascular system at rest, any level of activity above the resting level becomes more strenuous. At submaximal levels of exercise, heart rate increases of 10 to 20 beats are common in the deconditioned individual. In addition to an increase in the heart rate, the stroke volume tends to decrease, making the heart less efficient in delivering blood to the working muscles (Astrand, 1987; Shepard, 1987). Delayed recovery rates also indicate increased cardiac and metabolic stress. The return to baseline heart rate in the conditioned individuals occurs in less than 2 min and the systolic blood pressure returns to a resting level within 4 min. After 6 weeks of bed rest imposed on a healthy individual, it takes 3 to 6 min for the heart rate and and 5 to 7 min for the systolic blood pressure to return to preexercise resting levels (Astrand, 1987).

"Normal" aging is accompanied by a 1%-per-year decline in oxygen uptake starting at the age of 30 (Astrand, 1987; Shepard, 1987). It has been shown that oxygen uptake is improved with activity. There is less of a decrease in oxygen uptake in arm-chair rest versus bed rest. In one of the few studies of older men, maximum oxygen uptake decreased 15% after 10 days of bed rest (DeBusk et al., 1983). Oxygen uptake at submaximal levels of activity was approximately 10% less after bed rest despite a increase in heart rate. These oxygen uptake levels returned to their baseline within 1 month following resumption of daily activities. Interestingly, recovery rates were similar for subjects who participated in an aerobic exercise program as well as for those who just returned to their usual activities.

The cardiovascular system undergoes significant changes with bed rest. The alterations are noted even without activity by an increase in resting heart rate. Mere standing can be accompanied by orthostasis. Any level of activity stresses the heart, eliciting a greater heart rate and a diminished stroke volume. These factors contribute to the overall decrease in maximum oxygen uptake, resulting in decreased physical capabilities, decreased endurance, and lost function.

The cardiovascular consequences of chronic inactivity are similar to those seen in acute bed rest. Resting heart rates are higher. At submaximal activity levels, heart rate and blood pressure are greater than in physically fit individuals performing at the same intensity of exercise. Maximum oxygen uptake is lower than in individuals who exercise aerobically. The well-documented decline in maximum oxygen uptake with age is half as great in physically active individuals compared to inactive persons, for whom the recovery rate is prolonged. The biggest difference in the effects of acute versus chronic inactivity on the cardiovascular system is that the effects of long-term inactivity are cumulative. In other words, the longer an individual remains inactive, the more pronounced the cardiovascular changes are, and the longer it takes to return to a "healthy" preconditioned baseline.

EFFECTS ON THE SKELETAL MUSCLE SYSTEM. The skeletal muscle system of the body is the largest organ system by mass. It's physiological capabilities are closely related to levels of activity.

Alterations in skeletal muscle with aging and with inactivity resemble those observed with denervation. The classic cross-innervation studies of Buller, Eccles, and Eccles (1960) established the importance of the trophic influence on skeletal muscle function and demonstrated that the metabolic and physiologic profile of a muscle fiber (i.e., the fiber type) was primarily determined by the type of neural innervation (phasic or tonic firing pattern and other trophic factors) received. Adult skeletal muscle is composed of three distinct fiber types: type IIA (fast-twitch, high-oxidative fiber), type IIB (fast-twitch, low-oxidative fiber), and type I (slow-twitch, high-oxidative fiber). This heterogeneous fiber pattern is lost with aging, fibers becoming more homogeneous in respect to their physiological and metabolic profile.

It is well known that decreases in muscle mass occur with old age, with proximal muscles of the lower extremity particularly affected. This decrease in muscle mass is due to a decrease in both fiber number and diameter. No change in the number of motor neural fibers has been found, but the size of the motor unit decreases because of the loss of muscle fibers. The reported decrease in fiber number primarily affects the red oxidative fiber, the preponderance of evidence based on enzyme histochemistry and physiological properties suggest a greater loss in the fast type II fiber. The decrease occurs in both type IIA and IIB fibers such that the type IIB/IIA fiber ratio is unaltered with increasing age. As a result of this selective loss of type II fibers, the percentage of type I fibers increases from about 40% in 20- to 30-year-olds to 55% in 60- to 65-year-old individuals (Astrand, 1987; Shepard, 1987). With aging and with inactivity, then, we see a loss of lean body mass. The same changes are also observed in younger subjects on bed rest and in astronauts in a gravity-free environment (Ryback et al., 1971). Exercise positively affects body composition.

Bed rest imposes inactivity in a nonuniform way in muscle groups. Functionally, neck extensors and the antigravity muscles of the legs are the least exercised. Arm, back, and abdominal muscles may be used more frequently during positional changes and the basic activities of care. During several weeks of bed rest in young men, grip strength, abdominal, and back muscle strength did not show any discernible change (Astrand, 1987). A decrease of 6% in shoulder and arm flexor muscles was observed. The tibialis anterior (the muscle that pulls the foot up) decreased in strength by 13%, and the gastrocsoleus (the muscle group that pulls the foot into a ballerina position and assists in flexion of the knee) lost 20% of its strength. Muller ( 1970) reported a loss of approximately 1.5% per day during a 2-week period of bed rest. Most of the studies on the effects of bed rest on skeletal muscle have been done on younger subjects. The amount of strength lost by aged persons during bed rest has not been extensively studied. However, inactivity superimposed on the "normal" aging process previously mentioned is likely to have significant disabling consequences. The decrement in strength with aging is likely to be due partially to inactivity. Exercise programs have been found to improve strength in all age groups (Shepard, 1987).

The skeletal system functions to support, protect, and shape the body. Additionally, bone has the metabolic functions of blood-cell production and the storage of calcium and plays a role in acid-base balance.

Cortical thickening starts to decline at approximately age 35, decreasing by 20% in men and 30% in women in the eighth and ninth decades. Bed rest or a lack of weight-bearing activities produces bone loss. Astronauts have been shown to lose 4 g of calcium during 84 days of space flight simulation (Ryback et al., 1971). Conversely, exercise improves bone mineralization.

The most commonly known age-related change involving bone is calcium-related loss of mass and density. This loss ultimately causes the pathological condition of osteoporosis. Bone density is lost from within by a process termed reabsorption. As we grow older, an imbalance occurs between osteoblast activity, whereby bones build up, and osteoclast activity, whereby bone breaks down. Osteoclast activity proves to be the stronger. As one ages, a decline in circulating levels of activated vitamin $D_3$ occurs (Fujiswawa, Kida, & Matsuda, 1984). This causes less calcium to be absorbed from the gut and more calcium to be absorbed from the bones to meet body needs. In postmenopausal women, decreased estrogen levels influence parathormone and calcitonin to increase bone reabsorption, which decreases bone mass. Certain factors such as immobility, decreased estrogens, steroid therapy, and hyperthyroidism are known to accelerate bone erosion to pathological levels. Easily occurring fractures are the most common result (Kenney, 1982; Ham & Marcy, 1983).

Bone mass and strength decline with age. Osteoporosis is a major bone mineral disorder in the older adult. This bone loss has been characterized by decreased bone mineral composition, an enlarged medullary cavity, normal mineral composition, and biochemical normalities in plasma and urine. The rate of bone loss is about 1% per year for women, starting at age 30 to 35, and for men, starting at age 50 to 55. In elderly subjects, regions of devitalized tissue with osteocyte lacunae and Haversian canals containing amorphous mineral deposits have been described, indicating a change in the bone mass-to-mineral ratio. These have been identified as micropetrotic regions and are noted to increase in frequency in the skeleton with age. Thus, it is clear that the mineral content of bone qualitatively changes with age.

Qualitatively, osteoporotic bone exhibits a reduction in bone mass with a resulting decrease in bone strength. However, there is some evidence that alterations occur in the composition and structure of bone in the aged. Evans (1990) observed that the tensile strength of bone in man is related to the number and size of osteons. It has been found that bone from older humans have smaller osteons and fragments and more cement lines than younger bone. This would account for some of the reduced bone strength of the older bone specimens. The remaining difference in strength results from the geometric structure of the bone in its distribution per unit area as a response to environmental stress placed on the bone. According to Wolf's Law, bone is layed down in the direction of stresses it must withstand. In the absence of stress (i.e., bed rest or varying levels of inactivity), the composition of bone becomes diffuse rather than uniform and loses its tensile strength.

EFFECTS ON BLOOD VOLUME. Throughout life, red blood cells continue to be replaced after a life span of about 120 days. Some morphological changes do occur with aging. Red blood cells become slightly smaller and more fragile. However, blood volume is well maintained until approximately 80 years of age. In the absence of pathology, few changes are seen in the white blood cells and in the platelet count. What is lost with aging is the functional reserve to quickly accelerate the production of red blood cells when needed (Kenney, 1982). This inability is further accentuated by inactivity.

EFFECTS ON THE PULMONARY SYSTEM. In the pulmonary system, changes due to aging and changes associated with inactivity can be organized according to mechanical properties, changes in flow, changes in volume, alteration in gas exchange, and impairments of lung defense. Decreases in chest wall compliance and lung elastic recoil tendency are two mechanical properties that are altered with age. Increased calcification of the ribs, a decline in intercostal muscle strength, and changes in the spinal curvature (resulting from osteoporotic collapse of the thorasic vertebrae) all result in lower compliance and in increased work in breathing.

At normal lung volume, airway resistance is not increased; however, normal aging results in a reduction of maximum voluntary ventilation, maximum expiratory flow and forced expiratory volume in a second (alone and in relation to forced vital capacity). Though tidal volume remains fairly constant throughout life, vital capacity decreases while residual volume increases. Bed rest has a relatively small effect on pulmonary function in healthy subjects (Saltin et al., 1968). However, chronic inactivity may cause some reversible decrement in vital capacity, and exercise training leads to a more efficient respiratory function (Shepard, 1978).

Ventilation, diffusion, and pulmonary circulation are the three major components of the respiratory system that lose efficiency with age. There is an increased thickening of the supporting membranes between the alveoli and the capillaries, a decline in total lung capacity, an increase in residual volume, a reduced vital capacity, and a decrease in the resiliency of the lungs. It is difficult to separate completely pulmonary changes resulting with age from those associated with the pathology of emphysema or chronic bronchitis. Throughout a lifetime, exposure to occupational and environmental inhalants as well as cigarette smoke may result in chronic pulmonary changes and lung pathologies. These disease states closely parallel those of the aging process and also increase in incidence with advancing age (Zadai, 1986). "Normal" pulmonary aging includes loss of elastic tissue leading to expiratory collapse of the larger airways, difficulty with expiration, and dilitation of the terminal air passages (Cummings & Semple, 1973).

Aging and inactivity also affect the diffusion efficiency of the peripheral vascular system. Starting with the pulmonary system, impairment of gas exchange is illustrated by a reduced diffusing capacity of carbon monoxide, a lower resting arterial oxygen tension and an increased alveolar-arterial oxygen gradient. Aveolar surface area and pulmonary capillary blood volume diminish with age. As a result, the oxygen dissociation curve shifts to the left, which makes oxygen less available at the tissue level.

The ability to provide oxygen to working tissues diminishes with inactivity. Normal aging affects the cardiopulmonary system in a variety of ways, as already discussed, though in the absence of pathology, the heart and lungs can generally meet the body's needs. The most evident change in the cardiovascular and cardiopulmonary functioning with bed rest is that the reserve capacities are diminished. In other words, with any challenge, the body's demand for oxygen and perfusion may exceed available supply.

Of importance clinically in an older person is that normal changes with aging and a decreased level of mobility result in an impairment of pulmonary defenses. Cilia are reduced in number and those that remain become less strong. The "mucous escalator" and alveolar macrophages (the germ killers) are less effective in removing inhaled particulate matter. In the absence of physiological challenges, the system maintains fairly adequate defenses. However, an older individual who is chronically exposed to particle-ladened air in addition to inactivity (which in essence diminishes the efficiency of the lungs) will become at risk for pulmonary dysfunction. (Kenney, 1982; Wynne, 1979).

As previously mentioned in regard to bed rest, the postexercise recovery period following effort is prolonged. Among other factors, this reflects a greater relative work rate, an increase proportion of anaerobic metabolism, slower heat elimination, and a lower level of physical fitness.

EFFECTS ON CONNECTIVE TISSUE. Extremes of immobilization can lead to a decrease in joint range of motion secondary to connective tissue changes. There are many types of connective tissue in the body — loose, adipose, fibrous, and so forth. It is 'loose' connective tissue that functions to bind organs together while holding tissue fluids and permitting cellular-molecular diffusion. Loose connective tissue is located beneath most layers of epithelium and fills spaces between muscles (fascia). The most common type of cell in loose connective tissue is called a fibroblast. Fibroblasts work to produce protein fibers called collagen and elastin. (Goldman, 1979).

In youth, collagen fibers are strong and flexible. Collagen fibers are arranged in bundles that criss-cross to form fibrous protein in the body. As a person ages, there is an increased criss-crossing, or cross-linkage, of the fibers, resulting in more dense extracellular matrices. The collagen structure becomes more stiff as it becomes more dense. The increased density also impairs molecular movement of nutrients and wastes at the cellular level. (Ham, March, & Holtzman, 1983).

Structurally, elastin fibers also develop increased cross-linkage with age. Water and elasticity are lost. The elastin fibers become more rigid, may tend to fray and, in some cases, are replaced by collagen completely (Kenney, 1982).

The clinical significance of this increased cross-linking is seen in resultant collagenous contractures. Bonds between adjacent collagen strands can produce shortening and distortion of the collagen fibers. This shortening may result in contractures with a progressive restriction in tissue mobility (Hamlin, 1980). Collagen fiber contractures are tough and inelastic. Their bonds cannot be broken by mechanical stretching forces. Fibrinous adhesions have great clinical implications in working with the elderly. Fibrinogen, a soluble plasma protein is a normal molecular exudate within the capillary. When this substance passes through the capillary wall into the surrounding tissues, it is converted to strands of insoluble fibrin (Astrand & Rodahl, 1970). Fibrin strands can adhere to tissue structures and restrict movement of these structures. Normally, fibrin is removed as debris. With age the exudation of fibrinogen into the surrounding tissues is increased (Meyer, 1958). With reduced activity levels, complete breakdown of fibrin may not occur; the resultant accumulation of this substance restricts movement and possibly causes adhesions. Following an injury (traumatic or surgically induced), fibrinogen also accumulates at the site of tissue damage. If activity is limited, these strands can consolidate and create an adhesion (Pickles, 1983). Some decrements in flexibility can be reversed by exercise (Shepard, 1987). The most effective means of maintaining mobility is early intervention by means of bed exercises. What is not lost does not need to be regained. Prevention of contractures is of extreme importance in geriatric rehabilitation, and the only way to accomplish this is to maintain activity, even when bed rest has been prescribed for an aged person.

Other connective tissue that is also affected by aging and inactivity includes hyaline cartilage, elastic cartilage, and articular cartilage. Hyaline cartilage is found in the nose and the rings of the respiratory passages as well as in the joints. Elastic cartilage is found in parts of the larynx and the outer ear. Articular cartilage is found between the intervertebral discs, between the bones of the pelvic girdle, and at most articular joint surfaces (Hole, 1978). With aging, cartilage tends to dehydrate, become more stiff, and thin in weight-bearing areas.

Cartilage is formed when its cells are subjected to compressive (i.e., weight-bearing) forces in an environment of low oxygen concentration. Cartilage is a unique connective tissue in that it has no direct blood supply. Blood flow in adjacent bones and synovial fluid provide nutrients to the cartilage. A strong osmotic force attracts water with dissolved gases, inorganic salts, and organic materials into the cartilage, providing materials necessary for normal metabolism. The concentration of glycoproteins in the matrix of the cartilage determines the amount of fluid drawn into the cartilage. Normal aging is accompanied by a reduction in the amount of glycoproteins produced (Kaplan & Mayer, 1959) resulting in a decrease in osmotic attraction forces and impairment in the ability of the cartilage to attract and retain fluids.

Nutrients enter the matrix of the cartilage only when compressive forces are absent (Shepard, 1987). In a loaded or compressed state, fluid and nutrient substances are squeezed out. To provide regular movement of substances in and out of the cartilage, it is necessary that alternating application and release of compressive forces occur. Metabolites remain in the cartilage in the absence of compression. The presence of metabolites reduces the oxygen content, resulting in a reduction of the secretion of glycoproteins (Shepard, 1987). The destruction of the joint progresses in the absence of activity.

In synovial joints the articular surfaces are covered by hyaline cartilage. Lubrication at the interface of the hyaline cartilage is provided by the secretion of hyaluronic acid. Hyaluronic-acid molecules form a viscous layer covering the hyaline cartilage. Compression facilitates production of hyaluronic acid, ensuring continual lubrication of the joint during movement (Calliet, 1969). The secretion of hyaluronic acid decreases with age and in the absense of weight-bearing activity, thereby reducing the efficiency of the lubrication system of the joint (Palmoski, Colyer, & Brandt, 1980). Degenerative changes of the cartilage are not reversible and rehabilitation efforts need to be directed toward regular (but not excessive) compression and release of compression in the aging joint. Normal weight-bearing exercises are recommended to maintain cartilaginous health.

The cartilage that normally covers body joints thins and deteriorates with aging. This occurs especially in the weight-bearing areas. Because cartilage has no blood supply or nerves, erosion within the joint is often advanced before symptoms of pain, crepitation, and limitation of movement are perceived. Decreased hydration, reduced elasticity, and increased fibrous growth around bony prominances all contribute to increased stiffness and decreased functioning. Advanced stages of cartilage-joint deterioration is commonly known as osteoarthritis (Goldman, 1979; Kenney, 1982; Gardner, 1978).

Since some type of connective tissue exists almost everywhere in the body, the effects of aging superimposed on inactivity are widespread. Increased rigidity of collaginous and elastin fibers results in a greater amount of energy being needed to produce a given stretch. Skin becomes less elastic and more wrinkled. Lungs lose some recoil tendency, arteries become more rigid, and the heart becomes less distensible. Joints become more stiff, and decreased hydration in the intravertebral discs results in vertebral compaction and shrinkage of height. Cellular repair, nutrition, and waste removal are impaired (Kenney, 1982). All of these consequences of inactivity and aging have been shown to be preventable with regular exercise (Shepard, 1987).

EFFECTS ON BOWEL AND BLADDER FUNCTION. Lack of activity or deconditioning per se do not appear to directly impair bowel and bladder function, the effects of aging on which are discussed in chapter 2. Of note in the event of acute inactivity, however, is the increased incidence of constipation (Larson & Bruce, 1987). The effects of chronic inactivity are less clear. It is difficult to sort out physical changes solely related to inactivity from dietary and functional problems.

EFFECTS ON METABOLISM. The effects of bed rest on metabolic function include an increased excretion of calcium within the first 2 days of bed rest (Ryback et al., 1971). Perhaps indicative of skeletal changes, such excretion peaks in the fourth week of immobilization (Dietrick, Whedon, & Shorr, 1948). Calcium losses stabilize by the fifth week following the resumption of activity. Negative nitrogen balance can start by the fifth day of bed rest. This is indicative of protein degradation, primarily in the skeletal muscle. Following a return to activity, a return to normal occurs by the sixth week of exercise. Accelerated loss of calcium and nitrogen induced by bed rest has important implications with regard to the high incidence of osteoporosis and loss of lean muscle tissue with aging.

SUMMARY. It seems obvious from these body systems that the evaluation and treatment of hypokinetics is crucial in the total care of the elderly. Passive range of motion (PROM) or active-assistive range of motion (A-AROM) is appropriate even in the most immobilized patients to prevent the consequences of immobilization. Aging and inactivity are both associated with loss of lean body mass and a gain in body fat (Buskirk, 1985;

Shepard, 1987). A certain number of changes associated with aging are directly related to inactivity. Active aged individuals show lesser degrees of these changes, and exercise programs in sedentary aged persons have been shown to positively modify those changes associated with aging. Exercise has been shown to reverse the physiological changes of inactivity, including a return of cardiovascular and cardiopulmonary response to pre-bed-rest baselines, and a return of muscle strength and flexibility (Astrand, 1987). A mnemonic representation of the effects of bed rest is helpful in remembering the overall effects of inactivity on functional capabilities:

B   Bladder and Bowel incontinence and retention; Bedsores
E   Emotional trauma; potential Electrolyte imbalances
D   Deconditioning of muscles and nerves; Depression; Demineralization of bones
R   ROM (range of motion) loss and contractures; Restlessness; Renal dysfunction
E   Energy depletion
S   Sensory deprivation; Sleep disorders
T   Trouble with all systems

### Optimal Health

The third principle in geriatric rehabilitation is that of "optimal health." The great English statesman Benjamin Disraeli once said, "The health of people is really the foundation upon which all their happiness and their powers as a state depend." The World Health Organization defines health as a state of complete physical, mental, and social well-being, not merely the absence of disease or infirmity (World Health Organization, 1964). The existence of complete physical health refers to the absence of pathology, impairment, or disability. Mental health as defined by the World Health Organization would include cognitive and intellectual intactness as well as emotional well-being. The social components of health would include living situation, social roles (i.e., mother, daughter, vocation, etc.), and economic status.

In "normal" aging, we witness some cumulative biological, physiological, and anatomical effects that may eventually lead to clinical symptoms. As noted in the section on activity versus inactivity, some of these changes are associated with inactivity and are not purely a result of progressive aging. In light of this, a preventive approach to physical health should be in the foreground when addressing the needs of the aged. Preventing impairment and disability are key principles in geriatric rehabilitation. It is reasonable to assume that the health status of individuals in their 70s and in subsequent decades of life is not the best it has been. Thus, the desired health status for the aged should be focused toward preventing the complications that could result from that suboptimal health condition. In considering suboptimal health, then, the goal of geriatric rehabilitation should be to strive for the maximal functional and physical capabilities of the aged, keeping in mind an individual's current health status.

In reviewing the importance of promoting relative "optimal health" in terms of the musculoskeletal, sensory, or cardiopulmonary systems, an example of an aged woman with a hip fracture may help. The woman may be in suboptimal health and suffering from osteoporosis; however, we do not treat her *until* she fractures her hip. The resulting complications could include pneumonia, decubiti (bedsores) from bedrest, all of the changes previously noted in relation to inactivity, as well as the possibility of death. We need to intervene before illness or disability occurs. This intervention could include weight-bearing exercises to enhance the strength of the bone, strengthening exercises of the lower extremities to provide adequate stability and endurance, balance exercises to facilitate effective balance reactions and safety, education in nutrition, and modification of her living environment to ensure added safety and prevent her from falling.

Another excellent example of preventive intervention to maintain optimal health would be in the case of the aged individual suffering from diabetes. It is known that the sensory loss in the lower extremities that results from diabetes mellitus often predisposes the individual to ulceration of the foot. An ill-fitting shoe or a wrinkle in the sock may go unnoticed and lead to friction, skin breakdown, and ultimately a foot ulcer. If undetected, even the smallest ulcer may lead to amputation of a lower extremity. Screening of the foot during evaluation can prevent this devasting loss. Intervention includes teaching aged diabetics to inspect their feet or enlisting the aid of the family members or friends of individuals whose eyesight is failing; proper shoe fitting; and techniques for dealing with sensory loss (e.g., as temperature sensation diminishes, before taking a bath, the individual needs to test the water temperature with a thermometer, or have someone test it for them). With proper skin care and professional (podiatric) care of the nails and callouses, there is less likelihood that injury will occur. A therapeutic diabetic shoe (the P. W. Minor Thermold shoe, for example) provides protection and ample room for the forefoot and costs a fraction of what ulcer care does, not to mention hospitalization and rehabilitation for amputation (American Diabetic Association, 1988). The principle of obtaining relative optimal health in geriatric rehabilitation is not only cost effective but clearly leads to an overall improvement in the quality of life. Encouraging healthy behaviors such as decreasing obesity, minimizing stress, and not smoking while increasing activity could be the elements necessary in maintaining health and striving for optimal health as defined by the World Health Organization.

As health-care professionals involved in geriatric rehabilitation, we need to be good *evaluators* and *screeners*. We need to develop investigative skills to be able to detect minor problems before they become major. By using thorough assessment tools to evaluate physical, cognitive, and social needs, we can modify rehabilitation programs so they will truly improve the health and functional ability of our aged clients.

REHABILITATIVE MEASURES

Rehabilitation should be directed at preventing premature disability. A deconditioned aged individual is less capable of performing activities than one who is conditioned. For example, walking speed is positively correlated to the level of physical fitness in an aged person (Himann et al., 1988). When cardiovascular capabilities are diminished (i.e., maximum aerobic capacity), walking speeds are adjusted by the aged person to levels of comfort. Himann et al. (1988) found that exercise programs geared to improving cardiovascular fitness improved the speed of walking. The more conditioned the individual, the faster the walking pace.

If disease and physical disability are superimposed on a hypokinetic sequalae, the functional consequences can be disastrous. Pain often prevents mobility. For instance, the pain experienced by an aged individual with an acute exacerbation of osteoarthritic knee pain accompanied by inflammation of the knee capsule, may reflexively inhibit contraction of the quadriceps. Although the strength of the quadriceps may have been poor in the first place because of inactivity, the absence of pain still permitted this individual to rise from a chair or ascend shallow steps. Now, with the presence of acute pain, these activities cause severe discomfort and threaten the maintainance an independent lifestyle. In this situation, rehabilitation efforts should focus medically on reducing the inflammation through drugs or ice (administered by a physician or nurse); maintaining the joint's mobility during the acute phases by joint mobilization techniques of oscillation and low-grade passive range in addition to modalities such as interferential current to assist in reducing the edema and decreasing the discomfort (physical therapy); joint protection techniques and prescription of adaptive equipment, such as a walker, to protect the joint (occupational and physical therapy); and provision for proper nutrition in light of the medications being taken (through consultation with a pharmacist/dietician) and evidence that vitamin C is a crucial component in the health of the synovium (Palmoski, 1980); and social and psychological support (provided by social workers, psychologists, or religious personnel). These interventions to prevent the debilitating effects of bed rest highlight the need for an interdisciplinary approach when addressing geriatric rehabilitation.

Rehabilitation of the aged individual should emphasize (1) functional activity to maintain functional mobility and capability, (2) improvement of balance through exercise and functional activity programs (i.e, weight-shifting exercises, ambulation with direction and elevation changes, and reaching activities, to name a few), (3) good nutrition and good general care (including hygiene, hydration, bowel and bladder considerations, and rest), as well as (4) social and emotional support. It is important to optimize overall health status by implementing the concept of "independence." The more individuals do for themselves, the more they are capable of doing independently. The more that is done for aged individuals, the less capable they become of functioning on an optimal independent level and the more likely the progression of a disability. The advancing stages of disabilities increase vulnerability to illness, emotional stress, and injury. Aged persons' subjective appraisal of their health status influences how they react to their symptoms, how vulnerable they consider themselves, and when they decide they can or cannot accomplish an activity. Often aged persons' self-appraisals are reliable predictors of the rehabilitative clinician's evaluation of health and functional status, but such assessments may also differ in many ways. In older persons, perceptions of health status may be determined in large part by their level of psychological well-being and by whether or not they continue in rewarding roles and activities (Siegler & Costa, 1985).

Aged individuals' perception of their health status is an important motivator in their compliance with a rehabilitation program. One interesting study showed that even when age, sex, and health status (as evaluated by physicians) were controlled for, perceived health and mortality from heart disease were strongly related (Kaplan, 1982). Those who rated their health as poor were two to three times as likely to die as those who rated their health as excellent. A Canadian longitudinal study of persons over 65 produced similar results (Mossey & Shapiro, 1982). Over 3 years, the mortality of those who described their health as poor at the beginning of the study was about three times the mortality of those who initially described their health as good. Yet despite this apparent awareness among older persons of their actual state of health, the aged are known to fail to report serious symptoms and wait longer than younger persons to seek help. It is with this in mind that rehabilitation professionals need to listen carefully to their aged clients. It appears that, contrary to the popular view that older individuals are somewhat hypochondriacal, the aged generally deserve serious attention when they bring complaints to their caregivers. Their perceived level of health will greatly impact the outcomes of functional goals in the geriatric rehabilitation setting, whether it provides acute, rehabilitative, home, or chronic care.

Rosillo & Fagel (1970) found that improvement in rehabilitation tasks correlated well with the patient's own appraisal of her or his potential for recovery but not very well with others'. Stoedefalke (1985) reports that postive reinforcement (i.e., frequent positive feedback) for older persons in rehabilitation greatly improved their performance and feelings of success. This indicates that aged persons can improve in their physical functioning when modifications in therapeutic interventions provide feedback more often. Some research indicates that older persons with chronic illness have low initial aspirations with regard to their ability to perform various tasks (Nader et al., 1985). As situations in which they succeeded or failed occurred, their aspirations changed to reflect more closely their abilities. Older persons may have different beliefs about their abilities compared to younger persons (Prohaska, Pontiam, & Teitleman, 1984). When subjects were given an unsolvable problem, younger subjects ascribed their failure to not trying hard enough, while older subjects ascribed their failure to inability. On subsequent tests, younger individuals tried harder and older subjects gave up. This is of extreme significance in the rehabilitation potential of an aged person. If the cause of failure is seen as an immutable characteristic by the person, then little effort in the future can be expected.

Aged individuals may have a higher anxiety level in rehabilitation situations because they fear failure or are afraid of "looking bad" to their family or therapist (Eisdorfer, 1968). Eisdorfer found that if anxiety is high enough, the aged concentrate their efforts toward reducing the anxiety rather than accomplishing proposed tasks. Weinberg, Bruya, and Jackson (1985) found that subjects set their own goals for task achievement even if they are directed to adopt the therapist's goals. In another study, Mento, Steele, and Karren (1987) found that the best performance at difficult tasks, as many rehabilitation tasks are, occurs when the aged person sets a very specific goal, such as walking 10 ft with a walker. If the person simply tries to "do better," then performance is not improved as much. These are important motivational components to keep in mind when working with an aged client. Perhaps the therapeutic approach of the clinician may have the greatest impact on the successful functional outcomes in a geriatric rehabilitation setting.

### Physical Activity

Exercise programs have potential for improving physical fitness, agility, and speed of response (Shepard, 1987). They also serve to improve muscle strength, flexibility, bone health, cardiovascular and respiratory response, and tolerance to activity (Smith & Serfass, 1981). Evidence suggests that reaction time is better in elders who engage in physical exercise than in those who are sedentary (Stelmach & Worringham, 1985). In their findings, Stelmach and Worringham showed a positive correlation between individuals' ability to maintain their balance when stressed and their level of fitness. Initial test scores on reaction time were significantly improved following a 6-week stretching and calisthenics program in individuals 65 years of age and older. This has great clinical significance, given the increasing incidents of falls with age (an area discussed in more detail later in this chapter). In addition, exercise has been shown to provide social and psychological benefits affecting the quality of life and the sense of well-being in the elderly (McPherson, 1986). Intuitively it would appear plausible that an aged individual who is in better physical condition will experience less functional decline, maintain a higher level of independence, and benefit from the improvement in their perceived quality of life.

The risks of encouraging physical activity are small and can be minimized through careful evaluation. While it is not the purpose of this chapter to describe in detail all the exercise and activity programs that constitute "therapeutic" exercise, Table 7.2 summarizes therapies for the conditions seen most frequently in geriatric rehabilitation settings.

TABLE 7.2    Rehabilitation Therapies for Common Conditions

*Cerebral Vascular Accident (Stroke)*

Physical Therapy
Pregait activities (if individual is not ambulatory)
Gait training (if individual is ambulatory)
Provision of assistive ambulatory devices (quad cane, hemi-walker)
Ambulation on different types of surfaces (stairs, ramps)
Provision of appropriate shoe gear and orthotics
Education and provision of appropriate bracing
Range-of-motion, strengthening, coordination exercises
Proprioceptive neuromuscular facilitation
Bobath techniques to modify tone
Sensory Integration
Joint mobilization techniques (when appropriate)
Functional electrical stimulation (when appropriate)
Positioning and posturing (chair, feeding needs)
Family and patient education for home management
Occupational Therapy
Training in activities of daily living (grooming, dressing, cooking, etc.)
Transfer training (toilet, bathtub, car, etc.)
Activities and exercise to enhance function of upper extremities
Training to compensate for visual-perceptual problems
Provision of adaptive devices (reachers, special eating utensils)
Speech Therapy
Language production work
Reading, writing, and math retraining
Functional skills practive (checkbook balancing, making change)
Therapy for swallowing disorders
Oral muscular strengthening

*Parkinson's Disease*

Physical Therapy
Gait training
Provision for appropriate shoe gear and orthotics

Training in position changes
General conditioning, strengthening, coordination, and range-of-motion exercises
Breathing exercises
Training in functional instrumental activities of daily living
Proprioceptive neuromuscular facilitation/Sensory integration
Occupational Therapy
Fine/gross motor coordination of upper extremities
Provision of adaptive equipment
Basic self-care activity training
Transfer training
Speech Therapy
Improving respiratory control
Improving coordination between speech and respiration
Improving control of rate of speech
Use of voice amplifiers and/or alternate communication devices

### *Arthritis*

Physical Therapy
Joint protection techniques
Joint mobilization for pain control and mobility
Conditioning, strengthening, and range-of-motion exercises
Gait training
Provision of proper shoe gear and orthotics
Modalities to decrease pain and edema, and break up adhesions
Provision of assistive ambulatory devices (when appropriate)
Occupational Therapy
Range-of-motion and strengthening exercise of upper extremities
Splinting to protect involved joints, decrease inflammation, and prevent deformity
Joint protection techniques
Provision of adaptive devices to promote independence and avoid undue stress on involved joints

### *Amputees*

Physical Therapy
Fitting and provision of temporary and permanent prosthetic devices
Teaching donning and doffing of prostheses
Progressive ambulation
Provision of assistive ambulatory devices
Training in stump care
Wound care (when appropriate)
Provision of shoe gear and protective orthotic for uninvolved extremity
Instruction in range-of-motion, strengthening, and endurance activities for both involved and uninvolved
     extremities
Balance activities
Transfer training
Occupational Therapy
Teaching donning and doffing of prostheses
Training in stump care
Transfer training
Training in activities of daily living

### *Cardiac Disease*

Physical Therapy
Patient education
Conditioning and endurance exercises (walking, biking, etc.) Breathing and relaxation exercises

*(continued)*

Table 7.2 *(cont'd)*

Strengthening and flexibility exercises
Monitoring of patients' vital signs during exercise
Occupational Therapy
Labor-saving techniques
Improving overall endurance for participation in activities of daily living
Monitoring patients participation in activities of daily living

*Pulmonary Disease*

Physical Therapy
Patient education
Breathing control exercises
Chest physical therapy
Conditioning exercises
Joint mobilization of rib cage
Occupational Therapy
Training in labor-saving techniques
Monitoring of participation in activities of daily living
Improving endurance of upper extremities

*Low Back Pain*

Physical Therapy
Joint mobilization/stabilization
Modalities to decrease pain and improve tissue mobility
Strengthening and flexibility exercises
Instruction in proper body mechanics for lifting, sitting, and sleeping
Provision of proper shoe gear and shock-absorbing orthotics
Correction of leg length discrepancy (when appropriate)
Occupational Therapy
Training in labor-saving techniques

*Alzheimer's Disease*

Physical Therapy
Sensory integration techniques
Gait training (when appropriate)
Balance activities
Provision of proper shoe gear and orthotics
General conditioning exercises
Reality orientation activities/validation techniques
Occupational Therapy
Sensory integration techniques
Activities of daily living (grooming, feeding, etc.)
Reality orientation activities/validation techniques

*Hip Fractures*

Physical Therapy
Range-of-motion, strengthening, and conditioning exercises
Positioning
Progressive weight bearing and gait training
Provision of assistive ambulation devices
Provision of proper shoe gear, lift on the involved side and orthotics for shock absorption
Balance activities
Transfer training

Specialized exercise techniques such as PNF (proprioceptive neuromuscular facilitation), Bobath, and sensory integration techniques (see Table 7.2) are very useful in regaining and maintaining functional mobility and strength and improving sensory awareness in elderly individuals (Volicer & Fabiszewski, 1988). Though these therapeutic exercises vary in their application techniques, the concept of integrating sensory and motor function is consistent in each. These exercise techniques are methods of placing specific demands on the sensory-motor system in order to obtain a desired response. Facilitation by definition implies the promotion or hastening of any natural process — the reverse of inhibition. Specifically, the effect is that produced in nerve cells by the introduction of an impulse. Thus, these techniques, though highly complex and requiring specialized training, may simply be defined as methods of promoting or hastening the response of the neuromuscular mechanism through stimulation of the proprioceptors (Knott & Voss, 1968). The normal neuromuscular mechanism is capable of a wide range of motor activities within the limits of the anatomical structure, the developmental level, and inherent and previously learned neuromuscular responses. The normal neuromuscular mechanism becomes integrated and efficient without awareness of individual muscle action, reflex activity, and a multitude of other neurophysiological reactions. Variations occur in relation to coordination, strength, rate of movement, and endurance, but these variations do not prevent adequate response to the ordinary demands of life.

The deficient neuromuscular mechanism is inadequate to meet the demands of life according to its degree of deficiency. Response may be limited in aged persons by the faulty neuromuscular response previously discussed as a sequalae in the aging process, inactivity, trauma, or disease of the nervous or the musculoskeletal system. Deficiencies present themselves in terms of limitation of movement as evidenced by weakness, incoordination, adaptive muscle or connective tissue shortening or immobility of joints, muscle spasm, or spasticity. It is the deficient neuromuscular mechanism that becomes the concern of the rehabilitation team in a geriatric setting. Specialized exercise techniques are very useful in successfully retraining the neuromuscular system in the aged person. Specific demands placed on the patient by a physical or occupational therapist have a facilitating effect upon the individual's neuromuscular mechanism. The facilitating effects of these therapeutic exercises are the means used in physical and occupational therapy to reverse the limitations of the aged person (Knott & Voss, 1968).

### Safety Measures

A general measure to ensure the highest functional capacity should encourage early resumption of daily activities following trauma or acute illness. Safety measures to prevent falls and avoid accidents should include reinforcing the use of properly fitted shoes with good soles, low broad heels, and heel cups or orthotics to stabilize the foot during ambulation; stressing the importance of wearing prescription eye glasses; and teaching the staff and family about how to reduce potential hazards within the patient's living environment (i.e., decreasing the amount of furniture, fixing loose carpeting, obtaining a commode, and installing handrails around the toilet and tub areas and railings in the hallways as needed). (For further discussion of the use of adaptive equipment, see Chapter 9,

Work, Productivity, and Worth in Old Age.) Measures to safety-proof the environment will be examined more thoroughly later in this chapter.

### Pain Management

Pain management is a very important factor in geriatric rehabilitation. Pain is one of the most difficult pathophysiologic phenomena to describe. It can be defined as the human perception or recognition of a noxious stimulus. In geriatric rehabilitation we deal with two basic types of pain, acute and chronic. Chronic pain can be broken down even further into two subcategories, acute-chronic and chronic-chronic. Treatment of acute pain may include medications to reduce inflammation; ice, heat, or compression (also to reduce edema when present); rest; and gentle mobility exercises. (Low-grade oscillation techniques of joint mobilization are very helpful in pain relief and maintenance of joint mobility). Rarely are modalities such as ultrasound or electrical currents used in the acute pain situation of an aged individual, though they are widely used in acute sports-related injuries in younger populations. (High galvanic current reduces edema, interferential current neutralizes the tissue and assists in fluid removal.) The reasons for this are not documented, though this author's clinical experience teaches that the more conservative approaches of rest, ice, compression or elevation, and gentle exercise in combination with nonnarcotic analgesics, seem to be quite effective in treating acute pain in the older person.

Chronic pain is more frequently observed in the aged than in younger persons and is more difficult to control. Chronic pain may not always correspond with objective findings. It is well recognized that emotional and socioeconomic factors play a role in chronic pain. Tension and anxiety often lead to muscle tension and decreased activity, and a vicious cycle often results. Situational depression may exacerbate this type of pain. In management of acute-chronic pain (as in an acute osteoarthritic condition), treatment is similar to acute-pain management except for the inclusion of various modalities. For instance, ultrasound may be used to break up a tissue adhesion; interferential or high galvanic electrical stimulation may be used to break up adhesions, reduce swelling, and enhance the circulation to the painful area. Joint mobilization techniques are often employed to improve and maintain mobility. Nonnarcotic analgesics can be prescribed, but the aged are more susceptible to the cumulative effects as well as the side effects of these drugs.

Foot pain or discomfort from boney changes such as those induced my lifelong use of ill-fitting shoes, arthritic changes, or age-related shifting of the fat pads under the heel and the metatarsal heads can severely curtail the ambulatory abilities of the aged. Proper shoe gear and shock-absorbing orthotics that place the foot in a neutral position have been clinically observed to facilitate ambulation and prevent disability. Though few studies have documented the effect of reducing plantar foot pressures or altering the weight-bearing pattern of the foot during gait in aged individuals, this author has recently completed a study (unpublished) that clearly demonstrates a decrease in discomfort as a result of reduced pressure and alteration in the weight-bearing pattern of the foot, as well as an increase in walking distance and functional capabilities.

### Assistive Devices

Assistive devices such as a cane, a quad cane (a more stable four-legged cane), or a walker can also be prescibed to improve stability during ambulation and reduce the stresses on painful joints.

A wheelchair may be necessary for longer distances, in particular, for use outside the home, or when ambulation is no longer possible (i.e., in the case of a bilateral amputation or severe diabetic neuropathy). When possible, wheelchairs should be tailored to meet the specific needs of the aged individual. For instance, removable arms may be needed to enhance the ease of transfers, or when severe cardiac disease results in lower extremity edema; elevating leg rests may be prescribed for lower-extremity elevation. Likewise, if upper-extremity capabilities are limited by advanced rheumatoid arthritis or quadriplegia, an electric wheelchair will greatly improve the individual's capabilities of locomotion (Figure 7.1). Other considerations may be a one-arm manual drive chair for a hemiplegic,

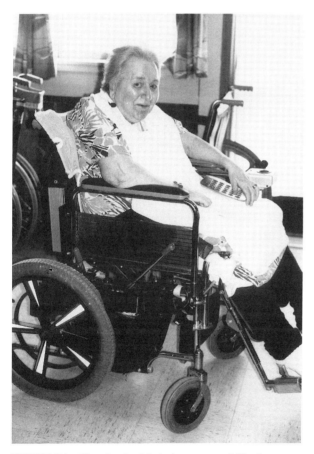

FIGURE 7.1   Electric wheelchair: improves mobility for severely disabled aged persons.

or a "weighted" chair to shift the center of gravity and improve the stability of the chair in transfers for the bilateral amputee. Health-care practitioners must work together to obtain the equipment that best suits the needs of the individual.

Proper positioning and seating for the aged individual who requires extended periods of sitting are required to decrease discomfort and keep pressures off of boney prominences, provide adequate postural support, facilitate feeding, and prevent progression of joint contractures and deformities (Figure 7.2). Many "geri-chairs" are on the market that address specific positioning needs. Arm chairs that provide assistance in rising from a seated position include higher chairs, which decrease the work of the lower extremities for standing, and electric "ejection" chairs that can be extended to bring the individual to a near-standing position. Functional assessment of the aged person is vital in the prescription of these specialized devices.

## SPECIAL CONSIDERATIONS IN GERIATRIC REHABILITATION

Although the present design of active rehabilitation programs, which involves learning and problem solving on the part of the aged individual, may not be realistic in severe

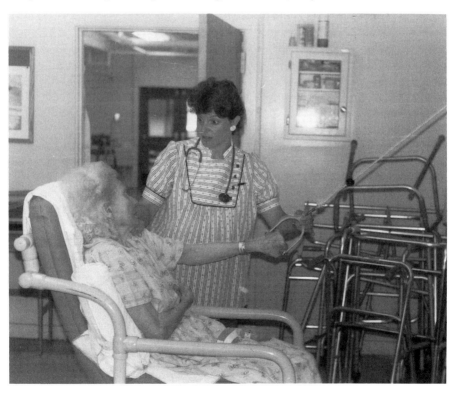

FIGURE 7.2    Proper positioning and seating facilitates function.

dementias such as that encountered in Alzheimer's disease because of impaired cognition, inability to learn new tasks, and difficulty in cooperating or participating in a regimented physical exercise program, functional capabilities can be maintained. Until the end stages of Alzheimer's, physical functioning remains relatively intact. It is the integration of movement, the motor planning (for instance, putting the sock on before the shoe), and the judgment required for safe functioning that becomes distorted.

The body communicates through its nervous system, which relays information and initiates motor activity. A breakdown in the system can lead to less efficient communication and a slowing of the body's responses. Thus it is important to consider the degenerative effects on the body of an aging nervous system. Neuromuscular changes with aging include deficits in coordination, strength, and speed of motion.

Changes in the sensory system with age provide less information to the central nervous system resulting from decreases in sensory perception. With loss of sensory input in combination with dementia of any degree, the aged individual is less able to assess the environment accurately, which leads to incorrect choices. Diminished hearing can also lead to incorrect choices because of inaccurately perceived communication.

As a result of normal aging, we will all experience changes in our ability to hear. For example, aged individuals experience a decreased ability to separate one sound or voice from background noises. Specific effects of aging on the auditory system include a diminished auditory acuity and poorer speech discrimination skills (Marshall, 1981). In other words, as the ear ages there is a greater distortion of auditory signals. In the aged person with dementia, these changes can add to confusion. Sensory losses and cognitive impairments, in addition to physical changes with age, need to be given special consideration in geriatric rehabilitation (specific interventions will be discussed in a later section, Adapting the Environment).

With aging there is a loss of neurons, as neurons are postmitotic cells and do not duplicate themselves (Gutman, 1972). This cell loss results in the narrowing of the convolutions and widening of the sulci in the aging brain. In fact, brain mass itself decreases by 10% to 20% by 90 years of age (Payton & Poland, 1983). The areas of the brain that show the greatest loss of neurons with "normal" aging are the frontal lobe (the area of cognition), the superior area of the temporal lobe (the main auditory area), the occipital area (the visual area), and the prefrontal gyrus (the major sensorimotor area of the brain) (Brody, 1979). A loss of neurons can be equated with a decrease in function if the losses are significant in any one area of the brain, and the rehabilitation of an elderly individual is directly affected by these changes. In the special case of Alzheimer's patients, the transcortical pathways are affected by the disease process and result in an inability to integrate activity. For instance, normally aging individuals know instinctively to alternate feet when walking. This may not be an automatic response of an individual with Alzheimer's disease, especially in the later stages of the disease. Compensation for cognitive, hearing, and visual decrements needs to be incorporated into rehabilitation programs (these changes will be readdressed in the section Adapting the Environment).

Diminished tactile sense often accompanies aging. Although vision and hearing are the predominant means of communication, touch is an important physical sensory communicator and should be considered when designing a rehabilitation program for aged patients. Information from receptors in muscles, joints, and the inner ear aid in movement and positioning. Decreased kinesthetic sensitivity owing to a general slowing and loss of receptor sensitivity with aging results in postural instability and difficulty in reacting to bodily changes in space.

Muscle strength determined by neurological function is defined by the rate of motor unit firing, the number and frequency of motor unit recruitment, and the cross-sectional diameter of the muscle (Lewis, 1985). The effects of the aging process on the neuromuscular system are seen clinically in deterioration of strength, speed, motor coordination, and gait. Muscular atrophy may be attributed to a decrease in the number of muscle fibers as previously described (McCarter, 1978). Other changes include a decrease in the clear differentiation of fiber type function (Moritani, 1981; Gutman & Hanzlikova, 1976). It has been suggested that muscle weakness in aging is a result of the replacement of skeletal muscle by fibrous tissue rather than free fat (MacLennan, Hall, & Timothy, 1980); however, there is great variability in loss of strength. Despite the obvious relationship between neuromuscular changes and loss of strength, disuse appears to play a very important role (Lewis, 1985). Changes in lifestyle as one ages apparently contribute to disuse of the muscles. As a result, aging changes of the muscle system closely parallel those discussed previously in the section on activity versus inactivity (Ragen & Mitchell, 1980).

Activity not only decreases but slows with aging and with disuse, and the aged exhibit slower reaction time. Nerve conduction velocity decreases at approximately 0.4% per year, starting at 20 years of age (Payton & Poland, 1983), but reaction time is a very complex response pattern to measure. The pathways involved include central nervous system processing, afferent nerve pathways, and the effector organ (muscles). Sensory stimuli and cognitive functioning are intimately involved in reaction time, and these factors must be considered when developing a rehabilitation program for the aged.

There are significant differences between the young and the old on tests measuring coordination and fine motor skills (Murray, 1975). An increase in "sway" as a normal balance correction, which diminishes the ability to maintain balance, is observed in the aged population. As a result, gait changes are observed. To compensate for the loss of balance, a wide base of support, allowing a greater distance between feet, is employed. Declines in sensory input because of inactivity also lead to sensorimotor deficits which alter gait in other ways.

Neurologic assessment must include psychologic factors and physiologic pathologies. The changes seen in the aging nervous system compound disabilities resulting from physiological or cognitive decline.

Musculoskeletal changes that occur with aging influence flexibility, strength, posture, and gait. Functional changes in lifestyle and activity add to these age-related changes.

Collagen, the supportive protein in skin, tendon, bone, cartilage, and connective tissue, changes with aging (Smith & Serfass, 1981), as the collagen fibers become irregular in shape as a result of increased cross-linking. This decreases the elasticity of the collagen fibers, decreasing the mobility of all the body tissues.

Inactivity too, has been shown to decrease muscle and tendon flexibility. Full immobilization in bed results in loss of approximately 3% per day of strength (Payton & Poland, 1983). Increased time spent in sitting significantly affects the body's flexor muscles, as adhesions are more likely to develop if the flexors of the body are maintained in a shortened position for extended periods of time. This has been observed in studies of astronauts, demonstrating the relationship between what we know to be the effects of aging, and those of disuse (Shepard & Sidney, 1987).

A decrease in lean muscle mass and changes in muscular function result from a variety of factors, including a decrease in efficiency of the cardiovascular system to deliver nutrients and oxygen to the working muscles and changes in the chemical composition of the muscle. Glycoproteins, which produce an osmotic force important in maintaining the fluid content of muscle tissues, are reduced in aging (Carlson, Alston, & Feldman, 1964). The inability of the muscle tissues to retain fluid, causes the hypotrophic changes observed in aging muscles, and there is a decrease in the permeability of the muscle cell membrane, making the cell less efficient. At rest, high concentrations of potassium, magnesium, and phosphate ions are found in the sarcoplasm, while sodium, chloride, and bicarbonate ions are prevented from entering the cell. In the senescent muscle there is a shift in this resting balance, with a decrease in potassium. Lack of potassium in the aging muscle reduces the maximum force of contractions generated by the muscle (Gutman & Hanzlikova, 1976). Clinically, tiredness and lethargy result from a depletion of potassium stores.

Decrease in total bone mass, or osteoporosis, is a characteristic change with age. Four times more women than men and 30% of women over the age of 65 years are osteoporotic (Payton & Poland, 1983). The older the person, and the poorer the nutritional history, ther greater the risk for this condition. Hormonal changes (as seen with menopause in women) and circulatory changes (as seen with decreased activity) also play a role. Though often asymptomatic, osteoporosis can be a major cause of pain, fractures, and postural changes in the musculoskeletal system (Lewis, 1985).

Balance, flexibility, and strength provide the posture necessary to ensure efficient ambulation. In aging, poor posture results from a decline in flexibility and strength, and from boney changes in the vertebral spine, resulting in less safe gait patterns. Gait is the functional application of motion. Changes in the gait cycle seen in aged include (1) mild rigidity (greater proximally than distally), producing less body movement; (2) fewer automatic movements with a decreased amplitude and speed (such as arm swing); (3) less accuracy of foot placement and speed of cadence (step rate per minute; (4) shorter steps because of changes in kinesthetic sense and slower rate of motor unit firing; (5) wider stride width (broad-based gait) in the attempt to enhance safety; (6) decrease in swing-to-stance ratio (improving safety by allowing more time in the double-support phase, i.e., when both feet are in contact with the ground at the same time); (7) decrease in vertical displacement, which is the up-and-down movement created by pushing off from the toes for forward propulsion, and the alternate heel strike (usually secondary to stiffness, a distinct push-off and heel strike are not observed in the aged); (8) decrease in toe-to-floor clearance; (9) decrease in excursion of the leg during swing phase; (10) decrease in the heel-to-floor angle (usually because of the lack of flexibility of the plantar flexor muscles and weakness of dorsiflexors); (11) slower cadence (another safety mechanism); and (12) decrease in velocity of limb motions during gait (Lewis, 1985).

Exercise is a physical stimulus that produces a metabolic increase above the resting levels of vital signs. In a healthy, young individual the cardiovascular system responds quickly to increase the metabolic rate by increasing heart rate, stroke volume (the amount of blood delivered to the system with each heart beat), and peripheral blood flow to deliver oxygen to the working muscles. In the aged, the response time of the cardiovascular system is delayed in restoring homeostasis when the level of physical activity has been increased (Shepard, 1987). The aged have a lower resting cardiac output and basal metabolic rate primarily because of age-related loss of lean body mass (Smith & Serfass, 1981) and inactivity (Shepard, 1978). Heart rate and stroke volume decrease 0.7% per year after 30 years of age, decreasing from approximately 5 L/min at 30 years to 3.5 L/min at 75 years. As exercise levels increase, this is manifested as reduced oxygen uptake (Ragen, 1980). In respiration there is a 50% decrease in the maximum volume of ventilation and 40% decrease in the vital capacity by the age of 85 (Payton & Poland, 1983). These limitations in oxygen transport capability translate directly into a reduced physical work capacity.

Understanding and managing patients' sensation of fatigue is essential in any exercise program. Fatigue, a word understood by everyone, lacks precise definition. Darling (1971) likened the concept of fatigue to the concept of pain. Both must be considered from physiologic and psychologic points of view. Physiologic types of fatigue include "muscle" fatigue from prolonged use of a muscle group, "circulatory" fatigue associated with elevated blood lactate levels during prolonged activity, and "metabolic" fatigue in which exercise depletes glycogen (energy) stores. General fatigue is related to more subtle factors like interest, reward, and motivation.

Given these definitions, it is easy to understand why a deconditioned person can experience fatigue. From a treatment perspective it is essential to determine what sensation the aged individual is describing as fatigue. Elevated vital signs and progressively weak muscle contractions suggest that rest is needed. A vaguer complaint of fatigue in the absence of these changes would not necessarily be a basis for reducing exercise. In fact, poor aerobic fitness may be related to an otherwise healthy aged person's complaint of fatigue (Kohl, Moorefield, & Blair, 1987).

In providing activity and exercise programs for the aged, "normal" aging changes in the musculoskeletal, neuromuscular, cardiovascular, and pulmonary systems will affect functional capacity. In addition, confusion, decreased sensory awareness, postural changes, cardiovascular limitations resulting from deconditioning, motivation, and perceived level of fatigue all affect the potential for rehabilitation and need to be assessed before activity or exercise programs are implemented. More specific exercise recommendations are included in the subsequent section on fall prevention.


NUTRITIONAL CONSIDERATIONS

Nutrition in the aged has been extensively addressed in Chapter 6, Nutritional Concerns and Problems of the Aged. Here nutrition is discussed only as it impacts on functional capabilities.

Just as a car needs gas in order to run, a human being needs adequate energy sources in order to function on an optimal level. Nutritional levels need close monitoring in relation to energy needs and functional activity levels. Increased feeding difficulties may be secondary to decreased appetite, poor oral status, visual or sensorimotor agnosia, cogni-

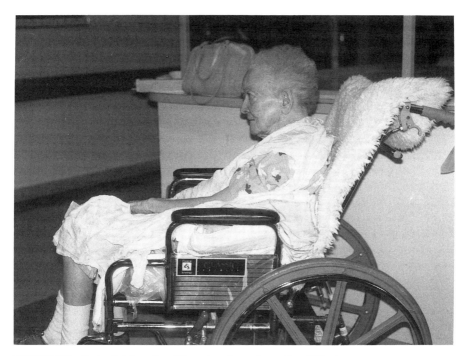

FIGURE 7.3    Postural deformity of thorasic spine makes eating difficult.

tive declines (decreasing attentiveness), and physical limitations. Environmental cues and adaptive eating equipment can often be employed to facilitate feeding. Postural considerations need to be addressed as well. A poor sitting posture can further decrease the ease of feeding by preventing upper-extremity movement or making chewing and swallowing difficult as a result of head position. For example, an elderly woman with severe osteoporosis and resulting kyphosis is at a postural disadvantage for feeding. Seated in an upright chair, her entire upper trunk will be forced forward and her face directed downward (Figure 7.3). Gravity only serves to allow the food to drop out of her mouth, especially if dentures are loose, she is edentous, or oral motor skills are compromised.

Specialized feeding programs may be necessary if there is neuromuscular involvement. For instance, an aged person sustaining a cerebral vascular accident may have difficulty swallowing or with mouth closure because of weakness in the muscles needed for these activities. In these cases, specialized muscle facilitation techniques can be employed to promote swallowing and facilitate mouth closure. By means of what is commonly termed a "dysphasia team," health professionals in nursing, dietetics, and speech, physical, and occupational therapy, the feeding needs of a neurologically impaired individual can be comprehensively addressed. In the geriatric rehabilitation setting this team is a vital component in obtaining maximal functional capabilities, promoting adequate nutrition through neuromuscular facilitation techniques, proper posturing and supportive seating, and adaptive eating utensils. Ultimately the goal of this team is to permit independent feeding by the aged person.

## FALLS

Falls are not part of the normal aging process. They are due to an interaction of underlying physical dysfunction, medications, and environmental hazards (Christiansen & Juhl, 1987). Poor health status, impaired mobility from inactivity or chronic illness, postural instability, and a history of previous falls are observable risk factors. The ultimate goals of rehabilitation are to combat the inactivity and loss of mobility that predispose the aged to falls.

Some of the ad hoc measures currently used to prevent falls — physical restraints and medications to reduce activity — are now suspected to increase the risk of falling (Christiansen & Juhl, 1987).

Medical conditions are often a cause of falling. A pathological fracture secondary to severe osteoporosis may result in a fall, possibly causing further fracture, or an arrhythmia may induce dizziness. Certain drugs, such as digoxin used in treating an arrhythmia, may also induce dizziness or fatigue (see Chapter 5, Drug Therapy in the Aged Patient).

The fear of falling is often a cause for inactivity. This is commonly seen in an individual who has sustained a previous fall. The guarding patterns that aged individuals use as a result of this fear (i.e., grabbing furniture that may not be stable or supportive) may in fact lead to further danger. Intervention by a psychiatrist or psychologist is often necessary to diminish this fear.

Functionally, limitations of range of motion, decreased muscle strength, joint mobility, coordination problems, or gait deviations can predispose an aged individual to falling. Specific strengthening and gait training programs assist in preventing falls by improving overall strength and coordination, balance responses and reaction time, and awareness of safe ambulation practices (e.g., freeing one hand for the use of a handrail when carrying packages up the stairs). Some individuals will have inadequate strength and balance to ambulate without an assistive device. Assistive ambulatory devices may also provide a safer mode for locomotion (Figure 7.4). Walking aids such as canes and walkers are beneficial for prevention of falls in some cases (Kalchthaler, Bascon, & Ouintos, 1978), whereas, in other cases they actually contribute to the cause of the fall (Tinetti, 1987). It is important to assess the appropriateness of the assistive device and ensure that the aged individual is using it properly. With proper instruction, the aged person can usually function safely within their environment without falling.

Gait evaluation is one of the most important components in fall prevention. The "get up and go" test is a method used often to test strength, balance, coordination, and safety during gait. Aged individuals are asked to get up out of a chair without using their hands, walk approximately 20 ft down the hall, turn around and come back to the chair, and then stand still. While they are standing still with their eyes closed, a gentle push on the sternum can be given to test righting reflexes. Finally, individuals are directed to sit down without the use of their hands. Upon completion, each component of the test is analyzed. For instance, the inability to arise from the chair without the assistance of the hands is indicative of hip-extensor or quadricep weakness. If step symmetry is absent (i.e., the individual is taking irregular steps), the cause can often be pinpointed just by observation. A leg length discrepancy may be present or the hip abductors may be weak. These alterations in anatomical structure or muscle status can easily be determined by close evaluation of the gait pattern.

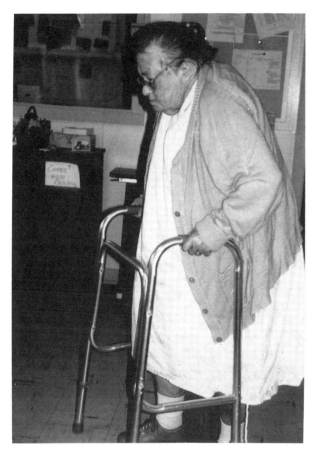

FIGURE 7.4    Ambulation with a standard walker.

Lower-extremity pain may also result in nonrhythmical steps as the individual attempts to avoid the painful extremity. A tendency to veer, lose balance, or hold on to surrounding objects may be indicative of dizziness, muscle weakness, or poor vision. While the individual is turning, loss of balance or a stiff, disjointed turn may alert the clinician to the possibility of neurological disorders such as Parkinson's disease or drug-induced muscle rigidity (often seen in aged individuals on Haldol).

With good basic patient and family education and modification of the environment to reduce hazards, it is possible to prevent falls through methods that do not undermine mobility or autonomy. It is important to identify and treat reversible medical conditions, as well as physical impairments in gait and balance. Many falls can be prevented through proper exercise to maintain strength, sensory integration techniques to promote all functional activites by improving balance and coordination, good shoes and orthotics to provide a proper base of support and gait training activities, and modifications to "safety-proof" the living environment.

Rehabilitation specialists play an important role in fall prevention. When disease states and medication responses are stable, an individualized program of safety education, environmental adaptations, lower-extremity strengthening exercises, balance exercises, and gait training should be implemented.

Safety education is an important first step in the prevention of falls. Many older individuals are not aware that they are at risk for falling. Often, simple instructions about environmental adaptations and encouraging a person to allow plenty of time for functional activities is all that is needed to facilitate their safety. Many aged people feel the need to rush to answer a phone or doorbell. They should be discouraged from doing so, because rushing could result in a fall. Caretakers and visitors should also be a part of the safety education process. They are often able to remind the person who is at risk for falling of the need for added precaution.

Aged persons who complain of dizziness during changes of position should be evaluated for postural hypotension. These individuals should be taught to change positions slowly and to wait before moving to another position in order to allow blood pressure to accommodate the change.

Any aged individual who has fallen is at risk for falling again. In fact, clustering of falls has been seen in some older individuals during the months preceding death (Gryfe, Aimes, & Ashley, 1977). Inability to rise or lack of assistance after a fall can have devastating consequences. In one study, half of the aged persons who lay on the floor for longer than 6 hours after a fall died within 6 months (Wild, Nayak, & Isaacs, 1981). Having a phone in every room may be a necessity for aged persons who live alone. A "buddy system" in which aged persons call each other regularly during the day is a means of "checking up" and allows early detection of a fall. Individuals at risk can also be provided with a device such as the "life-line" that summons emergency personnel by pushing a single button.

Eighty-five percent of all falls occur at home (Tideiksaar, 1987), most commonly on stairs (Droller, 1955; Archea, 1985), on the way to and from the bathroom (Ashley, Gryfe, & Aimes, 1977), and in the bedroom (Louis, 1983). Environmental evaluation and adaptation are required for those aged individuals who have fallen or are at risk for falling. Table 7.3 presents a safety checklist prepared by Tideiksaar (1987) for use in the home.

Safety evaluation should address such questions as: Are the carpets tacked down? Is the pathway from the bed to the bathroom obstacle free? Is there night time lighting? Additional environmental suggestions include adaptive equipment for the shower or bathtub (e.g., using a tub seat and a hand-held shower head can improve safety and independence while bathing). Adaptations may also be necessary to avoid falls en route to the bathroom. Individuals with urinary urgency, evening fatigue, or disorientation in the middle of the night should be encouraged to use a bedside commode.

The purpose of strengthening exercises in the prevention of falls is to provide adequate force in the lower extremities and trunk muscles for support of posture and control of balance. Some aged individuals will tolerate a progressive resistive exercise program. Others will derive greater benefit from a more functional approach to strengthening exercises. For example, practicing sit-to-stand movements and the reverse is a functional means of strengthening extensors and flexors of the lower extremities. Going up and down stairs one stair at a time requires less strength, range of motion, and balance than walking step

TABLE 7.3   Home Assessment Checklist for Prevention of Falls

*Exterior*

Are step surfaces nonslip?
Are step edges visibly marked to avoid tripping?
Are stairway handrails present? Are handrails secure?
Are walkways covered with a nonslip surface and free of objects that could be tripped over?
Is there sufficient outdoor lighting to allow safe ambulation at night?

*Interior*

Are lights bright enough to compensate for limited vision?
Are light switches accessible before entering a room?
Are lights glare-free?
Are handrails present on both sides of staircases?
Are stairways adequately lite?
Are handrails securely fastened to walls?
Are step edges outlined with colored adhesive tape and are they nonslip?
Are throw rugs secured with nonslip backing?
Are carpet edges taped or tacked down?
Are rooms uncluttered to permit unobstructed mobility?
Are chairs throughout home strong enough to provide support during transfers? Are armrests present?
Are tables (dining room, kitchen) strong enough to lean on?
Do low-lying objects (coffee tables, stools) present a hazard?
Are telephones accessible?

*Kitchen*

Are storage areas easily reached without standing on tiptoes or a chair?
Are linoleum floors slippery?
Is there a nonslip mat in front of sink to soak up spilled water?
Are chairs wheel-free, armrest equipped, and of the proper height to allow for safe transfers?
If the pilot light goes out, is odor strong enough to alert the person?
Are step stools strong enough to provide support?
Are stool treads strong, in good repair, and slip resistant?

*Bathroom*

Are doors wide enough to accommodate assistive devices?
Do door thresholds present tripping hazards?
Are floors slippery, especially when wet?
Are skid-proof strips or mats in place in tub or shower?
Are tub and toilet bars available? Are they well secured?
Are toilets low in height? Is an elevated toilet seat available?
Is there sufficient, accessible, and glare-free light available?

*Bedroom*

Is there adequate, accessible lighting? Are there nightlights and/or bedside lamps available?
Is the pathway from the bed to the bathroom unobstructed?
Are beds of appropriate height for safe transfers on and off?
Are floors covered with a nonslip surface and obstacle-free?
Can individual reach objects on closet shelves without standing on tiptoes or a chair?

*Adapted from Tideiksaar (1987)*

over step. A functional way to extend this activity, then, is to begin with one stair at a time and progress to step over step. Marching in place while standing can also strengthen lower-extremity flexors. This activity can be extended by asking the individual to hold the leg in flexion for a count of 3. During this activity, isometric strengthening also occurs in the extensors, abductors, and adductors of the stance leg. For safety, aged individuals should hold on to the back of a chair or the rim of the kitchen counter.

No matter which approach is selected for strengthening, the following precautions are recommended: (1) Many aged individuals have osteoporosis. Resistance and unilateral weight bearing may be excessive for them. It is possible to fracture an osteoporotic bone during strengthening exercises. (2) Many aged individuals have osteoarthritis. Isometric exercise may be less painful for them. Prolonging the amount of time that the contraction is held is an effective way to increase strength without adding external resistance (Lawrence, 1956). (3) It is especially important for aged individuals to avoid holding their breath (Valsalva maneuver) during exercise. Counting out loud helps to avoid this problem. (4) Aged individuals should be taught to monitor their heart rate during exercise.

Therapeutic exercises designed to improve balance are an important part of fall prevention. Balance exercises address three areas of posture control: response to perturbation, weight shifting, and anticipatory adjustments to limb movements (Horak, 1987). Individuals must be able to respond to an external perturbation such as a push to the shoulder or sternum with a postural adjustment that brings the center of gravity back over the base of support. The usual response to a lateral perturbation will be extension of the weight-bearing leg along with elongation of the trunk on the weight-bearing side. Flexion and abduction of the non-weight-bearing leg will also be seen (Bobath, 1978). A small backward force should stimulate the reaction of the dorsiflexors at the ankles and flexion at the hips, whereas a small forward push should be followed by plantarflexion at the ankles and extension at the hips (Woollacott, Shumway-Cook, & Nashner, 1986). Weight-shifting movements of the entire body during standing involve muscular activity similar to that used in response to a perturbation; however, during weight shifting, the muscle activation occurs voluntarily. Balance must also be controlled when a limb movement occurs, such as reaching with the upper extremity or swinging with the lower extremity. In this case, the postural adjustment actually occurs in anticipation of the limb movement, to prevent the center of gravity from moving outside of the base of support. For example, a forward movement of the arm should be preceded by ankle plantarflexion and hip extension. In this way, a small backward movement of the center of gravity counteracts the forward displacement caused by the moving arm. Practicing each of these activities — that is, response to perturbation, voluntary weight-shifting, and postural adjustments in anticipation of limb movement in standing — will help prepare the aged individual to use postural adjustment effectively during functional standing activities such as cooking, transfers, and ambulation. These activities are directed toward improvement of the motor component of balance.

Altering sensory conditions during balance activities encourages the aged person to attend selectively to support-surface or visual information. Balancing in bare feet with the eyes open or closed helps maximize the amount of somatosensory information that is available from the soles of the feet. On the other hand, balancing while standing on a piece of foam (Shumway-Cook & Horak, 1986) disrupts information from the sole of the foot and from the stretch receptors in the ankle muscles and forces the individual to practice using visual input to stabilize posture. Maintaining balance while turning the head from side to side and while nodding the head is also important. Many aged people report falling during head movements (Stout, 1978) or while looking up to hang curtains or change a lightbulb. Aged individuals should be instructed to use caution during upward head movements.

When an individual is unable to control standing balance and is about to fall, the normal response is protective extension of the arms or legs. Protective reactions such as arm extension and the stepping response should also be practiced. Upper-extremity protective extension can be practiced both forward and sideways against the wall, in the standing position (Carr & Shepard, 1987). Lower-extremity protective reactions should be practiced in standing in forward, sideways, and backward directions. Brisk and accurately directed limb extension is the goal.

Balance exercises can be incorporated into functional activities for the aged. Moving from sit-to-stand and from stand-to-sit are examples of controlled voluntary weight shifting. Shifting the trunk forward and back and from side to side while sitting are also examples of voluntary weight shifting. Voluntary weight shifting while standing with the individual's back to a wall is a safe way to facilitate control of balance. Dancing has also been recommended as a functional activity to improve balance for prevention of falls (Gabell, 1986). Postural adjustments in anticipation of arm movements can be practiced during functional activities by standing and reaching for objects on the kitchen or closet shelves. Reaching should be practiced in a variety of directions.

Ambulation requires weight shifting. Manual guidance during ambulation helps organize the time and direction of weight shifting (Carr & Shepard, 1987). Functional ambulation requires interaction with a variety of different support surfaces. Ambulation should be practiced on smooth as well as uneven surfaces and on levels as well as inclines, curbs, and stairs. Varying the amount of available light and background noise also stimulates realistic environmental conditions. If step lengths are irregular, footprints on the floor make good targets for foot placement. Manual guidance is also useful for regulating speed. A variety of speeds of ambulation are necessary for function. Challenging activities like crossing a busy street can be made less threatening if the aged individual practices with the therapist or caregiver.

Risk factors for falling among the aged suggest that falling should not be considered a normal concommitant of aging; rather, it should alert the health-care professional to the possibility of underlying disease or accelerated sensory or neuromuscular degeneration secondary to disuse. Secondary or multiple diagnoses; use of multiple medications, especially diuretics and barbituates; decreased vision and lower-extremity somatosensation; and decreased lower extremity strength all appear to contribute to balance and gait deficits, which in turn result in falling. Prevention of falling depends on addressing the specific problem area for each individual at risk. A team approach is the most effective intervention in preventing falls by the aged.

## ADAPTING THE ENVIRONMENT

The process of adapting to the environment, or of adapting the environment to the aged person, is especially important in geriatric rehabilitation. With decreased physiologic reserves, the aged person may not be able to engage in demanding activities. For instance, an older person who has suffered a stroke and who has underlying cardiac insufficiency may need to learn wheelchair mobility skills, and the environment will need significant modification. Doors may need to be widened, ramps installed, and counters lowered. Opportunities for obtaining new housing or adapting the present home may be restricted both by financial concerns and personal preferences.

The interaction between aged persons and their environment becomes increasingly precarious over time, involving the individuals' physical status, their living surroundings, and their social context. Of course, all persons interact with their environment. As one ages, however, physiologic reserves, underlying medical problems, affective states, and a host of other factors complicate this relationship.

The task of rehabilitation providers is to manipulate the environment to make it safer. Assistive walking devices or modifications of the home may be recommended. But even the use of these interventions is subject to variability in dealing with aging persons. The aged person with a disability may view such aids as unattractive or demeaning. Unlike eyeglasses, which allow individuals some choice in enhancing their appearance, walkers or chrome-plated grab bars may project an image of illness and disability. But older persons who have no qualms about home modifications may have difficulty finding someone who can install them. Some retired senior volunteer programs (RSVPs) have carpenters available for this purpose, but many communities are without such support services.

Any given physical and social context has the potential for facilitating or hindering the use of functional capabilities. Push-button controls placed at the front of a range assist aged individuals with low vision, whereas dials situated at the back of the range handicap them. Similarly, caregivers can enhance functional independence by providing aged individuals with adaptive equipment, such as plate guards, bath brushes with elongated handles, and sock aids, or they can promote dependence by feeding, bathing, and dressing the individual. Evaluation of the environment involves more than task analysis because the environment of concern is the one in which the individual actually lives and has to function, rather than a hospital or nursing home. Evaluation of physical space determines what architectural barriers safety and functional features exist, and the extent to which available equipment can be operated by the aged individual. Evaluation of the social context probes the availability of caregivers, their skills in rendering care and their need for training, their attitudes toward functional independence, and their experience in handling the burden of caregiving.

Aged persons with disabilities or physiological or anatomical changes resulting from inactivity and aging may experience memory loss, disorientation, decreased ability to perform normal physical activity, a diminished ability to remember details, difficulty in verbal expression, and impairment in judgment. Each of these factors is important when modifying the physical and social environment to meet the rehabilitation needs of the aged. Recent U.S. government hearings and reports suggest that certain social and organizational characteristics of institutions and the home setting can postpone the time when aged people become bedridden and require skilled nursing care (Alzheimer's: Report, 1984; Alzheimer's: Joint Hearing, 1984).

To prolong care at home it is reasonable for the direct caregiver to seek advice about practical strategies that could reduce confusion or injury on the part of the disabled aged. Environmental designs for aged patients have been studied, and several factors are consistently identified as environmental hazards, including poor illumination; inadequate color differentiation; cluttered furnishings and confused layout (e.g., a table fills a dimly lit hallway); bland, nondistinct textiles; unusual architectural features (such as split-level rooms); and insufficient climate control (Liebowitz, Lawton, & Waldman, 1979). Certain environmental features can be a threat to safety, produce anxiety, and amplify cognitive deficits (Weldon & Yesavage, 1982). Cohen (1984) found that behavioral approaches, (i.e., using environmental cues like color coding or labeling objects) has advantages over drugs in the treatment of cognitive impairments. Additional studies have emphasized that encouragement of independence, self-sufficiency, and social interaction is critical to prolonging cognitive functions (Reifler & Wu, 1982).

The aged individual's environment may have negative effects on their communication. Older people living alone are often isolated in home or community settings that allow few opportunities for successful, meaningful communication (Lubinski, 1981). Aged persons need an environment that stimulates and reinforces communication. Geriatric rehabilitation should encourage participation in a variety of activities that can serve as a basis for conversation and interaction. Socially stimulating environments within a hospital or a rehabilitative or long-term care setting can be provided by means of organized recreational and social therapies. This becomes more difficult in the home setting, though often resources such as church, community groups, or senior centers can facilitate social interaction. Meaningful conversation is a crucial component in enhancing and reinforcing cognitive functioning and a sense of well-being for the aged individual (Lubinski, 1981; Reifler & Wu, 1982).

Visual limitations such as farsightedness; decreased ability to adapt to changes in lighting conditions, requiring increased illumination to see; and an increased sensitivity to glare are not uncommon in the elderly patient (see Chapter 2, Physical Health Problems and Treatment of the Aged). Several changes normally occur within the aging eye that affect safety within their environment and need to be considered when adapting it. The lens of the eye begins to thicken and yellow, and the muscles that control dilation of the pupil weaken. The thickening of the lens and delayed pupil dilation means that the glare and reflections often encountered in the environment cannot be tolerated (Andreasen, 1985). In fact, the older eye needs approximately three times the amount of light to function adequately. The older person also has difficulty with depth perception and color differentiation which can interfere with ambulation (poor judgment in distance), the activities of daily living, and driving an automobile. Color vision deficiencies in the aged have been described by Andreasen (1985), who found that the aged individual has difficulty distinquishing between shades of blue-green, blue, and violet, and are unable to distinquish between two shades of a similar color. Aged persons maintain their ability to differentiate between brighter colors such as orange and red (Andreasen, 1985). Research has demonstrated the need for large pattern designs or solid bright colors in upholstery and textiles to enhance visability, interest, and appeal and to reduce the likelihood of bumping into or falling over furniture. Small patterns can produce blurring of vision and eye fatigue (Sharpe, 1974).

Independence can be facilitated by bright and sharply contrasting colors. Considering their poorer differentiation of similar colors, aged individuals will have trouble making their way in a poorly lighted livingroom with a blue carpet, light-blue walls, and lavender and blue-flowered furniture and draperies. Contrasting colors or better lighting (which is economically more feasible) would enhance safety in such a room. In hospitals and nursing homes, color coding walls and corridors with bright colors can help aged persons find their own room, bathroom, sitting room, and so on. Contrast is extremely important. Contrasting colors can eliminate the difficulty in making one's way along a stairwell or a dark, shadow-filled hall. Often color contrast can be accomplished through the use of fluorescent tape in shades of orange, lime green, or red.

Different colors have different effects on an individual's emotional state (Sharpe, 1974). The colors red, yellow, and orange have been associated with excitement, stimulation, and aggression (Sharpe, 1974). Red, which increases muscular tension and blood pressure, could be used as a visual stimulant to alert the elderly of environmental changes or hazards, such as stairs or level changes. Elderly individuals often need such warning signals. For those with dementia, however, soothing, warm colors, such as light oranges and blues, serve in their living quarters to enhance relaxation and comfort.

Higher, reasonably firm, supportive, comfortable chairs with high backs allow rising from a sitting position with minimal assistance. Wide arm rests, either wooden or metal, allow identification by touch when eyesight is poor or trunk rotation is limited. Aged individuals should always be instructed to feel the chair seat with the back of their legs before attempting to sit down.

Human beings have a great propensity for adapting to less than ideal conditions. The aged, particularly those with a severe disability, have much more difficulty in this respect. Sensory stimulation should be incorporated into every aspect of rehabilitation. Repetitive visual cues using graphics, color, and lighting encourage independence, thereby increasing pride and self-esteem.

Hellebrandt (1978) proposes a focus on the maintainance of good health and residual mental function, the latter through socialization and physical and recreational activities. The relationship between physical condition and behavior is particularly important in patients with dementia. Changes in environmental design can accommodate the "normal" physiological changes of aging and prevent the effects of functional disuse. A safe environment enables older persons to maintain their independence, improves their socialization, and enhances their performance of daily living activities.

CONCLUSION

Rehabilitation of the aged patient is one of the most challenging tasks for health-care professionals, who often difficult to separate the physiological aspects of aging and disability from cognitive changes when designing a rehabilitation treatment program. With increased knowledge, we may eventually succeed in altering the natural history of "normal aging." Until then, rehabilitation of aged individuals needs to focus on obtaining the maximum functional capacity within the care environment by simplifying that environment and providing activity to ensure that disabilities do not result from functional disuse. To maintain the highest level of functional ability for the longest amount of time, rehabilitative health-care professionals must treat decline in all sensory-integration and physical functioning capabilities of the aged individual. One of the most salient aspects of geriatric rehabilitation is the simultaneous management of multiple conditions. For the rehabilitation specialist, these conditions reflect multiple, and often multidimensional, impairments that complicate the activities of daily living and diminish functional capabilities. Rehabilitation is a process that is not determined by a specific diagnosis or the care setting in which services are provided but by multiple diagnoses and the aged individual's level of motivation. The primary goal of rehabilitation is to promote independent living, as defined by the aged themselves. When working with aged people, rehabilitation specialists need to be aware of the number of factors that make caring for them more complex, more challenging, and more fulfilling.

# REFERENCES

Alzheimer's disease: Joint Hearing before the Subcommittee on Health and Long-Term Care of the Select Committee on Aging and the Subcommittee on Energy and Commerce, House of Representatives, 98th Congress, first session. (1984). Washington, DC: U.S. Government Printing Office.

Alzheimer's disease: Report of the Secretaries Task Force on Alzheimer's Disease. (1984). Washington, DC: U.S. Government Printing Office. (DHHS pub. no. (ADM) 84–1323)

American Diabetes Association. (1988). *Direct and indirect costs of diabetes in the United States in 1987.* Alexandria, VA: Author.

Andreasen, M. K. (1985). Making a safe environment by design. *Journal of Gerontological Nursing, 11*(6), 18–22.

Archea, J. C. (1985). Environmental factors associated with stair accidents by the elderly. *Clinics in Geriatric Medicine, 1,* 555.

Ashley, M. J., Gryfe, C. T., & Aimes, A. (1977). A longitudinal study of falls in an elderly population: II. Some circumstances of falling. *Age and Ageing, 6,* 211.

Astrand, P. O. (1987). Exercise physiology and its role in disease prevention and in rehabilitation. *Archives of Physical Medicine and Rehabilitation, 68,* 305.

Astrand, P. O., & Rodahl, K. (1970). *Textbook of work physiology.* San Francisco, London: McGraw-Hill.

Baltes, P. B., & Schaie, K. W. (1986). On the plasticity of intelligence in adulthood and old age. *American Psychologist, 31,* 720–725.

Bobath, B. (1978). *Adult hemiplegia: Evaluation and treatment* (2nd ed.). London: Heineman Medical Books.

Bortz, W. B. (1982). Disuse and aging. *JAMA, 248,* 1203.

Bottomley, J. M. (1989). Rehabilitation of the Alzheimer's Patient. In J. Cummings & C. P. Miller (Eds.), *Alzheimer's disease: Treatment and long-term management.* New York: Marcel Dekker.

Botwinick, J. (1978). *Aging and behavior* (2nd ed.). New York: Springer.

Boyer, G. G. (1989). Vision problems. In P. Carnevali & B. Patrick (Eds.), *Nursing management for the elderly.* Philadelphia: J. B. Lippincott. 482–484.

Branch, L. G., & Meyers, A. R. (1987). Assessing physical function in the elderly. *Clinics in Geriatric Medicine 3* (1), 29–51.

Branch, L. G., & Jette, A. M. (1982). A prospective study of long-term care institutionalization among the aged. *American Journal of Public Health, 72,* 1373–1379.

Branch, L. G., Katz, S., Kniepmann, K., & Papsidero, J. A. (1984). A prospective study of functional status among community elders. *American Journal of Public Health, 74* (3), 266–268.

Branch, L., & Jette, A. (1981). The Framingham Disability Study: Social disability among the aging. *American Journal of Public Health, 71,* 1202.

Brody, H. (1979, November). Kliemer Lecture, Gerontological Society Meeting.

Bruce, R. A. (1984). Exercise, functional aerobic capacity, and aging — another viewpoint. *Medicine and Science in Sports and Exercise, 16,* 8–15.

Buller, A. J., Eccles, J. C., & Eccles, R. M. (1960). Interaction between motor neurons and muscles in respect of the characteristic speeds of their responses. *Journal of Physiology, 150,* 417–439.

Buskirk, E. R. (1985). Health maintenance and longevity: Exercise. In C. E. Finch & E. L. Schneider (Eds.), *Handbook of the biology of aging.* New York: Academic Press.

Butler, R. N. (1980). Current definitions of aging. In R. N. Butler (Ed.), *Epidemiology of aging* (pp. 7–8). Bethesda, MD: National Institutes of Health. (Publication No. 80–969)

Calliet, R. (1969). Mechanisms of joints. In S. Licht (Ed.), *Arthritis and physical medicine.* Baltimore, MD: Waverly Press.

Carlson, K. E., Alston, W., & Feldman, D. J. (1964). Electromyographic study of aging skeletal muscle. *American Journal of Physical Medicine and Rehabilitation, 43,* 141–152.

Carr, J. H., & Shepard, R. B. (1987). A Motor relearning programme for stroke (2nd ed.). Rockville, MD: Aspen.

Christiansen, J., & Juhl, E. (Eds.). (1987). The prevention of falls in later life. *Danish Medical Bulletin, 34* (Suppl. 4), 1–24.

Clark, B. A. (1985). Principles of physical activity programming for the older adult. *Topics in Geriatric Rehabilitation, 1,* 68–73.

Clark, G., Blue, B., & Bearer, J. (1983). Rehabilitation of the elderly amuputee. *Journal of the American Geriatrics Society, 31,* 439.

Cohen, G. D. (1984). The mental health professional and Alzheimer's patient. *Hospital and Community Psychiatry, 35*(2), 115–116, 122.

Commission on Chronic Illness: Chronic Illness in the United States (1957). *Prevention of chronic illness.* (Vol 1; pp. 285–311.) Cambridge, MA: Harvard University Press.

Cummings, G., & Semple, S. G. (1973). *Disorders of the respiratory system.* Oxford, England: Blackwell.

Darling, R. C. (1971). Fatigue. In J. A. Downey & R. C. Darling (Eds.), *Physiological basis of rehabilitation medicine.* Philadelphia: W. B. Saunders.

DeBusk, R. F., Convertino, V. A., Hung, J., & Goldwater, D. (1983). Exercise conditioning in middle-aged men after 10 days of bed rest. *Circulation, 68*(2), 245–250.

DeVries, H. A. (1971). Prescription of exercise for older men from telemetered exercise heart rate data. *Geriatrics, 26,* 102.

Dietrick, J. E., Whedon, G. D., & Shorr, E. (1948). Effects of immobilization upon various metabolic and physiologic functions of normal men. *American Journal of Medicine, 4,* 3–9.

Dinken, H. (1951). Physical treatment of the hemiplegic patient in general practice. In F. H. Krusen (Ed.), *Physical medicine and rehabilitation for the clinician* (p. 205). Philadelphia: W. B. Saunders.

Downs, F. (1974). Bed rest and sensory disturbances. *American Journal of Nursing, 74,* 434–438.

Droller, H. (1955). Falls among elderly people living at home. *Geriatrics, 10,* 239–244.

Duke University Center for the Study of Aging and Human Development (1978). *Multidimensional functional assessment: The OARS methodology.* Durham, NC: Duke University.

Eberl, D. R., Rasching, V., Rahlfs, V., Schwyzer, R., Fauchére, J. L., Tesser, G. I., & Chapman, M. W. (1976). Repeatability and objectivity of various measurements in rheumatoid arthritis. *Arthritis and Rheumatism, 19,* 1278–1286.

Eisdorfer, L. (1968). Arousal and performance: Experiments in verbal learning and a tentative theory. In G. A. Talland (Ed.), *Human aging and behavior.* New York: Academic Press.

Emes, C. G. (1979). The effects of a regular program of light exercise on seniors. *Journal of Sports Medicine, 19,* 185.

Enright, R. B., & Friss, L. (1987). *Employed care-givers of brain-damaged adults: An assessment of the dual role.* Unpublished manuscript.

Evans, C. E., Galasko, C. S., & Ward, C. (1990, March). Effect of donor age on the growth in vitro of cells obtained from human trabecular bone. *Journal of Orthopedic Research, 8*(2), 234–237.

Federal Council on the Aging. (1981). *The need for long-term care: A chartbook of the Federal Council on Aging* (U.S. Dept. of Health and Human Services Publication No. (OHDS) 81–20704). Washington, DC: Government Printing Office.

Fitts, R. H. (1980). Aging and skeletal muscle. In E. L. Smith & R. C. Serfass (Eds.), *Exercise and aging: The scientific basis.* Hillside, NJ: Enslow.

Fujiswawa, Y., Kida, K., & Matsuda, H. (1984). Role of change in vitamin D metabolism with age in calcium and phosphorous metabolism in normal subjects. *Journal of Clinical Endocrinology and Metabolism, 59,* 719–726.

Gabell, A. (1986). Falls in the elderly: Will dance reduce their incidence? *Human Movement Studies, 12,* 119.

Gardner, D. L. (1978). Aging of articular cartilage. In J. C. Brockehurst (Ed.), *Textbook of geriatric medicine and gerontology.* New York: Longman.

Goldman, R. (1979). Decline in organ function with age. In I. Rossman (Ed.), *Clinical Geriatrics* (2nd ed.). Philadelphia: J. B. Lippincott.

Granger, C. V. (1974). Medical Rehabilitation Research and Training Center No. 7 Annual Progress Report. Boston: Tufts University School of Medicine.

Granger, C. V., & Greer, D. S. (1976). Functional status measurement and medical rehabilitation outcomes. *Archives of Physical Medicine and Rehabilitation, 57,* 103–109.

Greenleaf, J. E., & Reese, R. D. (1980). Exercise themoregulation after 14 days of bed rest. *Journal of Applied Physiology, 48,* 72–77.

Griffin, S. J., & Trinder, J. (1978). Physical fitness, exercise, and human sleep. *Psychophysiology, 19,* 447–451.

Gross-Andrew, S., & Zimmer, A. (1978). Incentives to families caring for disabled elderly: Research and demonstration project to strengthen the natural support system. *Journal of Gerontological-Social Work, 1,* 119–135.

Gryfe, C. I., Amies, A., & Ashley, M. J. (1977). A longitudinal study of falls in an elderly population: I. Incidence and morbidity. *Age and Ageing, 6,* 201.

Gutman, E. (1972). *Age changes in the neuromuscular system.* London: Bristol.

Gutman, E., & Hanzlikova, V. (1976). Fast and slow motor units in aging. *Gerontology, 22,* 280–300.

Haines, R. F. (1974). Effect of bed rest and exercise on body balance. *Journal of Applied Physiology, 36,* 323.

Ham, R. J., & Marcy, M. L. (1983). "Normal Aging": A review of systems/the maintenance of health. In J. Wright (Ed.), *Primary care geriatrics.* Boston: PSG, Inc.

Ham, R. J., Marcy, M. L., & Holtzman, J. M. (1983). The aging process: Biological and social aspects. In J. Wright (Ed.), *Primary care geriatrics.* Boston: PSG, Inc.

Hamlin, C. R., Luschin, J. H., & Kohn, R. R. (1980). Aging of collagen: Comparative rates in four mammalian species. *Experimental Gerontology, 15,* 393–398.

Heather, A. J. (1960). *Manual of care for the disabled patient* (pp. 12–15). New York: Macmillan.

Hellebrandt, F. A. (1978). The senile dement in our midst: A look at the other side of the coin. *Gerontologist, 18,* 67–70.

Himann, J. E., Cunningham, D. A., Rechnitzer, P. A., & Paterson, D. H. (1988). Age-related changes in speed of walking. *Medicine and Science in Sports and Exercise, 20,* 161.

Hole, J. W. (1978). *Human anatomy and physiology.* Dubuque, IA: W. C. Brown.

Holloszy, J. O. (1983). Exercise, health, and aging: A need for more information. *Medicine and Science in Sports and Exercise, 15,* 1.

Horak, F. B. (1987). Clinical measurement of posture control in adults. *Physical Therapy, 67,* 1881.

Jones, E., McNitt, B., & McKnight, E. (1974). Patient classification for long-term care: User's manual. Washington, DC: U.S. Government Printing Office. (U.S. DHEW Pub. No. HRA 75–3107.)

Kalchthaler, T., Bascon, R. A., & Quintos, V. (1978). Falls in the institutionalized elderly. *Journal of the American Geriatrics Society, 26,* 424.

Kane, R. A., & Kane, R. L. (1981). Assessing the elderly: A practical guide to measurement. Lexington, MA: Lexington Books.

Kaplan, D., & Mayer, K. (1959). Distribution of alkaline phosphatase. *Nature, 183,* 1262–1263.

Kaplan, E. (1982). Psychological factors and ischemic heart disease mortality: A focal role for perceived health. Paper presented at the annual meeting of the American Psychological Association, Washington, DC.

Kasper, R. L. (1988). Eye problems of the aged. In W. Reichel (Ed.), *Clinical aspects of aging* (pp. 393–395). Baltimore, MD: Williams and Wilkins.

Katz, S., Ford, A. B., Moskowitz, R. W., Masucci, E. F., Rose-Innes, A. P., & Tralka, G. A. (1963). Studies of illness in the aged. The index of ADL: A standardized measure of biological and psychosocial function. *JAMA, 185,* 914–919.

Kenney, R. A. (1982). *Physiology of aging: A synopsis.* Chicago: Year Book Medical Publishers.

Knott, M., & Voss, D. E. (1968). *Proprioceptive neuromuscular facilitation: Patterns and techniques* (2nd ed.). New York: Harper and Row.

Kohl, H. W., Moorefield, D. L., & Blair, S. N. (1987). Is cardiorespiratory fitness associated with general chronic fatigue in apparently healthy men and women? *Medicine and Science in Sports and Exercise, 19,* S6.

Kumar, V. N., & Redford, J. B. (1984). Rehabilitation of hip fractures in the elderly. *American Family Physician, 29,* 173.

Kuriansky, J. B., & Gurland, B. (1976). Performance test of activities of daily living. *International Journal of Aging and Human Development, 7,* 343–352.

Lamb, L. E., Stevens, P. M., & Johnson, R. L. (1965). Hypokinesia secondary to chair rest from 4 to 10 days. *Aerospace Medicine, 36,* 755.

Larson, E. B., & Bruce, R. A. (1987). Health benefits of exercise in an aging society. *Archives of Internal Medicine, 147,* 353.

Lawrence, M. S. (1956). Strengthening the quadriceps: Progressively prolonged isometric tension method. *Physical Therapy Review, 36,* 658.

Lawton, M. P. (1972). Assessing the competence of older people. In D. Kent, R. Kastenbaum, & S. Sherwood (Eds.), *Research planning and action for the elderly.* New York: Behavioral Publications.

Lawton, M. P., & Brody, E. M. (1969). Assessment of older people: Self-maintaining and instrumental activities of daily living. *The Gerontologist, 9,* 179–186.

Lehman, J. F., Guy, A. W., & Stonebridge, J. B. (1975). Stroke: Does rehabilitation affect outcome? *Archives of Physical Medicine and Rehabilitation, 56,* 375.

Lewis, C. B. (1985). Aging: The health care challenge. Philadelphia: F. A. Davis.

Liebowitz, B., Lawton, M. P., & Waldman, A. (1979). Evaluation: Designing for confused elderly people. *AIA Journal, 2,* 59–61.

Linn, M. W. (1967). A rapid disability rating scale. *Journal of the American Geriatrics Society, 15,* 211–214.

Louis, M. (1983). Falls and their causes. *Journal of Gerontology and Nursing, 9,* 142.

Lubinski, R. (1981). Speech, language, and audiology programs in home health care agencies and nursing homes. In D. S. Beasley & G. A. Davis (Eds.), *Aging: Communication processes and disorders.* New York: Grune and Stratton.

Lubinski, R. (1981). Language and aging: An environmental approach to intervention. *Topics in Language Disorders, 1,* 4, 89–97.

MacLennan, W. J., Hall, M. R. P., & Timothy, J. I. (1980). Postural hypotension in old age: Is it a disorder of the nervous system or of blood vessels? *Age and Ageing, 9,* 25–32.

Marshall, L. (1981). Auditory processing in aging listeners. *Journal of Speech and Hearing Disorders, 46,* 226–238.

McCarter, R. (1978). Effects of age on contraction of mammalian skeletal muscle. In G. Kalkor & J. DiBattista (Eds.), *Aging in muscle* (pp. 1–22). New York: Raven Press.

McPherson, B. D. (Ed.). (1986). Sport and aging. *1984 Olympic Scientific Congress Proceedings* (Vol. 5). Champaign, IL: Human Kinetics.

Mento, A., Steele, R. P., & Karren, R. J. (1987). A metaanalytic study of the effects of goal setting on task performance: 1966–1984. *Organic Behavioral Human Decision Process, 39,* 52.

Meyer, K., Hoffman, P., & Linker, A. (1958). Mucopolysacchrides of costal cartilage. *Science, 128,* 896.

Miller, M. B. (1975). Iatrogenic and nursigenic effects of prolonged immobilization of the ill aged. *Journal of the American Geriatrics Society, 33,* 360.

Miller, P. B., Johnson, R. L., & Lamb, L. E. (1964). Effects of four weeks of absolute bed rest on circulatory functions in man. *Aerospace Medicine, 35,* 1194.

Moritani, T. (1981). Training adaptations in the muscles of older men. In E. L. Smith & R. C. Serfass (Eds.), *Exercise and aging: The scientific basis* (pp. 149–166). Hillside, NJ: Enslow.

Moskowitz, E., & McCann, C. B. (1957). Classification of disability in the chronically ill and aging. *Journal of Chronic Disorders, 5,* 342–346.

Mossey, J. M., & Shapiro, E. (1982). Self-rated health: A predictor of mortality among the elderly. *American Journal of Public Health, 72,* 800–808.

Muller, E. A. (1970). Influence of training and of inactivity on muscle strength. *Archives of Physical Medicine and Rehabilitation, 51,* 449.

Murray, M. P. (1975). Normal postural stability and steadiness: Quantitative assessment. *Journal of Bone and Joint Surgery. American Volume, 57*(A): 510.

Nader, I. M., Pallavicini, J., Legarreta, A., Mahaluf, J., Cumsille, F., Silva, C., & Vila, C. (1985). Level of aspiration and performance of chronic psychiatric patients on a simple motor task. *Perceptual and Motor Skills, 60,* 767.

Palmoski, M. J., Colyer, R. A., & Brandt, K. D. (1980). Joint motion in the absence of normal loading does not maintain normal articular cartilage. *Arthritis and Rheumatism, 23,* 325.

Payton, O. D., & Poland, J. L. (1983). Aging process: Implications for clinical practice. *Physical Therapy, 63,*(1), 41–48.

Pickles, L. W. (1983). Effects of aging on connective tissues. *Geriatrics, 38*(1), 71–78.

Prohaska, T., Pontiam, I. A., & Teitleman, J. (1984). Age differences in attributions to causality: Implications for intellection assessment. *Experimental Aging Research, 10,* 111.

Ragen, P. B., & Mitchell, J. (1980). The effects of aging on the cardiovascular response to dynamic and static exercise. In M. L. Weisfelt (Ed.), *The aging heart* (pp. 269–296). New York: Raven Press.

Reifler, B. V., & Wu, S. (1982). Managing families of the demented elderly. *Journal of Family Practice, 14*(6), 1051–1056.

Rikli, R., & Busch, S. (1986). Motor performance of women as a function of age and physical activity level. *Journal of Gerontology, 41,* 645.

Roscow, I., & Breslau, N. (1966). A Guttman health scale for the aged. *Journal of Gerontology, 21,* 556–559.

Rosillo, R. A., & Fagel, M. L. (1970). Correlation of psychologic variables and progress in physical therapy: I. Degree of disability and denial of illness. *Archives of Physical Medicine and Rehabilitation, 51,* 227.

Rubenstein, L. Z., Josephson, K. R., & Gurland, B. (1984). Effectiveness of a geriatric evaluation unit: A randomized trial. *New England Journal of Medicine, 311,* 1664.

Rusk, H. (1958). *Rehabilitation medicine* (pp. 40–44). St. Louis, MO: C. V. Mosby.

Ryback, R. S., Lewis, O. F., & Lessard, C. S. (1971). Psychobiologic effects of prolonged bed rest (weightless) in young, healthy volunteers (Study II). *Aerospace Medicine, 42,* 529.

Ryback, R. S., Lewis, O. F., Scwab, R. S., & Blum, K. (1971). Psychobiologic effects of prolonged weightlessness (bed rest) in young healthy volunteers. *Aerospace Medicine, 42,* 408.

Saltin, B., Astrand, P. O., Grover, R. F., Blomquist, C. G., Diamant, B., & Ekblom, B. (1968). Response to exercise after bed rest and after training. *Circulation, 38* (Suppl. 7), 1.

Schaie, K. W. (1984). Historical time and cohort effects. In K. A. McCluskey & H. W. Reese (Eds.), *Life-span developmental psychology: Historical and generational effects.* New York: Academic Press.

Schneider, E. L., & Reed, J. D. (1985). Modulations of aging processes. In C. E. Finch & E. L. Schneider (Eds.), *Handbook of the biology of aging.* New York: Academic Press.

Schoening, H. A., & Iversen, I. A. (1968). Numerical scoring of self-care status: A study of the Kenny self-care evaluation. *Archives of Physical Medicine and Rehabilitation, 49,* 221–229.

Seltzer, B., Rheaume, Y., Volicer, L., Fabriszewski, K. J., Lyon, P. C., Brown, J. E., & Volicer, B. (1988, February). The short-term effects of in-hospital respite on the patient with Alzheimer's disease. *Gerontologist, 28*(1), 121–124.

Sharpe, D. T. (1974). *The psychology of color and design.* Chicago: Nelson-Hall.

Shepard, R. J. (1978). *Physical activity and aging.* Chicago: Year Book.

Shepard, R. J., & Sidney, K. H. (1978). Exercise and aging. *Exercise and Sports Sciences Review, 6,* 1.

Shepard, R. J. (1983). Physical activity and the healthy mind. *Canadian Medical Association Journal, 128,* 525.

Shepard, R. J. (1987). *Physical activity and aging* (2nd ed.). Rockville, MD: Aspen.

Sherwood, S. J., Morris, J., Mor, V., Fabichowski, K. J., Chenoll, P. J., Fawson, W. W., & Cushan, P. I. (1977). *Compendium of measures for describing and assessing long term care populations.* Boston: Hebrew Rehabilition Center for Aged.

Shumway-Cook, A., & Horak, F. B. (1986). Assessing the influence of sensory interaction on balance. *Physical Therapy, 66,* 1548.

Siebens, A. W., Schmedt, J. F., Eckberg, D. L., Nixon, J. V., Pippen, J. J., Taylor, A. A., & Varghese, A. (1990). Hemodynamic consequences of cardiovascular deconditioning—Functional effects. *Circulation, 82*(4), 694.

Siegler, I. C., & Costa, P. T., Jr. (1985). Health behavior relationships. In J. E. Birren & K. W. Schaie (Eds.), *Handbook of the psychology of aging* (2nd ed.). New York: Van Nostrand Reinhold.

Siegler, I. C. (1983). Psychological aspects of the Duke longitudinal studies. In K. W. Schaie (Ed.), *Longitudinal studies of adult psychological development.* New York: Guilford Press.

Smith, E., & Serfass, R. (1981). *Exercise and aging: The scientific basis.* Hillside, NJ: Enslow.

Spiraduso, W. W. (1980). Physical fitness, aging, and psychomotor speed: A review. *Journal of Gerontology, 35,* 850.

Stelmach, C. E., & Worringham, C. J. (1985). Sensorimotor deficits related to postural stability: Implications for falling in the elderly. In T. S. Radebaugh et al. (Eds.), *Clinics of geriatric medicine* (Vol. 1., No. 3). Philadelphia: W. B. Saunders.

Stoedefalke, K. G. (1985). Motivating and sustaining the older adult in an exercise program. *Topics in Geriatric Rehabilitation, 1,* 78.

Stout, R. W. (1978). Falls and disorders of postural balance. *Age and Aging, 7,* 134.

Taylor, H. L., Henschel, J. B., & Keys, A. (1949). Effects of bed rest on cardiovascular function and work performance. *Journal of American Physiology, 2,* 223.

Tideiksaar, R. (1987). Fall prevention in the home. *Topics in Geriatric Rehabilitation, 3,* 57.

Tinetti, M. E. (1987). Factors associated with serious injury during falls by ambulatory nursing home residents. *Journal of the American Geriatrics Society, 35,* 644.

Trussel, R. D., & Elinson, J. (1959). *Chronic Illness in the United States: Vol 3. Chronic Illness in a Rural Area.* Cambridge, MA: Harvard University Press.

U.S. Department of Health, Education and Welfare. (1978a). *Working Document on Patient Care Management.* Washington, DC: U.S. Government Printing Office.

U.S. Department of Health, Education and Welfare. (1978b). *Long-term care minimum data set.* Preliminary report of the Technical Consultant Panel on the long-term care data set. U.S. National Committee on Vital and Health Statistics. Washington, DC: U.S. Government Printing Office.

Warshaw, G. A., Moore, J. T., & Friedman, S. W. (1982). Functional disability in the hospitalized elderly. *JAMA, 248,* 847.

Wechsler, D. (1972). "Hold" and "Don't Hold" tests. In S. M. Chown (Ed.), *Human aging.* New York: Penguin Press

Wedgewood, J. (1985). The place of rehabilitation in geriatric medicine: An overview. *Int. Rehabil. Med., 7,* 107.

Weinberg, R., Bruya, L., & Jackson, A. (1985). The effects of goal proximity and goal specificity on endurance performance. *Journal of Social Psychology, 7,* 296.

Weldon, S., & Yesavage, J. A. (1982). Behavioral improvement with relaxation training in senile dementia. *Clinical Gerontologist, 1*(1), 45–49.

Wild, D., Nayak, U. S., & Isaacs, B. (1981). How dangerous are falls in old people at home? *British Medical Journal, 282,* 266.

Woollacott, M. J. (1990). Changes in posture and voluntary control in the elderly: Research findings and rehabilitation. *Topics in Geriatric Rehabilitation, 5*(2), 1–11.

Woollacott, M. J. (1988). Response preparation and posture control: Neuromuscular changes in the older adult. *Annals of the New York Academy of Science, 515,* 42–53.

Woollacott, M. J., Shumway-Cook, A., & Nashner, L. (1986). Aging and posture control. *International Journal of Aging and Human Development, 23,* 97.

World Health Organization. (1964). Constitution of the World Health Organization. Geneva: Author.

Wylie, C. M. (1967). Gauging the response of stroke patients to rehabilitation. *Journal of the American Geriatrics Society, 15,* 797–805.

Wynne, J. W. (1979). Pulmonary disease in the elderly. In I. Rossman (Ed.), *Clinical geriatrics* (2nd ed.). Philadelphia: J. B. Lippincott.

Young, A. (1986). Exercise physiology in geriatric practice. *Acta Medica Scandinavica, 711,* 227.

Zadai, C. C. (1986). Cardiopulmonary issues in the geriatric population: Implications for rehabilitation. *Topics in Geriatric Rehabilitation, 2*(1), 1–9.

Zubek, J. P. (1963). Counteracting effects of physical exercise performed during prolonged perceptual deprivation. *Science, 142,* 504.

Zubek, J. P., & Wilgosh, L. (1963). Prolonged immobilization of the body: Changes in performance and in the electroencephalogram. *Science, 140,* 306.

# II

# Interpersonal and Societal Issues

Part II of the text addresses issues of the relationship of the aged to small and large groups of people and to society as a whole.

Chapter 8, The Ageing Family, is written by Frances Portnoy, a nurse, sociologist, and gerontologist. She builds a foundation of family structure, historical development, and cultural diversity. Upon this foundation she builds a discussion of the effects of family interaction, support, and stress on the aged. She also addresses a less commonly recognized phenomenon — the influence of the aged on family feelings and function. Finally, she explores ways of improving health and relationships for the aged and their families, recognizing the broadening range of options that current moral attitudes and cultural reality present.

Chapter 9, Work, Productivity, and Worth in Old Age, addresses the meaning for life of occupation, broadly defined. Margot Howe, an occupational therapist, looks at the emotional and social meaning of work in the lives of younger people; the significance of retirement and other loss of vocation with age; and the importance of gainful, volunteer, and avocational activity in the lives of the aged. Thus, the use of time and energy is seen as an essential aspect of emotional, social, and physical health. Howe not only describes the current distribution of activity patterns in the aged but makes recommendations for removing barriers to activity that would benefit the aged, their immediate social networks, and society as a whole.

Chapter 10, Ethical Issues at the End of Life: Death, Dying, and the Care of the Aged, explores ethical issues affecting the aged through the paradigm of dying and death. David Barnard, a medical ethicist and teacher of the medical humanities, presents basic concepts and terminology in ethics and some pertinent ideological debates. He then goes on to explore various aspects of death and dying and the ethical issues and actions related to them. The roles and needs of the aged, their families, caregivers, and society are all considered, including areas of competing interests. Although specific decisions and actions are determined by specific circumstances and responsible parties, values and outcome implications are clearly presented.

Chapter 11, Legal Issues in the Care of the Aged, deals with both protective and estate law. Thomas O'Hare, a specialist in mental health and probate law, addresses first the legal principles of responsibility and civil rights and discusses the circumstances under which these can be transferred from the aged to protectors. He reviews the legal actions that can be taken, the statutory and case law that determine these actions, and the issues yet to be adjudicated. Second, he points out important considerations in the preservation and allocation of aged persons' material assets. Then he details the preparations that can be made in anticipation of financial need, imcompetence, and death. The context for O'Hare's discussion is the rights, dignity, and well-being of the aged as counterbalanced by the interests of family, caregivers, and society.

In Chapter 12, Disability Trends and Community Long-Term Health Care for the Aged, Alan Jette, a physical therapist who researches and consults in social policy and practice in long-term care, looks first at trends in the size of the aged population and the reasons for them, and then reviews past and current social philosophy and government action as it relates to services to the aged and their long-term care needs. Finally, he makes both predictions and recommendations for meeting these needs in light of trends in the size of the aged population and changes in their capacities and incapacities. He highlights the considerable debate that has been engendered by this growing issue with its great moral, financial, and administrative implications.

Chapter 13, The Economics of the Health-Care System: Financing Health Care for the Aged Person, follows in many respects from the preceding chapters on family, work, ethics, law, and long-term care. Glen Koocher, public-policy consultant, and Diane Piktialis, sociologist and policy planner, trace the history of government responsibility and public and private financing of health care in general and for the aged in particular. The authors analyze crucial events such as the establishment of Social Security, Medicare, and Medicaid and their influences on health care; report more recent debates, actions, and choices in health care financing and provision; and review future possibilities. These large politico-economic facts are applied to the practical care of aged individuals.

In an interdisciplinary perspective on interpersonal and societal issues, David Satin notes the significance for medicine and psychiatry that society on a large scale and families, social groups, and communities on a small scale provide the help, support, and response the aged need. Because this population group suffers increasing limitations and develops special needs stemming from disease, disability, and loss of supportive resources in their lives, these social influences are especially important. Margot Howe, from an occupational therapy point of view, wonders whether the aged are flexible enough to adapt to their impairments as the times and the experience of cohorts of the aged change, or whether social conditions change so rapidly that they become unsupportive environments to people who have grown up under different conditions. Satin wonders how the aged fare in our affluent society, whose technology and morality change so fast that people and humanistic values are left behind.

Jennifer Bottomley's concern as a physical therapist is that in our current economic climate health care is reduced to treatment only after a disease occurs. For example, we do not provide shoes for the feet of diabetics who are at risk of ulceration, but we do provide prosthetic devices and shoes for those who have undergone amputation as a result of diabetes. Because people will be living healthier, longer lives in the future, prevention, or lack of it, will affect the economics of long-term care. Viewing the problem from the occupational therapist's perspective, Helen Smith looks at the health care of the aged that is centered in the home, where most of the aged live, in order to help them remain functional and independent. Home-centered health care is more likely to improve or maintain the existing quality of life and could be less costly than hospital- or clinic-based care.

Barbara A. Blakeney expresses concern as a nurse about the so-called "cost effectiveness" of what we in the health care field are attempting to do. And yet, as she points out, nursing is troubled that in our society today, a "cost-benefit" analysis clearly holds sway. Many policy makers and care providers emphasize the financial outlay and want the most care for the fewest dollars. However, we have not frankly addressed the issue of access to care. Since access and cost are likely to shape the way we look at health care in the future, we must critically address the standards for judging the success of health care and decide who should determine these standards. Satin warns that, in this process, social agencies and institutions, as well as individuals, can stereotype the aged, deciding that they all need this, or none of them need that, or that it's not worth investing other kinds of resources in the aged population.

Satin notes that both costs and benefits can be cast in other terms. There are costs of terms of loss of activity, loss of satisfaction in life, and loss of valuable and beloved people. There are benefits in terms of people being active and productive. Unquestionably, older people are living longer and remaining healthier in their late years. But if our societal policies continue to define them as nonproductive and forbid them to work and be productive, we are forcing a burden on the younger, productive population that we then decry. Instead, we could see the aged as productive members of society who help bear the burden of nonproductive members, some of whom are younger than the aged who could be productive workers. Indeed, many, if not most, economic issues turn out to be social policy issues. Ultimately, we are faced with the issue of how much aged people are worth in this society and how much society is willing to expend in the way of care, effort, concern, and respect, as well as money. Smith adds that too often we look only at work as being worthwhile. We must begin to define productivity and worth in terms other than just gainful employment, placing more value, for instance, in volunteerism, on which many hospitals and other institutions depend. The aged, who have such marvelous knowledge and experience, can be of great service in this area.

Blakeney concludes that obviously our society has not been able to articulate how much it values the aged . . . or maybe it *has* articulated this only too well. It's up to people in the fields of geriatrics and gerontology to address this issue in very clear and assertive ways.

# 8

# The Ageing Family

Frances L. Portnoy

Despite many changes in the form and definition of the American family, it would be incorrect to dismiss the family as a central force in the lives of most individuals throughout the life cycle. Shanas's (1979) contention that the contemporary family functions as an institution in which an individual can be appreciated, and find support and nurturance in an increasingly complex and impersonal society, still holds true. The family — defined broadly as a social unit in which biological, functional, legal, and other ties bind people to one another over time — continues to serve changing but nonetheless essential social and psychological functions.

Family structures other than the traditional nuclear family have become increasingly common. Young and old cohabiting couples, with or without children; gay and lesbian couples; and "blended families," the result of divorce and remarriage, think of themselves and function as "families." Demographic change, discussed elsewhere in this volume, has produced increasing numbers of multigenerational families, in which aged women outnumber aged men. As family members age, they take on new social roles and often experience physical, social, and personal losses. Although the majority of older people continue to function well, and are able to live independently, the proportion of those needing assistance increases with age. As this chapter will show, the family plays a critical role in providing support and assistance to older people.

## Coming to Terms

The readers of this chapter, if middle-aged or younger, probably have at least one living parent. The U.S. Senate Committee on Aging (1992) reports that 40% of those in their late 50s have at least one living parent, as do 20% of those in their early 60s, 10% in their late 60s, and 3% in their 70s. This indicates that most of us will have to come to terms with our feelings, attitudes, and responsibilities to our parents and aging relatives, as they age, decline, become more dependent, and eventually die. We may find ourselves in the middle, torn between responsibilities to ourselves, our children, and our parents. As the oldest generation more frequently ages into their eighth and ninth decades, the youngest cohort of aged — those 65 to 75 — may find themselves caring for the "oldest-old."

Taking on the responsibilities for the care of our aged parents can be rewarding and gratifying, fulfilling beliefs and values regarding the aged in the family. However, conflict may occur, rising from both the normal tensions that exist in every family and from those more deeply rooted conflicts that have their origin in early relationships. Silverstone and Hyman (1981), write that "when our parents age and begin to need assistance . . . old feelings, complex feelings come into play." We may feel love and compassion, but with economic and social stresses, we may also experience indifference, anger, fear, blame, and guilt.

Membership in a multigenerational family can bring rewards and pleasures, with parents and older relatives playing positive roles. Meyerhoff (1978) illustrates this, in describing a birthday celebration for the oldest member of a family:

> All those present were an extended family. . . . People applauded and recognized all the implicit messages, of continuity, of tradition, of respect for the older generations, . . . and responded to the sustained dramatization of the filial devotion and intense familism that characterized the whole ceremony.

The same adult children who value the aged person may step in too quickly to assist. In their eagerness, they rob their aged parents, still productive and eager to live independently, of their autonomy and choice. Most aged people can take care of themselves, and are capable of making their own decisions about what is best for them. Sometimes, adult children don't approve of their parents' decisions. In one instance, an 84-year-old woman who decided to marry her 89-year-old friend encountered disapproval from her children. They were fearful that she would end her life caring for a sick elderly man (Portnoy, private communication). Meyerhoff (1978) describes a situation in which a daughter wanted her mother to move from her apartment in a deteriorated neighborhood and come to live with her. But Basha, the mother, remonstrated:

> What would I do with myself in her big house, alone all day, no one to talk to. They don't like my cooking, so I can't even help with meals. . . . They don't keep the house warm like I like it. When I go to the bathroom at night, I'm afraid to flush. I shouldn't wake anybody up.

It may not always seem easy to communicate with aged parents. Edinberg (1987) suggests that children can learn to understand and deal with aged parents in confronting important issues that concern them. He describes communication strategies that can assist children and parents in discussing delicate questions about housing, legal and financial matters, health, long-term care, and other issues.

When the family situation becomes stressful, past experiences may return to haunt us. As the oldest in the family, we may have been expected to take on responsibilities, or as the youngest, been the last to leave. We may recall having been jealous of the favorite child, who somehow manages, even as an adult, to maintain that position. Despite our increasing contributions to caring for a parent, and no matter how hard we try, we are never able to acquire the affection we sought as children. As one woman said,

> I'm the meat and potatoes of my parent's lives, but my brother is the champagne. I'm around all the time, doing the ordinary, everyday chores . . . but he brings them some special treat (in his once a month visit). They can live on one of his visits for a week. (Silverstone & Hyman, 1981)

These feelings toward parents and parent figures are among the most intense and powerful one can experience. The individuals who form the intimate unit and who have offered support, protection, and nurturance are the recipients of complex feelings that often have a long and complicated history. The potential for conflict and even abuse always exists, heightened by the stressors associated with old age — chronic illness, the need for assistance, confusion, and loss — and those caused by social neglect — lack of economic resources, depression, and isolation (Pillemer & Wolf, 1986).

In stressful situations, long-harbored resentments and conflicts can be reawakened. In her short story, "Tell Me A Riddle," Tillie Olson (1961) describes the anger aroused when an aged couple confronts the problems of leaving the home they had lived in for many years.

> For forty-seven years they had been married. How deep back the stubborn, gnarled roots of the quarrel reached, no one could say, but only now, when tending to the needs of others no longer shackled them together, the roots swelled up visible, split the earth between them, and the tearing shook even to the children long since grown.

Of course older people, like people of other ages, are capable of manipulation, resentment, and hostility. They can be tyrannical and self-pitying and can act the martyr. Family histories and family wounds are not easily forgotten. Lifetime personalities do not change, nor do relationships that were angry, unfulfilling, or neglectful become suddenly comfortable and forgiving. The adult child must adopt a new perspective on their aged parents, as they come to need the kind of help they perhaps were not able to give their children when they were younger. It is difficult to reverse long-standing patterns of dependence and independence that characterize family relationships. For some spouses, the interdependence may be so strong that separation from or the death of one of the intimate partners is followed closely by the death of the other.

The adult children must not only come to terms with changes in the family and in the parents but must face their own aging, even as new demands are placed on them. Later in this chapter, we will discuss the extent to which this coming to terms is purely an individual or personal problem, or a more universal social issue demanding solutions in the social and economic spheres.

### The Family Structure

Each family group possesses a particular configuration that has some consistency throughout the life cycle. The members of a family form alliances and play significant roles in the ways the family solves problems, sets controls, and communicates. Minuchin (1974) describes family systems with different sorts of functioning, from one extreme, characterized by the "disengaged" family, in which there is scant order and authority, with weak bonds and little mutual dependence, to the other, defined by the "enmeshed" family, in which their is much involvement and mutual dependence among the members. Most families fall somewhere on a continuum between these extremes.

Increasing longevity and decreasing rates of fertility have changed the family structure from a pyramid, with few older people at the peak and larger numbers of children, grandchildren, and great-grandchildren at the base. Instead, the family structure is coming to resemble a narrow beanpole, consisting of multigenerational families, with fewer siblings and fewer peers within each generation (Bengtson, Rosenthal, & Burton, 1990).

As the family ages, there are inevitable shifts in the family "personality." Changes take place in individuals' functions and in their needs for emotional and physical support. Patterns of behavior and expectations that were useful in other developmental phases of family life may not be functional in new circumstances, such as the absorption of an older parent or grandparent into the household. The family balance can change when there are losses in membership because of chronic illness, institutionalization, and death. Reallocation of family functions and power must take place, requiring modification of familiar behavior patterns.

Aging couples often experience significant changes in relationships and roles. Retirement brings spousal couples into close everyday contact with each other at home, with a new sharing of tasks. Despite the increase in divorce and separation, many marriages are long-lasting, from an average of 28 years in 1900 to 43 years in the 1980s (Troll, 1986). In families with children, there is a long period in which the spouses are together after the children leave. Because they have a longer life expectancy than men and tend to marry men older than they are, women may expect to take care of and outlive their spouse. Most of these older women will live a third of their lives past child-rearing years and live as single women. Younger children will grow up in a family systems that includes mothers, aunts, grandmothers, and greatgrandmothers. Not as many of the aged will be male. The idealized portrait of the grandfather, fishing with the grandchildren is more of a wish than a reality. The family is more likely to visit with a grandmother who lives alone in elderly housing or who lives with one of her children.

According to the 1992 U.S. Senate Special Committee on Aging, 82% of older men, and 57% of older women live in families. Of those not living with a spouse 13% live with children, siblings, and other relatives. A substantial minority (38.8%) of the oldest-old, 85 and over, who live in the community live alone (Bould, Sanborn, & Reif, 1989). This does not indicate an absence of family involvement in the lives of these aged people, although Crimmins and Ingegneri (1990) note a decrease in family visiting and coresidence through 1984 that could be significant. For the most part, however, aged people with children tend to live near at least one of their children. Daily and weekly visits increase as the parents age, from 61% for the 65 to 74-year-old age group, to 73% for those aged 85 and older. 72% to 90% of aged people living along talk with a relative at least once in 2 weeks (Kane & Kane, 1986). The extended family structure is less common in the white population than for ethnic minority communities. A black elderly woman who heads a three-generation household is often cared for in later life by grandchildren or other foster children she has raised. Hispanic widowed women over 75 are likely to live with family members, and both groups are underrepresented in the institutionalized population. The diverse Asian population represents many countries of origin. With increasing acculturation and geographic mobility of younger generations, the elders may prefer to remain close to their familiar ethnic community. Values of filial piety, however, tend to remain strong (U.S. Department of Health and Human Services, 1990).

For those who are childless or have never married, other relatives or friends can compensate for the absense of a spouse or children. Gottleib (1989) claims that never married or lesbian women adapt positively to old age. In times of need, nieces and nephews, lovers and friends, substitute for family members. "These groups of women have had to manage on their own for most of their lives, and so have had to develop their coping skills . . . and their own support systems."

Women living with a spouse or in families, have significantly lower poverty rates than those living alone. Black aged women are most at risk, because of a long history of discrimination, reduced rates of marriage, and employment in low-paid occupations. The numbers of single older women continue to increase with widowhood and higher divorce rates. Divorce creates other complexities in the family structure. Children of divorced parents may experience family conflicts and the complicated logistics of caring for two parents not living together. The remarriage of a parent increases the pool of family members' children, parents, grandparents, and others in a new extended and "blended" family. When aged persons need assistance, they may call upon the new daughters- or sons-in-law, who are already responsible for caring for their own parents and who feel less obligation toward more recent additions to the family.

## CAREGIVING AND THE FAMILY

Rosalie and Robert Kane (1986) define long-term care as the "health, personal care and social services delivered over a sustained period to persons with functional impairments. These impairments compromise one's abilities to perform ordinary tasks of basic self care and independent living." In the United States, long-term care is provided primarily by and within families. The Kanes point out that when an aged family member needs assistance, the first resource is a family member, most frequently a daughter, daughter-in-law, and spouse. The care may involve some housekeeping chores, cooking, or laundry, or and it may involve considerable expense, time, and energy. With these efforts on the part of family, friends, and neighbors, most aged people are able to remain in the community. Three quarters of noninstitutionalized disabled older persons rely solely on informal care, and only 5% receive all their care from paid sources (Kane & Kane, 1986).

Despite social and economic influences that affect family caregiving, occupational demands, distance, and housing limitations, many families maintain the tradition of care of their aged parents. A woman of 37 from a suburban Italian family explains:

> We take care of our parents. Many of them live in and own a two family house, and the oldest son or daughter lives in an upstairs apartment. The grandchildren and greatgrandchildren are able to visit, and they help too. You would be surprised, but some of our parents are in their eighties and are still working. They did for us. We do for them. If a parent is sick, several children try to divide up the work of caring for them, but we keep our parents at home. (Portnoy, 1977)

Another woman in this same community expresses her concerns about the future and the difficulty of maintaining the old values:

> Some of the younger generation are finding it too expensive to live in this community and are moving farther out, to less costly suburbs. We are finding that the family group is dispersed. We want to care for our parents at home, but it has become increasingly more difficult. Before World War II, an Italian wife didn't work outside the home. But then wives began to work 3–11 shifts so the husband could be home with the kids. Although the husbands didn't believe in the wives working, we had to make ends meet. Today it's even worse. In the age group 35–50 most women work. And that's when caring for our parents becomes difficult. We also have to admit that values are changing. The further we get from the immigrant generation, the less the old family values hold. Perhaps we don't find the respect for the older generation we used to have. (Portnoy, 1977)

From the point of view of the older person, the changes and social pressures are not always understandable, and they represent a loss of certainty that the family will be a stable source of assistance. Meyerhoff (1978) describes the situation thus:

> The elders claimed that they had realized their most successful ideals in life by producing children who were educated, successful and devoted to them. They realize, they often say, that children must leave their parents, that they left their own families to emigrate. But the truth is that they counted family ties as the only completely trustworthy relationships. They occasionally reflected on this, asking, "Is this what our parents felt like when we left them? Did they deserve this? Do we deserve this?"

The care of the aged is primarily a female responsibility, both within and outside of the family. Most professional and nonprofessional caregivers are women. Of family caregivers 72% are women, with daughters comprising 29% and wives 29% (Kane & Kane, 1986). Women are undoubtedly socialized into caregiving roles from early childhood. Meyerhoff (1978) suggests that women are more prepared for the inevitable infirmities of old age and for the kinds of tasks that are required for in caring for the aged family member: "In her own world . . . the woman did a great many diverse tasks, all at the same time, always expecting to be interrupted, never finding full closure, but hastening from one activity to the next, watching her work become undone as soon as it was completed . . . incontinence of invalid people presented no surprises." Men, who more frequently take on caregiving roles as spouses and sons, are described by Lenard Kaye and Jeffrey Applegate (1989) as "Unsung Heroes."

Caregivers typically take on heavy responsibilities for care; one third serve as the sole provider. Four fifths of caregivers spend 7 days a week and on the average 4 hours a day on caregiving tasks. The care of the aged person in the family is not a short-term affair. One fifth of caregivers minister to the aged person 5 years or more. Care management, including finding assistance, coordinating services, shopping, providing transportation, and managing finances, is time-consuming and stressful. Personal care is expensive and difficult to maintain; many caregivers perform tasks such as bathing, dressing, toileting, and ambulating of the aged person (Select Committee on Aging, 1988).

For many, caregiving is a positive experience. People derive satisfaction and meaning in life from expressing feelings of love and concern and being useful. The author's father, in his 80s, offered neighborly assistance to aged friends who lived alone, dressing, bathing, and feeding them. He said, "As long as I live, I will help others." The Select Committee on Aging (1988) reports that a majority of caregivers feel that the aged person is company for them, and that they feel a sense of self-worth when they care for their loved one.

Although the work of caring may be difficult and stressful, when the aged person dies, the caregiver will mourn. Mrs. Long, 79, cared for her 93-year-old husband, who had gradually become incontinent and who could not walk, bathe, or feed himself without assistance. Mrs. Long "would balance her husband on her back and haul him into the bathroom . . . she cleaned up the many accidents and assuaged his feeling of humiliation. They shared many good moments. Mrs. Long felt this experience was the meaning for her whole life, that she had lived to take care of her husband when he needed her. When he died, she grieved for the loss and reminisced with fondness about their special relationship" (Bould et al., 1989).

In another situation, Mrs. Gold mourned the loss of the possibility of caring for her husband. Married 55 years, the two were very close, especially since Mr. Gold's retirement. One Thursday afternoon, Mr. Gold went for a walk to the bank and never returned. Mrs. Gold received a call from the police that her husband was dead on arrival to the local hospital. She was stunned and shocked and cried, "If only I could have taken care of him. This way I haven't had any chance to let him know how much he meant to me" (Portnoy, private communication).

In general, loss of cognitive abilities, confusion, and disruptive behaviors have a more significant impact on families than do the physical disabilities of the aged person. In cases where the disabled person progressively loses cognition, the caregiver often becomes more depressed and reports more health problems. Without sufficient support, other family relationships with spouse, children, and grandchildren are affected as the caregiver devotes increasing time and energy to the aged person. The competing demands of work and family exacerbate the burden of care. A rapidly increasing group of middle-aged daughters, daughters-in-law, and sons are simultaneously caregivers, parents, spouses, and workers. These competing obligations do not always reduce the amount of time devoted to caregiving; instead, caregivers take on added responsibilities and cut back on leisure time. This may have a major impact on the health of the caregiver. Just under one half of wives caring for their husbands and over half of caregiving husbands report their health as fair to poor (Select Committee on Aging, 1988). Almost half of married female caregivers of aged widowed mothers have previously helped an aged father before his death, besides assisting other relatives. The care of the mother is therefore an episode in an extended period of caregiving that can span decades. Despite the commitment to caregiving and the considerable sacrifice involved, many women feel guilty about not doing enough for their mothers (Gottleib, 1989).

It is not often recognized that caregiving can continue even when the aged parent is institutionalized. A 60-year-old woman writes:

> Cathy, my youngest sister, and I have been sharing the weekdays visiting mother. Cathy works part time 4 days a week, and I work 40 hours and often Saturdays too. Cathy went to see mother 4 days and I went the other 3. Well, Cathy has been terribly ill with a slipped disc and in traction. For more than a month, I have been going to the nursing home to see Mama every day, feed her, and do her laundry. Sometimes I don't think I can do this anymore, but I hope when Cathy is better I will be able to have a little more time for myself and my husband. (Portnoy, private communication)

Professionals should be aware of other types of strain created by non-traditional family bonds. An aged lesbian woman describes her fears when caring for her aged lover, "We worry about how we can be recognized as a couple if there should be hospital procedures. Red tape that may exclude all but 'immediate family,' one's spouse, but not one's lover. . . . I need to know how to take care of her. . . . I feel like I have a low grade fever emotionally. . . . I have crazy fits of crying" (Adelman, 1986).

## THE AGED FAMILY AND THE FUTURE

It is apparent that caregiving can have both a positive and a negative impact on and meaning for the family. Caro (1986) distinguishes between caregiving effort; the tasks required of the family; and caregiving burden, the negative consequences to the caregiver and the family of excessive burden. Such burdens can increase family conflict and in some instances result in abuse of the older person. Sager (1986) suggests that families may attribute their problems in caring for the aged person to their own inadequacy, rather than to the impact of social circumstances and the lack of adequate community support. The family then considers the burden of caring as solely an individual problem, not a social issue shared with others.

As Elaine Brody (1985) has noted, caring for a dependent aged parent is no longer a unique event, but an expected, normative experience for families: "Those societal changes that enabled us to increase our aged population also create new situations and demands on the family. Spouses, lovers, friends, children, and grandchildren, will, for the most part, provide most of the support and care for the aged in the family." Public policy regarding care of the aged however, has been governed by a fear that caregivers will give up care and substitute formal services if they are subsidized. Most research has found that the use of formal services does not reduce the amount of help offered by the family. Instead caregivers are enabled to assist the aged person in different areas, with an improved quality of life for caregiver and care recipient alike.

Caro (1986) asks if there should be public recognition that there can be a limit assigned to the caregiving effort reasonably expected of family members. Bould et al. (1989) suggest that the caregivers need for support should have equal weight with the care receivers need: "If more of the burden than already exists is shifted to the family, potential caregivers may be more reluctant to become part of the caregiving network. This could in the long run become self defeating public policy."

Despite the strains and changes in balance as the family ages, most families manage the life course and take on the major responsibilities of assisting family members as they age. Families make relatively modest demands on the formal service system, purchasing services only when the responsibilities of care become too heavy to bear. The goals of service provision should be to encourage maximal functioning and to develop systems that do not exhaust both the family and the aged individual. As Brody has stated, "Public policy which strengthens the family, will make the largest contribution to give meaning and quality to a longer life span" (Brody, 1985).

REFERENCES

Adelman, M. (1986). *Long time passing: Lives of older lesbians.* Boston: Alyson.

Bengston, V. C., Rosenthal, C. J., & Burton, C. (1990). Families and aging, diversity and heterogeneity. In R. H. Binstock & L. K. George (Eds.), *Handbook of aging and the social sciences* (3rd ed.). San Diego, CA: Academic Press, Inc.

Bould, S., Sanborn, P., & Reif, L. (1989). *85+ The oldest old.* Belmont, CA: Wadsworth.

Brody, E. (1985). Parent care as normative family stress. *The Gerontologist, 25,* 19–29.

Brody, E., Johnson, P., & Fulcomer, M. (1984). What should adult children do for elderly parents?" *Journal of Gerontology, 39,* 736–746.

Cantor, M. (1983). Strain among caregivers: A study of experience in the United States. *The Gerontologist, 23,* 597–604.

Caro, F. (1986). Relieving informal caregiver burden through organized services. In K. Pillemer & R. S. Wolf (Eds.), *Elder abuse: Conflict in the family* (pp. 283–296). Dover, MA: Auburn House.

Cicerelli, V. (1981). *Helping elderly parents: The role of adult children.* Boston: Auburn House.

Crimmins, E. M., & Ingegneri, D. G. (1990). Interaction and living arrangements of older parents and their children. *Research on Aging, 2,* 3–35.

Department of Health and Human Services. (1990). *Minority aging.* U.S. Public Health Service, Washington, DC.

Doty, P. (1986). Family care of the elderly: The role of public policy. *Milbank Memorial Quarterly, 64,* 34–75.

Edinberg, M. (1987). *Talking with your aged parents,* Boston: Shambhala.

Gottleib, N. (1989). Families, work, and the lives of older women. *Journal of Women and Aging, (1/2/3),* 217–244.

Kane, R., & Kane R. (1986). *Long term care: A review of the evidence.* Minneapolis, MN: Division of Health Services, Research and Policy, University of Minnesota Press.

Kasper, J. (1988). *Aging alone: Profiles and projections.* Baltimore, MD: The Commonwealth Fund Commission.

Kaye, L., & Applegate, J. S. (1989). *Unsung Heroes.* Bryn Mawr, PA: Graduate School of Social Work and Social Research.

Meyerhoff, B. (1978). *Number our days.* New York: Touchstone Books.

Minuchin, S. (1974). *Families and Family Therapy.* Cambridge, MA: Harvard University Press.

Mutschler, P. (1985). *Supporting families in caring for the elderly.* Waltham, MA: The Policy Center on Aging, Brandeis University, Working Paper No. 26. Unpublished manuscript.

Norris, J. (1988). *Daughters of the elderly.* Bloomington: Indiana University Press.

Olsen, T., (1961). *Tell me a riddle.* New York: Dell.

Pillemer, K., & Wolf, R. S. (1986). *Elder abuse: Confict in the family.* Dover, MA: Auburn House.

Portnoy, F. (1977). *Health care needs and health care services for the elderly in Newton, Massachusetts.* Newton, MA: Department of Health.

Sager, A. (1986). Mobilizing adequate home care resources: A mutual aid response to stress within the family. In K. Pillemer & R. S. Wolf (Eds.), *Elder abuse: Conflict in the family* (pp. 297–313).

Shick, F. (Ed.). (1988). *Statistical handbook on aging Americans.* Phoenix, AZ: Oryx Press.

Select Committee on Aging, U.S. House of Representatives. (1988). *Exploding the myths: Caregiving in America.* Washington, DC, U.S. Government Printing Office (Publication 100-665).

Shanas, E., & Sussman, H. (1981). The family in later life: Social structure and social policy." In R. Fogel, E. Hatfield, S. Kiesler, & E. Shanas (Eds.), *Aging: Stability and change in the family.* New York: Academic Press.

Silverstone, B., & Hyman, H. (1981). *You and your aging parent.* Westminster, MD: Pantheon Books.

Troll, L. E. (Ed.). (1986). *Family issues in current gerontology.* New York: Springer.

U.S. Senate Committee on Aging. (1992). *Aging in America: trends and projections.* Washington, DC: U.S. Government Printing Office.

# 9

# Work, Productivity, and Worth in Old Age

Margot C. Howe

The transition from the midlife years to old age and to very old age is gradual. The clinical problems of the aging are not sudden manifestations in the lives of older persons, though they may appear that way to clinicians who have just assumed the responsibility for diagnosis and intervention. The presenting problems have their origins in biological aging, disease processes, and psychosocial and environmental changes that occur over time. An interdisciplinary approach to health care appears ideally suited to deal with the complex problems encountered by aged persons.

Many Americans have been able to continue to enjoy productive and meaningful lives well into old age. They keep doing the things that they enjoy doing and that they find satisfying, and this gives them a sense of involvement in rewarding enterprises far into their later years. Others, through retirement or poor health, have lost the opportunity or the ability to engage in leisure or work activities, a factor that frequently leads them to experience depression, hopelessness, helplessness, confusion, and even results in death, according to some research studies. As Lewis (1983) explains:

> Old age is a time in which American society does not readily assign clearly defined roles. In fact, it is a time for permanent disengagement from two firmly entrenched social structures: the nuclear family and the occupational system. The older person actually loses a sense of who he is when terminated from the work force. No longer a teacher, chemist, or active parent, his identity suddenly vanishes, and he therefore becomes a person without a place. (p. 88)

Several theories of aging have been proposed to explain the behavior of the elderly once they have reached the age of retirement. Cummings and Henry (1961) formulated the disengagement theory, which suggested that elderly persons go through a gradual process of withdrawal from their roles in society to prepare for death. This theory sparked extensive controversy and has not been replicated with other groups of aged persons. Havighurst (1961) developed the activity theory, which stresses that continued activity from middle age into old age is desirable and has proved to be the best method for coping with growing old and maintaining adequate life satisfaction. Neugarten, Havighurst, and Tobin (1973) proposed the personality theory of aging, in which the individual's personality is considered to be the determining factor in predicting behavior as aging occurs. As individuals age, their behavior maintains consistency in personality traits, beliefs, and values. Individual personalities and preferences become increasingly important in determining life satisfaction. For example, persons who have had a cheerful and optimistic personality style throughout their lifetime will continue this way of behaving into old age, and their degree of life satisfaction will be influenced by this personality style.

Personal involvement in productive activity has been identified as a necessary ingredient in the successful and healthy transition to old age, and is positively correlated, in many studies, with high life satisfaction in later years. Indeed, productive activity supports health at any age. In children, such activity is usually called play; in adults, it is referred to as work or leisure activity. Fidler and Fidler (1978) state that human action is necessary and essential for human survival and growth. They go on to explain that the very action of "doing," or engaging in a purposeful activity, helps individuals adjust to, and be in accord with, their environment. Purposeful activity facilitates the ongoing adaptation process that individuals undertake in coping with the reality of their day-to-day surroundings.

In this chapter some of the salutary factors inherent in work will be discussed, along with the impact the loss of work can have on the health of a retiree. Work can be defined in many different ways. However, work usually carries the concept of purposeful effort to accomplish something, often with the implication of getting paid or rewarded for such effort. This definition is purposefully broad to include the work of homemakers and volunteers. Theirs is the ongoing work of everyday life that usually goes unpaid and socially unrecognized. Miner (1986) suggests that "Work can be defined as a 'job' which distinguishes work from other aspects of daily life, such as leisure, play, or socialization." He goes on to say that "at another level, work can be entitled a 'task,' suggesting a specific piece of work that requires hard effort and may permit pleasure and pride in accomplishing. 'Occupation' tends to denote a certain responsibility for an identity with work objectives and goals and further suggests contribution to a larger social enterprise." (p. 3)

The capability of the older adult to be productive in leisure or work activities is also examined in this chapter. The concept of productivity as defined here is related to work in that productivity pertains to the accomplishment, through work, of a given product or result. Productivity implies a sense of efficacy, an ability to produce the desired result through work. Looking at aging as a biological phenomenon, what are the physical factors in aging that may limit a person's productivity? Leisure activities are presented as a way of maintaining productivity during years of decreasing skills and abilities. The extent to which social worth and self-esteem are tied to productive activity will also be considered.

The final section of the chapter presents guidelines for clinical assessment and intervention with older individuals, using a case-study method. The discussion includes approaches to therapeutic activity that benefit the life satisfaction, social integration, mental health, the functional capacity of the aged.

## WORK

If we consider how work has been appraised by different societies throughout history, we find that it has been perceived and valued in different ways. In primitive societies work was such an integral part of everyday life that there was no special word for it (Neff,

1968). Among hunting-and-gathering tribes work was constant and necessary for survival. However, as societies expanded through the conquest of neighboring tribes, and enslaved the captured, slavery allowed the conquerors to do less work and to develop leisure activities. Work was seen as degrading and freedom from work was associated with high rank and status. The Greeks and Romans, for example, rejected physical work and valued mental activities. Then values changed again, and physical work was advocated as good and dignified by the monastery monks in the Middle Ages.

In Western culture work has been recognized as an important and valued activity. Work is commonly equated with having a job and receiving monetary payment in return. Webster's dictionary (1985) offers a broader definition of work when it states that "work is an activity in which one exerts strength or facilities to perform something," in order to achieve an objective or result. This definition will generally be assumed in this chapter.

Work is frequently the center of an adult's life. People tend to identify themselves in terms of their occupations or according to the institutions for which they work. In America, from early childhood, we play with toys that simulate work tools, we play at occupational roles, we make believe that we are teachers, firemen, mothers, and so forth. We are rewarded for a "job well done." Our educational system prepares students for jobs and teaches them the skills to do those jobs. We learn to take pride in work and to get satisfaction from the products or services that we have created. The work role is an important one. The change produced by work becomes a part of the person's identity and, according to Dooling (1979), a means of centering and discovering the self. Work and productivity are an essential part of life and contribute to the whole functioning of the individual. It is no wonder that some older adults face a difficult adjustment upon retirement and the loss of their role as worker.

An exploration of the qualities or functions inherent in work may help to clarify work's importance to individuals and the central role it plays in their lives. According to the theories of Friedman and Havighurst (1954), work has five universal functions: it provides income or reward, regulates life activities, determines status, presents opportunities for socialization, and provides meaningful life experiences.

Work provides income in the form of money or other economic gains. In this society, money is a major measure of worth. It is from this income that the physical necessities as well as the luxuries of life are obtained. Income also is deposited in savings and pension plans that will provide financial support during later life. For some people, work is unpaid but it provides other rewards, such as gratification, status, and recognition. In this category are homemakers, volunteers, creative artists, and others who perform unpaid work.

Friedman and Havighurst (1962) studied work groups and found that lower socioeconomic groups considered work as a means to earn income and acknowledged fewer extrafinancial meanings in work than did higher socioeconomic workers. They found that these differences in the meaning of work had implications for retirement in that workers who regarded work solely in terms of income looked more favorably on retirement than did those who stressed other meanings of work; the latter group preferred to continue working.

Work regulates life activities and structures time. It determines daily routines and schedules — the time to get up in the morning, meal times, times and lengths of vacations, and holidays. It even dictates the types of clothing worn on certain days and is associated with other lifestyle determinants. For example, some workers have an early dinner hour because they go to work early in the morning, while other groups of workers stay at the workplace until evening and hence have a late dinner hour. These differences in dinner hours may prohibit participation in certain societal activities. In their research comparing activity patterns of day- and night-shift workers, Rosenthal and Howe (1984), found differences in social activity patterns among workers in the same plant that stemmed from their work schedules on the job. For instance, as a group, night-shift workers participated in fewer social and community activities than did day workers. Their work hours precluded their participation in evening-hour recreational or sports activities. They couldn't even watch the same TV programs as did the day-shift workers.

Identification with a job or an occupation occurs as a function of work. Personal identity is more intense with an occupation than with a job, since an occupation denotes greater involvement and responsibility. People tend to define who they are by what they do. When asked to introduce themselves, individuals frequently state their names and where they work, or the nature of their occupation or job. In some cases the identification is with the institution or company for which they work. Some workers say, "I work for the government," or, "I work for the telephone company." Their identity is more with the company than with the job. Large, well-known companies have higher status and public recognition than do small companies. Identification, for others, may be with an esteemed figure such as their supervisor, teacher, or employer.

Social status is another factor related to work. Because of the complexity of our industrial society and continual changes in the demands of the work force, a division of labor has created distinctions in social status according to certain forms of work. Certain privileges are associated with a certain status. Workers identify with the status and privileges that go with their positions in the company. They may have their own office or their own parking place, or even be allowed to eat in the company dining room. These privileges enhance the workers self-esteem and sense of social utility or worth. They feel validated as contributing members of the work group.

For most workers, work provides opportunities to socialize and associate with other people. During the work day an employee comes into contact with many other people. Lunch hours and coffee breaks are frequently social times shared with coworkers. Social relationships within the work place are varied. Transactions occur between supervisors and subordinates, and in collaborative work relationships with peers. According to Miner (1986), "besides the opportunity to engage with other people in social give-and-take, work further provides other socially meaningful benefits. One gains recognition from others for good performance, thereby elevating self-esteen" (p. 11). These informal social contacts with fellow workers can become important sources of emotional support in times of illness or need. In formal organizations such as guilds, unions, and mutual-aid societies, workers have joined to help their fellow men and women. Through these groups they have provided better working conditions and have improved the lot of the aged worker. Unfortunately, for some types of workers — the self-employed, homemakers, and creative artists — these opportunities for socialization as part of the work place may be limited.

Opportunities for meaningful life experiences are available through work, which provides opportunities to measure achievement. This is particularly true for workers who take pride in their work and who enjoy it. The tangible results of work furnish numerous opportunities for testing and assessing abilities and degrees of success so that behavior can be adapted and adjusted in accord with desired outcomes. Hart (1947) observed that work involves a continuous adaptation to reality. Work involves such tasks as observing, measuring, perceiving, and copying, which, in turn, require attention, thinking, and the application of these to the situation at hand. Looking at the psychological aspects of work, Miner (1986) comments, "work promotes the exercise of autonomous ego functions and their integration in useful activity. Work achievement leads to the pleasures of competence, efficacy, and mastery" (p. 15).

Retirement — the separation of a worker from the work force because of age — involves the sudden loss of the attributes, or functions, of work, and consequently, adjustment to retirement involves basic changes in an individual's life patterns. When Social Security was initiated under President Franklin Roosevelt, age 65 was established as the age of retirement in the United States. Recent legislation has fixed this cutoff point between the working world and the world of retirement at the age of 70 and, in some cases, even beyond that. The age of retirement has been set, not so much on the basis of physiological changes due to aging, but rather on the basis of economic and political factors. For example, during the 1930s, when the Depression brought on massive unemployment, it was economically advantageous to require older workers to retire so that jobs would be available for younger workers. Although this is still advantageous today, age restrictions concerning employment have virtually been eliminated, largely on account of equal opportunity legislation.

The current trend toward industrial consolidation has increasingly made early retirement a popular practice. It is estimated that fifty years ago about half of the men over 65 were still working as part of the American labor force. Today that figure has dropped closer to ten percent. Many workers opt to retire at an early age, thus leaving more years of life before very old age and death. There is more energy available for the retired worker to adapt and adjust to postretirement life. With early retirement, workers may choose to start a second career or develop a hobby into gainful employment. According to Schmitthausler (1982), one out of every two retired Americans regret having retired, and many of those who have already retired are trying to return to an already tight labor market. Often the work they find is menial, part-time, and poorly paid. This situation contributes to the retirees' lowered sense of worth.

Despite their desire to continue working, compulsory retirement may leave retirees feeling deprived of status, income, dignity, and worth. Stevens' study (1979) of mortality rates among 4,000 people who had retired from a manufacturing industry, found a sharp increase of death occurring 3 to 4 years after retirement. The results suggested that this might be due to a postretirement depression related to joblessness, boredom, lowered income, and a sense of uselessness. These retirees may have lost their will to live.

Atchley's study (1977) of older people found that low morale was not directly connected with retirement but was influenced by such factors as health, family situation, personal factors, patterns of activity, and financial security. These factors could well have been aggravated by the stresses that retirement generates. Some people tend to grow more apprehensive of retirement as they approach retirement age. This apprehension may be related to other fears, such as loss of income, passivity, dependence, social isolation, poor health, and diminished sexuality (Ekerdt, 1976; Pelicier, 1978; Riley & Foner, 1968).

Reactions to retirement are varied and personal. Some workers view it as a justly earned right to do all the things they always wanted to do and never had time for. To others it is compulsory unemployment. The loss of a job can be difficult at any age, but under mandatory retirement the loss is "for the rest of one's life." A 69-year-old retired manager comments:

> As I see it, one of the big drawbacks to retirement is the big let down you feel. You feel out of the mainstream of things that used to matter a great deal to you. You suddenly realize a loss of self-esteem. You are no longer involved in making important decisions. After working so hard for so many years, suddenly nobody cares what you think anymore.

In the last decade both industry and community agencies have organized preretirement groups for older workers to help them cope with the changes that retirement will bring. These groups focus on planning for the future, settling finances, enjoying leisure activities, and possibly changing geographic location. The aim is to help group members replace the enrichment and functions that work provides with other activities. These groups are most beneficial when workers participate for several years before they retire so that behavioral changes can be accomplished before the actual retirement. Unfortunately, according to Beale (1982), only a minority of employed persons (10%) enter any type of preretirement program, and the majority of individuals do not think about retirement until they approach the event itself.

Research concerning the life satisfaction of older adults (Fulghum, 1983) shows an association between activity and a sense of well-being but also that individuals need the freedom to determine what their activity consists in and to schedule a routine for engaging in it. Individuals indicating a high degree of postretirement life satisfaction tend to maintain the same level of involvement they enjoyed in their preretirement years, though the types of activity they engage in may differ. It is the rate of activity rather than the specific nature of the activity that correlates with high life satisfaction. In a research study, Ray and Heppe (1986) found that happiness in the aged was related to the intensity of their commitment in a small number of activities and not to the numbers of activities pursued. Further, they found that activities with worklike qualities were more satisfying than other activities. Elliott and Barris (1987), too, conclude from their research that a positive relationship exists between the life satisfaction of the aged and the level of involvement they maintain in meaningful occupational roles. They found it was not so much the number of activities that led to high life-satisfaction ratings but, instead, a high level of involvement in a few activities.

PRODUCTIVITY

In the literature on industry and economics, the term *productivity* relates to the degree and effectiveness of utilizing labor and equipment, or to the work accomplished per unit of productive effort. Throughout this section a broader definition from Webster's Dictionary (1986) will be used: "The quality or state of being productive" (p. 938), with *productive* defined as "effective in bringing about" (p. 938). This definition will include nonindustrial production, such as the productivity of teachers, homemakers, artists, and so on.

The majority of older adults remain productive and maintain themselves in their communities. Fewer than 5% live in institutions, and 70% live in their own homes. They keep active and keep doing the things that they enjoy and that bring them pleasure. However, though they maintain strong ties with their families and friends, there is a pervasive sentiment that they are not a productive segment of the population. Lewis (1983) suggests that "by devaluing wisdom and experience, and emphasizing physical strength, dexterity, and the ability to constantly develop new ideas, society defines productive life in terms that automatically exclude older adults" (p. 1).

As we consider differing portrayals of the productive occupations of the aged, a question arises: Does the aging process cause changes in skill that directly affect the productivity of the aged? An attempt to answer this question produces rather conflicting information. First, there is controversy among biologists as to whether age-related changes are the result of intrinsic aging, wear and tear, or the consequences of injury or disease. Obviously, some biological changes can affect productivity. Components of the respiratory system show a loss of efficiency with age. In the cardiovascular system, the heart loses some of its capacity to respond to extra work. There is also a progressive increase in peripheral resistence to blood flow, causing the systolic blood pressure to increase. These factors, along with the respiratory changes, contribute to a decrease in endurance.

Changes in the skeletal system typical of the aging process include osteoporosis; collapsed vertebrae, causing a stooped posture; and osteoarthritis, resulting in stiffened joints. These lead to a decrease in mobility, efficiency, and capability of the organism. The nervous system also undergoes changes. Within the brain, loss of neurons causes atrophy of brain substance. Reaction time is increased. Components of the muscular system also change, resulting in muscular atrophy, hypotonia, and weakness. As muscular fibers degenerate, there is an increase of fat; as a result the muscle loses its ability to expand and contract (Hasselkus, 1974). This muscular deterioration can affect other bodily functions, such as respiratory efficiency and the ability to respond effectively at will, or in the case of a crisis.

Moreover, changes in the sensory system can affect the productivity of the older individual in a number of ways. The human organism gathers much of its information about the environment from the special senses of vision, hearing, touch, and smell. There are about 3 million people in the United States over age 65 who have either conductive or sensorineural hearing loss. Conductive hearing loss results in an inability to hear soft speech. Sensorineural hearing loss is the result of age-related neural degeneration, which brings about presbycusis, a gradual reduction in sensitivity to high-frequency sounds.

A change in vision can limit productivity through decreased mobility and poor orientation, as contact with the surroundings is dim, blurred, or limited. By age 65 about half of the population of the United States experiences a loss in visual acuity. A major characteristic change is the gradual loss of elasticity of the lens, which interferes with the process of accommodation, the ability of the lens to bring objects, from varying distances, into clear focus. The three most common age-related visual problems are cataracts, diabetic retinopathy, and macular degeneration.

As the skin ages, elasticity is lost and more pressure is needed to stimulate the sense receptors that are located underneath the skin. The loss of touch can severely restrict the ability of older people to use their hands in productive occupations. Without touch it becomes difficult to grasp and manipulate objects and tools, as the sense of touch gives clues regarding the amount of pressure needed to hold or release an object from one's grasp.

The gustatory and olfactory senses also seem to change with age. In old age the tongue contains only about half the taste receptors that were present in youth. Given that a good deal of taste sensation depends on the ability to smell, these two senses are closely interrelated.

The final sensory modality to be considered is kinesthesia, the ability to perceive changes in body position and body orientation. This ability also decreases with age. Changes are due to a variety of factors such as the decline in muscle tone and strength, disturbances of the vestibular system, decline in the neuromuscular functions that help control body position. The losses in brain neurons, including those of the cerebellum which effect balance, also relate to kinesthetic changes. The ability to control balance and body position is basic to activities such as walking, standing, and reaching. Effective use of arms and hands requires trunk stability. The planning and performing of a task depends on effective kinesthetic function. These age-related changes may be aggravated through drugs. Dizziness and loss of muscular control are common side effects of prescribed medications. These need to be carefully monitored to prevent overdosage or harmful drug-drug interactions.

None of these age-related changes in function occur suddenly; they occur gradually over a period of years. In the course of pursuing productive occupations the individual learns to compensate for one diminishing skill by relying more heavily on another. For instance, a person with failing hearing can use vision to supplement hearing loss with lip reading. It is usually only when several biological systems decline in function that the productivity of the aged person is seriously threatened.

As we continue to study the aging process, we may well discover that decrimental changes now attributed to aging may be the result of disuse. A decrease in muscular strength, for example, may be due to a sedentary lifestyle. A decrease in memory function may be related to a less stimulating environment among retirees. Distinguishing between problems caused by disuse and those caused by aging is important because the former are potentially reversible through therapeutic intervention. Problems caused by aging require a compensatory type of treatment.

The results of a number of research studies investigating the loss of motor and cognitive skills with age are inconclusive. Some show a decrease in the cognitive area of intelligence (as measured by standard IQ tests) and an increase in cognitive skills such as problem solving and "wisdom." Other studies indicate no decrease in motor skills with aging but do show a decrease in the speed of motor action. Motor strength and the capacity for physical exertion decrease, starting in the midadult years, in the form of lowered physical endurance. A U.S. Senate Committee on Aging position paper entitled "The Costs of Employing Older Workers" (1984) states that "chronological age is not related to any level of productivity," that "older workers maintain the capacity to learn and successfully apply new information," and that "when employees experience declining productivity, the declines are usually caused by factors other than age" (p. 40).

Leisure activities are those that are freely selected and engaged in by choice, and many retired persons are involved in productive leisure activities. One in four aged

Americans decide to do some kind of volunteer work in their communities. The type of activity chosen varies according to health, personality, and sociocultural background. According to Havighurst (1977), leisure activities perform three major functions: they give pure enjoyment, prepare one for the future by providing alternate areas of interest and productivity, and extend the limits of one's behavior. Productive leisure activities additionally provide a way for people to be of service to others, either through direct personal contact or through objects they have made which others can use or enjoy. Unfortunately, some people have been so involved with their work throughout their life, that they have never developed leisure interests they can turn to in retirement. This is particularly true for farmers, the self-employed, and homemakers, for whom "work is never done." These individuals may need to be taught the use of leisure time and how to derive enjoyment and satisfaction from such activities.

There is a continuum between work and leisure occupation. On either end of the continuum the conceptual definitions are clear. Work is tied to obligations to self, family, and society, and includes skills, roles, and responsibilities that are clearly outlined. In contrast to work activities, which must be done, leisure occupations involve activities a person chooses to do and involve minimum obligations to others. Between these two ends of the continuum is an area where definitions are unclear. Leisure differs from work in that it is not related to financial support, and is done in addition to, or in the absence of, self-supporting activities. Work activities do not have to involve paid employment, and what some people consider work, others consider leisure. It is the individual's own meaning of the activity that is crucial. For some individuals, work provides them with chosen, satisfying, creative experiences, in addition to financial support. There is frequently an overlap between work and leisure involvement among professional and career workers.

Leisure activities can be adapted to the interests, values, and capacities of the individual. Hall (1923) felt that leisure activities were effective in building or rebuilding productive skills when actual work activity might be too strenuous, not available, or not adaptable to the person's situation. As individuals become older or more involved with disease processes, leisure occupations may help them to accept reduced productivity. Interest in pursuing an activity will support an individual through the process of learning how to ask for help and how to instruct helpers to provide the assistance needed. Learning to ask for, and accept, assistance in a leisure activity is less threatening to individuals than in personal-care situations, where loss of autonomy and control is dreaded. Occupational therapists working in hospice programs have found graded activities helpful in maintaining a sense of control for dying individuals.

## WORTH

In a culture that is as work oriented and youth oriented as the United States, aged persons find themselves at a gross disadvantage in gaining recognition for themselves as a group. The wisdom of older age is not esteemed, nor is the perspective that age can bring to problem solving. Worth and esteem are very often attributed to a situation long after it has proved successful. Thus, frequently, worth and esteem are not conferred to the aged until they have died and can be judged in a historical perspective.

Self-esteem and self-worth can be connected to the worker role long after retirement. For instance, Julius, a builder, when asked about himself, gave a lengthy description of the architecture of the state capitol building and closed with the following words: "I laid the floor tiles in that building. Everyone said it was the most beautiful floor in the state at that time." Julius is 85 years old and the floor had been laid a half-century ago, yet he remembers having an important part in that enterprise. It still undergirds his feeling of worth as an individual many years later.

Dychtwold and Flower (1989) write of the emergence of a new "third age of man" in which the elderly will not be seen as social outcasts but as performing a unique role, that of providing feedback for society in the form of the "lessons, resources and experiences accumulated and articulated over a lifetime" (p. 347). As the population grows older, these researchers propose, the elderly will be valued for their wisdom, vision, and mature perspective.

Schilder (1950) did extensive studies on self-esteem and came to believe that self-esteem, or a sense of worth, was brought about, in part, by the sense of satisfaction or pleasure people experienced, and, in part, by society's response to their behavior. The former we will address as an intrinsic source of self-esteem and the latter as an extrinsic sense of self-esteem. For instance, if people listen to their favorite music or participate in a daily exercise that makes them feel good, feelings of self-worth are engendered by the activity itself — an intrinsic source of self-esteem. On the other hand, people might organize programs to provide transport services for seniors so they may attend symphony concerts during the winter months. The recognition they received from others in furnishing needed community services would be an extrinsic source of self-esteem.

Csikszentmihalyi (1975) studied the enjoyment that people received from engaging in activities that were subjectively motivated and found that these related to both work and play activities. He found that enjoyable activities provide a common experience, a satisfying feeling of creative accomplishment, which he called "flow." A state of flow is felt when the opportunities for action are in balance with the actors' skills. When the skills are greater than the opportunities, boredom results. When the opportunities are greater than the skills, anxiety and worry result. When experimental subjects were deprived of flow experiences, they reported feeling dull, angry, depressed, apathetic, and worthless. Many aged persons engage in activities that are subjectively motivated. These activities become an important source of their life satisfaction and self-esteem.

Whether persons are primarily externally or internally motivated, they need to engage in meaningful, satisfying activities, activities that build or maintain self-esteem. Boredom or meaningless "busy work" reinforce the aged person's feeling of being incompetent or worthless.

Abraham Maslow (1970) postulated five levels of human needs. As one level of needs is fulfilled, another level becomes important as a factor in motivating behavior. The first basic level of needs concerns physiological necessity; the second, safety; the third, love and belongingness; the fourth, self-esteem; and the fifth, self-actualization.

Using Maslow's theory, Tickle and Yerxa (1981a) found that aged people were motivated to engage in autonomous actions based on their living environments. The institutionalized aged who were studied had their physiological and safety needs met for them, thus removing these as primary motivators for active interaction with their environment; however, they were not motivated to satisfy their needs for love, belongingness, or self-esteem (the next levels in the hierarchy). On the other hand, a comparable research group, living in the community, who were participating in meeting their basic needs (physiological and safety needs), were motivated to satisfy the next level of needs (love, belongingness, and self-esteem) through active involvement in social and religious community groups (Tickle & Yerxa, 1981b). These studies suggest that aged persons who no longer participate in meeting basic needs lose the motivation to seek a more satisfying or worthwhile life.

Seligman (1975) also researched the phenomenon he called "helplessness" that develops in people who give up active involvement in the control of their lives. He found that helplessness sapped the motivation of people to initiate responses and disrupted their ability to learn. Unfortunately, aged persons are often placed in environments where they learn helplessness and lose their sense of autonomy and worth.

In an ethnographic research study of elderly Jewish people living in Venice, California, Meyerhoff (1978) vividly describes the lifestyle that enabled this group of aged to live long lives and to be satisfied with them into old age. She found two main factors contributed to the longevity and satisfaction of these people. First, they were able to tolerate a good deal of ambiguity. They were able to continue to live in a neighborhood that had undergone dramatic changes and to adapt their lifestyles to cope with them. For instance, because the streets were dangerous, group members frequently took taxis to the community center. Taxis were scarce and more expensive on holidays, so they moved the dates for celebrating holidays to a few days before or after each holiday, thus adapting the center calendar to fit their life needs. They even adapted their religious ceremonies to include more roles for women, as women in the group greatly outnumbered men. Thus both women and men participated in important ceremonial roles. Second, the group had a strong shared belief — not necessarily a religious belief — in the importance of Israel as a state for the Jewish people, and they wanted to help in supporting Israel. This shared value and belief gave them a strong reason to work together and gave them a sense of worth and effectiveness. Meyerhoff believed that this sense of effectiveness and worth contributed to the longevity of group members.

Many senior centers throughout the country provide opportunities for the aged to help each other. Although these programs are staffed by professionals and volunteers, the members themselves assume responsibility for many leadership and maintenance functions. Whether participation is tentative or enthusiastic, involvement in a successful, meaningful group task, can reaffirm an aged person's capabilities to be of help to others. This condition mitigates feelings of helplessness and worthlessness.

We indicated earlier in this chapter some of the benefits to the aged in continuing their engagement in productive activities. We must emphasize that the meaning or value of the activity to the people engaged in it is always of prime importance. An activity for the sake of being busy contributes little to people's sense of competence and worth. Activity is desirable and productive under three conditions: First, people must have a chance to choose how to occupy themselves so that they may become involved in activities that have meaning or value for them. Second, they need to be able to set their own time schedule for the activity. Finally, they need to have a part in structuring the environment in which they will carry out the activity. Unless the aged are given some degree of choice and control in planning and implementing their activities, they may experience them as demeaning, which may contribute to low self-worth. Being treated as dependent and childlike make people feel helpless and hopeless. According to Crepeau (1986), "'Being busy' promotes meaningless activities and therefore reinforces the concept that old people are dependent and need to be entertained." Moreover, she adds, "The atmosphere in an activity program should be one of support and safety so that the participants feel free to take risks they would not ordinarily attempt" (p. 203).

## INTERVENTION

Health in old age is a complicated concept that is much broader than the traditional medical framework acknowledges it to be, which defines it simply as the absence of disease. Essential to establish appropriate intervention, assessment of the health of the aged requires the consideration of a wide and sometimes overwhelming range of variables. The need to assess functional ability and to gain an understanding of the aged person's general well-being makes the task of assessment especially difficult. According to Kane and Kane (1981) "Measures of functional status that examine the ability to function independently despite disease, physical and mental disability, and social deprivation are the most useful overall indicators to assist those who care for the elderly" (p. 1).

As members of interdisciplinary teams, occupational therapists can contribute training and expertise in the assessment of independent living skills. Therapists' approach to assessment reflect their own convictions and values. The contribution of the aged person to the assessment needs to be affirmed, as the determination of the intervention plan should be a partnership endeavor. A systematic assessment of functional capacity is central to gerontic occupational therapy. By sharing perspectives and skills with team members, the occupational therapist may uncover ways of communicating and working with team members that will benefit both the aged person and the team. Information and expertise held by other team members will also benefit the assessment.

Three basic approaches can be used to evaluate the functions necessary for independent living:

1. Assessment of ability as well as incapacity or impairment in the activities of daily living, self-care, and use of leisure time
2. Assessment of lifelong activity patterns through the use of activity histories, interest checklists, social interaction measures, and activity configurations
3. Assessment of the biological parameters of function, such as range of motion, manual muscle strength, and endurance; the psychological dimensions of function, such as volition, memory, and learning ability; and the social dimensions of function, such as the availability of family and friends and other social resources

The assessment should determine:

1. The extent to which adaptive function is impaired by a disease process, an aging process, or disuse

2. The extent to which people engage in productive work or leisure activities, and information regarding their value systems and what is meaningful in their lives
3. The extent to which support systems are available to them: social, familial, professional, and financial

In making these evaluations with the aged, it is important to assess and interpret the results within the context of their normal life situations. The elderly have a history of experience with health-care providers, firm beliefs about health-care practices, and well-established health habits that will need to be considered in planning interventions.

Based on the assessment, an initial decision is made concerning the type of intervention that is deemed by the interdisciplinary team as potentially beneficial. There are two main types of therapeutic intervention: remedial and compensatory. If it is possible to remediate or cure an impairment, this type of intervention is undertaken. When remediation is not feasible, compensatory strategies are used. For instance, the reduced stature of aged persons with osteoporosis may be accommodated by lowering the furniture in the home. Intervention frequently involves a combination of remedial and compensatory approaches.

In some circumstances, intervention is needed to maintain function or to slow the progress of existing dysfunction. At other times, intervention may be directed to raising the level of occupational function:

> For example, many older adults failed to acquire leisure skills in their younger years. The development of leisure interests and abilities through occupational therapy aims at maintaining and challenging physical, mental, and social abilities and improving the quality of life of the older person. (Rogers, 1986, p. 120)

Early in this chapter we presented five universal functions of work and discussed the potential loss of these functions when a worker is faced with retirement. The following case study of Gregory N.* will illustrate the loss of function incurred following retirement as well as the role of the interdisciplinary health-care team in planning an intervention program.

Gregory N. is a 75-year-old man whose landlord asked for help in moving him to a safer and more appropriate place to live. Mr. N. was born in Russia, fled to Canada in 1919, and eventually came to Boston, where he rented a house and found work as a clerk. He developed a warm friendship with a woman and her family who lived next door, but otherwise shied away from people and organizations. Seven years ago Mr. N. retired, and has since occupied himself with reading and stamp collecting. He has suffered from bronchitis, hypertension, arteriosclerotic heart disease, and impaired hearing. He has "slowed down" lately.

Two years ago Mr. N's house was torn down as part of an urban renewal project, and he moved to a small, one-room apartment, over a bar, in a commercial district. He took with him as many of his possessions as he could fit into the room. Since then, he has stayed in his room and paid others to shop for the few things he needs. His diet consists largely of milk, wine, and crackers.

Mr. N. is a tall, distinguished-looking man with white hair and a long white beard. He was found lying in bed in a tiny room crammed with furniture, boxes, dirty clothes, and remnants of food. Cockroaches were everywhere, but Mr. N. did not notice them. He

---

*Adapted from Satin, D. S., & Nikolai, G. (1984). *A case study in geriatric health care.* Boston, MA: Harvard Medical School, Division on Aging.

looked clean but disheveled, wearing an assortment of pajamas and street clothes. His manner was polite but suspicious and rejecting. He reluctantly admitted that he had problems with illness, loneliness, and caring for himself. He knew vaguely where he was and who his visitors were, but not the date or the time of day.

Mr. N. stated firmly that he did not want treatment or better shelter, and only reluctantly agreed to call for help when he felt he needed it.

Several weeks later, Mr. N. phoned the team social worker because his landlord had raised his rent and he needed assistance in finding a cheaper room. Subsequently, the social worker and the occupational therapist visited Mr. N. to talk about subsidized senior housing programs and to make a preliminary evaluation of his potential for independent living and self-care. They then made a report to the interdisciplinary treatment team.

### Home visit with Mr. N. June 16, 1987:

The home environment was similar to that found on the previous visit. Mr. N. was sitting on his bed. His hair had been combed, but his attire was still a combination of bed clothes and street clothes. He was polite but distant, and reluctant to answer questions. He seemed to know who we were and that we had come in response to his phone call. He seemed vague, however and, at times, confused. He was agitated regarding his perceived need to move. Saving money was clearly the factor that motivated him to call for help, but he would give no information regarding his financial situation.

Upon understanding that housing might be available to him, depending on his ability to show that he could take care of himself in an independent situation, he seemed less agitated. When Mr. N. showed how he could put on a shirt, he demonstrated poor hand grasp and coordination, as well as shortness of breath from the exertion of the task. There was a mild intention tremor.

When asked about how he fed himself, he was vague and said someone brought him his food and that it was too dangerous to go out in the street. Reluctantly, he told about walking to the store when he first moved to this neighborhood and being followed, called names, and even accosted by a gang of boys. After that he never went out again. He is also not currently taking any medications, since he will not go to the drug store to refill his prescriptions.

When asked what he did during the day, he appeared unable to understand or answer. When asked specifically if he read during the day, he finally answered that it was too dark to read. When asked if he needed glasses to read, he got up and rummaged through a drawer, then a box, and finally said that he once had glasses but they are lost or stolen.

Mr. N's mind seemed to wander when questions were being asked, and they needed frequent repetition before a response was forthcoming. Even then he frequently needed to be reminded of the question. He was slow when responding, weighing each word carefully.

### Summary of the preliminary assessment of Mr. N:

1. Saving money appears to be the primary motivating factor to get help.
2. Muscular atrophy, hypotonia, and weakness are in evidence, probably due to disuse. Check out possible disease states as alternative explanations.
3. Fatigue and shortness of breath could also be related to disuse. Check out hypertension and arteriosclerotic heart disease as alternative explanations.

4. Mental confusion, poor attention, and impaired memory could be related to social isolation, lack of stimulation, or depression. Check out effects and extent of malnutrition, hearing and vision impairments, and possible alcohol abuse as alternative explanations.

**Tentative treatment plan for Mr. N. developed by the interdisciplinary team, June 16, 1987:**

1. Admit Mr. N. to a local hospital with a strong rehabilitation department. Goals of hospitalization are to do a thorough medical examination, provide adequate nutrition, and provide physical and occupational therapy to further evaluate physical and mental conditions. If disuse and social isolation are confirmed as the causes of the disabilities, through medical examination, Mr. N. would be transferred to a rehabilitation program to increase physical performance and endurance; to increase attention span and ability to concentrate; and to increase opportunity for engagement in meaningful and stimulating activity.
2. The social worker will collaborate with hospital and community agencies to find an appropriate housing program for Mr. N. upon his discharge from the rehabilitation program. Resources to obtain new glasses for Mr. N. will also need to be found.
3. The social worker or the occupational therapist will meet with Mr. N. to explain these plans to him and to enlist his approval and cooperation. These team members have been designated because they have established a relationship with Mr. N. Given the difficulty that he has had with interpersonal communication, consistent team contact is indicated. Other team members offered alternative plans for contacting Mr. N. should this approach prove unsuccessful.

The focus of therapeutic intervention for Mr. N. is to distinguish between problems that need immediate medical attention and those that present functional ramifications of medical conditions. Characteristically, older adults present multiple, and chronic, medical problems, each of which needs to be taken into account in assessing independent function and planning effective intervention. Dependency is one of the major fears of aged persons, and Mr. N. is no exception. He is independent, aloof, and resists help. The philosophy of a rehabilitation program is to minimize dependence and to set treatment goals for increased independent function in daily living skills. These include performance in self-care, work, and leisure occupations.

The performance problems experienced by aged persons are usually multidimensional, or biopsychosocial, as the case of Mr. N. illustrates. Although he may be hospitalized for medical evaluation, he is simultaneously coping with problems of mental confusion, poor eyesight, muscular degeneration, poor nutrition, generalized fatigue, social isolation, and a crisis in his living situation. Because of the biopsychosocial origins of Mr. N.'s problems, his rehabilitation program requires a multidimensional, or interdisciplinary approach. Nor will rehabilitation activities be limited geographically to the rehabilitation hospital. Daily living skills will have to be practiced in the home and community environment to which Mr. N. will be discharged. The goals for intervention are restoration of function, and if full restoration is not feasible, improvement may be possible through the use of compensatory measures as well as the services of community care centers.

CONCLUSION

This chapter has included extensive discussion of the role and value of work in contemporary society. Work organizes time, furnishes opportunities for important social interaction, fosters identification with a job or an organization, and provides meaningful life experiences that supply measurements for achievement as well as the pleasure of mastery. Retirement from the work force signifies the end of the worker role. However, in modern society, where so many people retire at a relatively early age, retirement no longer implies retirement from productive activities. We must look ahead to the time when productivity decreases because of age-related and illness-related losses of function. At that time, what will substitute for the qualities that work and work-related activities provide? This chapter has pointed to the benefits of maintaining a varied repertoire of leisure interests so that a few interesting activities can be adapted or graded to correspond with changing skill levels.

Finally, the poignant question of how an aged person is to maintain a sense of personal worth and self-esteem in today's work- and youth-oriented society needs to be addressed. This question relates not so much to the retirement-aged population but to the very old in our midst. As one 98-year-old woman commented recently, "When I look in the mirror, I see reflected the image of a very old lady — but inside of myself, I'm still sixteen." Perhaps a sense of worth is something that is built up over a lifetime, and the benefits of this self-esteem may be what adds satisfaction and meaning in old age. If this is true, people who work with the aged need to remember that each individual has a unique history. As aged persons, individuals' needs are also unique, and it is important to help them articulate them, value them, and respect them. Let us remember that today's aged persons were born a long time ago and that the standards and values on which they base their worth are the standards and values that are important to them.

REFERENCES

Atchley, R. (1977). *Social forces in later life: An introduction to social gerontology* (2nd ed). Belmont, CA: Wadsworth.

Beale, L. (1982). *Preparation for aging in national conference fitness in third age.* Ottawa Government Publication, Canada.

Crepeau, E. L. (1986). Activity programming. In L. Davis & R. Kirkland (Eds.), *The role of occupational therapy with the elderly* (pp. 199–207). Rockville, MD: The American Occupational Therapy Association.

Csikszentmihalyi, M. (1975). *Beyond boredom and anxiety.* San Francisco, CA: Jossey-Bass.

Cummings, E., & Henry, W. E. (1961). *Growing old.* New York: Basic Books.

Dooling, D. M. (1979). *A way of working.* Garden City, NJ: Anchor.

Dychtwald, K., & Flower, J. (1989). *Age wave: The challenges and opportunities of an aging America.* Los Angeles, CA: Jeremy P. Thatcher.

Ekerdt, D. J. (1976). Longitudinal change in preference age of retirement. *Journal of Occupational Psychology, 49,* 161–169.

Elliott, M., & Barris, R. (1987). Occupational role performance in life satisfaction in elderly persons. *O. T. Journal of Research, 7*(4), 215–224.

Fidler, G. S., & Fidler, J. W. (1978). Doing and becoming: Purposeful action and self-actualization. *American Journal of Occupational Therapy, 32,* 305–310.

Friedman, E. A., & Havighurst, R. J. (1954). *The meaning of work and retirement.* Chicago: University of Chicago Press.

Friedman, E. A., & Havighurst, R. J. (1962). Work and retirement. In S. Nosow & W. Form (Eds.), *Man, work, and society* (pp. 41–55). New York: Basic Books.

Fulghum, B. (1983). *Activity continuity and leisure satisfaction in retirement.* Unpublished masters thesis, Tufts University, Medford, MA.

Hall, H. J. (1923). *Occupational therapy: A new profession.* Concord, MA: Runford Press.

Hart, H. H. (1947). Work as integration. *Medical Research, 160,* 735–739.

Hasselkus, B. R. (1974). Aging and the human nervous system. *American Journal of Occupational Therapy, 28,* 27–18.

Havighurst, R. J. (1961). Successful aging. *Gerontologist, 1,* 8–13.

Havighurst, R. J. (1977). After work: Then what? In R. A. Kalish (Ed.), *The Later Years: Social Applications of Gerontology* (pp. 152–153). Monterey, CA: Brooks/Cole.

Kane, R. A., & Kane, R. L. (1981). *Assessing the elderly: A practical guide to measurement.* Lexington, KY: D. C. Heath.

Lewis, S. (1983). *Providing for the older adult: A gerontological handbook.* Thorofare, NJ: Slack.

Maslow, A. H. (1970). *Motivation and personality* (2nd ed.). New York: Harper and Row.

Meyerhoff, B. (1978). *Number our days.* New York: Dutton.

Miner, J. H. (1986). *Labor crowned with favor: The relationship of work to identity and self-esteem in old age.* Unpublished doctoral dissertation, Massachusetts School of Professional Psychology, Newton, MA.

Neff, W. S. (1968). *Work and human behavior.* New York: Basic Books.

Neugarten, B., Havighurst, R. J., and Tobin, S. S. (1973). Personality and patterns of aging. In B. Neugarten (Ed.), *Middle age and aging: A reader in social psychology.* Chicago: University of Chicago Press.

Pelicier, Y. (1978). The anticipation of retirement. *Annales Medico-Psychologiques, 136,* 453–456.

Ray, R. O., Heppe, G. (1986). Older adult happiness: The contributions of activity breadth and intensity. Physical and occupational therapy. *Geriatrics, 4*(4), 31–59.

Riley, M. W., & Foner, A. (1968). *Aging and society: Vol. 1. An inventory of research findings.* New York: Russell Sage Foundation.

Rogers, J. C. (1986). Roles and functions of occupational therapy in gerontic practice. In L. Davi & M. Kirkland (Eds.), *The role of occupational therapy with the elderly* (pp. 117–121). Rockville, MD: American Occupational Therapy Association.

Rosenthal, L., & Howe, M. C. (1984). Activity patterns and leisure concepts: A comparison of temporal adaptation among day versus night shift workers. *Occupational Therapy in Mental Health, 4,* 59–77.

Schilder, P. (1950). *The image and appearance of the human body: Studies in the constructive energies of the psyche.* New York: McGraw-Hill.

Schmitthausler, C. M. (1982). Paper on World Assembly on Aging. UU-UN Office, New York.

Seligman, M. E. (1975). *Helplessness: On depression, development and death.* San Francisco: W. H. Freeman.

Stevens, C. (1979, November 5). Aging Americans: Many delay retiring or resume jobs to beat inflation and the blues. *The Wall Street Journal,* pp. 11, 22.

Tickle, L. S., & Yerxa, E. J. (1981a). Need satisfaction of older persons living in the community and in institutions: Part 1. The environment. *American Journal of Occupational Therapy, 35,* 644–649.

Tickle, L. S., & Yerxa, E. J. (1981b). Need satisfaction of older persons living in the community and in institutions: Part 2. Role of activity. *American Journal of Occupational Therapy, 35,* 650–655.

U.S. Senate Committee on Aging (1984, September). *The costs of employing older workers.* Washington, DC: U.S. Government Printing Office.

Webster's Ninth New Collegiate Dictionary. (1985). Springfield, MA: Merriam Webster.

# 10

# Ethical Issues at the End of Life: Dying, Death, and the Care of the Aged

David Barnard

If, as Samuel Johnson observed, the thought of death wonderfully concentrates the mind, it is also true that the care of the dying presents in concentrated form many of the ethical issues involved in the clinical care of the aged person. Thus, while the focus of this chapter will be on ethical aspects of care for the dying, it will lay the groundwork for analysis of a broader range of problems, by discussing concepts and patterns of reasoning that will also serve in other contexts. (For discussions and bibliographic references on this broader range of problems, see Cassel, Meier, & Traines, 1986; Thornton & Winkler, 1988; Jecker, 1991.)

The fact that many significant issues in clinical ethics intersect in the decision making related to the dying is only one reason, however, that this topic is an appropriate context for a discussion of ethics and care of the aged. As described in Chapter 3, Emotional and Cognitive Issues in the Care of the Aged, dying and death are very stressful for patients, families, and caregivers. Tendencies toward denial, distancing, distorted perception, and interpersonal conflict make it especially important to have a clear understanding of the ethical dimensions of decisions that will have to be made in such an atmosphere.

In addition, for many aged persons the dying process itself has characteristics that make thoughtful anticipation of decision making critical. For many of the aged, death will be a gradual process following a prolonged period of increasing disability, even though the final terminal events may be sudden (e.g., respiratory or cardiac arrest, massive stroke), requiring urgent decisions about resuscitation, hospitalization, and the like. This combination of time to anticipate and plan with the possibility of sudden emergencies permitting no time for reflection makes it imperative that people understand alternatives and include all concerned parties in the process of evaluating possibilities and expressing needs and preferences. Finally, the sorts of interpersonal relationships and communication patterns among patients, families, and caregivers that facilitate optimal decision making about dying can help address other ethical problems as well.

This chapter will be divided into three main sections, corresponding to three major areas of ethical concern in relation to the dying: disclosure of information and talking about dying; refusing, withdrawing, or withholding life-sustaining medical treatment; and actively hastening death.

## DISCLOSURE OF INFORMATION AND TALKING ABOUT DYING

When Big Daddy, the autocratic Southern patriarch in Tennessee Williams's play *Cat on a Hot Tin Roof,* returns from an examination at the medical clinic, he triumphantly announces to his family that his trouble is nothing more than a spastic colon. Later that day, with the noise of Big Daddy's sixty-fifth birthday party in the background, the family doctor tells the truth to Big Daddy's son Brick: Big Daddy has inoperable cancer and does not have long to live. Stunned, Brick asks the doctor why he has lied to his father. "Professional ethics!" the doctor replies as he strides out of the room.

The ethics to which the doctor refers have a long history in medicine. Physicians have often tried to shield patients from bad news, either with outright lies, selective omissions, deliberate obfuscation with medical jargon, or overoptimistic prognoses of recovery. The main justification for deception is the doctor's obligation to protect the patient from harm. If patients hear the truth about a fatal prognosis, it is argued, they will give up hope and possibly die sooner or with more unhappiness than if they expect to recover; they may give up the will to live or even try to commit suicide; or they might refuse recommended therapy that, although not curative, might make them more comfortable and might even result in unprecedented reversal of their condition.

Three aspects of this ethic stand out: (1) it is based solely on prediction of future consequences to the patient, excluding any other criteria for determining proper conduct; (2) it assumes that the psychological impact of learning about one's likely death is either unequivocally harmful or that its harm outweighs any possible benefit; and (3) it is unilateral, that is, the decision as to what information to disclose to the patient is made by the doctor alone (sometimes in concert with relatives), without including the patient.

This unilateral, consequentialist ethic, based on the physician's own calculation of what action will most benefit the patient, is the oldest professional ethic in medicine. The Hippocratic Oath states, "I will apply dietetic measures to the benefit of the sick according to my ability and judgment" (Jones, 1923, p. 299). No mention is made here of the patient's judgment, or of the value of patients' participation in decisions regarding their care. Applied to the question of truthful disclosure, this ethic can be questioned from two points of view.

### *Predicting Harmful Consequences*

First, are physicians justified in predicting that the psychological effects of disclosing fatal diagnoses are overwhelmingly harmful to patients? Notice that this is both an empirical claim and a value judgment. The empirical claim is that patients are harmed when they receive bad news. The value judgment is that whatever level of harm is associated with receiving bad news is worse than that which might result from withholding it.

There are no significant data to support the empirical claim, even though physicians can often relate individual cases in which patients appeared to crumble emotionally upon receiving bad news, and family members occasionally urge physicians not to tell relatives the truth on the grounds that the patient "couldn't take it." Beyond the fact that physicians would normally consider it irresponsible to base therapeutic interventions on nothing more than anecdotal evidence, the anecdotal evidence itself is suspect. Research suggests that physicians have a greater fear of death, and greater difficulty talking about it, than the general population (Veatch, 1976). Moreover, families are understandably upset and fearful at the prospect of dealing with their dying relative. It is not hard to conclude from this that the presumption that patients will "not be able to take it" often represents the physician's and family's desire to avoid the difficult emotions of a frank discussion of dying with the patient, rather than an accurate assessment of the patient's emotional capacities. Indeed, when surveyed, patients have invariably indicated a greater desire for information — including information about fatal prognoses — than is predicted by physicians (Kelly & Friesen, 1950; Samp & Curreri, 1957).

What of the value judgment that the possible harm of receiving bad news outweighs the benefits of disclosure, or the harm of deception? Clearly, specifically *medical* expertise does not qualify one to assign priorities to the disadvantages and benefits for another person. For physicians or other professionals to assume that their technical expertise qualifies them to assess whether patients should experience the emotions of fear, anger, or grief that accompany fatal prognoses is either the inappropriate generalization of expertise from the technical to the moral sphere, or a rationalization of the desire to avoid the difficult emotional demands of communicating bad news (Veatch, 1976).

### *The Physician-Patient Relationship and Informed Consent*

Second, by directing professional attention entirely to the *outcome* of potential medical interventions, the consequentialist ethic ignores other aspects of medical practice that are morally significant. People are more than vehicles for the accomplishment of good outcomes. They are also centers of thought, feeling, and choice. Every person has a world of inner experience and continually discovers and creates personal meanings in the events of life. Illness is one such event. Rather than being random biophysical phenomena, illnesses are meaningful events in a biography. The choices they require about the seeking of help, diagnosis and therapy, and possible alterations in life plans, emerge from personal, social, and cultural contexts of meaning unique to the individual. The freedom to assign those meanings, and to act accordingly, is also of moral significance, independent of the outcome those actions produce.

For wisdom concerning the moral significance of individual freedom we can look to the writings of John Stuart Mill and Immanuel Kant. In *On Liberty,* Mill asserts:

> the sole end for which mankind are warranted, individually or collectively, in interfering with the liberty of action of any of their number is self-protection. . . . [t]he only purpose for which power can be rightfully exercised over any member of a civilized community, against his will, is to prevent harm to others. *His own good, either physical or moral, is not a sufficient warrant. He cannot rightfully be compelled to do or forbear because it will make him happier, because, in the opinions of others, to do so would be wise or even right.* These are good reasons for remonstrating with him, or reasoning with him, or persuading him, or entreating him, but not for compelling him or visiting him with any evil in case he do otherwise. To justify that, the conduct from which it is desired to deter him must be calculated to produce evil to someone else. The only part of the conduct of anyone for which he is amenable to society is that which concerns others. In the part which merely concerns himself, his independence is, of right, absolute. Over himself, over his own body and mind, the individual is sovereign. (Mill, 1977, p. 186, emphasis added)

According to Mill, respect for individual freedom is a necessary constraint on the obligation to produce beneficial consequences. Mill rejects the assumption that others — even those with "professional expertise" — may properly substitute their judgment for the considered judgments and choices of the affected individuals. In the first place, only the affected individuals can really *know* what is in their best interests. Therefore, respecting patients' preferences (assuming adequate understanding on their part) is required to guarantee the best outcome. But an even stronger justification for Mill's view is that, *regardless of the outcome, the protection of liberty to choose is morally required as an expression of the integrity and autonomy of persons.*

It is this point which Immanuel Kant emphasizes most clearly in his dictum, "So act as to treat humanity, whether in thine own person or in that of any other, in every case as an end withal, never as means only" (1949, p. 46). The injunction not to treat people merely as means to an end has two important implications. First, it forbids us to exploit other people by using them for the accomplishment of our own purposes. An obvious medical example is the conscription of unwitting or unwilling subjects for experimentation, when the results of the experiment have no promise of benefit to the subjects. (Kant's formulation would also prohibit unwitting or unwilling participation even when benefit *might* accrue to the subjects.) Second, we are forbidden to substitute our judgment of what ends a person ought to pursue for that person's own choice. Here, Kant is close to Mill. What distinguishes Kant's view, however, is that he emphasizes that such a substitution is wrong *not* because it may not produce the best outcome, but because it treats the person as a means rather than as an end, and violates our obligation to respect each person's absolute worth. This worth is most fully expressed through the person's autonomous choice of valued goals and life plans.

### Informed Consent

In medical practice, respect for self-determination is primarily achieved by means of patients' informed consent (Faden, Beauchamp, & King, 1986). By giving consent, a patient affirms that the goods envisioned by the professional, and the means to accomplish them, are in accord with the patient's own value system. The discussion of informed consent in the Ethics Manual of the American College of Physicians (American College of Physicians, 1984), captures this balance between promoting the patient's good and protecting freedom. It also underscores the point that respect for persons makes the *process* of medical care ethically important: how information is derived and shared, the nature of decision making, and the quality of interpersonal relationships:

> Truly informed consent is most apt to be achieved through effective personal communication within the physician-patient covenant; it is not achieved by perfunctory signing of a ("legal") consent form. The thoughtful clinician communicates with the patient in a warm, comfortable open manner that conveys his competence, loyalty, and respect for the patient, an attitude that engenders trust and confidence. Using language that can be understood, the physician endeavors to present to the patient and the family a basic understanding of problems they face together, and he makes it clear that the patient has the right to make the final choice in accepting or rejecting his proposed plan of diagnosis and treatment (p. 133).

Legal aspects of informed consent are discussed in Chapter 11, Legal Issues in the Care of the Aged, and will be dealt with again in this chapter in connection with patients

who refuse life-sustaining medical treatments. In the present context, the morally significant point is that a relationship based on respect for persons and informed consent
depends on the physician's truthful disclosure of information. It is inconsistent with such
a relationship for physicians to arrogate to themselves the choice of what information a
patient ought to receive.

Current medical practice is increasingly consistent with the ethic of truthful disclosure. While the doctor in Williams's play could point to the common practices of his day
to support his withholding the truth from his patient, a major shift has occurred in the
past two decades. In 1961, 88% of physicians responding to a survey published in the
*Journal of the American Medical Association* reported that they usually did not tell their
patients the truth about a diagnosis of cancer (Oken, 1961). A repeat survey in 1977
revealed a complete reversal, as 98% of physicians who responded reported the general
policy of telling the truth (Novack, Plumer, Smith, Ochitill, Morrow & Bennett, 1979).
Reflecting this shift, Avery Weisman (1967) writes, "The central question is not whether
to tell a patient about his dim outlook, but *who* shall tell, *how much* to tell, *what* to tell,
*how* to tell, *when* to tell, and *how often* to tell." (p. 664)

In other words, with the ethical issue resolved firmly in favor of being truthful, attention needs to be paid to the techniques and clinical behaviors required for the compassionate communication of bad news.

### Disclosure and Communication Skills

Although physicians' traditional concerns about the harmful impact of truthful disclo-
sures do not justify deception, it is still true that communicating — and receiving — bad
news is emotionally difficult. Professionals have an obligation to perform this task in a
way that takes account of the patient's emotional needs. Thomas Percival addressed this
issue in his *Medical Ethics* of 1803, with particular reference to the disclosure of bad
news:

> A Physician should not be forward to make gloomy prognostications; because they savour of
> empiricism, by magnifying the importance of his services in the treatment of disease. But he
> should not fail on proper occasions to give to the friends of the patient timely notice of danger
> when it really occurs, and even to the patient himself, if absolutely necessary. This office,
> however, is so peculiarly alarming when executed by him, that it ought to be declined when-
> ever it can be assigned to any other person of sufficient judgement and delicacy; for the
> Physician should be the minister of hope and comfort to the sick, that by such cordials to the
> drooping spirit he may smooth the bed of death, revive expiring life, and counteract the
> depressing influence of those maladies, which rob the philosopher of fortitude, and the Chris-
> tian of consolation. (Percival, 1803/1977, p. 22)

The striking point in this passage is Percival's suggestion that physicians delegate the
task of disclosure to others whenever possible. This is a twist on the idea that physicians
should tell others instead of the patient. Note that Percival occupies a middle position on
this: tell patients as a last resort, but tell them. In effect, he argues that patients should
learn the truth, but from someone besides the physician. Why?

Percival's reasoning goes to the heart of the connection between disclosure and the
physician-patient relationship. He argues that patients should be able to derive strength
and solace from their doctors, which requires that doctors not become associated with

death and hopelessness in the patient's mind. Bad news, Percival thought, would harm patients by contaminating physicians with the odor of mortality when their greatest therapeutic power lies in their association with vitality, health, and hope.

Percival's argument rests on the assumption that it is impossible to talk frankly about death and maintain hope at the same time. This is not necessarily true (Buckman, 1992). In the words of Howard Brody:

> If we were as good at listening to our patients as we are at telling them things, we would learn that hope is not automatically equated with survival. Hope means different things to different people; and hope means different things to the same person as he moves through different stages of his illness and his emotional reaction to it. The man who hoped for a cure for his arthritis may now hope that, on a good day, he can get in nine holes of golf. And, for those unfortunates for whom those who would keep them alive have truly become the "inquisitor" instead of the savior, hope may mean a pain-free and oblivious death. (1981, pp. 1411–1412)

Hope may mean the expectation of continued attention and love from others, adequate pain control, planning for the financial security of loved ones, and many other things that have meaning for individuals besides prolonging their lives. "When we talk to patients and find out what is really worrying them," Brody continues, "we can almost always give some realistic assurances" (p. 1412).

There will be many times when caregivers will be approached by relatives or friends with the request not to tell a patient the truth. The proper response to this request is to explore thoroughly and sympathetically with the family the reasons behind their request; to explain that the caregiver's primary responsibility is to the patient, and to maintain open communication in the caring relationship. Caregivers should point out that not only do most patients come to understand and know their situation despite efforts to deceive them, but that the damage to trusting relationships if and when the deception is discovered can be severe at the time when such relationships are most needed.

Finally, it should be pointed out that dying people need to make plans for their future care, particularly in an era when 80% of people die in institutions, and decisions need to be made regarding the application of medical technology in the last stages of life. Decisions about life-sustaining medical treatment have become increasingly complex as the technology, cost, and social impact of medical intervention have expanded, with particular implications for the aged (Office of Technology Assessment, 1987).

## DECISIONS TO LIMIT LIFE-SUSTAINING MEDICAL TREATMENT

The range of decisions that face the aged and their families and caregivers at the end of life are illustrated by the following cases.

### CASE 1

Mrs. Toivonen was 83 years old and had been confined to a nursing home for three years following a stroke. The stroke left her paralyzed completely on one side and unable to speak. She also had severe scoliosis of the spine, and spent her days curled up in bed. She had decubitus ulcers on her back and hip. She weighed 69 pounds.

For as long as her physician had cared for Mrs. Toivonen she had expressed dislike and distrust of doctors. She had refused hospitalization for most problems and had appeared to object to treatment of a pneumonia that had set in at the time of her stroke. She had been treated despite these objections, in the expectation that she would recover from her angry and depressed state. The pneumonia resolved; the paralysis and aphasia remained.

Mrs. Toivonen had one friend who expressed to the staff of the nursing home the hope that "there wouldn't be any heroics" if Mrs. Toivonen got sick again. Mrs. Toivonen's one relative, a niece in a distant state, had called to insist that "everything possible" be done for her aunt.

Once in the middle of the night Mrs. Toivonen's temperature rose to 103.5. When her doctor was called to the nursing home, the nurse on duty reported that Mrs. Toivonen had grown less and less responsive over the past several days, had hardly eaten, and had a cough. Mrs. Toivonen lay passively and without a sign of recognition as the doctor examined her. The doctor concluded that she probably had pneumonia. He debated his options: (1) transfering her to a regional hospital for a full evaluation, including many expensive tests, some of them uncomfortable and invasive, to determine for sure that Mrs. Toivonen had pneumonia; (2) starting an antibiotic and fluid therapy without further evaluation — on the assumption that she had pneumonia — thereby possibly staving off infection and death; (3) concluding that Mrs. Toivonen would prefer to be left alone to die, and providing only the sort of care that would keep her comfortable while she died (Hilfiker, 1983).

## CASE 2

Mr. Roberts, a 62-year-old machinist, was hospitalized for metastatic cancer. For many years he had suffered from disabling rheumatoid arthritis, requiring bilateral hip replacements. Two years before admission he had had a carcinoma of the colon resected. Since the resected nodes contained tumor, he had also received adjuvant chemotherapy, which he discontinued after a year because of severe vomiting. He felt well until a month before admission, when he developed abdominal and lower back pain, weight loss, and weakness. Evaluation at another hospital was inconclusive. When he developed progressive vomiting and urinary retention, he came to the emergency room. Evaluation revealed a hard pelvic mass. The patient had mild anemia and azotemia and slightly elevated liver function tests. A plain film of the abdomen showed a solid pelvic mass and bilateral hydronephrosis. A plain film of the abdomen showed colonic obstruction. An abdominal ultrasound showed a solid pelvic mass and bilateral hydronephrosis. Although there was no tissue confirmation, recurrent metastatic carcinoma was diagnosed. Treatment with narcotics and a nasogastric tube relieved his discomfort. Ureteral catheters allowed a diuresis, but the catheters fell out after two days. An oncology consultant recommended that neither chemotherapy nor radiation was likely to benefit Mr. Roberts.

Knowing the impossibility of treating his cancer, the patient and his family refused laboratory tests, antibiotics, transfusions, palliative surgery, and dialysis. They agreed to the use of pain medicine (morphine and an antiemetic parenterally around the clock), nasogastric suction, and intravenous fluids. His mind was clear, and he spoke openly and affectionately with his family about his approaching death.

Four days later Mr. Roberts requested that his doctors "speed up" his death. Although he was not in pain or discomfort, he said he had reached the limits of his endurance. He also was concerned about the costs of his hospitalization, since he had no insurance and had to spend his life savings before becoming eligible for Medicaid (Lo & Jonsen, 1980b).

The ethical issues in these cases revolve around decisions to limit medical treatment. Two basic questions are involved. First, what sorts of medical treatments may be withheld or withdrawn from dying patients, and for what reasons? Second, who should make these decisions? These questions will be addressed later in the chapter. A third question is raised at the end of Case 2: Is it ever morally permissible to act intentionally to shorten life, as opposed to withholding treatments that might prolong life? This will be the focus of the next section.

### Patient Refusal of Treatment: Questions of Competence and Informed Consent

Four reasons are commonly put forward to justify limiting medical treatment for the critically ill: (1) the patient refuses the treatment, (2) the treatment is medically futile, (3) the patient's quality of life is so poor as to make further life-prolonging efforts unreasonable, and (4) continuing treatment imposes unacceptable social or financial burdens (Lo & Jonsen, 1980a). The last three reasons assume more importance in the absence of clear direction from the patient.

In our society a consensus has developed that competent adult patients may decline any form of medical treatment, including treatments designed to prolong or sustain life (President's Commission, 1983a; Cantor, 1987; Emanuel, 1988; Weir, 1989). These decisions, and the respect accorded to the preferences of competent adults, may pertain to medical interventions such as hospitalization, cardiopulmonary resuscitation, treatment of infections with antibiotics, and, increasingly though still controversially, the provision of food and water (Lynn, 1986). Most of these interventions were refused by Mr. Roberts and his family in Case 2.

*Competence* is both a legal and psychiatric term. (For a discussion of the legal aspects, see Chapter 11, Legal Issues in the Care of the Aged.) It is also a term that is subject to abuse. For example, professionals may be tempted to interpret a patient's refusal of life-prolonging medical treatment as, in itself, evidence of mental incompetence. Perl and Shelp (1982) report instances of requests for psychiatric evaluation of patients on the grounds of refusal of treatment, when the real issue was a conflict in values between patient and staff, not the patient's mental status. Though it is important that the patient's competence be determined in all cases of treatment refusal (and, for that matter, in cases where treatment is accepted!), it is morally unacceptable to use a competency evaluation to coerce patients into accepting treatment simply because they have not agreed with the staff's interpretation of their best interests.

The key components of competence for medical decision making are:

1. The ability to appreciate that a decision is called for
2. The ability to understand one's medical condition and the likely consequences of alternative diagnostic or therapeutic actions or inaction
3. The ability to articulate the reasons behind one's choice

The last component — the patient's articulation of reasons — provides the basis for further discussion and clarification by professionals, in case the patient's refusal of care is based on misunderstanding, or is actually an attempt to communicate something else (Jackson & Youngner, 1979). For example, patients may express the desire to die when what troubles them most is the fear of abandonment and isolation. Patients may fear becoming a burden on relatives but not feel comfortable asking the relatives how they really feel. Patients may misunderstand the implications of various treatments and reject them on the basis of unrealistic, imagined expectations of side effects. Patients may be clinically depressed. Each of these states of mind can be addressed: fears of abandonment can be met with reassurance of ongoing commitments to provide comfort, company, and care; relatives can express willingness to continue caring for a patient, and can demonstrate efforts to obtain needed support services; groundless fears and expectations about treatments can be dispelled with factual information; depression can be treated medically and/or psychotherapeutically.

### The Importance of Open Conversation: Professional Advocacy and Patient's Decision

The patient's refusal of life-sustaining medical treatment should be seen as the stimulus for discussion and exploration. Professionals are obligated to present the medical facts as clearly and understandably as the situation (and inevitable prognostic uncertainty) permits. They are also obligated to be forceful advocates for continuing treatment if in their professional judgment such treatment carries a reasonable likelihood of benefit. If patients still refuse, professionals should attempt to assess not only the patient's competence to decide, but also the true meaning behind the patient's words. Whenever possible, misunderstandings and misconceptions should be clarified, groundless fears dispelled, and palliative treatments offered. Nevertheless, respecting people's self-determination requires that professionals not substitute their own values for those of patients. Patients' preferences to forego further treatment should be respected when they are based on a rational assessment of their situation, and express strongly held convictions about how to respond to the approach of death.

### Orders Not to Resuscitate

Especially in the high-technology environment of the modern hospital, cardiopulmonary resuscitation (CPR) has become routine practice for any patient who suffers cardiac or respiratory arrest. It is psychologically easier, and perceived to be ethically and legally safer, for professionals to apply CPR rather than to withhold it. Nevertheless, patients themselves often do not wish to be resuscitated (Bedell & Delbanco, 1984), and many groups of patients—particularly those with severely debilitating underlying illnesses—have almost no chance of surviving to hospital discharge even when CPR is successful in the short run (Blackhall, 1987).

Many patients fear that CPR will prolong their dying rather than contribute to their recovery or even to their enjoyment of their last days of life. Since most severely ill or debilitated patients who do survive CPR end up in intensive-care units, and many are dependent on respiratory support for long periods of time, these concerns are realistic. Moreover, patients with metastatic cancer (such as Mr. Roberts in Case 2) may well prefer the release of a fatal heart attack to a lingering, painful death from their cancer.

By its very nature, CPR cannot be debated and discussed at the time it is needed. Cardiac or respiratory arrests are emergencies requiring immediate action. In the absence of advance knowledge of the patient's preferences, professionals should opt for CPR in all patients who are likely to benefit medically, or when the effect of CPR is in doubt. If professional judgment is that the patient would not benefit, there is no obligation to attempt CPR unless the patient has specifically requested it. In that case, CPR should be offered, but physicians should review this decision periodically with the patient.

The best procedure is to ascertain patients' preferences in advance. Again, this requires open and full disclosure to patients of their underlying diseases, likely prognoses, the availability of CPR, as well as the likely outcomes of CPR in patients with their particular conditions. As discussed in the previous section, the preferences of competent patients should be respected when they are based on a thorough discussion and explanation of relevant medical factors.

Occasionally, family members will disagree with the patient's choice and request CPR against the stated wishes of the patient. In these cases the responsibility of the physician is to carry out the patient's wishes, explaining to the family that the physician's primary duty is to the patient.

Patients' preferences, and the reasons for them, should be clearly documented in the medical record. Decisions should be reviewed periodically as medical conditions change, or as patients change their mind (whichever initial preference they may have stated). Finally, it should be emphasized that the decision to withhold CPR in no way precludes other forms of aggressive medical care to treat the patient's illness or to mitigate symptoms. *Withholding CPR is compatible with continuing every other form of conscientious, aggressive medical care.* Patients should not fear, nor should professionals conclude, that a DNR (do not resuscitate) order is tantamount to giving up on the patient, or backing down from otherwise indicated treatments (Miles, Cranford, & Schultz, 1982).

The foregoing discussion assumes that patients are capable of participating in decisions about DNR orders. Frequently they are not. In that case, resuscitation decisions must be made by physicians, family members, or other surrogate decision makers. Guidelines for making these decisions will be the same as those governing all decisions to limit medical treatment for incompetent or otherwise nonautonomous patients.

### Nonautonomous Patients

The most vexing decisions concerning limitation of life-sustaining medical treatment are those involving patients who cannot express their own preferences. Whereas Mr. Roberts was fully involved in the decisions to withhold various treatments in Case 2 above, Mrs. Toivonen in Case 1 was incapable of expressing her own judgment about what treatment (or nontreatment) would be in her best interests. Because her physician could not restore her competence to participate in the decision, someone would have to make a judgment on her behalf. How should that be done?

The President's Commission for the Study of Ethical Problems in Medicine (1983a) suggests two approaches to decision making for incompetent patients, depending on the information available about the patients' previously stated wishes or values: *substituted judgment* and what the Commission calls the *best-interests standard.*

### Substituted Judgment

Substituted judgment requires surrogate decision makers to make choices patients themselves would if they were competent to do so. In respect for the diminished competence of patients, decision makers must make every effort to determine their values, preferences, and previously expressed wishes.

The relationship between patient and professional is an important arena in which to explore these matters. Indeed the quality of that relationship is the central factor in the ability to provide morally responsible care. The medical interview, conducted with sufficient rapport and time to permit thorough exploration of values and priorities, is an indispensable tool for establishing what Laurence McCullough (1984) calls the patient's "values history" — documentation of attitudes toward medical intervention, prolongation of life, and similar issues that may arise when the patient is no longer autonomous or communicative. McCullough rightly urges that the values history be sought with the same thoroughness and care that is devoted to past medical history, social history, and so forth. His recommendation applies to all patients, but especially to the aged, in whose care such issues can reasonably be expected to arise.

In Case 1 above, Mrs. Toivonen's physician could refer to Mrs. Toivonen's past statements concerning hospitalization and medical interventions, and to the reports from Mrs. Toivonen's longtime friend. Together, these sources suggested that, were Mrs. Toivonen able to participate in the decision, she may well have requested that no further medical treatment be given. The difficult question for her caregivers was whether this evidence was strong enough to justify decisions that would very likely hasten Mrs. Toivonen's death.

## Advance Directives

Increasingly, patients are being encouraged to provide some form of *advance directive* for their care should they lose the ability to communicate their wishes when decisions need to be made. The 1990 decision of the United States Supreme Court in the case of Nancy Cruzan (*Cruzan* v. *Director, Missouri Department of Health,* 110 S.Ct. 2841 [1990]), and the passage by the United States Congress of the Patient Self-Determination Act (PSDA) in the same year, have called special attention to the value of advance directives. PSDA, which became effective December 1, 1991, requires health-care institutions to provide patients on admission with written information about their rights under state law to provide instructions regarding medical treatment, their rights to refuse treatment, and their right to formulate advance directives. Institutions must ascertain whether the patient has such a directive and must record that information in the medical record. Although the implementation of this law, and the strengths and limitations of the various forms of advance directives, continue to be subject to debate (LaPuma, Orentlicher, & Moss, 1991; Wolf et al., 1991), public awareness of the advantages of open discussion and planning for end-of-life decision making has notably increased. (For further discussion of advance directives, living wills, durable power of attorney, and the related question of the appointment of a guardian to make decisions for incompetent patients, see Chapter 11, Legal Issues in the Care of the Aged.)

## The Best-Interests Standard

If reliable evidence of a patient's own preferences and values is not available, those making decisions on the patient's behalf should try to observe the best interests of the patient. This requires them to screen out competing interests of third parties, including financial hardship; the desire to be free of the psychological burden of caring for a dependent person; and needs for hospital bed space, transplantable organs, and the like. Then these decision makers must weigh the advantages and disadvantages of possible medical treatments:

1. Is the procedure medically indicated; that is, is it likely to accomplish a reasonable medical objective?
2. Does the procedure provide a benefit to this particular patient, in that patient's condition?
3. Does the procedure involve overwhelming or otherwise intolerable pain, restraint, or other burdens that outweigh the benefits to the patient?

The screening out of third-party interests does not mean such factors are irrelevant to medical decision making at the end of life. Patients themselves may well bring them forward to justify their refusal of further treatment. For others to base treatment refusal on these grounds, however, may leave incompetent, voiceless people vulnerable to discriminatory neglect or abandonment in order to meet the needs of others (Lo & Jonsen, 1980a).

### Considerations of Cost and Quality of Life

The aged are especially vulnerable to discrimination when surrogate decisions about life-sustaining treatment are based on quality-of-life judgments or calculations of cost. Both of these criteria are liable to express the biases of a youth-oriented culture that defines quality of life in terms of physical vigor, autonomy, and productivity. As Jerry Avorn (1984) has argued, the very terms of "cost-benefit" analysis, which seek quantitative measures of worth and value, are systematically biased against the aged, who have relatively short life expectancies and less anticipated income compared to younger patients with whom they are seen to compete for medical resources.

It is tempting to identify the costs of maintaining the aged on life-supports as the key to reducing large health-care expenditures in society. Daniel Callahan (1987) has argued that society should determine a "natural life span," beyond which resources would go only to alleviate suffering rather than to extend life. Resources could then be redirected to improving health care for younger patients as well as providing supportive, long-term care for the aged.

Callahan is careful to insist that if his recommendations are accepted by society, they would have to be implemented at the level of broad policies rather than as individual treatment decisions by physicians. This is a crucial point. Patients' trust in physicians could be seriously eroded if they came to expect that their care depended on the physician's calculation of the value to society of offering treatment for the patients' conditions. On the other hand, if society as a whole, through the normal political process, determined that particular services or treatments would be restricted by age (or some other nonmedical criterion), physicians could continue to be unequivocal advocates for the well-being of their patients while recognizing externally imposed constraints on available resources.

There are, however, further difficulties in Callahan's approach. One, which he himself acknowledges, is arriving at a broadly acceptable definition of a "natural life span" that does not fall victim to the same biases alluded to above in connection with judgments about quality of life. A second problem is reliably distinguishing medical treatments that alleviate suffering from those that extend life. Cardiopulmonary resuscitation is clearly life-prolonging, whereas administration of analgesic medication at the risk of depressing respiratory function clearly illustrates an effort primarily to relieve suffering. But what about surgery to remove a painful as well as life-threatening bowel obstruction in a patient with metastatic colon cancer? This is a major, expensive intervention that in turn could produce the need for more interventions in case of surgical complications. The distinction is easier to make conceptually than to put into practice.

Finally, Callahan may be mistaken in focusing on the high-technology interventions at the end of life as the real culprit in health-care costs. Although it is possible that the continuing rise in the aged population into the next century may change this, at present these interventions are not the major contributor to the problem of health-care expenditures. Rather, the costs associated with maintaining the chronically ill and debilitated aged are those that pose the greater fiscal challenge (Scitovsky & Capron, 1986). Indeed, providing adequate long-term care for the larger population of the aged who are *not* dying may well be more, rather than less, expensive in the long run. (For more detailed discussion of long-term care and the health-policy dimensions of care for the aged, see Chapter 12, Disability Trends and Community Long-Term Health Care for the Aged, and Chapter 13, The Economics of the Health-Care System. For a more thorough analysis of the ethical aspects of health-care policy, see, e.g., President's Commission, 1983b; Daniels, 1985).

For these reasons, the best interests of the individual patient constitute the ethically proper guideline for withholding or withdrawing care from nonautonomous patients. Though other criteria, such as the quality of life, or psychological and financial burdens, are morally acceptable when applied by the affected patients themselves, the possibilities of abuse and discriminatory neglect inherent in these criteria make them morally suspect when applied by third parties for patients unable to communicate for themselves.

### Institutional Ethics Committees and Decisions to Limit Treatment for Incompetent Patients

A resource for physicians, families, and other caregivers who must make treatment decisions for critically ill, nonautonomous patients is the formation of an institutional ethics committee (Kanoti & Vinicky, 1987; Cranford & Doudera, 1984). Usually composed of physicians from several clinical specialties, nurses, social workers, clergy, and others with specialized training in bioethics, the ethics committee may call upon the expertise required to verify diagnoses and prognoses for critically ill patients; make sure that all parties to a decision (physicians, nurses, other caregivers, family members, etc.) have the opportunity to present their perceptions and concerns; and apply moral reasoning to the case once all relevant facts have been taken into account. Most advocates of ethics committees recommend that they be advisory rather than take over the decision-making responsibility of the physicians and family members directly involved in the case.

## HASTENING DEATH BY ACTIVE KILLING OR ASSISTED SUICIDE

The request by Mr. Roberts and his family in Case 2 to withhold life-prolonging therapies is ethically noncontroversial: The available treatments were noncurative, Mr. Roberts's death was judged to be imminent regardless of treatment, and he participated fully and competently in the decision. From the point of view of respect for self-determination, and in light of the fact that physicians have no obligation to undertake futile interventions, the decisions to limit medical treatment for Mr. Roberts were fully justified.

What about Mr. Roberts's further request, 4 days later, that the doctors "speed up" his death? Given that no further attempts were to be made to extend Mr. Roberts's life, would it not be equally permissible to accede to his request to have his life ended more quickly? Is there any moral difference between agreeing to let Mr. Roberts die without medical intervention and acting intentionally to end his life? In the terms commonly used to pursue this debate, is there a moral difference between passive and active euthanasia, especially when both are apparently undertaken with the consent of the patient?

It is beyond the scope of this chapter to explore the vast literature on euthanasia that has attempted to answer this question (see, e.g., Kohl, 1975; Ladd, 1979; Horan & Mall, 1980; Rachels, 1986). Some of the key arguments, however, may be summarized as follows.

### Arguments in Favor of Active, Voluntary Euthanasia

Those who advocate active, voluntary euthanasia, that is, actions by physicians that are deliberately intended to kill the patient, argue that there is no moral difference between active and passive euthanasia. In either case, patients end up dying sooner than they otherwise would, either because a physician failed to do something that would have kept the patient alive, or because the physician did something — injected a lethal drug, for example — to bring about the patient's death. To stand by idly while a patient suffers an otherwise avoidable death from infection, dehydration, or respiratory arrest is no different, in other words, than actively killing the patient. If passive euthanasia is considered morally acceptable, then active euthanasia ought to be considered equally acceptable.

A second argument is that just as respect for the autonomy and self-determination of patients requires that professionals respect their refusal of treatment, so does respect for autonomy require professionals to allow patients to choose the time of their dying, in order to avoid agonizing pain, humiliating dependency, or financial ruin. No compelling state interest, according to this view, is strong enough to override the decision of competent individuals to end their own lives when their actions do not inflict significant harm to others (Engelhardt & Malloy, 1982).

A third argument is that prolonging life is only one moral obligation of health professionals. Relief of suffering is an equally significant obligation, and if the only way to end suffering is actively to shorten the life of the sufferer, then so acting is ethically permissible. To refuse to act is not only an unjustified, paternalistic substitution of professional values for those of the patient, but also potentially a cruel and inhumane prolongation of a patient's agony.

### Arguments against Active, Voluntary Euthanasia

Opponents of active euthanasia may well agree that active and passive euthanasia are similar *causally* but still deny that they are equivalent *morally*. The significant moral question is not simply whether the physician is the *cause* of a patient's death, but whether, at the time the patient dies the physician had a *duty* to save the patient's life (Clouser, 1977). As long as such a duty exists, whether the patient dies by omission or commission makes no difference: In either case the physician is morally to blame for failing to fulfill the duty to save. Killing and allowing to die would be morally equivalent. The important question is thus not whether allowing or causing to die are the same, but, rather, is there a point when the physician no longer has a duty to save?

As K. Danner Clouser (1977) argues, there may well be a point when medical therapy stops being beneficial and treatment becomes torture. Though the precise point of transition is hard to identify, when it is reached the physician no longer has the duty to save the patient's life. Since it is the physician's duty to save that makes killing and allowing to die morally equivalent, in the absence of that duty, allowing the patient to die by refraining from life-prolonging treatment is no longer the same as killing the patient. Killing, Clouser argues, would still violate the universal moral rule against homicide, while refraining from useless medical treatment would not.

At present, the position of the American Medical Association (AMA) on euthanasia reflects this reasoning. The AMA accepts passive euthanasia — the refraining from futile life-prolonging measures even at the risk of allowing death — while opposing any actions taken with the deliberate intention of hastening death (American Medical Association, 1986).

A second argument turns on the moral significance of intentions, as opposed merely to results, of actions. An act undertaken primarily to relieve pain that has as one possible (even foreseeable) outcome that the patient will die sooner, is morally different from an action taken primarily to end the patient's life. The best example is the administration of morphine to relieve pain. A dose sufficient to relieve excruciating cancer pain may depress respiratory function enough to hasten the patient's death. Opponents of active euthanasia would accept this risk and provide the pain relief but would oppose the same dose administered *with the sole intention of killing the patient.* The first act accepts the risk of death while still regarding intentional killing as a moral evil. The second act *intends* death, leaving the moral status of intentional killing in doubt (Dyck, 1977).

A related concern is that active killing in the case of dying patients may weaken traditional moral constraints on killing itself. Opponents of active euthanasia worry that a policy that sanctions active euthanasia, even in narrowly defined circumstances, could lead to abuse (Kamisar, 1958). As suggested above in connection with arguments about the quality of life and cost containment, the aged may be especially vulnerable to such abuse if traditional constraints on killing are loosened.

Finally, opponents of voluntary, active euthanasia question whether patients' requests for help in ending their lives are as clear-cut examples of autonomy and self-determination as advocates of active euthanasia assert. The cautions advanced by Jackson and Youngner (1979) in connection with patients' refusals of treatment apply with equal force to requests for active interventions to hasten death. "Autonomy" can be compromised by pain, fear, loneliness, and depression. Vigorous responses to these aspects of patients' suffering are a more constructive — and autonomy-enhancing — approach than actions to bring about the death of the patient.

### The Continuing Debate

The debate on active euthanasia and assisted suicide continues (Quill, 1991; Brock, 1992). In 1991, the citizens of Washington State defeated by a relatively narrow margin a referendum that would have permitted physicians to assist terminally ill patients in dying. In 1992, California voters defeated a law with similar intent but with fewer apparent safeguards against abuses. Similar citizens' initiatives are likely in the future.

Many people, especially the aged, remain more fearful of lingering pain and dependency than of the possible social dangers of modifying an absolute moral prohibition on killing. Many people in the general public fear that they will not be able to control their pain or suffering, and are not convinced by assurances from professionals that their caregivers can or will protect them from the ravages of painful, expensive, lingering death.

With the availability of effective pain control, and commitments by professionals and families to continuing attention to the emotional needs of dying patients, the fear, pain, or sense of worthlessness that lie behind many requests for active euthanasia are rarely beyond effective remedy. Instances in which active killing appears to be the only form of compassionate care for a dying person are thus also rare. (For a comprehensive treatment of supportive care for dying patients, see Doyle, Hanks, & MacDonald [1993]; see also Chapter 3, Emotional and Cognitive Issues in the Care of the Aged.)

Nevertheless, palliative care does not succeed in every case. We are therefore left with the need to formulate public policies that balance the evil of the uncontrollable suffering of some actual patients against the hypothetical but plausible evils that might result should we relax traditional prohibitions against active killing. The debate over assisted suicide and active voluntary euthanasia is primarily a debate over the nature and likelihood of those hypothetical evils, and over the reliability of the various safeguards that have been proposed to prevent them.

## REFERENCES

American College of Physicians, Ad Hoc Committee on Medical Ethics. (1984). American College of Physicians ethics manual (Pt 1). *Annals of Internal Medicine, 101,* 129–137.

American Medical Association, Council on Ethical and Judicial Affairs. (1986, March 15). Statement on withholding or withdrawing life-prolonging treatments. Chicago: American Medical Association.

Avorn, J. (1984). Benefit and cost analysis in geriatric care: Turning age discrimination into health policy. *New England Journal of Medicine, 310,* 1294–1301.

Bedell, S. E., & Delbanco, T. L. (1984). Choices about cardiopulmonary resuscitation in the hospital: When do physicians talk with patients? *New England Journal of Medicine, 310,* 1089–1093.

Blackhall, L. J. (1987). Must we always use CPR? *New England Journal of Medicine, 317,* 1281–1284.

Brock, D. W. (1992). Voluntary active euthanasia. *Hastings Center Report, 22*(March-April), 10–22.

Brody, H. (1981). Hope. *Journal of the American Medical Association, 246,* 1411–1412.

Buckman, R. (1992). *How to break bad news: A guide for health care professionals.* University of Toronto Press, Toronto, Canada.

Callahan, D. J. (1987). *Setting limits: Medical goals in an aging society.* New York: Simon and Schuster.

Cantor, N. L. (1987). *Legal frontiers of death and dying.* Bloomington: Indiana University Press.

Cassel, C. K., Meier, D. E., & Traines, M. L. (1986). Selected bibliography of recent articles in ethics and geriatrics. *Journal of the American Geriatrics Society, 34,* 399–409.

Clouser, K. D. (1977). Allowing or causing: Another look. *Annals of Internal Medicine, 87,* 622–624.

Cranford, R. E., & Doudera, A. E. (Eds.) (1984). *Institutional ethics committees and health care decision making.* Ann Arbor, MI: Health Administration Press.

Daniels, N. (1985). *Just health care.* New York: Cambridge University Press.

Doyle, D., Hanks, G., & MacDonald, N. (Eds.) (1993). *Oxford textbook of palliative medicine.* Oxford: Oxford University Press.

Dyck, A. J. (1977). An alternative to the ethic of euthanasia. In S. J. Reiser, A. J. Dyck, & W. J. Curran (Eds.), *Ethics in medicine: Historical perspectives and contemporary concerns.* (pp. 529–535). Cambridge, MA: MIT Press.

Emanuel, E. J. (1988). A review of the ethical and legal aspects of terminating medical care. *American Journal of Medicine, 84,* 291–301.

Engelhardt, H. T., & Malloy, M. (1982). Suicide and assisting suicide: A critique of legal sanctions. *Southwestern Law Journal, 36,* 1003–1037.

Faden, R. R., Beauchamp, T. L., & King, N. M. P. (1986). *A history and theory of informed consent.* New York: Oxford University Press.

Hilfiker, D. (1983). Allowing the debilitated to die: Facing our ethical choices. *New England Journal of Medicine, 308,* 716–719.

Horan, D. J., & Mall, D. (Eds.) (1980). *Death, dying, and euthanasia.* Frederick, MD: University Publications of America.

Jackson, D. L., & Youngner, S. (1979). Patient autonomy and "death with dignity": Some clinical caveats. *New England Journal of Medicine, 301,* 404–408.

Jecker, N. S. (Ed.) (1991). *Aging and Ethics.* Clifton, NJ: Humana Press.

Jones, W. H. S., trans. (1923). *Hippocrates* (Vol. 1). Cambridge, MA: Loeb Classical Library.

Kamisar, Y. (1958). Some non-religious views against proposed "mercy-killing" legislation. *Minnesota Law Review, 42,* 969–1042.

Kanoti, G. A., & Vinicky, J. K. (1987). The role and structure of hospital ethics committees. In G. R. Anderson & V. A. Glesnes-Anderson (Eds.), *Health care ethics: A guide for decision makers* (pp. 293–307). Rockville, MD: Aspen.

Kant, I. (1949). *Fundamental principles of the metaphysic of morals* (T. K. Abbott, Trans.). New York: Liberal Arts Press. (Original work published 1785)

Kelly, W. D., & Friesen, S. R. (1950). Do cancer patients want to be told? *Surgery, 27,* 822–826.

Kohl, M. (Ed.) (1975). *Beneficent euthanasia.* Buffalo, NY: Prometheus Books.

Ladd, J. (Ed.) (1979). *Ethical issues relating to life and death.* New York: Oxford University Press.

LaPuma, J., Orentlicher, D., & Moss, R. J. (1991). Advance directives on admission: Clinical implications and analysis of the patient self-determination act of 1990. *Journal of the American Medical Association, 266,* 402–405.

Lo, B., & Jonsen, A. R. (1980a). Clinical decisions to limit treatment. *Annals of Internal Medicine, 93,* 764–768.

Lo, B., & Jonsen, A. R. (1980b). Ethical decisions in the care of a patient terminally ill with metastatic cancer. *Annals of Internal Medicine, 92,* 107–111.

Lynn, J. (Ed.) (1986). *By no extraordinary means: The choice to forgo life-sustaining food and water.* Bloomington: Indiana University Press.

McCullough, L. B. (1984). Medical care for elderly patients with diminished competence: An ethical analysis. *Journal of the American Geriatrics Society, 32,* 150–153.

Miles, S., Cranford, R., & Schultz, A. (1982). The do-not-resuscitate order in a teaching hospital. *Annals of Internal Medicine, 96,* 660–664.

Mill, J. S. (1977). *On liberty.* In S. J. Reiser, A. J. Dyck, & W. J. Curran (Eds.), *Ethics in medicine: Historical perspectives and contemporary concerns* (pp. 186–190). Cambridge, MA: MIT Press. (Original work published 1859)

Novack, D., Plumer, R., Smith, R., Ochitill, H., Morrow, G., & Bennett, J. (1979). Changes in physicians' attitudes toward telling the cancer patient. *Journal of the American Medical Association, 241,* 897–900.

Office of Technology Assessment, United States Congress. (1987). *Life-sustaining technologies and the elderly.* Washington, DC: United States Government Printing Office.

Oken, D. (1961). What to tell cancer patients: A study of medical attitudes. *Journal of the American Medical Association, 175,* 1120–1128.

Percival, T. (1977). *Medical ethics.* In S. J. Reiser, A. J. Dyck, & W. J. Curran (Eds.), *Ethics in medicine: Historical perspectives and contemporary concerns* (pp. 18–25). Cambridge, MA: MIT Press. (Original work published 1803)

Perl, M., & Shelp, E. (1982). Psychiatric consultations masking moral dilemmas in medicine. *New England Journal of Medicine, 307,* 618–621.

President's Commission for the Study of Ethical Problems in Medicine. (1983a). *Deciding to forego life-sustaining treatment.* Washington, DC: United States Government Printing Office.

President's Commission for the Study of Ethical Problems in Medicine. (1983b). *Securing access to health care.* Washington, DC: United States Government Printing Office.

Quill, T. (1991). Death and dignity: A case of individualized decision making. *New England Journal of Medicine, 324,* 691–694.

Rachels, J. (1986). *The end of life: Euthanasia and morality.* New York: Oxford University Press.

Samp, R. J., & Curreri, A. R. (1957). A questionnaire survey on public cancer education obtained from cancer patients and their families. *Cancer, 10,* 382–384.

Scitovsky, A., & Capron, A. M. (1986). Medical care at the end of life: The interaction of economics and ethics. *Annual Review of Public Health, 7,* 59–75.

Thornton, J. E., & Winkler, E. R. (Eds.) (1988). *Ethics and Aging.* Vancouver: University of British Columbia Press.

Veatch, R. M. (1976). *Death, dying, and the biological revolution.* New Haven: Yale University Press.

Weir, R. F. (1989). *Abating treatment with critically ill patients: Ethical and legal limits to the medical prolongation of life.* New York: Oxford University Press.

Weisman, A. (1967). The patient with a fatal illness: To tell or not to tell. *Journal of the American Medical Association, 201,* 646–648.

Wolf, S., Boyle, P., Callahan, D., Fins, J., Jennings, B., Nelson, J., Barondess, J., Brock, D., Dresser, R., Emanuel, L., Johnson, S., Lantos, J., Mason, D., Mezey, M., Orentlicher, D., & Rouse, F. (1991). Sources of concern about the patient self-determination act. *New England Journal of Medicine, 325,* 1666–1671.

# 11

# Legal Issues in the Care of the Aged

Thomas F. O'Hare

Lawyers have traditionally dealt with the aged for the purposes of estate planning and administration. In recent years there has been an observable change in the attention given this "minority" by the legal profession. More and more, special-interest legal groups are springing up to represent the interests of the aged, and articles in legal journals and law reviews are addressing the problems of income maintenance, civil rights, political participation, and health care.

Just as lawyers and judges should refrain from attempting to practice medicine, so physicians and other clinical personnel should not make legal interpretations without the benefit of counsel. In recent years, health care providers have begun to seek input from legal consultants or risk management programs, as a means of better understanding the constraints and responsibilities of their profession. Society's interest in the provision of care for the aged is, in part, represented by legislative, regulatory, and judicial constructions, which health care providers cannot ignore, or simply acknowledge as a matter of "defensive" clinical practice. This chapter, while replete with admonitions, proposes that skilled legal consultation be viewed as an integral part of an interdisciplinary approach to the provision of care and treatment for the aged.

## COMPETENCE

Under the principles of ancient English common law, women, children, and idiots were conclusively presumed to be incompetent to manage their own affairs or make decisions for themselves. The modern trend is quite different. It is now an axiom of American jurisprudence that all persons of adult years are presumed to be competent to manage their own affairs. This legal presumption applies even to the infirm, the psychotic, the retarded, and others.

Though competence is a purely legal concept with no independent clinical significance, it has enormous implications for the medical treatment of those persons who reasonably might be presumed incapable of making informed decisions on their own behalf. For example, consider the issue of providing medical treatment of any kind. Legally, the relationship between physicians and patients is one of contract. Physicians offer diagnosis, care, and treatment; patients, if they accept the offer, promise to pay for, or to see to the payment for, the physicians' services.

Without the patients' knowing acceptance of the offer of treatment — that is, without "informed consent" — physicians have no authority to provide the treatment. To do so might amount to a technical battery, or an unconsented touching of another, though in certain, specific circumstances, most jurisdictions permit medical services to be provided in emergencies without fear of liability on the part of providers. (This is usually referred to as a "Good Samaritan" law.) An indispensable part of patients' capacity to accept or consent to treatment is their capacity to weigh the risks and benefits of the proposed treatments and to come to decisions based rationally on the available information. If patients cannot do this, they may be *de facto* incompetent.

Even though individuals may be incapable of offering informed consent to a proposed treatment, the legal presumption of competence continues to operate, and only a judicial determination may overcome the seeming stalemate. In most jurisdictions this is accomplished through guardianship or committee proceedings. Without such determination, even the most well-designed, benign treatment is commenced at the peril of the providers. Neither family members nor hospital administrators are legally empowered to substitute their consent for that of the patient.

At the heart of this concept of competence is an affirmation of the integrity of the individual. Competency, however, is not a term that can be subjected to precise legal definition. The courts examine it on a case-by-case basis. Gutheil and Applebaum (1982) have suggested that competence has to do with people's ability to manipulate available data in a manner that supports their decision-making process, as well as with their awareness and understanding of the nature of their situations and the issues confronting them. Judicial decisions are generally concerned with people's ability simply to manage their affairs. It might be more useful to consider whether individuals understand the probable outcome of their decisions or actions. If they do, then they are probably competent.

Competent decisions are not necessarily correct ones, or even, as one court put it, "medically rational." Many (if not most) individuals make decisions that are not in their own best interest from time to time. Such decisions do not make an individual incompetent, but merely unwise. Therefore, it should be clear that the test of competency is not whether patients or clients agree with a proposed course of treatment or plan for living. As long as they have an understanding of the potential risks and benefits of the various courses of action available to them, they are free to reject reasonable and appropriate proposals.

Another trend of modern guardianship law is to limit the findings of incompetency as much as possible, given the evidence. That is, individuals may be found competent to manage certain areas of their lives, and incompetent for other purposes. This requires that evaluations of competency be specific and that any conclusions be tailored to the needs and capacities of the people involved.

A major problem for all participants in competency proceedings is the reality of what may be termed fluctuating competency. The capacity to understand and retain information and to make reasoned personal decisions based on such information may ebb and flow, varying from day to day or sometimes from hour to hour. Courts and judges must be encouraged to assess a pattern of behavior over a period of time, and not allowed simply to take a "snapshot" of competency, based on a brief appearance before the court. Clinical personnel preparing testimony for competency proceedings should also take a "longitudinal" view of the individual's capabilities, forming their conclusions during any evaluation on the basis of available history as well as on their immediate impressions. This will usually permit the clinician more latitude in making "predictions" regarding future capacities.

### Testamentary Capacity

Thus far, we have considered only general issues of competency. Most jurisdictions make certain distinctions, differentiating competency to stand trial, for instance, from competency to make a will. Criminal-law issues such as criminal responsibility or competency to stand trial are beyond the scope of this chapter. Testamentary capacity is a major consideration for many elderly persons, however.

People are considered competent to execute their wills if they generally understand the nature and scope of their estates. If they are aware of their familial relationships, and if they understand that their legatees or devisees (recipients under their estate plans) need not share their estates in direct proportion to the closeness of their blood relationship, this probably meets the standards of that charming English phrase regarding recognition of the "objects of their bounty." Individuals are not required to leave their estate to their relatives, although most states provide that a surviving spouse is entitled to a statutory share, regardless of the wording of the testamentary instrument.

Testators must also be able to understand the substance of their estate. It is not necessary that they have detailed knowledge of accounts, investments, realty, or other assets, but rather that they generally understand the nature and description of such assets and the amount of money represented thereby.

If challenges are mounted to the allowance of wills, they may very well focus on the competency of the testator at the time of execution of the instruments. Since many families perceive inheritance to be a "right" and therefore object to a testamentary plan that slights or neglects their perception, such challenges are not uncommon. As a result, clinical personnel who have attended the testator may be asked to testify about the individual's competency. It is also the practice of many attorneys drawing up estate plans for aged persons to ask a clinical expert to conduct an evaluation and execute a contemporaneous affidavit regarding the testator's competency. In this context, competence is a much more narrowly defined concept than that involved in guardianship proceedings: Individuals may not be capable of managing their affairs but may be perfectly competent to approve a plan of distribution of their estates.

### INFORMED CONSENT

To understand the doctrine of informed consent, one must first understand its role in the developing law of health care. Given the difficulties the issue raises for many clinicians, it is ironic that the term first appeared in a brief submitted on behalf of the American College of Surgeons (Katz, 1981). Most clinical commentators have suggested that the doctrine of informed consent developed in an attempt to enhance patient autonomy, insight, and cooperation. They suggest that it has failed to achieve these goals and point to studies indicating that retention of information by the patient is very poor (Gutheil & Applebaum, 1982; Lidz et al., 1984; Rosoff, 1981). Thus the process of obtaining a satisfactory consent to treatment is often seen as a legal formality that has little or nothing to do with the success or failure of the treatment itself.

There is, perhaps, a more basic reason for the development of this concept. The modern contractual relationship between physicians and patients should be characterized by mutual understanding and agreement. Without such mutuality no valid contract exists, and without some other justification, such as public safety, imposition of treatment may expose clinicians to liability. Such liability may be predicated on breach of contract, tort (assault and battery), or professional misconduct.

Although the judicial history of informed consent is quite brief, there seems to be general agreement that valid consent must be (1) voluntary, (2) knowledgeable, and (3) competent. Each of these factors presents its own difficulties for clinicians.

1. Institutional settings, whether college dormitories or psychiatric wards, are inherently coercive, in that the individual is always expected to forfeit some degree of autonomy so that the institution may offer some directions common to the entire population. Without more, such coercion present in a clinical setting is not sufficient to vitiate an otherwise valid consent. On the other hand, if reprisals or restrictions are suggested as alternatives to compliance, the individual's consent may be invalid by reason of coercion.

2. It is always difficult for clinicians to know how much information should be shared with patients. The case law recognizes this difficulty but offers only general guidance. For example, in Massachusetts "a physician owes to his patient the duty to disclose in a reasonable manner all significant medical information that the physician possesses or reasonably should possess that is material to an intelligent decision by the patient whether to undergo a proposed procedure" (*Harnish v. Children's Hospital*, 1982, p. 243). In Rhode Island, "Materiality may be said to be the significance a reasonable person, in what the physician knows or should know is his patient's position, would attach to the disclosed risk or risks in deciding whether to submit or not to surgery or treatment" (*Wilkinson v. Vesey*, 1972, p. 627).

It is clear that disclosure should ordinarily include the nature of the patient's condition, the probability of both benefits and risks of the proposed treatment, and alternative courses of treatment (including no treatment) and their relative risks and benefits. In certain situations, a physician may have the privilege of nondisclosure, based on clinical determinations that disclosure would complicate the patient's condition or render the individual unfit for treatment. Such privilege "does not accept the paternalistic notion that the physician may remain silent simply because divulgence might prompt the patient to forgo therapy the physician feels the patient really needs" (*Canterbury v. Spence*, 1972, p. 789).

3. As already discussed, patients must be able to understand the available information and use it in ways that support their decisions. But even more, they must understand the probable consequences of their decisions and actions. Patients' decisions need not be "correct," and the test of their competency is not whether they agree with their attending clinicians.

If a patient has been adjudicated incompetent, then substituted consent to treatment must be obtained. In some cases this will mean that duly authorized surrogates (guardians, parent[s] of a minor) may offer consent. Here, the surrogates' consent must also be "informed." In other situations a court may approve a proposed plan of treatment and directly authorize the clinicians to proceed. Such authorizations may be based on an appraisal of the "best interests" of the patient, or on a conclusion regarding the "substituted judgment" of the patient (what the patient would choose, if competent to do so).

In any event, documentation of the consent of the patient or surrogates is legally advisable. At the same time, a reliance on the "magic" of a preprinted form developed by hospital counsel may be misplaced. Such a form or note in the patient's record is only an acknowledgment of a full and open discussion between clinicians and patients. It is not a substitute for such discussion and does not shift the burden of initiating the process from the physicians. It should also be pointed out that consent is freely revocable, and a patient's changes of mind must be respected, even if consent forms have been signed.

As a general rule, treatment that has a higher risk factor or is more intrusive requires a more detailed process of consent. The practical reason for this is that the liability exposure of the provider is in direct proportion to the potential for damage to the patient. This is also consistent with the entire doctrine of informed consent. The courts have been unwavering in pointing out that the decision to accept or decline medical treatment is essentially nonmedical. Thus, the process of seeking the patient's consent to treatment must address the needs of the patient but not necessarily those of the clinician.

The doctrine of informed consent is more than just a trap for unwary clinicians. It is a recognition that one of the most basic human rights is the right to control what happens to one's body. The practice of obtaining such consent from patients may be viewed as an interactive process rather than an isolated event. This maximizes the individuals' integrity and dignity and enhances their role and responsibility within the treatment relationship.

### Right to Refuse Treatment

The right to refuse medical treatment is a relatively recent legal phenomenon that has generated much controversy and confusion in the clinical professions. It appears, however, to be a natural outgrowth of the doctrines of competency and informed consent, as discussed above. It also has significant historical roots (Reiser, 1980).

The right to refuse treatment simply affirms the fact that treatment may not be imposed on people over their objections, or without their consent, except in certain circumstances. The issue commonly arises in the practice of psychiatry and in treatment of the aged, in which a patient's capacity to actively participate in treatment planning may be questioned. Nevertheless, the presumption of competency (discussed above) remains in effect even for persons who may be institutionalized. In most jurisdictions even involuntary commitment to a psychiatric facility does not, by itself, defeat the presumption that the individual is entitled to accept or decline proffered medical treatment (*Rogers v. Okin,* 1979; *Rennie v. Klein,* 1978).

There are two circumstances in which the patient's right to decline treatment may be overcome. First, if an individual has been adjudicated incompetent, the court may either authorize the guardians to consent to treatment, or it may directly authorize implementation of specific treatment plans. (The distinction between these two authorizations is discussed below in the section on guardianship.) In such cases, the finding of incompetency makes both consent to or refusal of treatment legally immaterial.

It should also be noted that certain state interests have been identified as "compelling" and may supersede the treatment (or nontreatment) preferences of the patients. Such interests include but are not limited to the preservation of life, prevention of suicide, maintenance of the ethical integrity of the medical profession, protection of innocent third parties, and orderly administration of the corrections system.

The second situation is more complex, involving a specific course of treatment and the presence of an emergency. Antipsychotic medications are often prescribed for their tranquilizing or sedating effects. Since the goal of such medications is to affect the mental processes of the patient, the courts have consistently held that their administration is a serious threat to the individual's right to privacy of thought and expression. Given the serious side effects that may occur with these drugs, many jurisdictions have declared their use to be "extraordinary," allowing involuntary administration only with court approval or for the purpose of ameliorating an emergency. *Emergency* has been defined by one court as "the occurrence or serious threat of extreme violence, personal injury, or attempted suicide" (*Rogers v. Okin,* 1979). If antipsychotics are to be administered in response to an emergency, they are to be considered a "chemical restraint" and their use limited to the present emergency.

It is quite common for low dosages of antipsychotics to be prescribed for their sedating effects on aged patients, particularly in nursing homes and other extended-care facilities. Too often, when confronted with the requirements of the law, attending clinicians in such facilities refuse to believe that the law applies to their efforts. They point out the staffing shortages and the disturbance to other patients when one or more of them is out of control. Unfortunately, these are the same justifications that have been heard and rejected by many courts that have decided cases arising out of both chronic and acute psychiatric facilities. Staff convenience is no excuse for involuntarily administering antipsychotic medications.

With the rapid growth of the public-interest bar and its increased attention to health care issues, it is not surprising to see its skilled attorneys turning their attention to the care of the aged. Obviously, clinicians treating the aged, particularly in institutional settings, must pay close attention to the issues of informed consent to treatment. Neither spouses, relatives, nor close friends have legal authority to substitute their consent for that of the patient, in most circumstances. If patients refuse treatment, particularly intrusive treatment such as antipsychotic medications, that refusal should be honored except in an emergency. The law provides alternative means of providing consent, either by direct authorization or by substituting the judgment of a guardian. Risk management programs and other continuing education for staffs of institutions that treat the aged should address these issues and provide appropriate means for resolution, while taking into account local laws, regulations, and procedures.

### Right to Treatment

An embryonic legal issue that should receive increasing attention is the purported "right to treatment." Essentially, this doctrine holds that those who have been committed (legally, or practically) to the care of the state are entitled to receive certain minimal services and treatments. The issue was first raised by Dr. Morton Birnbaum in an article in the *Journal of the American Bar Association* (Birnbaum, 1960). There are only a few reported cases that have examined this issue, but they may represent the tip of an immense submerged problem for health care providers.

One federal court has held that persons in state-run institutions for the retarded have the right to habilitation services and treatment designed to reduce the amount of restraint or seclusion necessary to care safely for them (*Youngberg v. Romeo,* 1982). In this case it was decided that the named plaintiff was not receiving services and treatment that might enhance his socialization skills and make it possible for him to learn to interact with others in a more appropriate fashion, thereby reducing the amount of restraints (chemical and physical) that were presently employed. Recognizing this "*Youngberg* principle," another federal case indicated that once a state "chose to house those voluntary residents, thus making them dependant on the state, it was required to do so in a manner that would not deprive them of Constitutional rights" (*Society for Good Will v. Cuomo,* 1984, p. 1246).

Limited to public institutions, such decisions are based on the government's obligations to those who are compelled by law or circumstance to depend on public services. The definition of "adequate" medical care has not yet been decided. Since the U.S. Supreme Court has not identified a *per se* "right to treatment," the courts have applied the analogous "conditions of confinement" doctrine. This states that the courts can intervene only when the conditions at an institution represent "a substantial departure from accepted professional judgment, practice, or standards" (*Youngberg v. Romeo,* 1982, p. 323).

Should it become fully operative, the doctrine of the right to treatment may cause great difficulty for those treating aged persons in any kind of institutional setting. In such settings it is not uncommon for the staff, and subsequently the patients, to accept as immutable the conditions and limitations of the patients. Innovative or aggressive programing and treatment may be forgone, and "management" may become the goal. In such situations, a strong case could be made that patients were *not* being accorded their constitutional right to treatment, compatible with "accepted professional judgment, practice, or standards."

The doctrine of the right to treatment is really an effort to establish minimal norms of care and treatment that may be expected by patients and their families. It may affect acute medical care, habilitation services, physical therapy, recreation opportunities, and social-service planning. Recognizing that common aspirations are often lost in a sea of bureaucratic and budgetary limitations, the doctrine affirms that the aged and the infirm are entitled to certain minimum levels of services as a result of both their reliance on the health care delivery system and the availability of those services in the health care community.

A word of caution may be appropriate at this point. Many clinicians and administrators, frustrated in their attempts to secure adequate funding for institutions or treatment programs, see the possibility of court-ordered funding increases as the answer to bureaucratic fiscal intransigence. They may consider the possibility of a "sweetheart" suit by patients or their advocates against them and their institutions for failure to provide constitutionally minimal levels of care and treatment. Such litigation is often termed friendly, because the goals of the litigants, in this case increased public funding, are mutually held by both plaintiffs and defendants, and the actual lawsuit may have been encouraged by the named defendants, who have been otherwise unsuccessful in obtaining such funding through the usual budgetary process. Although the desired outcome of increased funding and support may appear attractive, the reality is that such an outcome, as well as the process that precedes it, is not subject to precise control. Such litigation may result in the court involving itself in all aspects of institutional management, including treatment planning or admission/discharge policies. The potential loss of control over the administration of care and treatment should restrain enthusiastic participation in such litigation. Dr. Stonewall Stickney eloquently described his naiveté (and its subsequent loss) with regard to the administration of the public mental health system in Alabama. His experience argues strongly for caution in this area (Stickney, 1974).

## GUARDIANSHIP

In most jurisdictions the appropriate means for testing the legal competence of individuals and for providing surrogate decision makers (if patients are found to be incompetent) are guardianship proceedings. In the past 15 years this area of law has changed rapidly and dramatically. While guardianships were initially heard in the Courts of Chancery in 16th-century England, in a congenial, family atmosphere, such proceedings are now required to proceed in an adversarial fashion and constitute a significant threat to the autonomy of the individual, since persons under guardianship no longer have the right to vote, to marry, or to enter into contracts in their own names. Guardianship requires the serious attention of legislators and judicial officers and should not be taken lightly by family members or clinical caregivers.

As a result of the intervention of legal advocates for the disabled, new procedural and substantive safeguards are now in place in most jurisdictions. These include higher standards of proof of incompetence, provision of counsel for the alleged incompetent, and requirements for detailed findings of fact and conclusions of law on the part of the judge. Also, the trend toward tailoring the guardianship to fit the needs and capacities of individuals tends to avoid general decrees that rob wards of whatever potential they may retain.

### Considerations before Filing

Before initiating incompetency proceedings, family members (or clinical administrators) should consider several different issues. First, an evaluation of alternatives should be made. For instance, if management of the individual's property or assets is the primary question, is it possible to utilize a power of attorney, *inter vivos* (living) trust or conservatorship? (See later section on estate management.) Typically, a conservatorship deals only with management of the individual's property, whereas guardianship may involve management of the property, the person, or both. Obviously the latter is a more serious intrusion into an individual's sovereignty.

Family dynamics are further complicated when children of aging parents seek to become legally responsible for the management of their parents' lives. This may infantilize the parent, turning a lifetime of experiences and relationships upside down. Clinical professionals and attorneys should keep this in mind, exploring with the families alternatives that might meet everyone's needs. Failing that, families will need support as they redefine their relationships with each other.

Many times simple negotiations may go a long way toward problem resolution. Issues of property management or health care may be clarified by discussion and exploration, with the assistance and support of clinical and legal experts. In some cases it may be easier to persuade the aged individual that a third party should manage their property, someone who is not a relation and who is a professional, such as a bank trust officer, accountant, or attorney. Of course, such services would have to be compensated, which raises other issues.

Other considerations to be made prior to instituting proceedings include cost and timing. The primary cost in most proceedings will be the legal fees of counsel for the petitioners (family) and the respondent (patient). These fees may vary greatly, but most attorneys will likely bill at an hourly rate. Rates depend on the experience and expertise of the attorney, the location of his office, overhead, and the complexity of the litigation. In dealings with any professional, it is appropriate to gain a full understanding of what costs or fees will be charged and to seek comparative information from others. Total costs for prosecuting (or defending) a guardianship may run from several hundred to several thousand dollars, largely depending on the complexity of the issues and duration of the litigation.

It will often be important to move quickly for a determination of the respondent's competence because of medical or social conditions that will rapidly deteriorate to emergency status. Counsel must be apprised of this, and all parties must be prepared to move quickly. Ordinarily, an initial hearing may be held within a week to 10 days. In a true medical emergency hearings may be convened in a matter of hours, often right at the bedside of the patient. Full trials of permanent guardianships may not be heard for weeks or months, both because of crowded court dockets and because of notice and procedural requirements.

### Procedure

Judicial procedures vary from state to state and sometimes from court to court, though a number of actions are necessary or helpful in any jurisdiction. First, a petition must be presented indicating the nature of and reason for the proceeding. Names and addresses of all interested parties (which include the next of kin and heirs at law of the alleged incompetent) must be provided. All such persons must, at some point, receive notification of the proceedings and be given the opportunity to appear and be heard.

At least one physician will have to provide a certificate of opinion that the respondent is incapable of managing personal and/or financial affairs because of a specific disability or condition. It is often useful to supplement this certificate with an affidavit from the clinician, detailing the patient's history, condition, limitations, and proposed plan of care and treatment. This affidavit should be drawn with the assistance of the attorney representing the petitioners. If there is no opposition to the petition, the physician may not have to appear at the hearing. If, however, local procedures require it or if the attorney for the ward opposes the petition, the physician must be prepared to attend the hearing and give testimony. Again, this should be done in cooperation with the petitioners' counsel.

Many jurisdictions utilize the services of a *guardian ad litem*. This is usually an attorney who is appointed to act either as an advocate for the alleged incompetent or as an independent investigator for the court. Such individuals are not ordinarily empowered to substitute their judgment for that of the respondent but rather to gather and evaluate evidence and to provide recommendations for the court. It is important for everyone to understand fully the role and responsibilities of the various participants in such proceedings.

In most jurisdictions guardianship proceedings are not held before a jury. Since the roots of such proceedings are found in the Courts of Equity, the right to trial by jury does not apply. There is a trend, however, toward trying to amend this through legislation entitling guardianship respondents to jury proceedings, in which local procedures will govern.

The issues that must be decided in such proceedings are quite limited. First, a determination of the individual's legal competence must be reached. This will require not only expert opinion but direct testimony citing examples of behavior which support that opinion. In many situations, such testimony may only come from friends or relatives of the respondent, because they have had the best opportunities for observation. It should be noted that the modern impulse in guardianship proceedings is to permit findings that the individual may be competent for certain purposes and incompetent for others, thus preserving as much independence as possible. Such findings rest on the evidence submitted regarding the behavior of the respondent.

If the court finds that the respondent is incompetent, it will then examine specific issues, if necessary. Treatment issues will require relevant testimony and findings. Some courts distinguish "intrusive" treatments and require higher standards of proof. For example, one court has said that antipsychotic medications are as intrusive as electroconvulsive treatment or psychosurgery (*Rogers v. Commissioner,* 1983). As a rule of thumb, any medical treatment that is not routine should probably be described in detail, and specific authority should be sought prior to instituting the procedure.

When deciding such issues, the courts must know the risk–benefit ratio of the procedure or treatment and must reach a conclusion either about what the patients would choose if competent to do so ("substituted judgment") or about what is in the patients' best interest. The philosophical and procedural bases of either course of action are subtly different and should be understood by all participants. The principle of "best interest" seeks to determine what would best serve the needs of the incompetent, assuming that the individual would choose the course of treatment offering the best chance of recovery, comfort, or stabilization. According to the doctrine of substituted judgment, the courts must determine (as best they can) what the choices of the particular individual would be, based on life experiences, religious beliefs, and familial relationships. In the jurisdictions mandating substituted judgment, evidence must be submitted regarding all of these factors.

Finally, the court must decide who should be appointed to serve in this "fiduciary" capacity. Most commonly, petitioners and nominees will be friends or relatives of the incompetents. It is not uncommon, however, for family members to contest the appointment of a certain individual or for the court to find that the nominees would not be capable of appropriately discharging their duties. In guardianship proceedings, evidence regarding the fitness of the nominees must also be considered.

It should be remembered that guardianship proceedings are judicial in nature and thus, in the American tradition, adversarial. The attorneys representing the proposed wards are obligated to oppose the petitions for guardianship and to represent the wishes of their clients, if they can be ascertained. It would be unethical for such attorneys to reach conclusions regarding their clients' best interests and to represent that view, regardless of the clients' wishes. In many cases, counsel may be unable to ascertain the wishes of their clients, and this may be reported to the court. Still, the petitioners' cases must be proved, since alleged incompetents may not consent to the appointment of guardians.

After hearing the evidence, the court will make its findings and enter a decree. If there are limitations on the authority of the guardian, they should be noted on the decree, as should any special authorities. In some jurisdictions, the guardian will be authorized to consent to specific forms of treatment, whereas in others the court will authorize the implementation of a proposed treatment plan directly and will order the guardian to "monitor" such implementation. Often, the authority of the guardian will be limited in duration (temporary guardianship), or a date will be established, at which time the entire matter will be reviewed to determine whether guardianship is still necessary. Counsel should clearly advise all parties of their precise rights and obligations under the court's decree.

It should be noted that a guardianship is an "ambulatory" type of proceeding; that is, it is always subject to amendment or termination. If the ward's condition improves to the extent that competency is restored, in whole or in part, the conditions of the guardianship decree should be modified. A periodic review of the situation is often beneficial, and changed circumstances are easily drawn to the attention of the court.

### General Concerns

In many situations, the aged individual has outlived friends and family or may be estranged from them. This makes it difficult to identify someone to serve as guardian or conservator. Though the judicial model prefers a familial relationship between ward and guardian, that is often not possible.

Responses to this problem have included recourse to volunteer organizations, charitable corporations, public agencies, and "conscription" of the bar (whereby the judge "suggests" that an attorney appearing regularly in that court should volunteer to serve as guardian of the incompetent). Advocates for and caregivers of the aged should be aware of what resources are available in the community for provision of guardianship services for persons who have no family or friends willing or appropriate to serve.

Another widespread concern is the inordinate amount of time and public and private resources consumed by guardianship proceedings. This seems a particularly egregious state of affairs when the resolution of a particular treatment issue is unopposed and meets everyone's common understanding of what should occur. The judicial *imprimatur* is then little more than a rubber stamp. It is hoped that states will investigate alternative means to achieving this end, preserving all of the rights of the individuals involved while reserving utilization of meager judicial resources for those cases with a truly adversarial posture.

## DISCHARGE FROM CARE AND TREATMENT

One aspect of the relationship between physicians and their patients that is often neglected is the means by which such a relationship is terminated. This is particularly important at the end of a period of hospitalization. Current concerns regarding cost containment create pressures on hospital administrators to require that patients be discharged as soon as possible. Often discharge is perceived as precipitous, particularly with aged patients, who may not easily tolerate abrupt changes in their medical and living environments.

It is important to remember that physicians and treatment facilities may not abandon the care of an individual for whom they have assumed responsibility. Undertaking such responsibility acknowledges a relationship with special obligations to see that a patient's care is continuous, and not interrupted inappropriately. Abandonment of a patient is the refusal to continue providing care and treatment that is clinically indicated, the refusal to plan for continued treatment that meets the patient's needs, or the refusal to implement a referral for such continued treatment as may be clinically appropriate.

If a patient terminates treatment prematurely, it is necessary to document that this was done *against medical advice.* The patient should be asked to endorse a statement to that effect. If the hospital or clinician initiates terminating treatment, procedures should be established whereby the process is consistent and fair.

An essential component in terminating treatment is planning. With a hospitalized patient, the process should commence long before the anticipated discharge date. Planning should include medical, psychological and social-service considerations, and patients themselves should participate. In addition, the patient's family should be advised of the plan for discharge (with the patient's consent), and adequate notice of the discharge should be given to all interested parties. Objections to the discharge plan should be carefully considered and, if they cannot be resolved, should be referred to an officer of the hospital for review.

The increased pressures to terminate nonessential hospitalizations have caused several regulatory agencies, both state and federal, to specify safeguards for patient rights within the discharge planning process. These regulations may specify periods of required notice to patients or their families or require creation of discharge planning offices within a hospital. Clinicians and administrators are strongly advised to familiarize themselves and their staffs with any relevant regulations governing their practice. Failure to comply with such regulations may expose the hospital and the individual clinician to liability or sanctions.

## DEATH AND DYING

There is no more difficult issue with which the law and society wrestle than that of a death that might somehow be postponed. The law is a human process and an amalgam of societal experience and expectation. As such, it will always lag behind technological development. Nowhere is this clearer than when the law is confronted with the "penumbra where death begins, but life, in some form, continues" (*Barber v. Superior Court,* 1983, p. 1014).

The "right to die" is really a matter of the right to exercise some control over the manner of one's death. The philosophical and religious arguments surrounding this issue are beyond the scope of this chapter. It is enough to note that such arguments will continue for many years, as the courts are called upon to decide issues of brain death, "do not resuscitate" or "no extraordinary treatment" orders, living wills, or health care proxies.

The state — and therefore the law — has a strong interest in preventing suicide and preserving life (*Superintendant v. Saikewicz,* 1977) and thus an interest in establishing procedural guidelines for individuals, families, and clinicians who are facing the possibility of ending or limiting medical treatment that otherwise might prolong life in some form. One court reached the following conclusion:

> In certain, thankfully rare, circumstances the burden of maintaining the corporeal existence degrades the very humanity it was meant to serve. The law recognizes the individual's right to preserve his humanity, even if to preserve his humanity means to allow the natural processes of a disease or affliction to bring about a death with dignity. (*Brophy v. New England Sinai,* 1986, p. 635)

At the same time, the courts have avoided making assessments of the quality of the individual's life, realizing that such assessments might endanger the disabled, the retarded, or others who might not be able to articulate their own views regarding quality of life. There is obviously a delicate balance to maintain, and one whose boundaries are not rigidly defined. The state's reluctance mirrors society's uncertainty and demonstrates that the issue is not medical in nature, but moral and ethical.

The state's interest in preserving life wanes when the proposed treatment will not cure the affliction. The attention then turns to the cost to the individual of prolonging life. Courts have upheld "do not resuscitate" orders for terminally ill patients in many different circumstances (*Matter of Dinnerstein,* 1978). The removal of a respirator from a patient with amyotrophic lateral sclerosis (*Satz v. Perlmutter,* 1979), discontinuance of feeding by means of a gastrostomy tube in a patient with irreversible brain damage (*Brophy v. New England Sinai,* 1986), and removal of a nasogastric feeding tube in a quadriplegic who suffered continual pain (*Bouvia v. Superior Court,* 1986) have also been approved. It should be noted, however, that the courts will not order physicians or hospitals to undertake procedures that are contrary to their ethical beliefs.

Such cases usually involve all of the issues discussed earlier in the section on guardianship, as well as balancing any interests of the state against those of the individual. In making such determinations, one of the most important areas of evidence is that of the individual's wishes concerning the proposed treatment or procedure. If the person is incompetent at the time of trial, a "living will" or other recorded expressions of the individual's wishes regarding life-prolonging treatment or "heroic measures" will be examined as important pieces of evidence, even in states that have not enacted legislation permitting living wills. If no such recorded statements exist, then the manner in which that individual lived and behaved while competent may be examined through the testimony of acquaintances and family.

Recently, some states have enacted statutes allowing the creation of health care proxies. These are means by which individuals may nominate another to make any and all health care decisions for them at any time when they are incapable of articulating a competent decision. The decision of the nominee (proxy, or agent) should be followed by the clinician caring for the patient and will relieve that clinician of liability for failure to obtain the patient's informed consent to any procedure. It is advisable for *all* persons to consult with an attorney regarding the availability of such health care proxies.

## ESTATE PLANNING

Attorneys are generally on more familiar ground when asked to assist individuals in planning for the distribution and management of their estates. Even this nonmedical area, however, has become increasingly complex, given the realistic prospects of costly and extended care of the aged, together with evolving tax and reimbursement or insurance consequences. This is a highly technical area of the law requiring the services of experienced counsel. This chapter will only highlight certain issues strongly impacting the health care of the aged.

### The Living Will

Although legislation specifically authorizing the instrument known as the "living will" has been enacted in only a few jurisdictions, all recognize the validity of the concept. A living will is nothing more than the expression of an individual's wishes for medical treatment or for termination of treatment at a time when the individual may be incapacitated. It offers guidance to both the family and friends of the individual as well as to the clinicians responsible for care and treatment. It can also be influential in any court proceeding where the substituted judgment of the individual is in question.

### Durable Power of Attorney

Another useful device is the durable power of attorney, which allows people to appoint others to act in their behalf for almost any purpose. Drawn correctly, its authority will survive any later disability of its endorser. It may even be drawn so that it only *becomes* effective upon such disability. For example, people in the early stages of Alzheimer's disease may be competent to endorse such a power of attorney, giving their spouses (or anyone) full authority to act on their behalf should the disorder progress to the point where they are incapable of acting for themselves. This may obviate the need for guardianship at a later time, and save money, time, and pain for the families.

The durable power of attorney is primarily utilized for management of the business and personal affairs of the disabled individual. In addition, the durable power of attorney allows people to express their wishes regarding medical treatment or termination of such treatment, although unlike the living will or health care proxy, it is not usually enforceable with regard to health care decisions. While not binding, such expression will be given great weight by physicians and institutions faced with the alternative of termination or limitation of treatment and may offer the best possible evidence of the person's judgment before any court asked to authorize or withhold authorization of specific treatment for an incompetent person. Many attorneys will ask that a physician examine the individual at the time of execution of such durable power of attorney. An affidavit of that physician's opinion regarding the competence of the individual may then be attached to the document, eliminating many later challenges.


## MEDICARE/MEDICAID

Medicaid benefits presently depend on income and asset eligibility, and those persons whose income or assets exceed the minimum established by federal or state regulation will not qualify for coverage. Ironically, many older Americans are required to impoverish themselves to become eligible for the Medicaid program, which presently pays the costs of nearly three-quarters of all patients residing in intermediate or skilled-nursing facilities. For example, the current individual asset limit in Massachusetts is $2,000 (excluding the individual's residential home, automobile, and certain other specific forms of property). The person seeking eligibility for Medicaid benefits must "spend down" to that limit.

It may be useful to inject a brief political and philosophical note here. Some have suggested that financial planning for the purpose of minimizing the impact of this spend-down provision is tantamount to evasion of the law. However, the situation is analogous to consideration of the provisions of the Internal Revenue Code when planning investment strategies or estate administration. As Judge Learned Hand asserted many years ago: "Any one may so arrange his affairs that his taxes shall be as low as possible; he is not bound to choose that pattern which will best pay the Treasury" (*Helvering v. Gregory*, 1934, p. 810). Since estate planning has always been considered a legal sub-specialty of tax planning, there are no apparent ethical or legal inconsistencies in seeking to shelter assets within the appropriate sections of applicable law and regulations.

Further complicating the picture is the provision that transfers of assets to others within 30 months prior to application will continue to be counted as assets of the applicant, unless it is found that the transfers were not made for the purpose of qualifying for Medicaid. Handling assets clearly requires some anticipation and planning and is an area with which skilled legal counsel can help. As people age, they should be advised to carefully consider their financial and health care needs. This is often best accomplished by the joint assistance of an attorney and a social worker or other benefit specialist. Unfortunately, too often people wait until the need for intervention is acute, and little can be done about the 30-month "look-back" rule.

When a family member is diagnosed as suffering from a progressive disorder such as Alzheimer's disease, there is often sufficient time to accomplish sound financial and health care planning. It is important for support groups, clinical caregivers, and social service personnel to keep this in mind when working with the aging individuals or their families. Early referral can enable the planning of gifts, trusts, or other devices that may protect family assets and prevent the impoverishment of surviving family members, while ensuring that individuals will justly qualify for entitlements.

## ALLIED HEALTH PROFESSIONALS

This chapter has focused chiefly on physicians and their obligations and responsibilities rather than on the health care team as a whole. There are two reasons for this. First, historically the "deep pockets" (and professional liability insurance coverage) of physicians have provided attractive targets for plaintiffs' counsel. Second, there is a legal principle entitled "respondeat superieur" which dictates that the physician is at least jointly responsible for the acts or omissions of the members of a treatment team responsible for the care of the patient. One variant of this doctrine is referred to as "captain of the ship," whereby the physician is compared to the command officer who bears ultimate responsibility for the acts of subordinates.

With the increased professional organization of disciplines such as psychology, nursing, social work, and other health professions comes increased responsibility and, therefore, liability exposure. The independent licensing and practice of such professionals has blurred the traditional "command" lines referred to above. Although few cases have interpreted the independent liability of allied health professionals, they are subject to the same legal reasoning employed in the risk analysis of all medical practitioners. Tort liability requires a finding that there was a duty on the part of the professional toward the patient or client, that the duty was breached by action or inaction on the part of the professional, and that the patient was damaged as a proximate result of that breach of duty. The standards of duty are established by examining the standards of practitioners within the same discipline.

The coordinated interdisciplinary approach advocated in this book requires reconsideration of the legal analysis of individual liability. For example, the coordinator of a team treating an aged client may very well not be a physician, depending on the needs of the client. Clearly, such a coordinator does not supervise the team physician's practice of medicine, but may bear responsibility for appropriate referral and overall case management. The more autonomous the practice of the individual professional, the more likely it is that liability for negligent acts may be imposed on that individual (See Annas, Glantz, & Katz, 1981).

## CONCLUSION

This chapter was not designed to make lawyers out of clinicians. Its object was to sensitize persons involved with the direct care and treatment of the aged to some of the legal pitfalls and complexities involved. If it has raised more questions than it has answered, then it may encourage readers to consider consulting counsel or financial planners as part of a truly interdisciplinary approach in caring for their clients, patients, or family members.

The law is really a social process, best serving society when input is received from the broadest possible constituency. If clinical and academic personnel are reluctant to participate in the process of formulating new legal approaches to the problems facing the aged, lawyers, judges, and legislators will be forced to strive toward conclusions that may not appropriately address those problems. Fundamentally, ours is a participatory society, and educated persons should engage in those social processes where their skills and experience will serve themselves and others.

Persons who care for the aged in institutional settings should have the benefit of experienced counsel available for consultation and, if necessary, representation, as issues of informed consent to treatment and the treatment of terminally ill patients grow ever more complex, and the potential liability exposure for professionals and institutions increases. Risk management programs and frequent in-service programs for staff can help to reduce that exposure.

Many of the same issues face clinicians dealing with the aged in a community setting. Additionally, they often have the opportunity to anticipate problems and to help clients plan for their future and that of their families. Although most people don't enjoy considering the consequences of their dying process, it is a reality we all must face. The appropriate involvement of an attorney can assist aged individuals in organizing their affairs, in exercising some control over the manner in which they will be treated, and in managing and distributing their estates.

The clinician and the attorney need each other's expertise, if the aged are to be truly well served by either. If an interdisciplinary approach is to be valid, it must include all the professional disciplines that bear on the life of the subject.

## REFERENCES

Annas, G., Glantz, L., & Katz, B. (1981). *The rights of doctors, nurses and allied health professionals.* New York: Avon Books.

Barber v. Superior Court for Los Angeles County, 147 Cal.App.3d 1006, 195 Cal.Rptr. 484 (1983).

Birnbaum, M. (1960). The right to treatment. *American Bar Association Journal, 46,* 499.

Bouvia v. Superior Court for Los Angeles County, 179 Cal.App.3d 1127, 225 Cal.Rptr. 297 (1986).

Brophy v. New England Sinai Hospital, 398 Mass. 417, 497 N.E.2d 626 (1986).

Canterbury v. Spence, 464 F.2d 772. (D.C.Cir.), cert. denied, 409 U.S. 1064 (1972).

Gutheil, T. G., & Applebaum, P. S. (1982). *Clinical handbook of psychiatry and the law.* New York: McGraw-Hill.

Harnish v. Children's Hospital Medical Center, 387 Mass. 152, 439 N.E.2d 240 (1982).

Helvering v. Gregory, 69 F.2d 809 (1934).

Katz, J. (1981). Disclosure and Consent in Psychiatric Practice: Mission Impossible? In C. K. Hofling (Ed.), *Law and Ethics in the Practice of Psychiatry.* New York: Brunner/Mazel.

Lidz, C. W., Meisel, A., Zerubavel, E., Carter, M., Sestak, R. M., & Roth, L. (1984). *Informed consent.* New York: Guildford Press.

Matter of Conroy, 98 N.J. 321, 486 A.3d 1209 (1985).

Matter of Dinnerstein, 6 Mass.App. 466, 380 N.E.2d 134 (1978).

Regan, J. J. (1985). *Tax, estate and financial planning for the elderly.* New York: Matthew Bender.

Reiser, S. J. (1980). Refusing treatment for mental illness: Historical and ethical dimensions. *American Journal of Psychiatry, 137,* 329.

Rennie v. Klein, 462 F. Supp. 1131 (D.N.J., 1978).

Rogers v. Commissioner of Mental Health, 390 Mass. 489, 458 N.E.2d 308 (1983).

Rogers v. Okin, 478 F. Supp. 1342 (D. Mass., 1979).

Rosoff, A. J. (1981). *Informed consent.* Rockville, MD: Aspen.

Satz v. Perlmutter, 362 So.2d 160 (Fla., 1979).

Society for Good Will to Retarded Children v. Cuomo, 737 F.2d 1239 (2d Cir., 1984).

Stickney, S., (1974). Wyatt vs. Stickney: The Right to Treatment. *Psychiatric Annals, 3,* 11.

Superintendent of Belchertown State School v. Saikewicz, 373 Mass. 728, 370 N.E.2d 417 (1971).

Wilkinson v. Vesey, 110 R.I. 606, 295 A.2d 676 (1972).

Youngberg v. Romeo, 457 U.S. 307 (1982).

# 12

# Disability Trends and Community Long-Term Health Care for the Aged

Alan M. Jette

*The society which fosters research to save human life cannot escape responsibility for the life thus extended. It is for science not only to add years to life, but more important, to add life to years.*

*Annals of Internal Medicine, 1939*

### THE GRAYING OF AMERICA

Society's increasing concern for the long-term care of its aging population is not surprising once one examines the demographic changes that have occurred in the United States during the 20th century (Figure 12.1). At the start of this century, the U.S. population

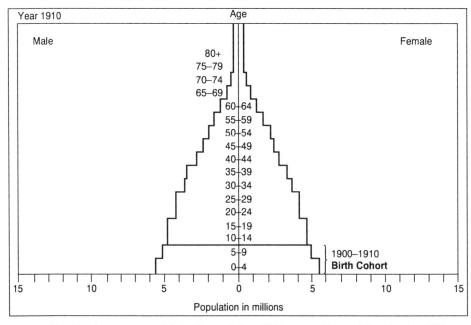

FIGURE 12.1   Age structure of the U.S. population: 1910 census. (Adapted from Soldo, 1980)

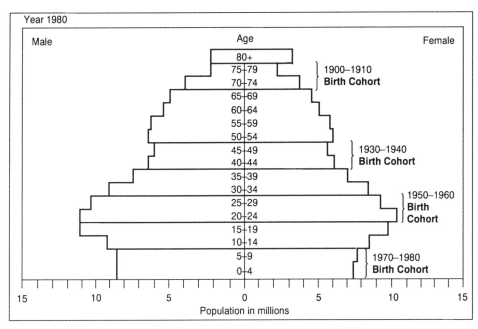

FIGURE 12.2    Age structure of the U.S. population: 1980 census. (Adapted from Soldo, 1980)

experienced very high fertility and immigration rates, along with substantial infant and adult mortality rates. Consequently, the U.S. population pyramid, as Figure 12.1 illustrates, was fairly broad at its base, with a very narrow apex. At the turn of the century, approximately 4% of the U.S. population was 65 years of age or older (Soldo, 1980).

Figure 12.2 illustrates the very dramatic changes that have taken place in the composition of the U.S. population throughout this century. We see the very large baby boom of the post–World War II period represented by the 1950 to 1960 birth cohort followed by smaller birth cohorts over the past 20 years. Changes in fertility rates coupled with the increasing longevity of earlier birth cohorts accounts for the increasing percentage of older adults in U.S. society. By 1980, the estimated 25.5 million older Americans made up just under 11% of our population (Soldo, 1980). By the year 2030, some project that the proportion of the U.S. population age 65 and older will approach the 20% mark (Soldo, 1980).

Table 12.1 illustrates the dramatic improvement in the life expectancy from birth of the U.S. population during the 20th century. If we look at the most favorable case, white females, life expectancy at birth has increased from 49 years at the turn of the century to just under 80 years as of 1978. Similar but smaller increases are seen for nonwhite women and men of both races.

This expanding aged population was a major impetus to the passage of the 1965 amendments to the Social Security Act which introduced Medicare into the U.S. health care system. Some have referred to the 1965 Social Security amendments as "the first revolution in care of the aged" (Brody & Magel, 1984). The environment within which Medicare was

TABLE 12.1    Life Expectancy of U.S. population
at birth, by race and gender: 1900, 1950, 1978

| Race and Gender | Life Expectancy at Birth | | |
|---|---|---|---|
| | 1900 | 1950 | 1978 |
| White | | | |
|   Men | 47 | 67 | 70 |
|   Women | 49 | 72 | 78 |
| Nonwhite | | | |
|   Men | 33 | 59 | 65 |
|   Women | 34 | 63 | 74 |

passed was one in which the number of aged was approaching 20 million, or 10% of the total population. Of those elderly, one of six was hospitalized at least once a year, with lengths of stay twice as long as for people under 65 years of age (Brody, 1987). In the 15 years between 1950 and 1965, the average cost of an inpatient hospital day almost tripled (Health Insurance Association of America, 1985), placing the aged and their families at risk of economic catastrophe. Since the introduction of Medicare aged Americans have enjoyed considerable access to acute-care services and important protection from economic catastrophe from acute illness (Brody, 1987). In 1977 Medicare paid 84% of the acute hospital costs of those 65 years of age and older (Fischer, 1980).

## THE GRAYING OF THE GRAY

Even more important than the continuing increase in the proportion of the population that is aged are the changes in the distribution of those 65 years of age and older. At the midpoint of this century, 68% of our elderly population were 65 to 74 years of age, 27% were aged 75 to 84, while only 5% were 85 years of age or older. By the turn of the century, the portion of the elderly population 65 to 74 years of age will approach 55%, with a corresponding increase in the 75- to 84-year-old cohort, but, and most important, the 85-and-older cohort will approach 12% of the aged population. We are observing an aging of the aged in American society because of a striking increase in the life expectancy of adults who reach age 65 (Soldo, 1980; Rosenwaike, 1985).

In 1935 someone entering the age cohort 65 years of age and older could expect to live an average 12.5 additional years of life. By the year 2000, depending on what happens to current mortality trends, those approaching age 65 can expect (on average) up to 20 additional years of life (Fuchs, 1984).

Between now and the year 2000 the proportion of the U.S. population aged 65 or older will continue to swell, especially the oldest cohort of those 85 years of age or older. Mortality rates of this 85-and-older cohort are decreasing faster than any other aged group. The absolute numbers of this cohort and the percentage of the population it makes up are increasing at an astounding rate. Between 1960 and 1980 the oldest old increased by over 40% among all persons 65 and older. By 2040, 12,834,000 adults in the United States will be 85 and older (Rosenwaike, 1985).

These dramatic improvements in life expectancy after age 65 can be attributed in large part to the reduction in mortality from the major chronic diseases. Age-specific death rates due to heart disease and cerebrovascular accidents, two of the leading causes of death for adults, have shown dramatic changes in the adult U.S. population. From 1965 to 1980 we have experienced a 2% to 2.5% drop per year in these age-specific death rates due to heart and cerebrovascular disease for all the aged subgroups. Why death from these causes has plummeted is not well understood. Many attribute much of the reduction to a combination of better control of hypertension; medical innovations such as open heart surgery; and changes in lifestyle affecting diet, smoking, and exercise (Fuchs, 1984).

## DISABILITY TRENDS IN AN AGING POPULATION

The dramatic demographic changes occurring in U.S. society today have a correspondingly important impact on the prevalence of disability in the aged. In contrast to common belief, to be aged in our society is not necessarily to be beset with numerous and complex disabilities. Life after age 65 is not a period inexorably marked with massive physical deterioration (Jette & Branch, 1981). Nevertheless, the increasing life expectancy of those reaching age 65 has affected the prevalence of functional disability in this population. The National Health Interview Survey provides national estimates of the level of functioning of the noninstitutionalized aged in the United States. In 1981 approximately 20% of those 65 years of age and older living in the community reported some restrictions in their mobility. There are similar findings with respect to restrictions in the major daily activities such as performing one's job, doing household chores, or carrying out other major life activities. Forty-three percent of those 65 and older report some limitation in amount or kind of major functional activity (Figure 12.3) (National Center for Health Statistics, 1982). When disability figures such as these are viewed for all elders 65 years and older, the majority of elders appear to be functionally well. For most, the

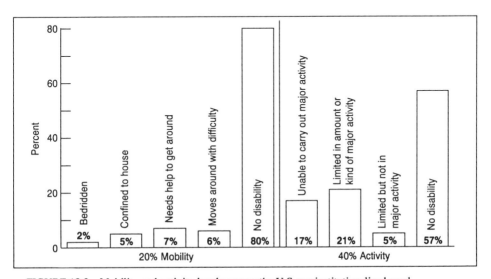

FIGURE 12.3   Mobility and activity levels among the U.S. noninstitutionalized aged.

TABLE 12.2   Prevalence of Disability in Basic ADL[a] and Instrumental ADL[b] in Adults 65 and Over, United States

| Disability | Ages | | |
|---|---|---|---|
| | 65–74 | 75–84 | 85+ |
| Needs help in one or more Basic ADL | 5.3% | 11.4% | 34.8% |
| Needs help in one or more Instrumental ADL | 5.7 | 14.2 | 40.0 |

[a]Basic ADL include walking, going outside, bathing, dressing, using toilet, getting in and out of a bed, or eating.
[b]Instrumental ADL include shopping, doing routine household chores, preparing meals, or handling money.

later years of life are characterized by substantial physical ability and functional independence. Is the prevalence of physical disability not increasing as our population ages, or are these disability data inaccurate? The problem lies in viewing the elderly as a homogeneous group of individuals above the age of 65.

A different picture emerges when we examine disability estimates within subgroups of the aged. The data in Table 12.2 from the same National Health Interview Study of adults 65 or older in the United States illustrate the increase in prevalence of disability in three aged subgroups: the young old (65–74), the old (75–84), and the old old (85+) (National Center for Health Statistics, 1982). Disability levels include basic activities of daily living (Basic ADL) — walking, going outside, bathing, dressing, using the toilet, getting in and out of bed, and eating — and instrumental basic activities of daily living (instrumental ADL) — shopping, doing routine household chores, preparing meals, and handling money. Disability was defined as needing help in or not performing one or more of the activities listed. In the young-old cohort approximately 5% has some level of disability in basic ADL. Prevalence of disability doubles in the 75- to 84-year-old cohort (11.4%) and approaches 35% of those 85 years or older. A very similar trend is seen in the prevalence of disability in instrumental ADL: 40% of those 85 years of age or older need help, compared with 5.7% of those 65 to 74 years old. Clearly, a substantial proportion of the oldest cohort of our aged population (the one growing at the greatest rate) are estimated to be disabled in one way or another, and this trend is expected to continue well into the next century.

These well-understood demographic changes in our population, coupled with the less understood disability trends, are the basis for society's increasing concern and long overdue attention to the long-term care of its heterogeneous aged population.

## LONG-TERM CARE OF THE DISABLED AGED

As the needs of our aging population continue to change through the end of this century and into the next, many have begun to call for a "second revolution in the care of the aged" to address the emerging and intensifying long-term care needs. As T. F. Williams, former Director of the U.S. National Institute on Aging, has affirmed: "While current and projected increases in the number of older Americans symbolize a stunning triumph of survivorship, this tremendous achievement carries with it the responsibility to insure the health and well-being of the elderly to the fullest extent possible and to forestall the development of premature disability and dependence" (Williams, 1983).

Since the advent of Medicare and Medicaid, the increasing demand for acute medical intervention for an aging population is one that our society is well able and willing to satisfy. As Brody has noted:

> An elaborate system of third party pay is available for many of the secondary and tertiary procedures that make up the heroic effort that is an integral part of hospital care. This, in turn, is backed up by an extensive media program that focuses on medical "discoveries" and "firsts." Potential hospital patients expect advanced medical technology and procedures as a result of the conditioning to which they have been subjected. (Brody & Persily, 1984)

In our increasingly disabled aging population the demand for chronic care services is of a very different nature than acute care and has very different objectives. The needs of our aging population increasingly include long-term care, often with continuous support services provided by a different cadre of personnel. In this chapter, *long-term care* is used as a generic term to describe one or more services provided on a sustained basis to individuals whose functional capabilities are chronically impaired in order to maintain them at their maximum levels of psychological, physical, and social well-being. Those served may reside in their own homes or in some type of institutional facility (Brody, 1984).

The growing demand for long-term care today is, in part, instigated by existing third-party payment systems that insist on the discharge of hospital patients no longer requiring acute medical care. The Diagnosis Related Group (DRG) prospective payment system, for instance, reinforces the need for prompt hospital discharge. Increasingly, these discharge procedures are becoming the mechanisms by which the patient, family, hospital, and support service agencies negotiate for the continuance of care, which frequently is long-term care.

Long-term care as a philosophy or belief system espouses ambitious goals that are also different from those found in acute care. Callahan and Wallack (1981) have put forth five major long-term care goals:

1. Rehabilitation or maintenance of maximum functional independence of individuals at all times, even in the face of limitations in activity or deterioration of functions.
2. Humane care for persons who are functionally and permanently dependent.
3. Utilization of the least restrictive environment.
4. Death with dignity for individuals in the dying process.
5. Prevention of avoidable medical/social problems.

The resources used to achieve long-term care goals are traditionally organized into formal and informal support services. The formal services are those provided by government or private agencies as illustrated in Figure 12.4. These services are delivered by a wide range of professional and technical personnel such as nurses, rehabilitative therapists, social workers, homemakers, and personal-care aides, among others. The phrase "long-term care" emerged to describe the formal system of government and agencies needed to provide the continuum of sustained help dictated by chronic, disabling disease, though attempts to define it were not made until the late 1970s (Brody, 1987).

Well before the term "long-term care" came into use, the family, the major element in the elder's informal care network, was making the shift from providing episodic, short-term acute care to providing ongoing, long-term care to the disabled elder. Indeed, as E. Brody (1985) has stressed, it is the family that invented long-term care. Contrary to the

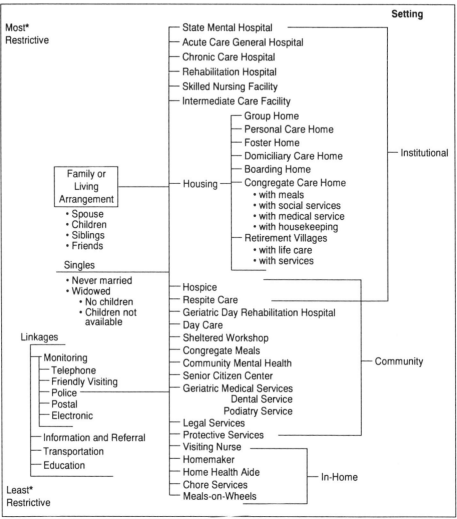

FIGURE 12.4   Array of long-term care services. (Adapted from Brody & Masciocchi, 1980)

persistent myth that institutionalization of the aged in U.S. society reflected "dumping" or abandonment, providing care for a dependent elderly parent has become a normative experience for individuals and families, and, in some cases, exceeds their capacities. Again, as Brody so pointedly notes, "the irony of the myth is that nowadays adult children provide more care and more difficult care to more parents over much longer periods of time than they did in the good old days" (Brody, 1985, p. 21).

The Health Interview Survey of 1979, for example, indicates that 73% of the disabled community aged rely exclusively on family and friends for their assistance (National Center for Health Statistics, 1979). Another 16% receive help from both informal and formal care givers (Soldo, 1980). Such estimates have been confirmed in other population samples as well (Branch & Jette, 1983).

The reliance on informal long-term care providers is, in part, due to the large proportion of disabled aged who live in the community. At any one time there are perhaps twice as many impaired aged being supported at home by spouses and children (9% of the aged) as there are in nursing homes (5% of the aged) (Mindel, 1979; Callahan, Diamond, Giele, & Morris, 1980).

A second important reason for the disabled aged's reliance on informal sources of long-term care is the serious limitation in existing reimbursement policy. In contrast to the acute-care needs of aged patients, which are supported largely by third-party payment, the second, long-term stage of care is given short shrift by the formal reimbursement system in the United States. Medicare, Medicaid, Blue Cross, and commercial insurance carriers afford little financial support for long-term care services. In 1977, for example, Medicare paid only 2% of nursing home costs, private insurance covered about 1%, while Medicaid paid nearly 48%. Nursing home residents and their families shouldered the burden of more than 48% of out-of-pocket nursing home costs (Leutz, Greenburg, Abrahams, Prottas, Diamond, & Greenburg, 1985).

Occasional support of noninstitutional services by Medicaid, as well as the other public programs as the Older Americans Act[1] have been insufficient to create an adequate and coordinated non-institutional, formal long-term care system (Kane & Kane, 1987). No single organization is responsible for the care of clients across the whole system, and the separation of the acute- and chronic-care systems works against the interdependent nature of the services being given. Many hospital patients could be cared for more appropriately in nursing homes if beds were available and properly staffed. Moreover, patients who are admitted to the hospital from home could be cared for at home if providers could be reimbursed for services provided in the home setting.

There is general agreement that the societal response to the needs of the individual and the family for long-term care has been inappropriate and inadequate. Societal concern, as in previous reactions to human catastrophe, is usually economic, not social. Some fear that long-term care will become an endless progression of expensive in-home and nursing home care. The corollary to this perception is the fear of the abdication of the family from its informal care-giving responsibilities if formal services are provided.

The lack of societal support for long-term care services has led to a lack of efficient and effective delivery systems that would encourage health professionals to work together efficiently and effectively. The underdevelopment of home- and community-based chronic-care services and the fragmented arrangements for managing the care of aged clients across the full range of acute- and chronic-care services have become major problems in meeting the emerging long-term care needs of our population.

Although a more integrated approach to long-term care makes obvious sense in terms of health care, both government and the private insurance industry are fearful of reimbursing a broader range of services because of the possibility of increased costs. This fear stems largely from concern over the "add-on" effect — the creation in the community of *new* long-term care cases that would begin to receive formal services despite their lack of need of nursing-home care. The fear of a substantial shift from the provision of predominantly informal long-term care to the formal long-term care system has greatly hindered efforts to develop a more efficient and effective formal system of long-term care. The magnitude of shift from informal to formal sources of long-term care, the cost of such a shift, and its desirability to society remain areas of considerable debate and controversy. Fortunately, a number of recent research demonstrations have begun to yield data on these and other important questions about expanded community-based long-term care.

## DEMONSTRATIONS OF COMMUNITY LONG-TERM CARE

Continuing concern over expanded public financing of formal community long-term care has led to a series of community demonstration programs. Although these programs are extremely diverse with respect to the interventions tested, the evaluation design, and populations served, most share a common goal of testing whether or not community long-term care, including nonmedical services and formal case management, can substitute for nursing home or hospital care. The underlying, guiding hypothesis is that long-term care for chronic, disabling conditions will cost less if the disabled person receives care in the community or at home rather than moving permanently into a nursing home. The common objective is to substitute community care for nursing home care whenever appropriate. Meeting this objective was expected to reduce long-term care costs and improve the overall quality of the lives of aged persons. Case management[2] and an expanded package of community services are the key program elements of these demonstrations. This discussion focuses on a few of the major publicly funded programs whose findings are consistent with other investigations. More detailed reviews are available elsewhere (Weissert, Cready, & Pawelak, 1988).

### Medicare Home-Based Waiver Programs

In the early 1980s the Health Care Financing Administration (HCFA) funded an evaluation of five community-based Medicare waiver demonstration programs that shared the objective of examining the impact of community care on traditionally covered health service use (Capitman et al., 1986). The five projects were (1) the New York City Home Care Project (Horowitz, Brill, & Dono, 1984), (2) the Long-Term Care Project of North San Diego County (Hill & Pinkerton, 1984), (3) Project OPEN (Sklar & Weiss, 1983), (4) the South Carolina Community Long-Term Care Project (Blackman, Brown, & Leaner, 1985), and (5) the OnLok Community Care Organization for Dependent Adults (Ansak & Zawadski, 1983).

All five projects assumed that by offering expanded case-managed community long-term care services, use of services traditionally covered by Medicaid and Medicare, such as nursing home care and hospital care, would change. All of the projects incorporated case management as an administrative service that directed clients' movement through a series of involvements with the formal long-term care system, while integrating formal and informal service provision wherever possible. The five demonstrations were in highly diverse communities and differed in terms of major elements of intervention design and evaluation. San Diego, Project OPEN, and South Carolina used randomized study groups; New York used a nonequivalent comparison group design; while OnLok attempted a matched comparison group design.

Although the provision of expanded case-managed community care was intended to alter the use of traditionally covered Medicare or Medicaid services, only in the cases of home health services under Medicare in San Diego and nursing home care under Medicaid in South Carolina were significant impacts observed.

The South Carolina project appeared to reduce significantly the number of nursing home days reimbursed by Medicaid, whereas the San Diego project reduced the number of Medicare-reimbursed home health visits. The San Diego home health reductions, however, were more than offset by the use of comparable waiver services.

Capitman suggests that the lack of impact on nursing home use in projects other than South Carolina may be attributable to the low rates of nursing home use. In contrast to South Carolina, where 52% of participants used nursing homes, rates of use in the other projects was very low. In general, the five projects were also not successful in significantly reducing hospital use reimbursed by Medicare.

South Carolina's success at attempting to divert nursing home applicants to community settings as part of a preadmission screening and case-managed alternative service suggests that targeting community services to aged persons at high risk of using or needing institutional care may be a key variable if home care is to be a substitute for institutional care. But even where projects were not successful in reducing institutional service use, they did meet real service needs and fostered better maintenance of function or quality of life.

### The Channeling Demonstration Programs

The U.S. Department of Health and Human Services began the National Long-Term Care demonstration, known as channeling, based on the premise that multiple resources and services could be provided and coordinated at the local level through a single organizational entity (Carcagno, 1986). The channeling program attempted to test rigorously the premise that comprehensive case management of community long-term care could contain the costs of expanding formal long-term care for the disabled aged and improve the outcomes for elderly clients as well as the family members and friends who care for them. The specific goal was to enable the disabled aged to stay in their homes when appropriate rather than enter a nursing home.

Channeling was designed to serve severely impaired older persons who required long-term care services for an extended period of time and who, in the absence of channeling, were at high risk of being institutionalized in a nursing home. For these high risk aged, the objective of channeling was to substitute services provided in the community — both formal services and the informal care provided by family and friends — for nursing home care, wherever community care was appropriate. This substitution, in turn, was intended to reduce costs and improve the overall quality of life of its clients and their informal caregivers.

To achieve the objective of managing the health care of the disabled aged at risk of nursing home placement while limiting the resources used, the channeling program included two models: the basic case-management model and the financial-control model. Both models shared a set of core functions, which included:

- Outreach, screening, and eligibility determination aimed at attracting frail aged persons to channeling
- Assessment, care planning, and service initiation by formal case managers
- Monitoring and reassessment for as long as the frail aged remained in channeling

The basic case-management model tested the premise that the major barrier to getting appropriate community long-term care to the aged was not lack of financing for services but lack of information about and ability to obtain and manage services under the existing service system. Case management was designed to determine needs and help arrange and coordinate services under the existing system.

In the financial-control model, service access and use were addressed through expanded service coverage, a funds pool, and the delegation of authorization power to case managers. These first two expanded elements were designed to allow the purchase of community services not covered under existing government programs and the use of existing public funds irrespective of the aged's categorical eligibility. Authorization power gave case managers the ability to determine the amount, duration, and scope of services paid for from the funds pool.

Evaluation revealed that the channeling programs clearly increased community service use by the impaired aged, not because of the substitution of community for nursing home care (as was originally hypothesized), but because of increased use among other aged persons living in the community. The bulk of these services consisted of in-home care, particularly personal-care and homemaker services. Despite the success in targeting services to an extremely frail population, channeling did not identify a population at high risk of nursing home placement and thus did not substantially reduce nursing home use. The channeling population was frequently hospitalized and made heavy use of physicians and other medical services. The costs of expanding case management and community services in the channeling sites were not offset by reductions in nursing home or other institutional costs. Channeling resulted in a net increase in costs of approximately 18% when compared to the care of the impaired aged who served as control clients.

The channeling programs did achieve a number of important patient outcomes. Evaluation results clearly show that this program reduced unmet needs of its clients, increased their confidence in receipt of care, and increased their overall satisfaction with life. In addition, it increased the informal caregivers' satisfaction with service arrangements and with their lives. However, it did not affect the impaired clients' functioning or mortality rates among participants.

The results of the five HCFA Medicare waiver demonstrations and the channeling demonstration projects are generally consistent with those of other community care demonstrations (USGAO, 1982; Kemper, Applebaum, & Harrigan, 1987; Skellie, Mobley, & Cohen, 1983; Birnbaum, 1984), which have generally found insufficient nursing-home and other institutional cost savings to offset the increased costs of expanded case management in community services to populations at relatively low risk of entering a nursing home.

### Hospital-Based Demonstrations

The difficulty in identifying and enrolling a population at high risk of entering nursing homes is a major reason for the increased costs of channeling and other community-care demonstrations. The need to target services more effectively to clients at high risk of requiring institutional care led the Robert Wood Johnson Foundation to undertake the Program for Hospital Initiatives in Long-Term Care, which was cosponsored by the American Hospital Association and the National Governor's Association. This was an attempt to stimulate hospitals, which treat an aged population at high risk of needing nursing home care, to seek a broader role as health centers rather than restrict themselves to acute-care medicine. This 4-year demonstration project involving 24 hospitals is one of the first major attempts to involve hospitals systematically in providing long-term care to the aged.

Massachusetts General Hospital (MGH) was 1 of 24 not-for-profit, voluntary, or public hospitals that participated in the Robert Wood Johnson Foundation's Program for Hospital Initiatives in Long-Term Care. MGH Coordinated Care targeted its demonstration efforts toward the frail hospitalized older person in need of long-term care and at high risk of negative outcomes following acute hospitalization. The major objectives of the MGH Program included (1) maximizing patients' functional recovery following discharge from the hospital, (2) maximizing the use of community long-term and primary care following discharge; and, subsequently, (3) minimizing hospital readmission and nursing home placement, thereby reducing the overall costs of health care provided to these high-risk individuals.

The essence of MGH Coordinated Care's intervention was case management provided by two long-term care coordination teams each staffed by a nurse, a social worker, and consultant geriatrician. Each coordination team was based within the MGH Social Service Department and worked to (1) identify, enroll, assess, and provide coordination services to eligible hospitalized frail elders soon after admission to hospital; (2) collaborate closely with the MGH discharge planners and community-based health and social-service professionals to develop and implement an optimal posthospital long-term care plan; and (3) monitor, reassess, and respond quickly to problems that developed throughout the demonstration period following discharge from the hospital. Once enrolled, participants were eligible to remain in the program throughout the length of the demonstration.

MGH Coordinated Care was designed to test the underlying premise that a major problem in sustaining appropriate long-term care for high-risk elders was a lack of information about the patient's needs and available services as well as an inability to access and manage the appropriate mix of services available to elders under the existing acute- and long-term care financing systems in this country. Coordination and systematic efforts were believed to be necessary for the appropriate orchestration between acute and long-term care required for efficient and effective long-term care.

The MGH coordination teams were designed to systematically assess needs, develop care plans, help arrange for, and coordinate the provision of these services and provide ongoing monitoring of each patient. MGH admission cards were reviewed daily to identify potential participants. Following chart review to confirm eligibility criteria and a discussion with the patient's attending physician, one team member invited eligible elders to enroll in the demonstration and sought their informed consent. Soon thereafter team members began a comprehensive patient and family assessment to determine postdischarge needs. All participants received an inpatient geriatric assessment from the program's consultant geriatrician; the results were shared with the patient's attending staff and discussed with the other coordination team members.

Soon after the patient's discharge, the coordination team conducted a visit to the patient's home and held a case conference with community professionals involved in the patient's care to coordinate ongoing care planning. Once a patient was reestablished in the community, the primary coordinator maintained close contact with the patient, family members and friends, as well as involved professionals to monitor and reassess the patient's ongoing needs and to ensure the continuation and appropriate modification of each patient's long-term care plan.

To evaluate the extent to which MGH Coordinated Care objectives were met for the 200 demonstration patients, the project's evaluation team enrolled and monitored 101 high-risk comparison patients admitted to MGH from local communities similar to those from which the Coordinated Care participants were drawn and who met the same eligibility criteria used to screen for demonstration participants. Elders in the comparison group received a limited evaluation from members of the MGH Coordinated Care evaluation team at hospital discharge, 6 and 12 months following enrollment.

As hypothesized, a significantly greater proportion of Coordinated Care patients received home health visits during the year following enrollment. Sixty seven percent of Coordinated Care patients received one or more visits during the first 6 months of the demonstration, compared with 39.8% of comparison patients during the same period. Use of home health care dropped precipitously for both groups in the second follow-up period, with 20% of Coordinated Care patients receiving one or more home health visits, compared with 9.9% of Comparison patients (Table 12.3). There were no statistically significant group differences in use of outpatient care during the 12-month follow-up period.

The Coordinated Care intervention did not appear to alter hospital readmission experience in the 12 months following enrollment (see Table 12.3). Eighty-seven percent of Coordinated Care patients and 91.6% of Comparison patients experienced one or more hospital days during the 6 months after initial assessment. Hospital readmissions dropped substantially for both groups during the second 6 months with 27.6% and 26.3% of Coordinated Care and Comparison patients, respectively, experiencing one or more hospital days. On average, Coordinated Care patients used 22.9 hospital days during the first 6 months and 6.2 days during the second 6 months following enrollment in the project. Patients in both groups experienced just over 5 hospital days, on average, during the 12 months prior to enrolling in this demonstration.

These findings hold true in multivariate analyses controlling for the influence of age, medicaid status, sex, and disability levels on health-care utilization (Jette et al., 1988).

## REFOCUSING THE GOALS OF COMMUNITY LONG-TERM CARE

Past community long-term care demonstrations suggest that expanding publicly financed community long-term care does not reduce aggregate costs, and it is likely to increase

TABLE 12.3   6- and 12-Month Health Care Utilization for MGH Coordinated
Care and Comparison Patients

|  | 6-Month Utilization | | 12-Month Utilization | |
|---|---|---|---|---|
|  | Coordinated-Care Patients ($n = 154$) | Comparison Patients ($n = 83$) | Coordinated-Care Patients ($n = 234$) | Comparison Patients ($n = 80$) |
| *Number of home health visits*[a] | | | | |
| None | 33.1% | 60.2% | 79.8% | 90.0% |
| 1–5 | 14.9 | 4.8 | 4.4 | 1.2 |
| 6 or more | 52.0 | 35.0 | 15.6 | 8.7 |
| *Number of outpatient visits* | | | | |
| None | 11.7 | 18.1 | 11.2 | 17.5 |
| 1–5 | 22.1 | 19.2 | 17.1 | 20.0 |
| 6 or more | 66.2 | 62.7 | 71.6 | 62.5 |
| *Number of hospital days* | | | | |
| None | 13.0 | 8.4 | 72.4 | 73.7 |
| 1–5 | 8.4 | 16.9 | 7.4 | 8.7 |
| 6 or more | 78.6 | 74.7 | 20.2 | 17.6 |
| *Number of skilled-nursing-home days* | | | | |
| None | 98.7 | 98.8 | 97.8 | 97.5 |

[a]$p \leq .05$

them – at least under the current long-term care service system, which already provides some community care. The one exception, the South Carolina project, suggests that it may be possible under some conditions to expand public financing of community long-term care without increasing aggregate public costs. The bulk of evidence suggests that costs are likely to rise with increased public financing of community long-term care. This is because it is difficult to identify and serve only those at high risk of nursing-home placement, difficult to effect large reductions in placement rates, and costly to provide the level of community care that may be appropriate.

The available evidence also suggests that providing increased formal long-term care will not cause wholesale substitution of publicly financed formal services for care provided by family and friends. Although some substitution in the area of instrumental activities of daily living may occur, the degree of substitution is small and much less than some have feared.

The findings from recent community-care demonstrations raise many questions about the traditional argument of cost savings as the justification for expanded community long-term care. Kemper et al. (1987) suggest the community long-term care demonstrations should change the nature of the debate around expanding community services for the frail aged. Given most of the current evidence, expansion of community services will need to be based not on its cost savings but on its benefits to the disabled elder and the family and friends who care for them. The debate thus will move to address how much community care society is willing to pay for, who should receive these publicly financed services, whether the availability of family and friends affects eligibility for services, and how a more efficient system should be designed to deliver these services more effectively.

## NOTES

1. The Older Americans Act, passed in 1965 by the U.S. Congress, clarified the responsibilities of the state and federal governments in concern for older Americans. Subsequent amendments have authorized funding for senior centers, congregate and home-delivered meals and other supportive services for the aged, established a National Clearing House for Information on Aging and established research and training grants in aging.

2. The term *case management* as used here includes multidimensional functional assessment and reassessment, care plan negotiation and periodic revision, and service arrangement, monitoring, and, where appropriate, planning for termination from the program. For a more extensive discussion of case management, see Capitman, Hoskins, and Bernstein (1986).

## REFERENCES

Ansak, M., & Zawadski, R. (1983). OnLok's CCODA: A cost-competitive model of community based long-term care. San Francisco: OnLok Senior Health Science.

Birnbaum, H., Barke, R., Swearingen, C., & Dunlop, B. (1983). Implementing community-based long-term care: Current findings of Georgia's alternative health services project. *American Journal of Public Health, 72,* 353–358.

Blackman, D., Brown, T., & Leaner, R. (1985). Four years of community long-term care project: The South Carolina experience. *Pride Institute Journal, 3,* 30–49.

Branch, L., & Jette, A. (1983). Elders' use of informal long-term care assistance. *Gerontologist, 23*(1), 51–56.

Brody, E. (1985). Parent care as a normative family stress. The Donald R. Kent Memorial Lecture. *The Gerontologist, 25,* 19–29.

Brody, S. (1984). Health Services: Need & Utilization. In S. Brody & H. Persily (Eds.). *Hospitals and the aged: The new old market* (p. 25). Rockville, MD: Aspen.

Brody, S. J. (1987). Strategic planning: The catastrophic approach. *Gerontologist, 27*(2), 131–138.

Brody, S. J., & Magel, J. R. (1984). DRG — The second revolution in health for the elderly. *Journal of the American Geriatrics Society, 32,* 676–679.

Callahan, J., Diamond, L., Giele, J., & Morris, R. (1980). Responsibility of families for their severely disabled elders. *Health Care Financing Review, i*(3), 29–48.

Callahan, J., & Wallack, S. (1981). Major reforms in long-term care. In Callahan, J., & Wallack, S. (Eds.), *Reforming the long-term care system: Financial & organizational options.* Lexington, MA: D. C. Heath.

Capitman, J., Hoskins, B., & Bernstein, J. (1986). Case management approaches in coordinated community-oriented long-term care. *Gerontologist, 26*(4), 398–404.

Carcagno, G. J., Applebaum, R., Christianson, J., Phillips, B., Thornton, C., & Will, J. (1986). The Evaluation of the National Long-Term Care Demonstration: The Planning and Operational Experience of the Channelling Projects. Mathematica Policy Research Inc., Princeton, NJ.

Fisher, C. (1980). Differences by age group in health care spending. *Health Care Financing Review, 1*(4), 65–90.

Fuchs, V. B. (1984). "Through much is taken": Reflections on aging, health and medical care. *MMFQ Health & Society, 62,* 143–166.

Health Insurance Association of America. (1985). Source book of health insurance data 1984–85. (No. 1A). Washington, DC: Author.

Hill, D., & Pinkerton, A. (1984). Final report: The long-term care project of North San Diego County. San Diego, CA: Allied Home Health Association.

Horowitz, A., Brill, R., & Dono, J. (1984). Delivery of medical and social services to the homebound elderly: A demonstration of inter-system coordination. New York: New York City Department of the Aging.

Jette, A. M., & Branch, L. G. (1981). The Framingham Disability Study. II: Physical disability among the aging. *American Journal of Public Health, 71,* 1211–1216.

Jette, A. M., Daniels, A., Deutsch, S., Fister, S., Murphy, P., O'Brien, J., & Walker, S. (1988, November).

Does hospital-based long-term care coordination improve function and change health service use? Presented at the American Public Health Association Meetings, Boston.

Kane, R. A., & Kane, R. L. (1987). *Long-term care: Principles, programs & policies.* New York: Springer.

Kemper, P., Applebaum, R., & Harrigan, M. (1987, summer). Community care demonstrations: What have we learned? *Health Care Financing Review, 8*(4). Baltimore, MD: U.S. DHHS Health Care Financing Administration.

Leutz, W., Greenburg, J., Abrahams, R., Prottas, J., Diamond, L., & Greenburg, L.: Changing Health Care for an Aging Society. Lexington, MA: D. C. Heath.

Mindel, C. (1979). Multigenerational family households: Recent trends and implications for the future. *Gerontologist, 19*(5), 456–463.

National Center for Health Statistics (1982). Current estimates from the National Health Interview Survey: United States, 1981. *Vital and Health Statistics* (Series 10, No. 141). Department of Health and Human Services.

National Center for Health Statistics (1979). *Health interview survey, 1977, 1979.* Washington, DC: U.S. Department of Health, Education and Welfare.

Rosenwaike, I. (1985). A demographic portrait of the oldest old. *MMFQ Health & Society, 63,* 187–205.

Skellie, A., Mobley, G., & Cohen, E. (1983). Cost-effectiveness of community-based long-term care: Current findings of Georgia's alternative health services project. *American Journal of Public Health, 72,* 353–358.

Sklar, B., & Weiss, L. (1983). Project OPEN: Final Report. San Francisco: Mounty Zion Hospital and Medical Center.

Soldo, B. J. (1980). America's elderly in the 1980s. *Population Bulletin, 35,* 1–48.

United States General Accounting Office (1982). The elderly should benefit from expanded home care but increasing those services will not ensure cost reduction. (Report No. GAO IPE-83-1). Washington, DC: Author.

Weissert, W., Cready, C., & Pawelak, J. (1988). The past and future of home- and community-based long-term care. *The Milbank Quarterly, 66*(2), 309–388.

Williams, T. F. (1983). Comprehensive functional assessment: An overview. *Journal of the American Geriatrics Society, 32,* 637–641.

# 13

## The Economics of the Health-Care System: Financing Health Care for the Aged Person

Diane S. Piktialis
Glenn S. Koocher

The health-care system for older Americans is financed by a complex, multitiered system of government insurance programs, private supplemental coverage, and, frequently, substantial direct out-of-pocket payments by the aged and their families. Caring for the aged invokes not only a diffuse and often uncoordinated medical delivery system but also a maze of similarly sounding yet very different payment programs, such as Medicare, Medicaid, and medigap insurance. The aged and their families may confront not only deductibles, coinsurance charges, and gaps in coverage for essential services but a labyrinth of rules, regulations, and paperwork that may vary from state to state. It is no wonder that the aged, their families, and health-care providers find the economics of health-care reimbursement and delivery perplexing, intimidating, and infuriating.

The health-care delivery and financing system is also difficult to manage. Medical care emerged after World War II as a predominantly private, autonomous institution dominated by independent physicians and hospitals. It has developed as an emergency response and acute-care system in which priority has been given to curing acute medical problems at hand rather than investing in promoting wellness, preventing disease, or meeting the needs of those with chronic illnesses. Both providers and insurers have worked within this framework.

Health care was financed historically in the United States through a service-driven incentive system that rewarded providers of care for the volume of treatment they delivered. More frequent office visits, lab or X-ray exams, or lengthy hospital admissions all triggered higher payments to doctors, hospitals, and the rest of an extensive provider network. The health-care financing system grew as a creature of both the emergency-response, acute-care model and this "fee-for-service" reimbursement system that evolved out of respect for the traditions of private medical practice.

Meanwhile, many who lacked the ability to pay for private health services benefited from an informal system of free care by practitioners who considered such "charity" a part of their social responsibilities. This was supplemented by government-sponsored health programs, largely at the community or county levels, various state-sponsored programs for the severely mentally ill, and the Public Health Service. However, because of the informal nature of charitable services and limits on public spending for health services prior to 1965, care was not universally available to those who lacked the ability to pay or access to the caregiver.

Before the "Great Society" antipoverty programs of the 1960s, patients paid a substantial portion of their own health-care bills. With the introduction of the federal Medicare program, this burden was relieved significantly. The aged paid 65% of their health care expenses in 1950 (White House Conference on Aging, 1982), but with Medicare, the figure fell between 10% and 12% in 1966.

Prior to the advent of Medicare, management and cost controls were rare and often considered inappropriate to the medical field, and research into health-care financing was in its infancy. Whereas European nations adopted national services as means of controlling their limited resources, the health-care financing system in the United States was developed to use public funds to foster and accommodate, rather than reform or restructure, the private provision of medical care.

With Medicare and Medicaid, America's public health priorities were stated boldly to expand accessibility to health care for older and poor people. This philosophy was reemphasized in 1972 with the extension of Medicare to disabled individuals and patients with end-stage renal disease. However, some significant cost-sharing provisions of the 1990 budget reconciliation law, which aimed at reducing expenditures and increase revenues, including higher monthly premiums, demonstrated an emerging shift in government policy, whereby Medicare beneficiaries would shoulder more of the burden of overall costs.

The policy objectives to improve access to and quality of care for the aged have been substantially achieved. In 1964, 72% of low-income older Americans had seen a physician within the previous 2 years, compared with 82% of wealthier patients. By 1979, the gap had closed, as 86% of both groups had been treated by a doctor. Along with improvements in preventive care and technology, life expectancy grew by 2.5 years during the first 20 years of Medicare. However, the national health bill grew substantially as a result. In 1966 Medicare paid out $824 million; in 1984 it paid out $35.5 billion.

The acceptance of a major federal role in medical financing for the aged triggered a dramatic escalation in health-care costs by expanding accessibility to care, supporting an increase in the number of providers, and underwriting new technologies that improved prospects for longer life. Between 1950 and 1980, an average day in the hospital became five times more costly.

The demands on the health-care system and the federal budget also increased as the over-65 group became a progressively larger segment of the population. Elders account for more than 30% of the overall national medical bill, although they comprise about 12% of the population at large. Advances in technology, in drug, radiological, and cancer treatments, and in transplant surgeries, together with improved access to services, have also impacted the cost of care by introducing readily available, if not expensive, therapies and broadening their availability, thereby extending further the lives of older people.

In response to these financial pressures, powerful health-care cost containment measures were introduced in the 1970s, aimed principally at reducing more costly acute inpatient care and channeling treatment to interventions considered more appropriate and efficient and to less expensive, outpatient services. Gradually, other federal policies have been implemented, including the practice of "cost shifting," which transfers a larger responsibility for financing care onto the aged. For example, 1980s legislation encouraged older Medicare-eligible workers to defer federal coverage and elect employer-based health coverage as the primary insurer until retirement.

These cost-conserving trends have had the dual effect of reducing the responsibility of government and, in many cases, shifting the burden to private insurers to finance days in the hospital; at the same time, this trend expanded the burden of health-care payment and delivery to individual patients and their families, who must now manage in the community and at home. Most health insurance programs, including Medicare, impose some degree of shared payment responsibility for outpatient care, requiring older people to assume a greater burden of this expense. Twenty years after the Medicare amendments were added to the Social Security Act, elders found themselves paying 15% of their income for health care, edging past the portion paid in 1965 before the law was passed (U.S. House of Representatives, 1985).

Despite more than twenty-five years of Medicare and Medicaid, health-care financing and delivery remains largely misunderstood. Most families are caught unexpectedly in the web of coordinating services, transporting patients to providers, arranging for care at home, processing the necessary paperwork for reimbursement for covered services, and shouldering substantial direct expenses. Few anticipate these responsibilities, discovering their obligations of time and resources only after a medical crisis has hit. Exacerbating this situation is the general absence of public or private insurance options for the aged to cover their routine physical examinations and checkups on one hand, and many chronic or long-term services, particularly nursing-home care, on the other. Except for Medicare-risk health maintenance organization programs, which frequently offer certain preventive services, and Medicaid coverage, which is broad in scope, routine and wellness services and chronic or long-term care remain the responsibility of the patient.

Presently five principal sources of financing are available to the aged. America's health-care bill for the aged is divided among Medicare (45%); private insurance, including Medicare supplements (11%); Medicaid (13%); other public sources, including the Veterans Administration (6%); and patients and their families (26%) (Prospective Payment Assessment Commission, 1987).

In this chapter we will explain how health care for the aged is financed in the United States, describe the programs that support the cost of medical services for them, and explain how the aged and their families can deal with the growing responsibility of assuming a significant burden of care with their own resources.

## MEDICARE AND MEDIGAP INSURANCE

### History

In 1965 the Medicare amendments to the Social Security Act established a system of hospital and medical insurance for people over 65. In 1972 eligibility was extended to certain disabled individuals and victims of end-stage renal disease (requiring kidney transplant and dialysis treatment). Divided into two parts, Medicare provides basic but far from complete hospital and medical coverage financed by a combination of payroll taxes, premiums, general government revenues, and shared patient payments in the form of deductibles and coinsurance charges. The subsequently repealed 1988 catastrophic-care amendments added an income tax surcharge to Medicare-eligible individuals, the first Medicare financing provisions based on the ability-to-pay. This provision was one of the most unpopular, and the response of older persons shook the political system, driving part of the repeal initiative.

Hospital insurance, or Part A, is provided free to most eligible individuals and covers inpatient care and follow-up care in a skilled nursing facility. Supplementary medical insurance (SMI), or Part B, requires a monthly premium and reimburses professional providers and patients for many inpatient and outpatient services related to the diagnosis and treatment of medical problems. In most cases, the Part B premium is deducted directly from the monthly Social Security benefit (pension) check.

With the Medicare amendments, government policymakers sought to construct a program that would establish basic health insurance for the aged and avoid some of the pitfalls that beset the old-age pension system established 30 years earlier. President Franklin D. Roosevelt, in signing the Social Security Act, proclaimed it would provide "some measure" of security for the aged, after shelving more ambitious income maintenance programs and a scheme for a state-administered, but federally funded, health insurance system (Schottland, 1970). The law left room for private retirement plans and individual savings to supplement modest federal retirement benefits. Despite these intentions, many business leaders and working Americans failed to respond to voluntary incentives and did not invest in company pension plans or long-term individual savings. As a result, as many as one out of three of the aged presently relies on Social Security as the sole source of income, while two thirds depend on the monthly checks as the principal financial resource.

Medicare was designed to preclude similar systemic flaws by establishing a series of meaningful incentives and important roles for government, workers, employers, commercial insurers, hospitals, and physicians.

By providing the options of direct reimbursement to physicians or billing patients directly rather than filing claims with fiscal intermediaries on a "participating" basis, the Medicare program respected the preferences of many doctors to conduct independent practices and manage medical offices without unreasonable intrusion of government. (See later discussion of balance billing.)

By allowing hospitals to participate in selecting state-sited fiscal intermediaries to administer the program and by creating a source of financing for an underserved aged population in need of inpatient care, the medical community was reassured and participated widely in the Medicare program.

### Financing and Structure

The Medicare program is administered by the Health Care Financing Administration (HCFA), a unit within the U.S. Department of Health and Human Services. Thus a major role for government involves overall administration and regulation, management of the Social Security Trust Funds, collection of payroll taxes, and, in certain cases, contributions of general treasury revenues.

Individual workers contribute to Social Security Trust Funds through the payroll tax, set at 7.65% from 1990 to 2000. Under the Federal Insurance Contribution Act (FICA), worker contributions are matched by employers (self-employed persons pay both worker and employer portions) and deposited in the Old Age Survivors Trust for monthly pensions for retirees or dependents (5.6%); the Disability Insurance Trust for disabled worker pensions (0.6%); and the Hospital Insurance Trust, which finances part of Medicare (1.45%). Hospital Insurance, also known as Medicare's Part A, is available without charge to people over 65 who are eligible for Social Security or Railroad Retirement Act benefits through covered employment. Spouses of eligible workers are also eligible as are certain divorcees and dependents. Not all aged, therefore, are eligible for Social Security and Medicare. Among them are individuals who worked in state and local governments or for certain academic, religious, and nonprofit employers who, until 1986, were not mandated to participate in the Social Security system. Although many did elect to participate in Social Security payroll deduction programs, others, including government employers, elected alternative public pension programs and health insurance plans for retirees. Others who may not be eligible are individuals who have not worked during their lifetime and recent immigrants, including certain resident aliens. However, these aged may be eligible for Medicaid (see the section on Medicaid).

Medicare-eligible individuals must enroll on their own within 3 months before or after the month in which they turn 65. Those who elect to work beyond age 65, the "working aged," may elect to continue with employer group health insurance and defer enrollment into Medicare until retirement. Others who are not eligible for Social Security (less than 3% of the population) may purchase Part A coverage for a substantial monthly fee.

Medicare beneficiaries also enroll in supplemental medical insurance (SMI), known as Medicare Part B, although the "working aged" may defer this coverage until retirement. SMI may be purchased separately by those who are not eligible for Part A.

Medicare B requires payment of a monthly premium that is, in most cases, deducted automatically from Social Security pension checks. These contributions are combined with general treasury revenues of the federal government into a fourth Social Security Trust Fund.

In addition to government, worker, and employer roles in financing care for the aged, the significant deductibles, coinsurance charges, and gaps in coverage created a substantial Medicare supplement market for the private insurance industry. These Medicare supplements, called "medigap insurance," are available under various brand names from many health insurance providers across the country and offer the aged a further opportunity to insure themselves against significant, but not all, out-of-pocket expenses for medical care.

### Benefits and Coverage: Medicare A

Hospital insurance under Medicare covers inpatient room and board, nursing care, and other hospital services care for an unlimited period. Physician services are usually covered under Part B. The inpatient deductible was set originally at $40 in 1966 but, with annual adjustments, grew to $676 by 1993. Until 1987, when the deductible charge was tied to a medical expense index, it was based on the cost of an average day of hospitalization for a Medicare beneficiary. Medicare inpatient coverage is limited to 60 days of full coverage, after the deductible charge, and 30 days of 75% coverage. An additional 60 "lifetime reserve days" are also available for which the patient must pay a substantial daily copayment.

Inpatient care in a mental health hospital is treated differently and is limited to a lifetime maximum of 190 days.

Medicare A will also provide up to 100 days in a properly designated and certified skilled-nursing facility (SNF) for posthospital rehabilitation requiring a highly skilled level of care. There is an initial coinsurance charge for each of the first 20 days equal to one eighth of the inpatient deductible. It is important to note that Medicare-covered SNF care is considered substantially different from the less intensive services of intermediate level and custodial care facilities. Many of these intermediate and custodial facilities, commonly called nursing homes, offer what is regarded by many family members as skilled-nursing care. However, they remain uncovered by Medicare.

### Home Health Care

Also included in Medicare A are home health benefits and hospice care. Home health services are provided to patients by agencies offering skilled-nursing care or specified therapeutic services under plans supervised by physicians. Deductibles and coinsurance charges do not apply. However, medical eligibility criteria for reimbursement under Medicare are strict and require the patient to be in need of skilled-nursing care. Many patients with long-term and chronic-care needs are not eligible because they fail to meet these criteria.

### Hospice

Hospice services are offered through agencies providing care to terminally ill individuals and their families on a 24-hour basis as they are needed. The categories of services include inpatient care, respite care, routine and continuous home care, and certain prescription medications. Eligibility requirements call for a life expectancy of no more than 6 months, but benefits can be extended based on medical necessity.

### Medicare B

Supplementary medical insurance (SMI) covers a broad range of outpatient care, including physician services necessary for the diagnosis and treatment of medical problems. However, benefits exclude routine physical examinations and checkups. In most cases, Medicare B will reimburse to a provider or patient 80% of "reasonable" charges after applying a $100 calendar-year deductible.

Mental health services are again treated differently, and outpatient benefits have been expanded in recent years, but a substantial copayment of up to 50% is required.

Medicare does not generally cover prescription medications outside the hospital except in rare instances for certain immunosuppressant drugs or for injectable drugs in limited cases of osteoporosis.

In particular, Medicare B benefits include:

- Therapeutic or diagnostic physician services in the hospital, outpatient units, physicians' offices, or at home
- Outpatient mental health care
- Nonroutine podiatry care
- Anesthesiologist, radiologist, and pathologist services (inpatient radiology and pathology are covered 100%)
- Diagnostic lab tests, including X-rays
- Kidney dialysis treatment and supplies
- Radiology therapy
- Ambulances
- Rental or purchase of medically necessary durable medical equipment, such as hospital beds, wheelchairs, walkers, or prosthetic devices (except for teeth)
- Outpatient physical therapy, up to $500 per year
- Pneumococcal and hepatitis B vaccines
- Mammography screening

Outpatient physical therapies, including speech therapy, and mental health services are capped at preset limits. Some medigap plans extend coverage and certain states enforce mandated benefit legislation, which efforts expand service limits modestly. However, patients in need of physical or mental health rehabilitation often experience exhaustion of benefits before a course of treatment can be completed and must utilize their own financial resources to pay. In some cases, notably mental health services, treatment may go uncompleted.

### Coverage for Prescription Drugs

The 1988 catastrophic-care amendments expanded coverage for prescription medicines through a separate system of deductibles and coinsurance payments. These benefits were rescinded before they could be implemented when the entire catastrophic package was canceled in late 1989. As a result, coverage for outpatient prescription drugs remains severely limited.

### Qualified Medicare Beneficiary (QMB) Program

Originally part of the Medicare Catastrophic Care Act, the QMB Program was expanded in 1989 to apply to Medicare beneficiaries with incomes at or below federal poverty levels. Under the program, eligible Medicare beneficiaries are exempt from Medicare premiums, deductibles, and coinsurance. The Medicaid program absorbs the cost. Effective 1993, exemptions from Medicare premiums only are extended to those whose incomes are within 100–200% of poverty. This eligibility will be expanded to 120% of poverty by 1995.

### Balance Billing

Under Medicare there are two options for payment of physicians. Doctors and other authorized providers may elect a direct method of billing called "assignment," wherein charges are submitted directly to the fiscal intermediary on behalf of the patient and any reimbursement is made directly to the physician or appropriate clinician. Patients are responsible for a coinsurance charge equal to 20% of the Medicare fee (50% for outpatient mental health services), although frequently medigap insurance will cover this balance. In accepting assignment, physicians and other providers agree to accept the Medicare "allowed" charge as the maximum allowable fee.

Physicians who elect to refuse assignment are not bound to accept Medicare reimbursement as full payment and may require payment in full directly from the patient in advance of processing Medicare claims. Effective in September 1990, however, physicians were required to file the Medicare Part B claim forms for their patients whether or not they accepted assignment or limited their fee to the Medicare approved charge. The patient must still file the Medicare supplementary insurance claims for the portion that Medicare does not cover. Occasionally, physicians will file these claims as well. In certain states where the medigap insurer is also the officially designated Medicare "fiscal intermediary" (meaning that the insurer processes Medicare claims for the federal government), there may also be an automatic "piggy-backing" process whereby the intermediary processes the Medicare claim and automatically forwards it to the medigap plan for co-processing. Other medigap insurors may also participate in the "piggy back" process as a convenience to their policy holders.

Also, providers who do not accept assignment are free to charge patients amounts in excess of the allowable charges for Medicare. However, federal law limits the amount above and beyond the Medicare-allowed charge that providers can assess patients. (The figure was 115% in 1993.)

This practice is called balance billing. About 30% of all Medicare claims were filed on an unassigned basis prior to the September 1990 claims-processing changes and the implementation of the limits to the size of balance bills.

Winning the right not to accept assignment and, accordingly, to "balance bill" the patient was critical to obtaining the support of physicians across the nation and securing the political compromises that facilitated the passage of the Medicare amendments in 1965 (Marmor, 1973). Recently, federal lawmakers have considered mandating that all physicians accept Medicare assignment and have measures implemented with the goal of increasing physician compliance (e.g., limits to the size of balance bills, requiring physicians to file claims, favorably treating reimbursement for participating physicians, etc.). Nonetheless, the aged are frequently presented with unexpected "balance bills" for the uncovered portion of service from physicians and other providers they believed were "covered by Medicare." These may require substantial out-of-pocket payments.

Recent federal legislation requires nonparticipating physicians to notify patients in advance of any procedure when charges will exceed $500. In addition to the federal statutes and regulations, state legislation has been considered to limit or prohibit balance billing of Medicare patients, but these measures have been implemented only in a few states.

Overall, Medicare is principally a hospital and physician reimbursement program. Inpatient care absorbs between 60% and 65% of overall benefit payments, but skilled-nursing facilities collect only 1%. Physicians receive about 25%. Outpatient facilities collect about 6% of Medicare payout, and home health agencies receive 3 to 4%.

### Uncovered Services

Excluded from Medicare coverage, in addition to routine examinations, are many over-the-counter and wellness promotion products and routine supplies frequently used by the aged. Also excluded are hearing and vision testing, reimbursement for hearing aids and eyeglasses (although certain prosthetic lenses are covered for certain eye surgeries), and most dental services. Elective cosmetic surgery is also not covered.

Medicare provides no coverage outside the territorial United States, except in very limited situations. Medigaps may fill in.

Most significantly, Medicare does not cover long-term or custodial care, or the services of a family member. It is for these categories of care that most of the aged and their families incur substantial out-of-pocket responsibilities. Long-term care will be addressed in a later section.

### Medigap Insurance

Medicare supplementary insurance, more commonly known as "medigap" coverage, is purchased by two thirds of all aged Americans. Plans may vary substantially in terms of price, benefits, and paperwork requirements. In an effort to establish minimum requirements for medigap insurance, Congress authorized the setting of optional minimum standards under the "Baccus Amendment" (PL 96–265) to prevent abuse in the marketing and advertising of supplementary coverage (General Accounting Office, 1986b). Based on the Omnibus Budget Reconciliation Act of 1990, these standards were strengthened. Criteria established by the National Association of Insurance Commissioners were incorporated in the Baccus Amendment were influential in establishing ten nationally standardized medigap plans. As a result, in most cases, medigaps will be consistent in benefit structure from state to state although premium costs may vary widely by insurer.

Most medigaps will cover the initial inpatient deductible and reimburse subscribers for the 20% coinsurance charges under Medicare B for most covered services. Coverage for the $100 Part B deductible is also available from some of the standardized supplemental plans, as are benefits for preventive care, prescription drugs, out-of-country care, and home care.

Although most inpatient facilities process medigap insurance claims for the hospital deductible, coinsurance, and other expenses, responsibility for obtaining reimbursement for the beneficiary share of medical services under the Part B program frequently falls upon patients. This may be confusing to the aged who do not generally distinguish between Part A and Part B benefits; who do not comprehend the complexities of the 20% coinsurance provisions, the reduced mental health coverage, or balance billing; or who are ill at ease with claim forms.

Certain medigaps extend coverage in varying degrees to prescription drugs and out-of-country care (see above). Although some subscribers confuse skilled-nursing facilities with nursing homes, medigap plans do not provide reimbursement for custodial care or for services required over a long period of time.

Between 65% and 75% of the aged have medigap coverage of some form, including Medicaid, but the proportion of individuals over 80 without supplemental coverage

(27%) is higher than those aged 65 to 69 (17%; General Accounting Office, 1986b). Important determinants of retention of medigap coverage include income, education, race, and self-perceived health status.

Because of the great fear of catastrophic illness and bankruptcy among the aged, some of them purchase duplicate medigap policies, effectively paying twice for the same coverage from different insurers. This is unwise but understandable, considering the barrage of powerful medigap advertising and the confusion among the aged about the health-care financing system.

### Indemnity and Dread-Disease Policies

Some indemnity and dread-disease insurance plans are also used by the aged to serve as medigaps. Indemnity plans pay a preset daily cash benefit to patients based on length of hospital stay or other preestablished criteria. These benefits are usually paid regardless of any other coverage available. Although some of the aged may use these indemnity payments to cover hospital or medical bills, others use them to replace lost income during illness, pay the expenses of spouses at home, or build a cash reserve for home care following discharge.

Dread-disease policies limit benefits exclusively to specific illnesses, such as cancer. Because of the comparatively low ratio of dollars paid out to premiums collected, or "benefit ratios," among certain plans and the fact that Medicare and medigaps provide substantial coverage for treatment of these diseases, some states have banned dread-disease policies.

In addition to private insurer medigap offerings, health maintenance organizations (HMOs) have begun to offer programs to Medicare beneficiaries. These programs will be addressed later in a discussion of alternative health delivery systems.

### Coverage for Public Employees

Until the mid-1980s, most employees of federal, state, and local governments were excluded from the Social Security System and ineligible for Medicare. Recent changes in law have required these workers to participate in the Medicare program, although the public pension system has been left separate and distinct from Social Security. However, government retirees who are not eligible for Medicare are generally covered by the Federal Health Employee Benefit Program or state-authorized group health insurance. Recently, as a cost control device, states have encouraged retired government workers to enroll in Medicare if they are eligible through previous or part-time private sector employment, or through their spouse.

### Impact of Federal Cost-Control Initiatives

Recent federal cost-containment and Medicare management programs have had a direct impact on how health care is financed, particularly for out-of-pocket expenses. The most significant of these changes were the introduction of stronger utilization controls and, in 1983, the prospective payment system (PPS), including the Diagnosis Related Group

(DRG) program of hospital reimbursement. Moreover, a movement toward research-based relative value scales to rate physician payments and standardize reimbursements to doctors based on the complexity and severity of the procedures involved was implemented in the early 1990s.

As early as 1972 a national system of professional standard review organizations (PSROs) was established to include physicians in the monitoring of medical care to assure both appropriateness of treatment and quality of health services. By 1982, these groups were replaced by peer review organizations (PROs), whose powers were expanded to include preadmission screening of certain elective inpatient treatments, prior approval of other procedures for appropriateness of site, and review of quality-of-care issues, including inadequate service and premature discharge.

Recognizing that cost-containment measures could impact the quality of care, numerous federal, state, and private studies have begun to examine such issues as patient satisfaction, length of stay, effectiveness of discharge planning, availability of home-based support services, hospital readmissions, and postdischarge morbidity and mortality.

In the meantime, a system of 470 diagnosis-related groups of illness, or DRGs, was established to reimburse hospitals on a prospective basis. Under the prospective payment system each DRG category triggers a preset reimbursement to the hospital for an inpatient stay falling within certain broad outlier limits. Thus, hospitals are reimbursed by Medicare with a predetermined amount regardless of length of stay under most circumstances. DRGs are determined by individual category and are designed to reflect the average cost of caring for patients suffering from the illness in each group. For example, DRG reimbursement for cardiac surgery is greater than payment for an appendectomy.

Each DRG also has an "outlier" limit to ensure that extraordinarily lengthy stays generate more equitable payment to the hospital. After this point is reached in an exceptionally long inpatient stay, the fixed prospective payment is supplemented by an additional reimbursement. This protects the hospital from absorbing all the costs of an extended stay.

With the establishment of DRGs, service-driven incentives that evolved over many decades under the "fee-for-service" system were reversed. Hospitals were no longer reimbursed on the basis of the volume of service they provided. Proponents of the DRG system argued that fixed, diagnosis-based prospective reimbursements stimulated efforts to eliminate waste and maximize efficiency as hospitals responded to the new system. Advocates for the aged, including prominent members of Congress, cited instances of discharges of patients "quicker and sicker" than before. DRGs and other utilization review measures shortened hospital stays for the aged and increased reliance on outpatient and home-based care. With shorter inpatient stays covered by Medicare Part A, a greater volume of follow-up care was required in outpatient Part B services in which 20% of copayment expenses were borne by the aged and their families. Moreover, uncovered home health needs imposed even greater financial obligations.

Between 1980 and 1985, covered inpatient days under Medicare fell from 3,908 per 1,000 beneficiaries to 2,875. SNF days also dropped from 309 to 280. In the meantime, home health visits increased 94% and outpatient physical therapy services grew 103%. Hospital outpatient department service volumes grew 27%, reflecting the movement away from inpatient care. Physician services per patient increased less dramatically but significantly at 8% (General Accounting Office, 1987).

### Other Cost-Containment Proposals

Various proposals and initiatives have been developed to help reduce federal budget obligations for Medicare or to manage and control health-care costs for the aged. Among them are increasing the SMI premium beyond the 25% share of program costs (the premiums were legislated at higher rates by the Omnibus Budget Reconciliation Act of 1990), raising the Part B deductible beyond the present limit (the deductible was raised from $75 to $100 effective January 1, 1991), expanding the prospective payment concept by folding anesthesiology, radiology, and pathology fees into basic DRG, developing a DRG system for physician reimbursement, and imposing coinsurance charges on home health services.

Other recommendations seek to restructure the health-care system by expansion of managed care and health promotion, including the Medicare-risk HMO program, reviewed later in this chapter.

### MEDICAID

Medicaid, the antipoverty program of medical assistance for low-income individuals, is administered by states under federal guidelines. Financing is shared between the state and federal governments based on the services states elect to provide. Because it is frequently administered at the state level by human or social-service or welfare agencies, Medicaid is widely perceived as a "welfare" program. As a result, many aged who have lived a lifetime of independence and who wish to avoid the stigma of the "welfare" label do not apply for Medicaid coverage.

Like Medicare, Medicaid was established in 1965 as part of the Social Security Act. For various reasons it is often confused with Medicare. Medicaid enrollment, however, is not restricted to the aged but is accessible to low-income people of all ages, including the disabled. Medicaid eligibility for the aged falls into two categories tied to income and available assets: "categorical" and "medically needy."

### Eligibility

The "categorically eligible" aged include those who meet criteria for federal cash assistance under the Supplemental Security Income (SSI) program, established under the Social Security Act and administered by the states. SSI, the successor to the former state and federal Old Age Assistance programs, assures a minimum income to elders, blind, and disabled individuals. Cash payment benefits may vary from state to state. Medically needy individuals are those with some limited financial resources, but not enough to pay for medical care. Certain assets are not included in determining eligibility. These include the principal residence, automobile, household goods, personal effects, and limited life insurance designed to pay for burial expenses. Both monthly income limits (which vary from state to state) and maximum allowable asset allowances (about $2,000 for individuals, $2,700 for couples) define eligibility. Medical expenses may be deductible from total income calculations in order to determine eligibility. When a Medicaid-eligible aged person is institutionalized, the assets of the patient and spouse may be divided equally up so the spouse remaining in the community may retain a minimum amount which is adjusted annually (this amount was $13,740 in 1992). States have the option of extending the share to as much as $68,780 (as of 1992) in order for the spouse remaining in the community to retain an equitable portion of the economic resources without jeopardizing health coverage.

In many cases, states will encourage the purchase of medigap insurance and include those premiums among deductible health expenses.

There is duplication and overlap among insurance and public financing plans beyond the appropriate Medicare/medigap coupling. About 8% to 13% of Medicare beneficiaries are also enrolled in Medicaid (Prospective Payment Assessment Commission, 1987). It is not uncommon for individuals who are eligible for Medicaid to carry a medigap plan simultaneously. In some states it may be necessary to incur a medigap premium expense in order to reduce residual income to the Medicaid eligibility limit.

### Benefits

Medicaid features a two-tiered benefit program. The first tier is a mandated basic services program of inpatient hospitalization, skilled-nursing facilities, outpatient services, physician care, lab and X-rays, and home health in addition to services at rural health clinics. Family planning, nurse midwife services, and early screening and exams for those under 21 are also covered.

States may elect to offer a second layer of services including prescription drugs, eyeglasses, dental care, adult day care, inpatient psychiatric services, physical therapy, and intermediate-care facilities. These are services of great value to the aged, most notably intermediate-level nursing homes, which are covered only partly or not at all by Medicare. Nominal cost sharing by beneficiaries is permitted for this second level of Medicaid benefits.

It is estimated, however, that 64% of poor older Americans are not eligible for Medicaid, and 20% of all aged have no health insurance coverage beyond Medicare (Prospective Payment Assessment Commission, 1987).

The growth of the elderly population and the nursing-home census covered by Medicaid has had a serious financial implication for states that share the burden of cost. Many state policymakers have called Medicaid a "budget buster," growing at a seemingly unmanageable rate. Initiatives to attach the value of homes of Medicaid recipients upon death or to implement managed-care initiatives to hold down costs are being considered along with overall limitations upon benefits.

## OTHER PUBLIC PROGRAMS

In a limited number of cases, hospital and medical benefits may be available from the Veterans Administration (VA), special state programs for uninsured or impoverished patients, and local hospital and clinic programs. In addition, valuable supportive social services may be available through the national network of Area Agencies on Aging under the provisions of the Older Americans Act and state or local units on aging.

Among these are valuable home based social services designed to prevent inappropriate institutionalization.

### Veterans Administration

Inpatient, outpatient, mental health, and long-term care services, including institutional care, are available from VA facilities for honorably discharged veterans, including those over age 65. Family members or dependents are generally not eligible for services. Treatment for those with military service-related medical problems and certain disabled individuals receiving a VA pension is usually provided without charge.

For other veterans of military service means tests are applied to determine if patient copayments are required. Income eligibility and net worth guidelines are more generous than in the case of Medicaid. Copayments for hospitalization and outpatient care are modest even for those not eligible for free services. VA facilities include acute inpatient and chronic disease hospitals, outpatient care centers, and long-term care institutions. The number of veterans is expected to reach 9 million by 2000, including two out of three males over age 65 (Wetle, 1988).

## PRIVATE OUT-OF-POCKET FINANCING

Despite high public expectations and perceptions, Medicare covers only about half of health costs for the aged. As many as two out of three Americans erroneously believe their existing insurance will pay the cost of long-term illness (Louis Harris & Associates, 1986). Nearly four out of five believe Medicare will cover nursing-home care (Rice & Gabel, 1986). Though the proportion of hospital bills paid by Medicare is high, coverage for outpatient care, is less substantial. Prior to the introduction of the first stage of the ill-fated catastrophic-care provisions of Medicare, most of these expenses fall into five categories: Medicare Part B premiums, Medicare deductibles and coinsurance charges, Medicare supplementary insurance premiums, balance billing, dental care, and prescription drugs. To maintain some initial control over public expenditure, the architects of Medicare excluded most forms of routine care and other frequent expenses that would have been costly and difficult to control. Medicaid was established as a final "safety net" to protect the aged from going without necessary care, but only after they had depleted most of their financial resources.

Among those noncovered services for which the aged must pay directly are routine physical examinations, hearing and vision testing, hearing aids, eyeglasses, and most podiatric care.

Although it is a form of health insurance, the medigap premiums represent not only an of out-of-pocket expense but a means of passing through to the aged costs shifted from Medicare. When the cost of financing care increases, medigap insurance passes the added expenses on to subscribers in the form of higher premium charges. For example, in 1983 radiology and pathology services were shifted from Medicare Part A to Part B, where the then $75 deductible ($100 as of 1991) and 20% cost-sharing obligation were required from patients or from their medigap insurance. Furthermore, starting in 1983, the working aged were given the option of remaining in employer group health plans, shifting away from Medicare and onto private insurers some responsibility for the cost of health care for aged workers. As a result, medigap insurers lost these younger, lower-risk aged from their overall subscriber population. This left a greater percentage of advanced aged to finance a more severe medigap risk pool, and premiums were forced up as a result.

In addition, families confronting chronic illness or long-term care institutionalization incur substantial costs for home health providers or nursing-home expenses. It is estimated that in 1991 about 43% of the $60 billion annual nursing-home bill was paid directly by patients or their families (U.S. House of Representatives, 1993). They shoulder 60% to 80% of the burden of long-term care needs, including home-delivered services (White House Conference on Aging, 1982). The long-term care dilemma will be explored in detail later in this chapter.

With out-of-pocket costs of the aged growing at rates significantly higher than income, considerable public attention has been focused on addressing catastrophic costs of health care of the aged. In addition, recent initiatives in managed-care alternatives, including HMOs, have been developed. These will be discussed below.

LONG-TERM CARE FINANCING

The increasing number of aged with chronic impairments has accelerated the need for long-term care services. The incidence of chronic impairments increases with age, and an estimated 5.9 million Americans over 65 suffered from some limitation associated with a chronic condition (U.S. Senate Special Committee on Aging, 1991). It is also estimated that one in four older Americans will enter a nursing home. Moreover, the proportion of individuals residing in long-term care institutions increases dramatically with age. For example, about 2% of those aged 65 to 74 reside in nursing homes, 5% to 6% of those aged 75 to 84 do so as well, but 22% of those 85 and over are institutionalized.

Overall long-term care costs were estimated to reach $76.6 billion by 1992, of which $66.3 billion was for nursing-home care. Consumers paid 41% of this institutional care. Projected costs for nursing home care alone are estimated at $92.9 billion in 1995 and $147 billion by 2000 (American Association of Retired Persons, 1993).

Contrary to popular belief and the expectations of patients and families, Medicare covers very little of the cost of services needed for chronic care. Moreover, the since-rescinded Medicare catastrophic-care legislation never included meaningful long-term care benefits, but much of the public at large conceived that it did. Neither Medicare nor medigaps pay for long-term nursing-home or home health care. In 1984 Medicare paid only 2% of all nursing home costs. Medicaid is the major payer of long-term care, absorbing nearly one half of all expenditures, but, as already noted, there are stringent income and asset eligibility standards.

The process whereby individuals deplete their assets to reach the Medicaid eligibility level is called spending down. In the process of "spending down," families ultimately bear about one half of all long-term institutional-care expenses and, frequently, the aged are impoverished before the Medicaid program provides assistance. Private long-term care insurance has been emerging as one solution to this dilemma. Yet these insurance policies, to be discussed later, currently pay an insignificant 1% of the total long-term care bill.

## THE NEED FOR NEW APPROACHES TO LONG-TERM CARE FINANCING

The aged and their families face substantial financial risks for long-term care expenses. Nursing-home care represents their largest single out-of-pocket health-care cost.

The problem of paying for long-term care has been exacerbated by public and private programs that have been designed primarily to cover skilled medical care for acute illness, as previously described. Little coverage has been designed for the costs associated with chronic conditions afflicting the aged (Willing & Neuchler, 1982). Those payment sources that do exist (e.g., Medicaid) favor provision of benefits in nursing homes despite the preference of many aged to remain at home or in noninstitutional settings. Moreover, a combination of spiraling health-care costs and a substantial federal deficit have made policymakers reluctant to implement new benefits to address chronic illness and long-term care needs. Finally, existing benefit programs, particularly Medicare and Medicaid, are poorly coordinated, creating access and continuity-of-care problems for the aged. These biases toward acute care and institutional services, as well as the overall poor coordination among programs are well documented (Piktialis, 1986).

### *Impact on the Aged and on Family Caregivers*

The impact of current long-term care financing on the aged and their families is often catastrophic. The magnitude of the burden can best be seen in the case of the Alzheimer's disease patient. Three case studies follow. These cases, prepared by the Massachusetts Chapter of the Alzheimer's disease and Related Disorders Association, Inc., are hypothetical, but are considered typical.*

### CASE 1

Mrs. F, a widow whose sole source of income is Social Security, resided in a small, rent-controlled building with no relatives nearby. Her only son, a merchant mariner, lived in Seattle. Her brother lived in Florida, and her sister and brother-in-law, both in poor health, were an hour away by automobile, although they spoke almost daily by telephone. Mrs. F had friends in the neighborhood and often visited the senior center.

Mrs. F first became confused at age 81 after the death of her husband but was able to

---

*Case study material was prepared in 1985 by the Massachusetts Chapter, Alzheimer's Disease and Related Disorders Association under the supervision of Executive Director Joan Hyde.

maintain herself with little outside help for 2 years. Then she began to lock herself out of her apartment, forgot to pay several utility bills, and experienced difficulty shopping and cooking. At first, her friends helped, but her accusations and hostility led them to stop. Eventually, a neighbor and a staff member at the senior center helped her apply for and receive some case management and home-care services, including home-delivered "meals on wheels."

These arrangements had only been in effect 3 months when Mrs. F slipped on an icy street and fell. She was taken to the hospital and found to have only minor injuries. However, as she was agitated and confused, she was admitted, evaluated, and diagnosed as having senile dementia of the Alzheimer's type.

The hospital discharge planning department reviewed the case with her case manager and discharge to a nursing home was arranged. However, Mrs. F remained in the hospital for 5 days, 2 beyond that necessary for diagnosis. This was necessary to complete paperwork and find an available bed for a Medicaid-funded patient.

Mrs. F remained in the nursing home until her death 5 years later.

## CASE 2

Mr. and Mrs. S owned their own home and had $65,000 in savings when Mr. S was forced to take early retirement at age 63 because of increased confusion and forgetfulness at work. For the first 2 years after his retirement, Mr. S was able to stay home alone during the day while Mrs. S was at work. During this period, he was evaluated and followed at an outpatient unit of a major hospital, where he was diagnosed as having Alzheimer's disease. In order to take him to the doctor and to check on him more frequently at lunch time, Mrs. S began to take progressively more time from work and, finally, like her husband, had to retire earlier than planned.

At first, Mr. S could be left alone for 2 or 3 hours at a time. However, by the end of her first year at home, Mrs. S found that she was housebound round the clock, as he had become increasingly confused. Not eligible for home-care services, she hired a series of companions and nurses' aides through agencies and friends at an average cost of $6 per hour to provide respite care. Their children took turns staying with Mr. S on Sunday afternoons. At first, needed respite care totaled 8 hours per week. This rose slowly until, at the end of 2 years, Mrs. S was paying for 16 hours a week for service, not only for respite, but increasingly to assist her in the care of her husband.

Five years after onset of the disease, Mr. S could no longer dress, shave, or bathe himself, and he was occasionally incontinent. He began to have difficulty walking. It required two people to bathe and dress him properly in the morning and to get him through the difficult early evening hours, when he tended to become agitated and had difficulty eating dinner. Mrs. S then hired two workers, one for mornings and the other for evenings, to assist her in caring for her husband. The evening worker came two additional afternoons each week so that Mrs. S could go out. One of their children came Saturday afternoon, and the other came on Sunday.

After a year of this, Mrs. S hurt her back while struggling to help her husband from the toilet and was confined to bed for 2 weeks with medication. Her children took time off from work to stay with them but, by the end of the week, it was clear she would not be able to continue to care for her husband at home. At that point, the family arranged to place him in a nursing home.

On the advice of her attorney, Mrs. S had transferred half her savings from their joint account into her name. She had used $15,000 to pay for home care. His remaining $25,000, along with his pension and government benefits paid the first year and $12,500 of the second year which was spent in the nursing home, and Medicaid picked up the remaining $5,500. At the end of his second year in the nursing home, Mr. S died at age 71.

## CASE 3

Mrs. P was a widow living in her own modest home supported by SSI and a small pension. Her married daughter lived nearby. When, at age 68, she became markedly confused and forgetful, her daughter and son-in-law insisted she come to live with them. They arranged a durable power of attorney, helped her sell her house, and built an addition onto their home, providing Mrs. P with her own bedroom and bathroom. After paying for the addition, which her son-in-law built, in part with his own labor to keep down costs, her life savings, including the proceeds from the sale of her house, totaled $70,000.

Before leaving for work in the morning, her daughter helped her dress and left a prepared lunch. The 12-year-old twin grandchildren returned from school at 3:00 P.M. and were instructed to stay with their grandmother until the return of their parents. Although Mrs. P often forgot where she was, she was calmed by calling her daughter at work and seemed generally satisfied with her new living arrangements.

However, after a year in the house her behavior became more unmanageable. Her family decided to consult a physician. After several attempts to get a definitive evaluation, Mrs. P was diagnosed as having Alzheimer's disease.

Her daughter then cut back her work schedule so she could dress and feed her mother in the morning and allow herself one day each week to complete all the extra housework, arrange appointments with doctors, and make telephone calls related to her mother's condition. However, after Mrs. P let water boil out of the kettle for the second time while left alone at lunch, her daughter arranged for a neighbor to prepare the noon meal in her home every day. All expenses other than lunch delivered by a neighbor were paid by her daughter and son-in-law. Meanwhile, her assets had grown to $80,000.

After a year of strain on the family, the daughter found a day care center for her mother. The cost, including transportation, consumed the entire income from Mrs. P's government and pension checks, but this care allowed the daughter to return to work on a full-time basis. After 2 years in day care, Mrs. P fell and fractured her hip. She spent 2 weeks in the hospital, where she could not learn to use a walker. After consultation with the family and the day care center, Mrs. P was discharged to a nursing home as a private-paying patient, where she remained until her death 2 years later. By that time, her savings were nearly depleted, and her daughter was looking into application for Medicaid.

The prevalence of financial devastation is thought to be widespread among all aged. A recent House Select Committee report presented two Massachusetts studies that showed a strong likelihood of impoverishment among the aged with chronic, disabling illnesses (U.S. House of Representatives, 1985). These studies found that 46% of those aged 75 and over would be impoverished after only 13 weeks in a nursing home, while 63% of those aged 65 to 74 would reach the stage of poverty within the same period. Both studies found that spouses of patients placed in nursing homes experienced impoverishment within a similar period of time.

## FINANCING ALTERNATIVES FOR LONG-TERM CARE

Given the absence of either a public or private financing system to protect the aged against the costs of long-term care, policymakers have begun to address the issue of how to finance such long-term care. However, the public has become increasingly confused as various proposals have been put forth to address "catastrophic care needs," which, in fact, expand coverage only to acute and, typically, hospital-based services. Thus there is a distinct difference between highly publicized "catastrophic care" provisions of Medicare that were ultimately rescinded and other proposed legislation and proposals to address the catastrophe faced by families burdened with the real costs of long-term, chronic care for aged relatives.

### Expansion of Existing Programs

Some have suggested financing long-term care through a substantial expansion of existing public programs. The Harvard University Medicare Project recommended expanding Medicare to cover nursing-home care, while at the same time, expanding covered benefits for outpatient mental health and home care (Harvard Medicare Project, 1986). This proposal also addresses new payment mechanisms, including premiums and other payments from beneficiaries, payroll taxes, and general government revenues. Among frequent items before Congress has been a proposal initiated by the late Rep. Claude D. Pepper (D. Fla.) and his successor legislative advocates for the aged to establish a Medicare program covering long-term care. In spite of many proposals, federal and state policymakers continue to be preoccupied by fiscal constraints, and public long-term care benefits that extend beyond those services already covered in part by Medicare are unlikely in the near future.

### Long-Term Care Insurance

Others have looked to private, long-term care insurance as a solution to paying for chronic care for the aged. The U.S. Department of Health and Human Services (DHHS) has suggested private long-term care insurance as a mechanism for financing catastrophic costs and controlling Medicaid expenditures (U.S. Department of Health and Human Services, 1986). The consolidated Omnibus Reconciliation Act of 1985 (COBRA) created a special task force to study this approach. Nevertheless, private long-term care insurance is likely to remain only a partial solution for some time to come because few insurers offer policies, and costs are prohibitive for most older persons (Piktialis, 1986).

By 1991 the number of policies sold was about 1.7 million (William M. Mercer, Inc., 1991). However, a study released by the Families USA Foundation estimated that only one of six older persons could afford to purchase a policy from private insurors (National Report on Work and Families, 1990).

Those private insurance policies currently on the market provide limited coverage and often have very restrictive waiting periods before reimbursement begins, exclusions for preexisting conditions which limit payments, prior hospitalization requirements, and other limitations to reduce risks to insurers. Moreover, insurers have been and will continue to be reluctant to enter this market because of rating and actuarial problems, adverse selection, uncertain market demand, and government regulatory issues (Piktialis, 1986). With little experience on potential utilization of nursing-home and other long-term care benefits under a private coverage system, it is difficult to predict accurately the extent to which these policies will be required to pay for services.

Even if private insurance became widely available, it has been estimated that private policies will still show only a modest impact on home health and Medicaid expenditures because they will be expensive (Weiner, 1987).

The total cost of long-term care is so great that many have suggested that no one payer can or should assume full responsibility for it (Piktialis, 1986; Sommers, 1987). This responsibility must be shared by the public and private sectors through multiple sources, including personal savings, family resources, private insurance, and state and local assistance. Sommers (1987) has suggested, as a guiding principle, a model whereby the federal government assumes a position of leadership in setting policy, but in a way that encourages, rather than supplants or undercuts, state or private innovations.

The resolution of this financing dilemma is yet to be seen. Undoubtedly, it will involve the cooperation of government, the insurance industry, the aged community, and the public at large. Meanwhile, it is likely to surface in many other health-care debates, particularly as catastrophic care captures greater public attention.

## CATASTROPHIC HEALTH INSURANCE

Beginning in 1986, public interest in insurance plans that would safeguard against the costs of catastrophic illness among the aged soared in the United States. President Ronald Reagan endorsed a report of the Department of Health and Human Services Secretary, Dr. Otis Bowen, proposing insurance for catastrophic health-care costs (U.S. Department of Health and Human Services, 1986). This initiated a legislative process that lead to the adoption of the Medicare Catastrophic Coverage Act of 1988. However, debate around catastrophic care obscured important differences in the definition and scope of the problem. Sommers (1987) has likened the push for catastrophic coverage to the excitement that surrounded the debate for a national health insurance in the late 1960s and early 1970s.

Issues that highlighted the policy deliberations on long-term care included: (1) whether the protection should be provided for long-term care in addition to acute care; (2) the scope of expanded acute-care services to be included; (3) whether coverage should extend to all aged or only to elders in low-income categories without Medicare supplementary coverage; and (4) financing the expanded program.

The scope of the 1988 legislation was limited and failed to address many concerns of those seeking to cover meaningful levels of long-term care. The term *catastrophic* has confused the public at large. Where Medicare coverage now extends to those acute-care services for catastrophic illness, that program does not protect the aged and their families from the financial catastrophe of having to shoulder the burden of long-term, chronic illness and nursing-home institutionalization.

The recission of Medicare catastrophic benefits and the subsequent escalation of long-term care costs has led to pessimism over the ability of the federal health care reform initiative, a major effort of the Clinton Administration, to incorporate long-term care benefits.

## MANAGED CARE: THE HMOS AND OTHER ALTERNATIVES

In the early 1980s, public policymakers began to examine alternative health-care systems to rectify the multitude of problems that made the Medicare and Medicaid programs ineffective in meeting the needs of the aged: the fragmentary nature of both programs, coverage limitations, and a bias toward institutional services that created problems of availability and continuity of care (Schlag & Piktialis, 1987).

### Health Maintenance Organizations

Reflecting a trend in federal health policy, the health maintenance organization (HMO) was promoted. The HMO combines both a prepaid health insurance plan and a comprehensive array of health-care providers. In an HMO, providers are under contract to deliver specific health services to enrolled members for a prepaid, fixed payment. Providers are, therefore, at economic risk and do not have incentives to provide unnecessary care.

Early proponents of HMO programs for the aged argued that these health plans were better suited to provide care to an older population than the traditional health-care system (Bonnano & Wetle, 1984; U.S. Senate Special Committee on Aging, 1981). Commonly, the aged rely on multiple health programs requiring treatment by different types of health professionals. The HMO can provide a delivery system offering a continuum of care, a single delivery source, and better coordination of services. The financial incentives to control costs may support the use of less intrusive and costly interventions that, in some cases, may be beneficial for older patients (Bonnano & Wetle, 1984). Centralized patient information allows the monitoring of polypharmacy, the prescribing of multiple medications that is necessary for many aged. HMOs may also function as a focal point for coordination with other acute- and nonacute-care providers in the community and may promote access to an even broader continuum of care for the aged (Schlag & Piktialis, 1987). Finally, HMOs have been promoted by cost-conscious federal and state policymakers since they have historically been considered a more efficient health-delivery system than traditional fee-for-service medicine in terms of cost and provision of services (Beebe, Lubitz, & Eggers, 1985).

Despite the support among many segments of the health-care community, HMOs have played an insignificant role in health care of the aged until recently because Medicare reimbursement policies were considered inadequate to the HMO industry. Between 1978 and 1985 the HCFA developed several demonstration projects to test prospective capitation, and, by March of 1985, about 300,000 Medicare beneficiaries were enrolled as HMO members.

These experiments were considered successful enough that, in February 1985, the federal government issued regulations under the Tax Equity and Fiscal Responsibility Act of 1982 (TEFRA, PL 97–248), allowing HMOs nationwide to offer Medicare programs under federal contracting standards. On April 1, 1985, the final regulations implementing TEFRA became effective, and by late 1987, more than 150 HMOs had Medicare programs enrolling over 850,000 members. Though this indicates significant growth over prior years, Medicare enrollment in HMOs is still limited to about 3% of the aged population. Expansion of prepaid health programs for the aged is expected well into the 1990s.

As HMO programs have received increased attention, policymakers have raised concerns about whether they can fulfill earlier expectations. The single most important policy issue is how well HMOs can balance quality and the cost of health care. Since providers must deliver specific services for a fixed, prepaid amount, they do not have incentives to provide unnecessary services. The HMO, however, must protect against providing too few services as well, and it should provide its members with ready access to the services they need (Schlag & Piktialis, 1987). A second problem is the belief that many HMOs are "skimming" by consciously recruiting and enrolling from among the healthiest aged.

Dangers previously hypothetical became real when the largest Medicare HMO program, International Medical Centers (IMC) in Miami, was fraught with scandal. In 1986, IMC was found to be $22 million in debt, plagued by bad management, and providing inferior care to its 135,000 Medicare members (Stevens, 1987). While the HMO industry and HCFA claimed this was an isolated case, Congress has passed special legislation to tighten controls over HMOs. One measure would prohibit inappropriate incentives to physicians that reward doctors financially for inappropriately limiting patient utilization. Another brought HMOs under Medicare peer review programs that were under supervision of federally authorized professional review organizations (PROs) and had, up to that time, monitored fee-for-service inpatient care.

Perhaps a greater deterrent to HMO growth is widespread dissatisfaction among the managed-care plans with the level of federal reimbursement to Medicare programs. U.S. Healthcare, for example, a large independent practice-model HMO based along the Northeast Corridor, withdrew its unprofitable Medicare HMO programs from the New Jersey market area in 1988.

Reimbursement is based on the average cost of providing services in the same areas as the HMO, adjusted for demographic characteristics of Medicare beneficiaries in each individual program. This payment is called the adjusted average per capita cost (AAPCC). The HMO receives 95% of the AAPCC and is expected to achieve its 5% savings through efficient management of care. Once in the program, many HMOs have discovered that caring for the aged costs far more than they had anticipated. Moreover, reimbursements were trimmed further through the implementation of the Gramm-Rudman budget-balancing reductions that impacted federal programs across the board. Ten HMO programs, with a combined Medicare membership of over 30,000 members, had dropped out of the program by mid-1987 (Stevens, 1987).

The federal government has recognized that reimbursement issues may hold the key to the success of Medicare HMO programs on a national scale and is attempting to support growth of Medicare HMOs by correcting flaws in the AAPCC formula. In fact, the Bush administration began serious consideration of a 100% AAPCC reimbursement formula in 1990 and directed Edmund Moy, Director of the Office of Prepaid Health Care, to make a demonstrative effort to reach out to HMOs and preferred-provider organizations (PPOs) to identify concerns and propose a mutually agreeable solution.

*Other Alternatives*

In addition to HMO alternatives, the federal government is encouraging other forms of pre-payment for medical care because of the potential for cost containment (Davis & Rowland, 1986). For example, the Reagan administration considered a controversial Medicare voucher proposal that was characterized by some as the logical expansion of the current HMO program. Another proposal would have expanded the types of health-care providers eligible to receive prepaid reimbursement to include private insurance companies and preferred-provider organizations. (PPOs are similar to HMOs in that they rely on elements of managed care to control costs. However, PPOs vary in that they allow members to receive care outside the authorized provider network, but at a lower rate of reimbursement.)

An additional proposal still under development in 1988 was called the Employer At Risk program, which would provide prepayment to employers for retiree groups. These last two options have features commonly considered "managed care." For example, they allow providers an opportunity to share in financial risk and savings in return for controlling the providers that treat patients and manage the volume of medical services.

Regardless of the particular form it takes, Medicare prepayment is likely to grow beyond the present scope of HMO programs and to affect providers and the aged in ways similar to HMOs. Other financing alternatives that have been studied to date include the development of social/health maintenance organizations (SHMOs), which incorporate long-term care services into the prepaid comprehensive health format.

Continuing-care retirement communities (CCRCs), which combine residential settings and social services, have seen significant growth in recent years, although the cost of such developments have put them out of the reach of most aged.

Financing alternatives have also included the establishment of individual medical accounts (IMAs), similar to individual retirement accounts (IRAs), with the provision that funds could be withdrawn to pay for health-care expenses. Critics of this format have noted that one result of IMAs could be oversaving since most people will not experience a costly extended stay in a nursing home (Rivlin & Weiner, 1988).

Finally, conversion of home equity into funds for health-care costs for the aged has been explored.

## QUALITY OF CARE: A GROWING CONCERN

Increasingly, health care in the United States is being described as private business (Relman, 1987). Pressures to contain costs emanate from insurers and third-party payers, both government and private. At the local level, physicians and hospitals are being forced to act more businesslike in order to survive financially. This transformation has been supported by the federal government as the best method for allocating health-care resources and containing costs.

Relman (1987) has noted the impact of economic imperatives on the doctor-patient relationship. A physician faces the difficult task of caring for patients who are viewed as customers by business entities with which the physician has ties. The interests of the patient and priorities of the business world are often not congruent.

Practicing medicine in this financial climate raises inevitable questions about quality of care. At the heart of the debate is the ability of the health-care provider to assure high quality now that economic incentives have been introduced into the clinical arena. Many unresolved questions remain and are the subject of considerable ongoing study. Will physicians afford Medicare patients the same access they provide others? Will older patients be rushed out of hospitals in an effort to keep costs under DRG allowances in order to generate excess revenues? Can HMOs maintain high quality in a managed-care setting under a capitated payment scheme? Are providers accurately describing the advantages *and* disadvantages of HMOs to all prospective members? Will federal budget crises undermine quality of care in the Medicare program by forcing reductions in services, lowering reimbursement to providers, and discouraging physicians and others from caring for the aged?

Threats to quality of care for the aged also raise important ethical issues. Wetle (1985, 1987) has suggested a taxonomy of such issues relevant to geriatric care which includes the individual, family, service providers, and the health-care system as a whole. She describes numerous "assaults on autonomy" of the aged. Autonomy is defined as "the individual's right to make decisions which are voluntary or intentional, and not the result of coercion, duress or undue influence" (Wetle, 1987). Examples of ethical issues faced commonly are: failure to discuss a full range of clinical options with older persons; exclusion of the older person from clinical decision making; involvement of children in decision making as having priority judgments when parents may still be competent to decide; and establishment of a lower priority for treatment for the aged patient.

Particularly germane to a treatment of the economics of health care are those value judgments that impact on the system's level and provide the framework for social policy. For example, they influence the allocation of resources within the health-care system and affect the enactment and enforcement of laws and regulations governing the health-care system (Wetle, 1985).

Health-care financing in the United States is at a turning point. Public opinion and government policy will determine whether the current commercialism will continue. Already, many experts are predicting a return to more active government involvement in regulation (Fuchs, 1987; Ginsberg, 1987). At stake is the preservation of the advances gained in access to health care for the aged resulting from Medicare, Medicaid, and the extension of those programs.

Within the realm of possibility is the crafting of an even better financing system that can add rationality to arrangements that have proved inadequate as the age structure of American society has changed. Such a system of the future should be based on clearly defined policies that reflect societal values accurately. However, it is difficult to establish consensus among the public at large as to what these values should be when such a large portion of the population fails to perceive that problems of financing, service delivery, access to caregivers and providers, and quality of services exist.

CONCLUSION

The system of health-care for the aged is financed by a complex array of public and private insurance programs and, frequently, by the aged and their families. Identification of problems in this financing is not a new phenomenon. Coverage limitations, poor coordination of services between programs, access problems, and substantial out-of-pocket costs are discussed widely in the literature and are real problems faced daily by the aged, their families, and clinicians. While a lengthy discussion of health-care economics and financing programs may seem far removed from clinical geriatric issues, it provides an important framework for understanding how financial arrangements can affect patient management, as evidenced in the case studies presented in this work.

## REFERENCES

American Association of Retired Persons. (1993). *The AARP public policy agenda: Toward a just and caring society* (p. 191). Washington, DC: Author.

Beebe, J., Lubitz, J., & Eggers, P. (1985). Using prior utilization to determine payments to Medicare enrollees in health maintenance organizations. *Health Care Financing Review, 16,* 27–50.

Bonnano, J. B., & Wetle, T. (1984). HMO enrollment of Medicare recipients: An analysis of incentives and barriers. *Journal of Health Politics, Policy and Law, 9,* 41–62.

Commonwealth of Massachusetts. (1985). *The Governor's Committee on Alzheimer's Disease: Final Report.* Boston, MA: Author.

Davis, K., & Rowland, D. (1986). *Medicare Policy: New Directions for Health and Long Term Care.* Baltimore, MD: The Johns Hopkins University Press.

Easterbrook, G. (1987, January). The revolution in medicine. *Newsweek,* 40–74.

87's the year for action of health care catastrophe. (1987, March). *AARP News Bulletin,* p. 1.

Fuchs, V. R. (1987). The Counterrevolution in Health Care Financing. *The New England Journal of Medicine, 316*(18), 1154–1156.

General Accounting Office. (1986a). *An aging society — Meeting the needs of the elderly while responding to rising federal costs.* (p. 38). Washington, DC: General Accounting Office.

General Accounting Office. (1986b). *Medigap Insurance — Law has increased protection against substandard and overpriced policies.* Washington, DC: General Accounting Office.

General Accounting Office. (1987). *Medicare and Medicaid: Effects of recent legislation on program and beneficiary costs.* Washington, DC: General Accounting Office.

Ginsberg, E. (1987). A hard look at cost containment. *The New England Journal of Medicine, 316*(18), 1151–1154.

Louis Harris & Associates, Inc. (1986). *Problems Facing Elderly Americans Living Alone,* Report for the Commonwealth Fund, Commission on Elderly People Living Alone. (pp. 3–5). New York: Author.

Harvard Medicare Project, (1986). *Medicare coming of age: A proposal for reform.* Center for Health Policy and Management & Division of Health Policy Research and Education, Harvard University, Cambridge, MA.

Kennel, D. (1985). *The role of Medicare in financing the health care of older Americans.* Report Prepared for the American Association of Retired Persons. Washington, DC: IFC Incorporated.

Manton, K., & Liu, C. (1986). *The Future Growth of Long Term Care: Trends and Projections.* Report of AARP to U.S. Senate Special Committee on Aging. Washington, DC: American Association of Retired Persons.

Many elderly can't afford long term care insurance. (1990, February). *The National Report on Work and Family.* Washington, DC.

Marmor, T. R. (1973). *The politics of Medicare.* (revised American ed., pp. 70–81). Hawthorne, NY: Aldine.

William M. Mercer, Inc. (1991). *Long term care insurance: An emerging employee benefit* (pp. 1–3). New York: Marsh & McLennan.

Piktialis, D. (1986). Private long term care insurance: A partial solution. *Journal of Azheimer's Care and Related Disorders. 1*(1), 37–43.

Pollard, M. R., & Paradise, J. (1987), Medicare physician participation. *Health Affairs, 6*(2), 107–120.

Prospective Payment Assessment Commission. (1987). *Medicare prospective payment and the American health care system — Report to the Congress* (pp. 63–73).

Relman, A. (1987). Practicing medicine in the new business climate. *The New England Journal of Medicine, 316*(18), 1150–1151.

Rice, T., & Gabel, J. (1986). Protecting the elderly against high health care costs. *Health Affairs, 5,*(3), 7.

Rivlin, A. M., & Weiner, J. M. (1988). *Caring for the disabled elderly. Who will pay?* (pp. 16–20). Washington, DC: The Brookings Institute.

Schlag, W., & Piktialis, D. (1987). Health maintenance organizations and the elderly: The potential for vertical integration of geriatric care. *Quality Review Bulletin, 13* (4), 140–147.

Schottland, C. I., (1970). *The Social Security program in the United States.* New York: Appleton Century Crofts.

Sommers, A. (1987). Insurance for long term care, *The New England Journal of Medicine, 317*(1), 23–28.

Stevens, C. (1987, May). Why HMOs are dumping Medicare. *Medical Economics,* pp. 54–59.

U.S. Department of Health and Human Services. (1986). *Catastrophic illness expenses. Report to the president.* Washington, DC: Author.

U.S. House of Representatives, Committee on Ways and Means. (1993). *Health care resource book* (pp. 57–63). Washington, DC: US Government Printing Office.

U.S. House of Representatives Select Committee on Aging. (1985). *America's elderly at risk, a report.* Washington, DC: U.S. Government Printing Office.

U.S. Senate Special Committee on Aging. (1981). *Medicare reimbursement to competitive medical plans: Hearing before the Special Committee on Aging.* Washington, DC: U.S. Government Printing Office.

U.S. Senate Special Committee on Aging. (1991). *Aging America: Trends and projections* (pp. 146, 175). Washington, DC: U.S. Department of Health and Human Services.

Weiner, J. (1987). *Modeling long term care insurance for the elderly: The case of private insurance.* Paper presented at a conference on long term care insurance, San Antonio, TX.

Wetle, T. (1985). Long term care: A taxonomy of issues. *Generations, 10*(2), 30–34.

Wetle, T. (1987). *Ethical Issues.* Unpublished paper, Division of Health Policy Research and Education, Harvard University, Boston.

Wetle, T. (1988). The social and service context of geriatric care. In J. Rowe & R. Besdine, (Eds.), *Geriatric medicine* (2nd ed.). Boston: Little, Brown.

White House Conference on Aging. (1982). *Final Report of the 1981 White House Conference on Aging.* (Vol. 1, pp. 68–86). Washington, DC: U.S. Government Printing Office.

Willing, P., & Neuschler, E. (1982). Debate continues on future of federal financing of long term care. *Hospitals, 56*(13), 61–64.

# III

# Theoretical Issues of Interdisciplinary Education and Practice

Part III of the text presents theory, technique, and values that apply to geriatric health care in general.

Chapter 14, The Interdisciplinary, Integrated Approach to Professional Practice with the Aged, develops models of working relationship among the health care disciplines. David Satin, a geriatric and community psychiatrist, explores the factors that affect how professionals relate in geriatric practice and the ways these relationships influence the care professionals give. He presents a range of working relationships and clinical examples. Finally, he discusses the costs and benefits of the interdisciplinary model and the settings in which it is worthwhile, at the same time identifying the characteristics of health professions and health care institutions that facilitate or impede interdisciplinary practice.

Chapter 15, Developing the Interdisciplinary Team, examines the characteristics critical to team development and functioning, and proposes methods of dealing with them. Benjamin Siegel, a primary-care physician, speaks from his experience with a variety of health care teams to give practical recommendations about their inner workings as well as how to make such teams more effective and durable.

Chapter 16, Attitudes, Values, and Ideologies as Influences on the Professional Education and Practice of Those Who Care for the Aged, addresses the beliefs and perspectives that drive health care professionals. Lisa Gurland, nurse, social worker, psychologist, and clinical health care consultant, presents a careful analysis of motivations and then applies it to research findings about differences between health care disciplines and practitioners in differential clinical settings. She reminds us forcefully that these personal perspectives influence the health care the aged receive in major and very practical ways, and raises unsettling concerns over how health care decisions are made.

As part of an interdisciplinary perspective on theoretical issues of interdisciplinary education and practice, Jennifer Bottomley, a physical therapist, notes that, in keeping with our goal throughout this book, we continue to address disease, treatment, and people from a holistic point of view. We look at the interdisciplinary team as an effective model for treating people in this manner, dealing with the multiple changes in people's internal systems that occur with aging and helping the aged achieve their highest level of functioning.

David Satin offers the physician and psychiatrist's observation that clinical caregivers and institutions, like other segments of society, are motivated by attitudes, values, and ideologies. We must become aware of the way these affect what we teach, practice, and encourage in students, patients, and colleagues, and in the ways we direct and license other professionals to practice. The education of health care professionals clearly has a role to play here, as well as the policies of caregiving institutions in promoting and implementing forms of disciplinary working relationships that provide the best care for the aged. Professional societies and legal entities, as guardians of accrediting standards, licensing regulations, and evaluation of clinical practice, are responsible for implementing quality controls that promote the best kind of practice, which, in our opinion, must include an interdisciplinary component.

Satin continues that, aside from attitudes, values, and ideologies, the way professionals work together affect the way we conceptualize the aged and their health problems, and the kind of care we give. The structure of caregiving institutions powerfully influences the way professionals in these settings work with one another as well as the kind of care they give. The policies, practices, organizational hierarchies, and even the architecture of health care institutions have great impact on what can and cannot be done and on what collaboration among professionals is encouraged or discouraged. Therefore, it behooves professionals and caregiving institutions to pay attention to these working relationships and change detrimental influences to create the most effective environments for delivering health care. Helen Smith, as an occupational therapist, adds the observation that health care disciplines need to be more flexible in communicating and exchanging information. Through interdisciplinary courses students from different disciplines have the opportunity to work together and become aware of one another's skills, and graduates want and expect to practice in an interdisciplinary fashion. This has an impact on the way health care workers interact and on the health care system as a whole. Margot Howe, also from occupational therapy, agrees that, because of the multiplicity of problems the aged present, they are prime candidates for interdisciplinary team treatment.

# 14

# The Interdisciplinary, Integrated Approach to Professional Practice with the Aged

David G. Satin

"Interdisciplinary" is a recently popularized concept that has different meanings in various health education and practice settings. Many training programs and treatment agencies describe themselves as "interdisciplinary." Funding agencies may make support contingent on the use of an interdisciplinary model, and grants are given to study or teach an interdisciplinary approach to health care issues.

Despite all the apparent enthusiasm and rationale, there is serious question about what is actually taught and practiced. The term "interdisciplinary" is used to refer to a wide variety of practices involving more than one health profession (Ducanis & Golin, 1978). It may be applied to a project to which several departments have subscribed only for appearances and in which they do not, in fact, collaborate; to a program in which the various professions are polite to one another while they pursue their separate activities; or to the attention and discussion that a mixed professional group gives to reports by disciplinary subgroups. Conversely, a variety of terms are applied to the same type of activity, sometimes interchangeably or in combination in the same discussion. "Interdisciplinary," "multidisciplinary," "collaborative," and "team" are the more commonly used terms (Holm, 1978). Overall, it is very often hard to discern what characteristics of the activity the terms refer to, and to distinguish and label significant variations in practice.

Though much has been discussed and written about the preparation for interdisciplinary activities and their accomplishments, remarkably little attention has been given to a detailed understanding of the interdisciplinary approach to education and practice itself. If this approach is distinct and valuable, it is imperative that those who wish to practice it define it clearly, relate it to other collaborative approaches to health care, understand what is required to implement it, and determine appropriate applications. It is instructive that, in talking of team development, Rubin and Beckhard (1972) observed that

> Some conscious program that helps team members look at their particular goals, tasks, relationships, decision-making, norms, backgrounds and values is essential for team effectiveness. It is naive to bring together a highly diverse group of people and to expect that, by calling them a team, they will in fact behave as a team.

We here propose a conceptual framework clearly defining a range of model working relationships among disciplines, and, in the process, contrasting the interdisciplinary model with others. We also discuss applications of the various models—both their advantages and problems.

## CLARIFYING CONCEPTS

### Discipline

The term "discipline" is used to denote a profession or occupation whose knowledge, skills, practices, and values allow it to make a contribution distinct from that of other disciplines and whose theory, practice, and terminology is sufficiently different from those of other disciplines that serious effort is required to communicate and collaborate with them. Thus nursing and occupational therapy are examples of different disciplines. Major specialties within a single profession also may represent different disciplines, such as psychiatry and pediatrics within medicine. Minor differences in focus within the same profession, such as child and geriatric psychiatry, would not be considered separate disciplines, since they share a common foundation, and practitioners in both fields readily understand each other and interchange practices.

### Spheres of Competence

Disciplines have areas of competence (Devitt, 1970; Heilman, 1977). While the differences among them are real, it is from their historical traditions in relating to one another that disciplines derive their names, customs, and experiences. In addition, their self-interests spur them to claim and defend exclusive theoretical and practice territories for the sake of reinforcing identity, preserving status, safeguarding job opportunities, and maintaining economic security. However, in reality a range of expertise characterizes each discipline, as outlined in Table 14.1.

It is useful to conceptualize spheres of *primary competence*, in which one discipline

TABLE 14.1   Spheres of Disciplinary Competence

*Primary Competence*
Unique or superior expertise shared by few disciplines
Expert and sole practitioner or one of few practitioners
Sole consultant or trainer or one of few consultants and trainers

*Secondary Competence*
Useful expertise equaled by other disciplines
Effective practitioner
Problems referred to and training gained from discipline(s) with primary competence

*Tertiary Competence*
Little expertise
Not a practitioner except to give rudimentary help in emergencies
Refer all cases to disciplines with secondary or primary competence

has unique, or near-unique, expertise; functions as the sole or one of few practitioners; and acts as consultant and trainer to other disciplines practicing in this area. For example, psychoanalysis has primary competence in depth psychotherapy and personality change, social work has primary competence in the mobilization and coordination of community resources, and occupational therapy has primary competence in the evaluation and enhancement of the activities of daily living.

There are also spheres of *secondary competence,* in which several disciplines are effective but do not have the greatest expertise, and consult or refer special problems to a discipline or disciplines with primary competence when appropriate. For example, psychiatry, social work, clinical psychology, and pastoral counseling have secondary competence in ventilative and directive counseling; physical therapy, occupational therapy, and nursing have secondary competence in building physical strength and skill; and social work, pastoral counseling, and community/social psychology have secondary competence in advocacy.

Finally, there are spheres of *tertiary competence,* in which many disciplines have very little expertise and defer to those with secondary or primary competence, except when the latter are not readily available and temporary aid must be provided. For example, internal medicine, nursing, and physical therapy have tertiary competence in surgery; medicine, physical therapy, and pharmacy have tertiary competence in finding community resources; and psychiatry, social work, and pastoral counseling have tertiary competence in the analysis and reduction of physical dysfunction.

## A SPECTRUM OF MODELS OF DISCIPLINARY WORKING RELATIONSHIPS

Multiple disciplines with overlapping areas of competence when working with people, problems, or projects that have interdependent needs, may interrelate to varying degrees. Table 14.2 presents a proposed spectrum of disciplinary working relationships in order to designate significantly differing models.

### Unidisciplinary Model

According to the unidisciplinary model, each discipline plans, learns, and practices alone, without consideration of the nature of any other discipline. In some cases the unidisciplinary practitioner is not even aware of the existence of some other disciplines. Members of the discipline develop professionally within it; individual development of interests, competence, and professional relationships outside the discipline are considered idiosyncratic and nonprofessional. This model is common in private individual or single-discipline group clinical practice, and in many disciplinary education programs and institutions.

### CASE 1

Jules Vieillard, an 88-year-old, divorced man, lives alone in elderly housing. He complains that his vision has become poor. During an office visit, a private ophthalmologist takes a thorough history of his visual problems, asks briefly about recent hospitalizations and med-ications, performs a thorough eye examination and refraction, and recommends a slight change in his eyeglass prescription. The ophthalmologist does not take professional interest in or responsibility for Mr. Vieillard's recent confusion, suspiciousness, fearfulness, and accusations; recurrence of his chronic blood disease (polycythemia) and erratic contacts with the hematologists in his community hospital clinic; the concern of the police, public health social worker, and housing development manager; and the fact that eviction proceed-ings have been initiated and the local geriatric psychiatry program is involved.

## Paradisciplinary Model

According to the paradisciplinary model, each discipline plans, learns, and practices alone, but with knowledge of the involvement of other disciplines (although not their training, areas of competence, and professional roles). Reports or data may be exchanged, but the disciplines feel no need to relate to each other's practices or to share activities. Again, peo-ple develop professionally within their disciplines. This model is common in multidepart-

TABLE 14.2    A Spectrum of Models of Disciplinary Working Relationships

*Unidisciplinary*
Segregated disciplinary roles
Unaware of/uninterested in other disciplines
Plan, learn, and work alone
Competence, role, and identity developed within the discipline

*Paradisciplinary*
Segregated disciplinary roles
Aware of other disciplines but not their roles
Courteous but plan, learn, and work alone
Competence, role, and identity developed within the discipline

*Multidisciplinary*
Segregated disciplinary roles
Understand other disciplines and their roles
Plan together
Assign tasks by discipline
Learn and work alone, avoid intrusion on others' territories
Competence, role, and identity developed within the discipline

*Interdisciplinary*
Overlapping and flexible disciplinary roles
Understand other disciplines and their roles
Plan together
Assign tasks by competence — disciplinary, personal, and situational
Learn and work in combinations determined by tasks and participants
Competence, role, and identity modified by experience, interests, and contact with other disciplines

*Pandisciplinary*
A single disciplinary role spanning the areas of competence relevant to the field of endeavor
Concerned with other disciplines only as contributors of training in their areas of competence
Pandiscipline assumes all tasks
Plan, learn, and work alone
Competence, role, and identity developed within the discipline

mental hospitals and clinics, and in multispecialty group clinical practices in which patients are referred from one unit to another, accompanied only by a referral note or medical record.

## CASE 2

Anna Del Vecchio, an 86-year-old widow, is brought by her family to the General Internal Medicine Clinic of a prestigious teaching hospital so that their mother/grandmother might get the best of care. Here brittle diabetes mellitus is diagnosed and careful treatment and monitoring are undertaken. A full examination reveals dense cataracts in both eyes. Consequently, she is also referred to the ophthalmology clinic, where the diagnosis is confirmed. After review of the medical record one of the cataracts is removed with the latest laser procedure, and an artificial lens implanted, thus improving her ability to function. It is noted that her hearing, too, is impaired. Consequently, she is referred to the otology clinic, where careful evaluation reveals otosclerosis and mild sensorineural impairment. A hearing aid is tried, found beneficial, and fitted for permanent use. When the family reports to the medical clinic that Mrs. Del Vecchio has become withdrawn, irritable, and has made a feeble suicide attempt, she is referred to the geriatric psychiatry clinic, where a major depression is diagnosed. She is admitted to the inpatient psychiatry unit for observation and treatment with mood-elevating medications as well as individual and family psychotherapy. Thereafter, she has regular appointments (at varying intervals) at the general internal medicine, ophthalmology, otology, and geriatric psychiatry clinics, where notes are entered in her centralized medical record, with the record delivered to each clinic in time for her appointment.

### Multidisciplinary Model

The multidisciplinary model is most often misidentified as "interdisciplinary." The various disciplines intend to integrate their efforts on behalf of their patients and projects. They meet, share information, plan the approach to the problem, and decide who will be involved and what their contributions will be. However, the separate disciplines learn substantially alone except for peripheral experiences gained while coordinating with other disciplines. Work tasks are assigned strictly according to traditional concepts of disciplinary role. Each discipline practices independently, careful not to intrude on the identified territories of the others. Again, professional development takes place within the individual disciplines.

Most geriatric consultation teams function in this way, with team members performing the professional functions traditionally or institutionally identified with their disciplines. The traditional child psychiatry team is similar, with the psychiatrist treating the child, the social worker providing casework counseling to the parents, the psychologist administering and interpreting psychometric tests, and, in hospital, the nurse supervising daily activities and medications.

## CASE 3

Serious questions of dementia and spouse abuse have been raised about George and Alma Senior, a married couple in their 80s. The community agency social worker who has been working with them refers them to the highly regarded outpatient geriatric consultation team of a large academic research and referral hospital. An intake interview is completed by the geriatric nurse/team coordinator. Her report is discussed at the next team meeting and, after comments by some team members, the geriatric internist/team leader sets up a schedule of evaluations, designating team members to tasks for which their disciplines are approved by the hospital's professional credentialling committee: The Seniors are examined physically by the geriatric internist; referred for blood and urine laboratory studies to both the hematology and chemistry laboratories; referred to the diagnostic radiology department for CT scans of the head, which are routinely obtained for research and clinical purposes; interviewed about family, financial, and housing characteristics by one of the social workers assigned part-time to the team; and sent to the Geriatric Neuropsychology Research Project for a battery of neuropsychological and personality tests and a sociocultural survey that this project has developed for research and clincal purposes. The Seniors are put on the roster of cases to be discussed and, at the scheduled team meeting, team members present their findings; the reports of affiliated laboratories, departments, and units are paraphrased; and the Seniors' various problems and treatment approaches for them are tabulated. Finally, the nurse/team coordinator prepares a summary report, the internist/team leader countersigns it, and it is forwarded to the Seniors' local physician. The referring community agency social worker learns that the evaluation has been completed and receives fragmented impressions of its results from the Seniors during a home visit.

### Interdisciplinary Model

As indicated previously, the term "interdisciplinary" has been applied to many endeavors involving more than one discipline or subspecialty of a single discipline. In its stricter usage, the term defines the model of disciplinary working relationships in which learning, planning, and practice are all informed by an understanding of the overlap of disciplinary competence and the interrelationship of health issues (Blakeney, Bottomley, Howe, & Smith, 1988; Bottomley, Blakeney, O'Malley, Satin, Smith, & Howe, 1990).

The disciplines learn together. They meet to evaluate the problem to be dealt with, goals to be achieved, and interventions that will achieve these goals. Tasks are assigned not only on the basis of disciplinary competence but also personal expertise and the needs and circumstances of the problem being addressed. Disciplines may work individually or jointly. Moreover, roles and task assignments are not rigid but may shift as new needs are addressed or new resources brought into play. Administrative roles, too, are are assigned on the basis of competence and availability rather than disciplinary tradition (Satin, Barnard, Jette, & Howe, 1985). Finally, in this model disciplinary practice and identity are not confined within the disciplines of origin. They change and grow through exposure to other disciplines, experience, deepened insight into professional needs and practice, and encouragement of the talents and interests of individual professionals.

### CASE 4

The visiting nurse brings Molly Alter, a 78-year-old widow living alone in a second-floor apartment, to the attention of the neighborhood health center's geriatric service because her bizarre complaints have concerned and alienated her neighbors, her son, and the local police. The nurse attends a service meeting, where she describes Mrs. Alter's cataracts, hearing impairment, osteoarthritis, arteriosclerotic heart disease, many medications, loneliness, and hallucinations and delusions about a neighborhood boy breaking into her apartment, as well as her children's frustration in trying to help her while fulfilling their obligations to their own families and jobs. It is decided that the importance of Mrs. Alter's religious tradition in her life makes the pastoral counselor the person most likely to gain access to her to assess the situation and introduce other caregivers. The internist, occupational therapist, and pharmacist then visit together to evaluate her health status, functional capacity, and medication usage and effects, and to estimate her needs and plan helping interventions. The physician and pharmacist collaboratively develop a choice of medications and dosing regimen that will meet this patient's unique metabolic and behavioral needs. The occupational therapist teaches the internist and nurse about certain activities essential to the woman's successful functioning in her environment, the methods for strengthening them, and the assistive devices that will support them. The internist, nurse, and psychiatrist jointly develop goals and protocols for Mrs. Alter's physical and psychiatric care. The internist and nurse coordinate the contributions of other professionals and agencies. The social worker and pastoral counselor collaborate in increasing her social activities and supports. The pharmacist, physical therapist, psychologist, and nutritionist provide consultation in their various areas of primary competence to the other staff members. Case review and evaluation meetings are held every two weeks and include all service members. In the process, modification, expansion, and redirection of efforts are suggested to many of the service members. Decisions are made to obtain further services and staff training from an architect (regarding modification of the physical environment) and an attorney (regarding conservatorship, designation of a health care proxy, and the drawing of a will and trust).

### Pandisciplinary Model

Some educators have seen geriatrics/gerontology as a unitary discipline distinct from others, rather than an area of subspecialization within the traditional clinical disciplines. They conceive it as encompassing the areas of competence of social research and planning; education, advocacy, and governmental influence; as well as applied therapeutic evaluation and intervention. The implication is that this discipline has "primary competence" in all areas of aging, the geriatrician/gerontologist being the most expert trainer, consultant, and practitioner in the field. A significant and growing number of education programs — at bachelor's, master's, and doctoral levels — have been developed to prepare professionals in this discipline. Their charters and descriptive materials proclaim their innovation, authority, and leadership.

In the pandisciplinary model a single disciplinary role spans all areas of competence relevant to the field of aging and, in a sense, is segregated from the traditional clinical disciplines. Other relevant disciplines are understood only in terms of their contributions of training in those areas of their competence applicable to the pandiscipline. In the process of education, students of the pandiscipline and other disciplines may learn together from teachers of various relevant disciplines. However, the pandiscipline plans and works alone except as other disciplines may have preempted governing, administrative, legal sanctioning, or caregiving roles. Theoretically all tasks may be assigned to any member of the pandiscipline based on availability. Individuals who happen to have special interests or competence may be informally recognized.

## CASE 5

The gerontology service is called in by concerned neighbors and the city public health nurse to help Margaret Crone, a 78-year-old woman who lives as a recluse in her small house, eats little, is suspicious and intolerant of well-wishers who look in on her, and refuses medical care when ill. Her husband will no longer tolerate her unreasonable and nasty behavior and recently divorced her. Her children visit weekly to help with chores but are intimidated and helpless about changing the situation. A gerontologist has Mrs. Crone's son arrange access and evaluates her mental status, medical condition, nutritional state, and predominant needs and concerns. The gerontologist also surveys the house in terms of its accessibility and safety for Mrs. Crone and how it has been maintained. On the basis of this comprehensive evaluation, the gerontologist determines that the son should assume guardianship in order to facilitate care and arranges the services of an attorney who has the legal standing to carry this through. A geriatric psychiatrist must be recruited for the licensure and hospital staff appointment needed to arrange civil committment to the psychiatric unit in a community hospital for psychiatric, neuropsychological, and medical evaluation and prescription of antipsychotic medication. The gerontologist provides ongoing guidance and support for the children in arranging the necessary services for Mrs. Crone, provides supervision and guidance for her, arranges for home help to assist with bathing and homemaking during a brief return to her home after hospital treatment, and arranges for admission to a nursing home for long-term structured and supervised living.

## IMPLICATIONS

Geriatrics is certainly one of the fields in which multiple areas of competence are needed for the following reasons: The aged are more likely than other populations to have multiple health needs. The various systems related to health—physical, cognitive, emotional, interpersonal, and material—are probably more exquisitely interdependent and interresponsive than is the case with most other age groups. Because multiple health care disciplines and institutions are likely to be involved with the care and support of the aged, it is important to understand and structure the working relationships among these health disciplines—in the interests of the care of the aged patients, the effectiveness and satisfaction of the practitioners, and the preparation and competence of students in the health professions.

Three characteristics account for the differences among the working relationship models and the continuum along which they all lie: the awareness of and extent of knowledge about other disciplines, the degree to which the disciplines plan together, and role segregation. In the unidisciplinary model individuals know little or nothing about other disciplines and do not work with them. In the paradisciplinary model practitoners are little more involved, relating merely through the courteous exchange of information. In the multidisciplinary model participants know much about and plan extensively with other disciplines. However, it is important to note that in all these models the disciplines are strictly distinct and isolated: disciplinary roles are segregated conceptually and preserved operationally, and practitioners learn and work essentially alone (though other disciplines may contribute visiting lectures or ancillary services). It follows from this that competence and identity are developed entirely within the respective disciplines.

It is interesting to note that the pandisciplinary model, at the opposite extreme of the spectrum, is no different from the above models; if anything, it is among the most isolationist. The pandiscipline is distinct from the other, traditional disciplines. It may consider itself the *true* discipline in geriatrics and gerontology, and the others more or less dabblers in the field. Its very omnicompetence discourages learning, planning, and working with other disciplines, which can only contribute to its development and facilitate its work by providing legal sanction or institutional *entrée*. It knows of other disciplines only through these facilitating relationships. Because it is omnicompetent, work roles are assigned *within* the discipline and thus *by* discipline. By the same reasoning, competence and identity develop within the pandiscipline.

Several objections may be raised to this conception of a pandiscipline. First, there is serious question as to whether any one discipline can encompass in effective depth the expertise that is necessary to deal with the range of needs encountered in health care, especially with the aged. Second, a new discipline must prove its worth and establish its viability in both academic and practice environments in a way that (geriatric) subspecialties in established disciplines need not. Third, pride, suspicion, and self-interest are as powerful in the health field as in any other, and a new disciplinary competitor will face many institutional obstacles and much collegial opposition from established disciplinary empires (Satin, 1987). In all fairness it must be said that the "pandiscipline" of geriatrics/gerontology is new and tentative enough that a spectrum of transitional forms may exist. Various attempts at implementing it educationally and in clinical practice may involve much more interaction and overlap with other disciplines than this ideal model portrays.

The interdisciplinary model is qualitatively different from the others. First, it most consciously recognizes and conscientiously implements the overlap in spheres of competence among the disciplines. On one hand, it recognizes the unique and indispensable contributions of the various disciplines. On the other, it capitalizes on their interrelationship. Second, in comparison with the other models, interdisciplinary education and professional practice entails the most intimate and flexible working relationship among disciplines. Third, the interdisciplinary model entails the most extensive knowledge of the preparation, expertise, and responsibilities of other disciplines, respect for them, and an interest in sharing tasks and learning with them. Fourth, it is the only model in which tasks are assigned not solely by discipline, but by competence determined also by the personal characteristics of team members and the demands of the project at hand and its environment (Satin et al., 1985). Fifth, in interdisciplinary practice participants are flexible about the assignment of clinical, teaching, and administrative roles on the basis of the needs of the situation and the capabilities of the participants. Finally, it is the only model of disciplinary working relationship in which competence and identity are not developed solely within the parent disciplines but are also influenced by professional experience, personal talents and interests, and, most significantly, by contact with other disciplines. Thus, professional identities are more flexible and open to change. It should be noted that this extradisciplinary involvement and influence is one of the aspects of the interdisciplinary approach that is most threatening to the traditional (unidisciplinary) perspective on professional education and practice, posing the threat of loss of loyalty to the disciplinary group and adulteration of the disciplinary tradition.

The interdisciplinary educator must be able to articulate and demonstrate that it is both safe and beneficial to *share* knowledge and skills with other disciplines. It is even more important to make students comfortable in *accepting* knowledge, skills, and values from other disciplines and incorporating them into their own professional practices. It is critical that educators be secure enough in their disciplinary identities to demonstrate that they can modify them in response to education from other disciplines. (Whether disciplinary identity must be instilled before exposure to interdisciplinary sharing can be fruitful, or whether openness to interdisciplinary sharing must be built into disciplinary identity early is an issue addressed in detail elsewhere [Satin et al., 1985].) Students look to faculty as role models. Through exposure to demonstrations of their teachers' responsiveness to other disciplines, students will learn to be open to opportunities for enriching growth. Alternatively, exposure to faculty examples of closed and defensive reactions to other disciplines can teach rigid defensiveness; posessiveness of roles, jobs, and patients/projects; and the fear of destabilizing loss of professional identity (Bufford & Kindig, 1974).

If interdisciplinary education and clinical practice are complex and demanding, why be burdened with them? Why not opt for the simplicity, tradition, and security that comes with unidisciplinary education and practice?

One benefit is that the interrelationship of expertise and disciplines in interdisciplinary education and practice matches the interdependence of health needs and resources that the health professional will face, especially in working with the aged. For students an interdisciplinary education involving professionals from various disciplines illuminates problems from multiple perspectives and may lead to solutions tailored to the patients and problems being addressed and, perhaps, even to more creative solutions. For the interdisciplinary clinical practice team this model brings to bear all the professional expertise called for, with the opportunity to integrate it in planning, teaching, evaluation, and intervention. This provides more effective health care and, consequently, more benefit to the patients and problems and to society.

The interdisciplinary approach, with its openness to new learning and interaction, also makes for a creative environment. In addition to the immediate benefits to the patient, for the practitioner this makes for professional growth and satisfaction and often compensates for the complexities of the task, the burden of work, and inadequate material reward.

The costs of an interdisciplinary approach are significant. Much time and energy are required of multiple participants to arrange to meet, learn, and work together. Aside from time demanded of faculty, students, or practitioners, the effort to mesh differing schedules is considerable. Many institutions express appreciation for the interdisciplinary principle but cannot spare the staff or time to engage in it, and many individuals are too busy and prefer to invest in more traditional and secure disciplinary endeavors.

Example 1. A teaching hospital studies problems in patient care in its emergency ward (E.W.). The study committee reports:

> of particular concern was the identification of underlying significant areas of conflict within and between the Medical Staff, Nursing Service, and Administration. These areas of conflict exist not only within the confines of the E.W. but also between the members of the various disciplines in the E.W. and their presumed confreres in the various in-hospital units. . . . [There was] an underlying perception of everyone that their individual efforts to improve patient thru-put [would] inevitably be stymied by the inefficiencies of others. . . . [One suggested solution is to] better define certain areas of hazy responsibility among and between various services in order to hopefully improve overall patient care as well as the working relationships within the hospital staff (Ad Hoc Committee on Emergency Services, 1984).

In true *multidisciplinary* fashion, this was to be done by giving senior medical, surgical, and subspecialty residents (physicians) additional authority. The restructuring of the emergency ward and its staff along the lines of an interdisciplinary model was rejected implicitly as too costly in staff numbers and time, and too foreign to the institution's traditional staff roles and hierarchy.

A second cost is the change required in organizations and individuals unprepared for or unsympathetic toward interdisciplinary endeavors. Thinking through or attempting to introduce interdisciplinary education reveals how much administrative structure, policies, and procedures are geared to unidisciplinary education and practice. In addition, patterns of thinking and practice of administrators, faculty, and students are based on a single discipline. Introducing the interdisciplinary approach requires renovation of major portions of the curriculum, the educational institution, and thinking patterns.

Example 2. A large university embarked on a demonstration project in developing an interdisciplinary curriculum in mental health. Individuals from 11 programs were enthusiastically dedicated to the project. However, departments and schools varied from passive acceptance to hostile skepticism, both because of the inability to understand or value the concept of the interdisciplinary approach, and for fear of losing students, faculty, funding, and university support. And many in the university administration feared the political tensions and policy changes that would be entailed. In the end the suspicion, competition, and self-interest of individuals and programs caused the project to deteriorate into unidisciplinary education — much to the relief of the university administration and many of its "participating" units (Satin & Saxe, 1979).

Example 3. A multidisciplinary clinical internship program was subverted by a special interest group which felt that the original broad goal of shared clinical training was only a convenient means for gaining funding for advocacy of its special interest (Satin, 1987).

Not the least cost is the effort and discomfort individuals must undergo in reevaluating their own and other disciplines. This leads them to struggle with the limits of their competence and disciplinary identity. Interdisciplinary education and practice challenge traditional values, organization, and practices. After considerable experience with interdisciplinary education, Harris (1978) has observed the following:

Change, no matter how slow, is always viewed with skepticism and some fear, is frequently resisted, and, unless carefully controlled and programmed, may be disruptive. Change that necessitates such careful attention to the integration of patient-care goals and educational direction carries the potential for even more disruption, fear, and skepticism.

Example 4. A prestigious geriatric education center embarked on a study of its parent Division on Aging's "interdisciplinary" geriatric clinical and teaching teams. However, it quickly canceled the study as "disruptive of professional relations" when it found that the disciplinary working relationships in the teams and projects were actually either paradisciplinary or multidisciplinary rather than interdisciplinary and that highlighting these relationships and suggesting changes threatened vested interests and hidden agendas of high-status disciplines (especially medicine) and individuals (Satin, 1987).

Certainly the interdisciplinary model of working relationships is mandatory in specific situations. A situation involving multiple influences and processes calls for the involvement of multiple disciplines with their various areas of primary and secondary competence. Complexity and uncertainty of approach and outcome call for the creativity and flexibility of the interdisciplinary model. Participants must have expertise in their own disciplines; security in their areas of competence; self-esteem; openness to and enthusiasm for new learning; and readiness for professional growth. The institutions that control sanctions, staff time, and material resources must be both understanding and supportive in order to provide a viable environment. And material resources must be available and reliable. As many of these factors of authority and resources as possible should be under the control of the interdisciplinary project to protect them from inevitable changes in personnel, commitment, and resources in outside institutions.

In contrast, projects involving few factors, clear and familiar goals and means, and personnel and governing institutions oriented toward well-established disciplines and practices do not justify the costs and effort of an interdisciplinary approach — unidisciplinary, paradisciplinary, or multidisciplinary models may be effective and economical.

## CONCLUSION

The clarification of the working relationship among professionals from various disciplines inevitably identifies their educational and clinical practices. This can be welcome or embarrassing, but certainly it makes it possible to consider clearly the current status and alternatives in any given institution or program. The purpose of this chapter has been to define the interdisciplinary approach and discuss some of its benefits to help identify current practices in any program, consider alternatives, and implement desired changes. This perspective may also be useful in research into the recruitment of personnel, training, administration, and working relationships in geriatrics and other health care fields.

Perhaps the interdisciplinary model of education and practice is more complex and costly than others, but its special advantages in matching health needs with helping interventions far outweighs the cost. And it fosters unparalleled excitement and enrichment of professional practice and growth. This approach is most appropriate where multiple needs, systems, and disciplines interact. Surely geriatrics and gerontology are prime examples.

## REFERENCES

Ad Hoc Committee on Emergency Services (1984). Report and proposals. Internal report, Massachusetts General Hospital, Boston.

Blakeney, B. A., Bottomley, J. M., Howe, M. C., & Smith, D. H. (1988). Teaching a functional approach to assessment. In United States Department of Health and Human Services and United States Department of Education (sponsors), *Rehabilitation and geriatric education: Perspectives and potential.* McLean, VA: The Circle, Inc.

Bottomley, J. M., Blakeney, B. A., O'Malley, T., Satin, D. G., Smith, H. D., & Howe, M. C. (1990). Rehabilitation and mobility of older persons: An interdisciplinary perspective. In S. Brody & L. G. Pawlson (Eds.), *Aging and rehabilitation. II: The state of the practice.* New York: Springer.

Bufford, J. I., & Kindig, D. (1974). Institute for team development—The next two years. In H. Wise, R. Beckhard, I. Rubin, & A. L. Kyte (Eds.), *Making health teams work.* Cambridge, MA: Ballinger.

Devitt, G. A. (1970). *Commonalities of curricular objectives in the preparation of nurses, physical therapists, occupational therapists, and therapeutic dieticians at the baccalaureate level.* Unpublished doctoral dissertation, University of Pittsburgh, Pittsburgh, PA. Dissertation Abstracts No. ADG 71-16183.

Ducanis, A. J., & Golin, A. K. (1978). *Interprofessional perceptions in the interdisciplinary health care team.* Paper presented at the Association of Schools of the Allied Health Professions, Miami.

Harris, J. ( 1978). Interdisciplinary health education: A case study of fact and fancy. *Journal of Community Health, 5,* 357.

Heilman, M. E. (1977). *Identification of certain competencies needed by health care personnel in order to function as a health care team.* Unpublished doctoral dissertation, University of Pittsburgh, Pittsburgh, PA. Dissertation Abstracts No. ADG 78-09588.

Holm, V. A. (1978). Team issues. In K. Allen, V. A. Holm, & R. Schiefelbusch (Eds.), *Early intervention: A team approach* (pp. 99–115). Baltimore, MD: University Park Press.

Plovnick, M., Fry, R., & Rubin, I. (1972). *Managing health care delivery.* Cambridge, MA: Ballinger.

Rubin, I., & Beckhard, R. (1972). Factors influencing the effectiveness of health teams. *Milbank Memorial Fund Quarterly, 50,* 317.

Satin, D. G., Barnard, D., Jette, A., & Howe, M. (1985). Teaching an integrated, interdisciplinary approach to geriatrics: A solution to babel. Presentation at the Association for Gerontology in Higher Education, Washington, DC.

Satin, D. G. (1987). The difficulties of interdisciplinary education: Lessons from three failures and a success. *Educational Gerontology, 13,* 53.

Satin, D. G., & Saxe, L. (1979). Complexity of process and role in the evaluation of an interdisciplinary mental health education program: The deacon's masterpiece. *Evaluation and Program Planning, 2,* 285.

# 15

# Developing the Interdisciplinary Team

Benjamin S. Siegel

As is clear from the earlier chapters in this book, the nature of modern health care – with its increasingly sophisticated technology, its many professionals with new and expanded roles, and its complex nature, encompassing physical, psychosocial, cultural, ethical, legal, and economic issues – requires an interdisciplinary team approach to solve problems and provide optimum health care, and this is especially true for the aged. This chapter will discuss the complex issues of team functioning, including professional relationships, organizational structure, and environmental supports. In addition, it will provide a framework for thinking about the nature of effective teamwork and how it may be developed. Finally, our discussion will turn to a review of some of the educational interventions that can be implemented by health-care organizations to improve the effectiveness of the interdisciplinary team.

## A HISTORICAL PERSPECTIVE

One of the earliest records of interdisciplinary health care comes from ancient Indian medicine. The Vedic period, around the ninth century B.C., marked the peak of Indian medicine, and the writings of one of the foremost Hindu physicians, Susrata, describes the physician working in collaboration with the holy man and astrologer to assist the king in battle. The doctor's role is to identify any poisons in the camp by using very careful inspections. The holy man, through prayers, wards off evil influences. The astrologer, consulting the stars, suggests specific sacrifices to prevent harm to the king's army (Margotta, 1967). In medieval England, physicians and barber surgeons practiced quite independently. However, when a woman patient needed to see the physician or barber surgeon, the midwife was required to serve as an intermediary for the patient. Thus, the doctor and midwife formed a health team (Margotta, 1967). In 13th-century Italy, the first public pharmacies were established in monasteries and in the courts of rulers. They later became private and there physicians frequently consulted with the pharmacists and even saw patients with them (Margotta, 1967).

In more recent times, one of the earliest interdisciplinary team programs for the aged was established at Montefiore Hospital's Home Health Team in Bronx, New York (Wise, 1972). In 1948, the hospital administrator wanted to provide home care for chronically ill patients (mostly aged) who no longer needed hospitalization but were not entirely well. The hospital embarked on a comprehensive home support system, using a health-care team. Homemaking support services that addressed dealing with nutrition and daily living were to be provided by family members. The team members included a public health nurse, an internist, a social worker, a physical therapist, a team secretary, and an automobile driver. Because of the lack of experience with teamwork, the team used a hospital model: the nurse as leader and team coordinator, the physician making weekly rounds, and other members of the team in a consulting role.

The first published description of a non-hospital-based health team was by George Silver, MD (1963) in a demonstration project, also at the Montefiore Hospital. In this project, the goal was to provide team-based primary-care services for 150 families selected randomly from a prepaid group practice associated with the hospital. In this project the team consisted of an internist, a pediatrician, a public health nurse, a social worker, and a team secretary. A psychiatrist, psychologist, and health educator were available for consultation to the team and to the families. The team provided all of the primary health care to these families and met periodically to address health maintenance and preventive aspects of health care. The project was a huge success; in general patients and providers were highly satisfied with the new arrangement for primary-care services.

One of the negative conclusions of the project's report was that the social worker's role was the most difficult to integrate into the team because of the different perceptions and values of the social worker compared to others on the team. In this project social workers were to care for the emotional and psychiatric concerns of their clients; however, the long-standing (professional) dichotomy between mental health and conventional health services was brought to bear: Many patients, especially those of lower socioeconomic status, would not readily accept a social worker as a primary-care provider. To introduce a family to a social worker implied acknowledgment of a disturbed family situation. Families tended to respond more positively to the nurse, who was involved in health teaching and family counseling, and so the nurse took on many of the functions of a social worker. In addition, the research noted that the social workers tended to respond more negatively and with more pessimism to solving health problems than the nurses, who tended to be more optimistic. It was also difficult to reorient the social worker, whose traditional training was in problem solving and psychopathology, to accept a primary preventive role with many healthy families. Finally, the social worker was viewed as a consultant or specialist by other team members and therefore divorced from everyday problems.

Since that time there have been numerous programs fostering interdisciplinary team care, and a number of universities and teaching hospitals have devised curricula, instituted in-service training, and designed experiments to investigate the effectiveness of health-care teams in relation to patient health status and improved quality of care. A description of these programs is presented at the end of this chapter.

As explained in Chapter 14, The Interdisciplinary, Integrated Approach to Professional Practice with the Aged, which provides an excellent definition of the various levels of collaboration (interdisciplinary, paradisciplinary, multidisciplinary, etc.) and describes the theoretical advantages and disadvantages of each, the essential difference between the multidisciplinary and interdisciplinary models is that of overlapping roles.

Both models share information and collaborate to develop health-care plans. Only in the interdisciplinary model, however, is there an overlapping of roles that leads to the ideal form of teamwork, including interdependence, reciprocity of influence, and the hoped-for synergy among team members.

## THE COMPLEXITIES OF INTERDISCIPLINARY TEAM CARE

In an excellent book by Ducanis and Golin (1979), the complexities of interdisciplinary health care are carefully spelled out. These issues, which will be discussed in detail in this chapter, can be summarized as follows:

1. The health-care team obviously must involve two or more individuals in order to be a team.
2. The team members should be in communication with each other, whether face to face or by some other form of communication.
3. There is an identifiable leader, although in many teams leadership is a function rather than the role of a particular person, based on status or profession.
4. Teams function within and between organizational structures and thus the organizational, institutional, and environmental support is crucial to the optimal functioning of teams.
5. Even when the roles of the professional are defined and the nature of the task identified, there may be, and usually is, conflict of goals, overlap in disciplines, and uncertainty about who does what.
6. In well-working teams, there tend to be protocols of operation, both for providing medical care (content) and operational guidelines about *how* the team works together as a team (process).
7. Teams have unique personalities and personal values that are sometimes consonant and at other times conflict with the personalities and values of their members. Team members obviously have different personalities, perceptions of roles, and concerns about status and power, all of which influence team functioning.
8. Team members, because of their different professional backgrounds, bring varied theoretical approaches and professional values to the task. For example, medicine's general goal is to cure illness, whereas nursing's theoretical and professional credo is one of concern for the activities of daily living and provision of care and comfort. (This is not to say that physicians are unconcerned about the care of the patient, but the dominant theme of medical training and practice is the cure of illness.)
9. The team is usually client centered, the client is being defined, at once or together, as the individual, the family, the social grouping, or the entire community.
10. The team is as task oriented as possible.

Obviously, in a health-care program, the work of the team is to provide health care. However, because the team works at an interdisciplinary level, the members of the team must make a commitment to their functional tasks within the context of a team. This requires the team, or various members, to plan how they wish to provide care, to decide who does what task, and to resolve whatever conflicts, differences in values, and different perspectives each team member may have. Because the team must devote some time and energy to sorting out these "team maintenance" issues, it cannot be task oriented all of the time. On the other hand, too much time and energy on team maintenance issues is generally cost inefficient.

## TEAM SIZE AND COMPOSITION

Team size is an important issue, but no hard-and-fast rules exist for determining ideal size. It is obvious that the greater the number of team members the greater the number of possible relationships that must be maintained to ensure good communication and effective joint problem solving. Thus, with three members of the team there are 4 possible relationships, but with a six-member team there are 15 possible relationships. Optimal or ideal size follows the physiological or architectural principle "Form follows function." The structure of the team is dependent on the specific goals or tasks of the team. That is, the team should be made up of only those people who would be interdependent in their approach to a particular problem or task and who would influence each other's behavior and activities. Thus, in a large health center serving the aged, where there is a geriatrician, psychologist, pharmacist, public health nurse, and occupational and physical therapist, and a nutritionist, not everyone needs to meet all the time to "team up." Often, high-quality health care is provided without the requirements of teaming. In fact, there are so many roles and differing health problems and resources available that it is probably best not to define the members of the team rigidly but define them in relation to the health problem, the treatment modalities available, and the available resources, both financial as well as psychosocial and medical. Indeed, flexibility and overlap of functioning is required, especially when many health-care goals tend to be uncertain or ambiguous.

As there are many different team models functioning, there is much debate and discussion in the literature (Siegel, 1974) about the mix of people who should work together as a primary-care team in an overlapping role and who should be consultants. For example, should the physician provide the primary-care services or serve as a backup to the nurse or community outreach worker? The alternative primary-care team structures that have been suggested include the following:

1. Physician, nurse, and community health worker
2. Physician, nurse, community health worker, and social worker
3. Physician and nurse practitioner
4. Nurse and community health worker (home health aide)
5. Nurse and psychiatrist
6. Nurse, physical therapist, and occupational therapist
7. Physicians, physician's assistants, nurses, and nursing assistants
8. Physician, nurse, and social worker
9. Physician, social worker and physical therapist, secretary, and automobile driver

Other professionals such as the pharmacist, dietician, dentist, clergy, psychologist, audiologist, rehabilitation expert, and indigenous community healer sometimes serve as consultants and sometimes are members of the primary-care team.

For example, Kane (1975) in her review of over 200 health-care teams found disciplines combined in 162 different ways. Thus, there is no perfect or ideal mix of professionals constituting "the team." Indeed, team composition is predicated on the range of the patients' problems: The needs of the patients are matched as closely as possible to professionals whose expertise and unique contributions can make a difference (Campbell, 1987).

## THE PATIENT AND THE TEAM

Clearly the relationship between the entire team and the patient is different and more complex than the dyadic professional–patient relationship. From the patient's perspective there may be uncertainty about which member of the team the patient should consult for which purpose. With multiple team members, repetition of history and multiple visits to the health center or office may be necessary. The patient's relationship with a team tends to be less intense and perhaps more impersonal than with a single provider, who attempts to provide much of the primary-care services. The aged seem to respond better to this decreased intensity. When the patient has a relationship with a team, there is the possibility of less dependency and more autonomy on the part of the patient. On the other hand, emotionally troubled or "borderline" patients may provide different information to different team members, resulting in conflicting or confusing data. Many of these patients manipulate team members for self-serving needs. Patients differ in their compliance with team recommendations, so teams often struggle with the issues of allowing the patient to become an active member of the team for decision-making purposes. Sometimes, the health problems of the patient and family can become so complex that the members go off in multiple directions without coordination, which leads to "comprehensive fragmentation" rather than integrated care. On the other hand, given the variety of personalities on the team, the patient may be able to choose which team member is most compatible in a relationship, independent of the professional role of the health provider. Occasionally, if the team is working well, the values of team members may shift from concerns about the patient to the psychological needs of the team members, and thus the team itself may become more important to the members than the patient or the health problem.

Just as team members may differ in their attitudes, values, and ideologies (AVI) patients also differ in their AVI as they interact with the health-care system. Because many of the aged enter the health-care system in crisis, little is known firsthand about their personality structure, belief system, and understanding of health care. The health-care AVI of the patient are often overlooked when the team formulates its treatment plan. This can result in noncompliance, mutual distrust, and ineffective treatment. What a patient needs from professionals besides competent advice and treatment is acknowledgment of the patient's AVI configuration and its integration into the treatment plan. If patient's have only a rudimentary knowledge of health care, then the team members must educate them and help them formulate a personally meaningful AVI configuration relevant to their health-care needs.

## INSTITUTIONAL SETTING

The organizational framework in which the health team works is a critical factor in determining its success or failure.

At the organizational level many important questions arise. For instance, does the administration support the concept of the team approach? From a fiscal perspective, teaming requires time that would otherwise be used to deliver services, which is not revenue generating. Also, is there support for team maintenance? Is the organization a profit or nonprofit one, and how does this affect the value of the teamwork? Issues of hierarchy and bureaucratic lines of power, authority, and communication may inhibit teamwork. For example, if a professional has a conflict with another, does one seek out the supervisor who, in turn, must seek out the supervisor of the other professional and arrange management meetings, propose a change in job description, and so on, so the professionals can work together in a more harmonious way, or is there support in management for professionals to work out conflicts themselves?

It is important to communicate organizational goals and values to the team members. Issues such as the conflict between curative services and preventive services, given limited resources, and how much of each service can be delivered, need to be clearly communicated to the team in order for it to develop priorities and work schedules. How, and by what criteria, does the administration evaluate the effectiveness of the services provided by the team? How much is productivity alone the measure of effectiveness of health care as opposed to time spent with the patient or family addressing psychosocial, family, cultural and ethical issues, which may not be reimbursable, valued, measured, and rewarded by the health-care organization? If team members are having difficulty in their teamwork, to what degree does management provide help, support, and time away from service to support the improvement of team functioning? How do various institutional settings differ in their unique attitudes, values, and ideologies and how does this affect those of the different team members and the functioning of the team.

As one way to ensure effectiveness at the interdisciplinary team level, organizational structures such as the matrix organization have been proposed (Beckhard 1972), in which the administrative-support and supervisory professional systems are organized as *managed teams* around issues of organization and delivery of health services and around the technical and qualitative professional issues that support the delivery system as a team rather than as individual specialties. This creative alternative way of organizing an institution will be explored in depth in the following discussion.

TEAM DEVELOPMENT

In reviewing the experience of health-care teams, it is clear that some very important lessons have been learned about team development and team functioning.

1. Having all the best and brightest professionals at the same place and same time does not necessarily make an effective team.

2. Not every patient or family needs a team at all times or at any time. If teamwork is required, not all members of the team are required to solve problems or to implement care plans. Thus, team membership shifts and changes as the nature of the problem changes.

3. There may be some patients or families in which the health-care problems are so complex that the team could spend hours agonizing over what to do. After a certain amount of time, it is useful to decide that only certain goals can be achieved and that

there are limits to any intervention, whether medical, nursing, physical therapy, occupational therapy, or psychosocial. Continuing to obsess over complex issues eventually becomes a waste of time and energy. The team must focus on what is possible to accomplish within the limits of the available resources and what is ethically appropriate.

4. Many professionals realize that it is fun practicing on a team. It provides a richer professional experience and allows for alternative perspectives on problem solving and planning. With painful issues such as termination of life supports, the diagnosis of chronic illness, death and dying, team members can be a source of comfort and support to each other.

5. Of all of the potential team members, the physician has probably the greatest difficulty in working on an interdisciplinary team. There are a number of factors associated with this phenomenon. There is great status and power given to the physician (and given up by other health professionals to the physician). Physicians have had little exposure to interdisciplinary training experiences either in medical school or in residency training. Moreover, both the overriding concern about taking responsibility for medical decision making and the threat of malpractice have inhibited physicians' willingness to share the patient or share decision making with non-physicians as equal members of the healthcare team. Many physicians do not realize that nurses, social workers, and theologians who do pastoral counseling must carry malpractice insurance as well. Because of their lack of preparation for teamwork, it may be best for team functioning that physicians not be designated as team leaders. Physicians are still free to make medical decisions and maintain medical responsibility without assuming leadership. For a full discussion of leadership issues, see Team Dynamics.

6. It takes time to develop well-functioning teams. Many estimate full team development takes 6 months to a year, and educational programs have been devised (Rubin, Plovnick, & Fry 1975; Plovnick, Fry, & Rubin 1978) to assist in team development. The team usually begins in a mood of excitement and commitment and denial of or smoothing over of conflict; later as the team develops, conflict is sure to surface and must be addressed and resolved or the team will fall apart. There is no team that does not experience some conflict.

7. Finally, health-professional schools spend very little time or attention to team theory or practice (consider, in contrast, professional football), which requires 30 to 40 hours of weekly practice for a 2-hour game. It is the rare health-professional school that places students on teams during their training.

To understand team development we need to address team *process* rather than team *content*. By content, we mean the provision of physical therapy and nursing, pharmaceutical, medical, and social services to patients and their families. Team development deals with *process issues* — that is, how the team is organized; how goals are established; how roles evolve; how problem solving, decision making, and conflict resolution are managed; and how the leadership functions. In other words, *how* a team works is as important as *what* it does to provide health care.

These issues and others are always present. How they are managed or dealt with determines the efficiency and effectiveness of the team in providing service, which is its ultimate goal. The degree to which the team knows, understands, and deliberately deals with process issues ultimately determines the success or failure of the team.

In the following section, we will first examine the dynamics of health team interaction and then suggest organizational structures that help support the interdisciplinary approach to health care.

TEAM DYNAMICS

A particular model (Rubin & Beckhard, 1972; Plovnick, Fry, & Rubin, 1978) has been very helpful in conceptualizing the dynamic process of team development, and it can be used to evaluate team effectiveness. This model describes four key elements of team process, each of which can by analyzed critically: goals, roles, procedures, and interpersonal issues (GRPI). Team members can learn to develop the skills to become proficient in learning and reviewing these elements. When professionals come together as a interdisciplinary team for whatever purpose, these four elements provide a strong basis for team development before any of the work (content) of health care begins.

This model also assumes a hierarchy of importance for team effectiveness: *goals* are the most important, and interpersonal issues the least important. This is not to say that interpersonal issues on a team are not a concern. However, with respect to team effectiveness, many issues that appear on the surface to stem from personality conflicts, personal values, or just plain personality differences may in fact originate in the other elements, such as goal or role conflicts, but are perceived as interpersonal issues.

After each of the key elements have been described, suggestions for ways in which the team can deal with each of these elements will be given. Five to seven meetings of approximately 1 to 2 hours are required for team development and can be adapted from programed texts available to any health professional or administration interested in team development (Rubin, Plovnick, & Fry, 1975; Plovnick, Fry, & Rubin, 1978).

*Goals*

A team has a special purpose. In health care it can be very complex, depending on the problem. How much energy should be spent on specific curative services, and how much on preventive and health maintenance services? What about psychosocial issues? What are the specific goals of the team vis-à-vis the patient, the family, or the community? How clearly are these goals defined? Can the team accomplish the goals with the given resources, and to what degree? Who defines these goals? Is there agreement or conflict about these goals either among the team members or the patients and their families? How much commitment on the part of the team members is there in carrying out these goals? Once accomplished, how are these goals measured? By whom? How do the team goals relate to the goals of the institution or organization which the team is a part? How do the team goals relate to the personal goals and values that each team member brings from the professional and personal perspective? A social worker and a physician may disagree about a particular plan of treatment, and a nurse and nutritionist may have other alternative suggestions. How goal decisions, conflicts, and ambiguity are dealt with by the team is probably the most important element of team development and needs to be decided on before the other elements of the model are examined.

Because of the complex nature of providing interdisciplinary health care to the aged, with improved technology; the pressure to limit costs; the variety of health personnel; the differences in attitudes, values, and beliefs of the provider, patient, organization, and society (for example, in terms of willingness to pay), team goals can never be perfectly defined, and all of the critical information about a patient or family can never be completely obtained. In reality, interim or limited goals need to be established and agreed upon. After an attempted treatment intervention, new data about the effectiveness of the intervention will readjust a particular goal and the overall health-care plan. Thus, the process of establishing team goals is always open, changing, and needs to be renegotiated frequently. Using such an open problem-solving approach to setting team goals is crucial.

Briefly, this problem-solving process defines a particular problem, with as much pertinent data as possible, develops hypotheses and alternative plans to meet the problem, and tests these plans against what is considered to be reasonable outcomes. The plan most likely to achieve the goal is identified and implemented. The results of the implementation are then reevaluated, leading to either a solved problem or a problem at another level of definition and the setting of new goals.

Two aspects of goal implementation can be isolated: goal setting and the management of goal conflicts.

GOAL SETTING. All team members should formulate general statements of what the care mission or goal of the team is in their view or what the goal of care is for a particular patient or family. As views are shared openly, as they must be, perceived conflicts over power, prestige, and professional status will surface and a process of addressing some of them will begin. The ideal is that all members of the team have equal input. Brainstorming — sharing all ideas no matter how impractical, without any discussion or criticism at first — is a useful way for all members of the team to feel empowered to act as equals.

Because proposed goals tend to be very broad, idealistic, and "fuzzy," as individual goals are shared, a priority list should be drawn up by the team, who will then examine them to see if they can be expressed as *performance goals*; that is, team members will determine, based on available evidence, whether particular goals could be achieved. For example, it is too general a goal for the team to provide psychosocially sensitive health care. Perhaps this could be redefined to state that, in order to provide psychosocially sensitive care, the health team must gather psychosocial data, understand the patient or family's cultural and economic background, and determine what the patient perceives as personal health goals. Once the performance goals have been established, the team then needs to address team goals in order of priority and discuss whether resources are available to achieve them.

MANAGING GOAL CONFLICTS. Since different professionals will have differing views about what the mission or goal of the team is or what the patient or family needs are, there will always be differences of opinion. Such conflicts need to be managed openly. There are four different ways to manage goal conflicts, each with different costs to the team.

1. Negotiate a compromise among conflicting views. Sometimes the process of negotiation leads to improved understanding and a new goal everyone can live with. Effective

negotiation enables those in conflict to agree to carry out all or part of the plan. Sometimes, if the team does not handle conflict well, certain members of the team will assent to the goals but silently subvert the plan. Negotiation is probably the best approach to take to goal conflict unless additional resources made available to the team permit conflict resolution or some part of the organization is willing to change without resolving differences.

2. Do nothing about the conflict and cope as best one can. Sometimes this works but more often this strategy leads to a demoralized staff and to decreased effectiveness of team members.

3. Team members quit the organization or are fired because of the conflict. Each of these choices is costly to the team and organization but is sometimes necessary. If this happens frequently, it may be that the organization needs to look carefully at its hiring and selection policy. It may be that the goals and attitudes, values, and beliefs of the organization are not being effectively communicated to prospective employees or that the selection process is not sensitive to the different attitudes, values, and beliefs of new personnel. If the team selects and educates its own members, their untimely loss may be prevented.

4. Change the nature of the system. Sometimes because of lack of resources, a particular problem cannot be solved. For example, there are not enough home health aides, or interpreter services are lacking to help with a new population of Spanish- or French-speaking clients. In such a situation, the conflict can be dealt with at the organizational level rather than at the team level. Though this often creates friction, the effects of changing the system may lead to more permanent changes in the organization and a more effective team — through the hiring of more home health aides or an interpreter, for example. One inner-city health center hired an anthropologist to conduct an ethnographic study to determine how a particular ethnic group could be served by a neighborhood health center.

### Roles and Role Negotiation

A role can be defined simply as what one does to get the job done. Roles are also defined by professional training experiences, patient expectation, and public perception. For practical purposes, we define *role* here as the set of expectations health team members have of each other to achieve the goal or mission of the team. Though specific enough to formulate a job description, such expectations of (i.e., role definitions) must be flexible enough to meet demands not necessarily anticipated by a rigid job description.

One of the key elements of interdisciplinary team care is interdependence and bilateral influence of behaviors. Roles, according to the GRPI model, cannot be established on a team unless the goals have been established or agreed upon. To achieve a particular goal, the health professionals all decide what their specific roles are and what they need from each other to achieve the goal. Roles are therefore defined as the set of expectations that each has of the other. For example, in order for nurses to help aged people with their diabetes management, nurses need to obtain information about medication and side effects from those they expect to have it, namely a physician or pharmacist. Needing data about foods that affect blood sugar or data about a patient's social functioning, nurses will consult a nutritionist or social worker, respectively. In addition, nurses, as all members of the team, have demands originating from the organization about productivity, allocation of time, and so on, that serve to define their roles.

The multiple demands and needs of various team members, patients, families, and organizations can create a number of problems related to the concept of roles.

ROLE CONFLICT. Should professional X or professional Y provide the service if both can do it equally well? For example, should the nurse or physician counsel the patient with diabetes? Should the nurse, physician, social worker, or psychiatrist deal with the emotional response of the patient and family once diabetes has been diagnosed? Should the nurse or nutritionist begin to evaluate and deal with the dietary changes necessary to manage the diabetes? Besides confusion in disciplinary functions, role conflict may also be an expression of rivalry, job insecurity, or overlapping values of professional societies. (For further discussion of these questions, see Interpersonal Issues).

ROLE OVERLOAD. In some instances a professional is asked to do too many tasks and cannot do them all within the constraints of available resources. This overload may be due to lack of time, energy, or interest or to emotional investment rather than professional investment or may stem from multiple authorities and obligations within the organization.

ROLE AMBIGUITY. Sometimes in carrying out a particular task, uncertainty arises about how to achieve goals. Lack of knowledge can lead to duplication of effort and wasted resources. It can also increase stress, lead to rebellion on the team, subversion of effort, and general demoralization. For example, if social workers do not understand the religious or cultural belief of patients, they are less effective in counseling them about how to adapt to a particular illness. Or certain foods may have important meaning to a particular patient based on cultural beliefs. If the management of an illness, such as diabetes, or hypertension, requires attention to the diet, health-care providers should have knowledge of the health beliefs of the patient as it affects their food intake.

ROLE NEGOTIATION. Role conflict, overload, and ambiguity can be managed effectively in an open team meeting through the process of role negotiation. This process requires team members to share their expectations of other members in relation to their own roles in a clear and open way. Expectations can be defined as describing *what* new behaviors are expected and *why* to achieve the overall goal. Role expectations should also be stated in such a way as to minimize accusations or cause defensiveness. As these expectations are shared and negotiated, explicit "role contracts" are developed that can then be reviewed and evaluated each time there is a problem with roles. As team members interact to define their roles and carry them out, the usual experience is that role negotiation does not clarify every aspect of a working relationship among team members. Thus conflict, uncertainty, or ambiguity will *predictably* arise. Team members should learn to identify these role problems early so that they can be managed, rather than later, when they usually cause greater conflict and much personal pain, invariably leading to decreased team effectiveness. For an excellent article on role negotiation, see the work of Harrison (1973).

## Procedures

The emphasis up to now has been on the "what" — the goals — and the "who" of teams. We now look at the "how" of our subject: the various procedures necessary for appropriate team functioning. Knowledge of these procedures is important and useful. If team members can identify problems in the way the team functions, then team members can propose alternative ways of solving these problems and improve procedures. Each one can be discussed, managed, and dealt with by the team at their regular team meeting.

According to the GRPI team development theory, procedures should not be discussed until the goals and roles have been established and clarified. Such procedures include decision making, leadership, conflict resolution, team norms, and communication patterns. The effectiveness of the coordination of care in a team setting depends on agreement by the team about the use of procedures, for example, about how decisions will be made, who will be the leader in carrying out certain decisions, how team meetings will be run, how to solve problems and conflicts, and how to understand how team norms affect the behavior of team members.

DECISION MAKING. Decision making can be broken down into two sub-elements: (1) the actual decision making and (2) the allocation of decision-making responsibility. An effective decision by any team has two important criteria: (a) In solving particular health problems, each decision should be one of high quality and logical soundness, which quality usually derives from the goals of the health team. (b) The effectiveness of each decision is judged by the degree to which team members are committed to the decision once it is made.

The team can arrive at a decision in a number of ways. Some teams require that all members unanimously and wholeheartedly agree to support the decision. A slightly less stringent stipulation is consensus, involving broad discussion of all the alternatives, though team members in the end commit themselves to carrying out the decision. Majority rule, whereby most members of the team agree to the decision but a certain number do not entails the greater likelihood that some will not be committed to carrying out the decision. Dictatorial decision making is executed by a single leader without much discussion and with no collaboration or alternative problem solving. As in majority rule, in dictatorial decision making there is less likelihood of the decision being implemented as well as greater likelihood of its being sabotaged. Dictatorial decision making works only when the team has agreed to this approach in advance of the actual decision making. Sometimes, for example, in a surgical operating room, decisions appear to be dictatorial, but it is obvious from the nature of the work that dictatorial decision making must be used to complete the surgery efficiently and with good quality. Surgical teams have accepted this way of decision making as appropriate for their kind of teamwork.

Finally, there is the "*plop effect*," the least effective way to make a decision. In this approach, a team member simply offers a decision on a particular problem before any problem solving by team members has been initiated or before any of the other team members are ready to make a decision. For example, without any discussion, one team member may declare: "Mr. X needs a homemaker." This procedure hardly ever works and is usually rejected outright by team members. Before arriving at a decision as to whether a homemaker may be useful or not, the team usually discusses all of the medical and psychosocial problems of the patient and is pretty clear about goal and role issues. The care plan, which may include a homemaker, is usually part of a much more comprehensive set of goals and is not a simple goal in isolation. The most effective teams use unanimity or consensus in their decision making, whereas the least effective use majority rule and dictatorial methods. Not only is the "plop effect" not effective, but those who persistently use this procedure have not really understood the nature of good decision making in the context of the GRPI model.

In allocating decision-making responsibility, it is important for the team to be clear about *what* decisions they are trying to make, with particular attention to each phase of the problem-solving process. In addition, it is important to decide *who* should be involved in the decision-making process: that is, it is necessary to recognize who has information about the decision, who has the relevant expertise, and who will be required to implement the decision once it is made. Participation in decision making leads to greater acceptance and commitment to carry out decisions. *How* people are involved in the process is another dimension. Team members are *directly* involved in decision making because they have the medical information, are medically responsible for or have an important relationship with the patient, or are experts in a health area important for patient care (for example, the clergy). Others on the team need to be *consulted* before the decision is made but are not necessary for direct decision making. Still others need to be *informed* about the decision after it has been made. Finally, one person on the team needs to *manage* the decision. This role can be performed by anyone on the team. Managing the decision becomes an important coordinating responsibility after the decision has been made.

For example, a 76-year-old woman has just developed diabetes. She is alert, competent, and can understand what is happening to her. She also has a good understanding of diabetes thanks to the team nurse. The physician in this case needs to be directly involved in the decision for appropriate medication; the dietician also needs to be directly involved to help with the appropriate diet; the occupational therapist who has been working with the woman in a geriatric day-care center should be informed of any decisions; and the social worker may need to be consulted ahead of time to see how much involvement or direct care is necessary. Finally, someone on the team, in this case, the team nurse, because of a close relationship with the family and knowledge of the family's cultural heritage, is probably in the best position to manage the team members and coordinate the care between the physician, the dietician, social worker, and occupational therapist.

Because of the multiplicity of decisions that take place all the time, the team may wish to adopt decision charting as a way to keep track of what the decision is, who is involved and how the involvement takes place. *Decision charting* is a formal grid or flow chart that identifies a decision and all the people that are directly involved, consulted beforehand, or informed, and finally the manager of the decision. Decision charting can serve as the team "memory" and may be an important part of the medical record (Plovnick, Fry, & Rubin, 1978).

LEADERSHIP. Leadership as a procedure is very important for effective team functioning. All teams have leaders and, traditionally in health care, because of status and power, the physician has been considered *the* team leader. However there is nothing, a priori, in the physician's training or for that matter any of the other health-care providers' training that requires a particular professional to be the leader of the team. Leadership in this model is considered a functional role that any team member can take responsibility for. Thus, instead of one person on the team assuming the role of the leader because of tradition, power, or status, this should be considered an action to help the team function better. So we can speak of *acts* of leadership performed by any team member. Moreover, many teams have "spiritual leaders" whose presence provides support and nurturing to all members. Although the leader of the team is given the responsibility of calling the meeting, setting the agenda, and so forth, there are leadership *tasks* each team member can fulfill to help the team maintain its effectiveness. The function of leadership is to enable the group to accomplish its goals, to help maintain a good working relationship, and to ensure a productive team climate. Leadership tasks (Likert, 1961) can be divided into two types as follows.

1. *Goal-oriented leadership.* Acts that focus the team, allowing it to accomplish its stated purpose effectively and efficiently are said to be goal oriented and include the following:

   a. Initiating discussion and providing clarification of a particular problem
   b. Seeking more information and offering new ideas or information
   c. Opinion seeking and opinion giving
   d. Coordinating
   e. Evaluating
   f. Suggesting alternative courses of action
   g. Energizing and providing psychological support
   h. Assisting in procedures such as distributing materials, arranging seating, recording suggestions and group decisions, completing decision charting, and so on.

2. *Team-supportive leadership tasks.* Acts that support the team, foster effective teamwork, and indirectly lead the group include:

   a. Encouraging others' point of view
   b. Elaborating on others' contributions
   c. Harmonizing or mediating differences between other team members and thus relieving tension in conflict situations
   d. Compromising when conflict occurs and yielding to maintain team harmony
   e. Accepting other team members' points of view
   f. Seeking group reactions and testing to see if the team has a clear perception of roles, goals, and decision-making strategies

Thus, leadership is not one person dependent solely on status or prestige for its effectiveness but conceptually consists of many "acts of leadership," which taken together facilitate team functioning while paying attention to the emotional climate of the team. There can be, and usually are, multiple acts of leadership performed by all team members. Some teams rotate formal leadership for running team meetings, to encourage team members to develop leadership skills, and to share leadership responsibility. Leadership is also involved in managing health care once decisions are made by the team.

CONFLICT RESOLUTION. Conflicts are inevitable in all interdisciplinary teams. They arise because of differences in professional perspectives and differences in the values and goals of team members. Conflicts are also common because the outcome of health-care intervention is usually uncertain and not always predictable. Health-care team members are always weighing risks and benefits in the care provided to patients and their families. Complicating these issues are ethical questions concerning what is the right action, what is beneficial for the patient, from whose perspective, who decides, and so on. The ideal approach to conflict resolution is similar to all problem-solving approaches. Alternative views, values, and goals are shared openly and discussed fully. This ideal of open discussion and negotiation is usually only partially realized because most people do not wish to confront conflict. Early in the life of a team most team members quickly smooth over differences of opinion. It is common for team members to misinterpret a goal or role conflict as an interpersonal one. An open approach that includes renegotiating goals and roles and considering alternative solutions prevents conflicts from being perceived as personality issues originating from one of the team members. To resolve conflicts effectively, the team must commit itself early in its life to open and nonjudgmental conflict resolution.

TEAM NORMS. Norms can be defined as unwritten rules of behavior that have a strong impact on the way in which people behave on a team. Agreeing to openness about conflicts, assuming they will occur, and dealing with them openly are very critical norms of behavior. Agreeing to start meetings on time, allowing everyone to speak, rotating the formal leadership of meetings, and confronting emotional problems are other important norms in the life of a team.

Norms tend to develop early and become very powerful influences on behavior. Once established, they are difficult to change. Oftentimes it is only when a new team member joins that the team becomes aware of its norms. When the new member breaks one of these unwritten rules of behavior, they become painfully apparent. Norms themselves should be discussed and modified as the team looks at its procedures.

COMMUNICATION PATTERNS. Finally, it is crucial for the team to examine communication patterns, such as who speaks first, and most often, and to ask if this is related to status or power. Is communication face to face, or is there separation by physical or geographic barriers? Is communication unidirectional or multidirectional? Do all team members involved in a particular problem contribute? How and whether team members communicate information will affect the decision-making process and, ultimately, the outcome of care. Careful observation of communication patterns can provide clues to the issues of leadership, power, and influence on a team (Kolb, Rubin, & McIntyre, 1971).

### Interpersonal Issues

Interpersonal issues comprise the final element of the GRPI hierarchical model of team interaction. This is a crucial element, yet the most difficult to address effectively. As previously stated, the team model has issues of conflict, uncertainty, and ambiguity built into it. The effective team, however, develops mechanisms to deal with these issues through an "open systems" approach; that is, issues are recognized and discussed openly, and alternative methods are suggested and decided on in an organized manner. If the first three elements in the team model — goals, roles, and procedures — are fully understood, only then should the team concentrate on the interpersonal issues as the possible *source* of the team's problems. In fact, a majority of conflicts that seem to stem from interpersonal issues or personality conflicts most often reflect an uncertainty about the other elements of team functioning. Interpersonal issues and conflicts are usually present in all human systems.

Sometimes, however, people just don't get along, and this is indeed an interpersonal or interprofessional issue that the team must recognize and address. The team must realize, too, that to change a person's personality, behavior, or deeply held professional values is a most difficult task, but it can also be very meaningful for the person as well as the organization. The choices facing the team, or management, include encouraging professional help, for example, through an organizational consultant to the team or psychotherapy for the individual or members of the team; permitting team members to transfer to other teams; or allowing members to quit the organization. These last measures are painful and usually not taken unless other interventions have been tried first, since such actions can affect the emotional climate of the entire team. Quitting is the most costly of all. It is obviously important, as new personnel are hired, that attention be directed to the personality style of the new member and to the degree of "psychological fit" that might exist between the person, the team members, and the norms of the organization.

Using this model of team interaction, the members can begin to organize themselves, build themselves into a team, and maintain themselves through regular team meetings throughout their existence. All team members should become skilled in team process, be able to diagnose where a given problem may dwell, and deal with it. There are, in fact, some teams that appoint a member at each meeting to be the "process consultant" who will reflect on team process during the meeting or interrupt when necessary to clarify process issues. Like the formal leadership role, this can also be a rotating role. Other health teams have hired outside consultants or have made use of educational programs for team development referred to in this chapter (Wise, Beckhard, Rubin, & Kyle, 1974; Rubin, Fry, & Plovnick, 1978; Plovnick, Fry, & Rubin, 1978; Rubin, Plovnick, & Fry, 1975).

## THE MATRIX ORGANIZATION: A WAY TO SUPPORT TEAM CARE

In order for interdisciplinary teams to function effectively, there are important organizational structures which must be in place to support the workings of the team (Beckhard, 1972). Most health-care programs are not organized around the concept of the interdisciplinary team as the functional unit of service. Most community-based health-care organizations incorporate the traditional structure found in most hospitals, which are staffed by directors, formal administrators, and heads of departments and based on disciplines such as medicine, nursing, and social services, with the support of a laboratory, a pharmacy, and so on (see Figure 15.1). But in highly structured organizations there is often little

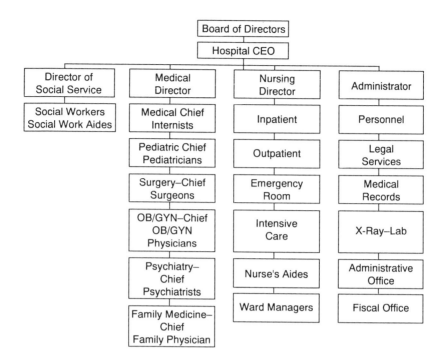

FIGURE 15.1   Traditional hospital hierarchical structure.

collaborative communication among health-care providers from dissimilar professions. Professions tend to relate best with members of their own discipline. In the hospital, goals are fairly well defined: Take out the appendix, cure the infection, complete the neurological diagnostic evaluation, and so forth. The psychosocial value and ethical issues, though important, seem secondary to the goal of hospitalization, and certainly not the basis of reimbursement to the hospital. Diagnosis Related Groups (DRGs) have now mandated a specific number of days of hospitalization for each medical episode, based on the norm of the expected medical evaluation and medical outcome. Little consideration is thus given to the complex psychosocial, cultural, or familial circumstances of the patient. There is good reason to believe that a patient's health problem cannot be completely dealt with if psychosocial issues are not addressed as well.

Interdisciplinary teams providing health care to the aged must be organized, flexible, and able to address the complex psychosocial, rehabilitative, and community-resource issues in addition to the complex medical problems facing the aged daily. These teams, as the main units of service to the aged, cannot function without support from the parent organization, usually the hospital. Yet the traditional hospital organization has developed to support professional departments and specialized services and cannot support the integration of services required by the interdisciplinary team. Such structures support administrative planning, but little attention is given to the planning of health-care professionals. How often have organizations encouraged professionals to stop seeing patients in order to discuss how services are being carried out and the quality of those services? Hospitals need to develop systems to support the work of the team, allowing, for instance, sufficient time and appropriate places for team meetings with sufficient administrative support for those meetings, recognizing team development and maintenance as an important activity, and offering training to professionals in teamwork.

The formal leadership of such organizations must address a number of key issues to make practice effective. The major problems are how the leadership can:

1. Help the teams with their basic work: diagnosing and treating complex health problems.
2. Provide an organizational structure that reflects the work of the team.
3. Deal with the human problem of health-care providers with different roles, backgrounds, and values who must collaborate to solve the problems of patients and their families.
4. Locate authority and develop competence so that decisions are made by those with the best information and by those closest to the problem.
5. Build information systems to ensure that all health-providers have the best available information.
6. Build linkages between providers and members of support systems in the organization, for example, between those purchasing supplies, those in charge of short- and long-range planning, those carrying out quality evaluation, and staff responsible for priority and goal setting for the entire organization.
7. Develop adequate educational programs to disseminate information about treatments; the social conditions of patients and their families; and the unique culture of the community that the teams and the organization are serving. In addition, organizational leadership should provide opportunities for team members to acquire skills in team development, leadership and membership, goal setting, role negotiation, conflict resolution, and so forth.
8. Keep a staff with a variety of backgrounds and values motivated and working together (Beckhard, 1972).

A concept in organizing administrative structures to support the interdisciplinary team has evolved in recent years: the *matrix organization* (see Figure 15.2 [Wise, Beckhard, Rubin, & Kyle, 1974; Beckhard, 1972; Tichy, 1977]). In this structure, teams as a whole report to an administrative leader (the unit manager), who is responsible for the acquisition of supplies, data collection, program planning and evaluation, and the allocation of resources for the team, such as space, supplies and equipment. The unit manager reports to the director of administration for organizationwide planning and evaluation.

The second part of the matrix concerns the technical resources and professional capabilities. The heads of all the professional departments join together with the director of administration to form a management team including the unit managers, which is responsible for supporting the professional staff by providing information, technical resources, and quality-crae control, and maintaining professional standards. For example, the management team may wish to conduct cost-benefit studies; update the provider staff with the latest technology through educational programs; and keep a staff with different backgrounds and values energized, motivated, and working together. The team nurse, in this

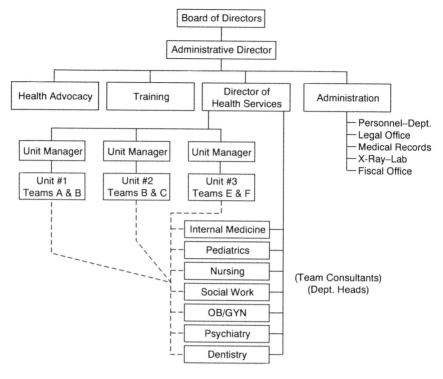

Adapted from Rubin, Plovnick, and Fry, 1978.

FIGURE 15.2  Matrix organization.

structure, will be able to go directly to the chief of medicine to obtain the latest treatment approaches for the aged patient with diabetes, or consult with the head of social services about community resources for such a patient, without going through the director of nursing first. Thus the administrative and support systems must be as flexible as the health-care team itself in order to support the work of the team. Such an organizational structure is effective and necessary because there are interdependencies in caring for the aged that no simple hierarchical structure or departmental structure can allow for.

Thus the essence of this management structure is to provide support to the basic teams, who in turn provide all of the care and decide on priorities as teams. The matrix organization permits and encourages fluidity of communication among professionals by supporting the basic decision-making work of the team at the team level rather than at the supervisory, or administrative, level.

According to this organizational structure, the role of the interdisciplinary team in the organization may change as new functions are added to their responsibilities. For example, the institutional goals and the allocation of resources can be defined jointly by the team and the administration. The team may decide on particular priorities based on patient need, with the administration defining the limit to the resources available. The team could be entrusted with monitoring the quality of health care with consultation and support from administration. If there are a number of functioning teams, they may wish to establish a peer review mechanism to evaluate each other's quality of care. Education and in-service training programs could be important team functions. Team members from different professions could evaluate potential new members and review professional qualifications and the degree of psychological fit with the rest of the team. Teams could set up protocols for management of patient care based on the team's assessment of patient need. Finally, the team could also be the basic unit to train the health-care professionals of the future.

Thus, the administrative leaders in a matrix organization function as educators and facilitators of the health-care team and allow the team to function as independently as possible. Professional specialists set quality standards and can make themselves available as consultants to address specific technical, medical, and psychosocial problems. Equally important, the interdisciplinary team needs support and encouragement from top administrators to be able to receive the resources essential to the process of teamwork and team development.

## EFFECTIVENESS OF INTERDISCIPLINARY TEAM CARE FOR THE AGED

Recently, the recognition of the need to integrate services in an interdisciplinary fashion has meant improved services for the aged. In Milwaukee in 1978 (Fisk, 1983) two central city hospitals joined to develop a geriatric clinic to be coordinated, comprehensive, and interdisciplinary. Acute care was provided in a 24-bed special geriatric unit, and the services of a 174-bed nursing home were incorporated into the unit. An outpatient clinic, clinics in community centers, housing projects, retirement homes, a senior citizen's center, a home-care program, and six outreach centers were also established. Team members included physicians, serving in all three locations, geriatric nurses, rehabilitation therapists, a home health aide, a social worker, a nutritionist, and a recreation therapist. This model has yet to be evaluated, but it represents an attempt to build an interdisciplinary network and to link tertiary care, nursing-home care, community clinics, and outreach into one organizational structure.

In the inpatient setting, geriatric evaluation units, or assessment teams, have been established to plan, evaluate, and offer consultation to ensure the most effective care of the aged. These teams have been set up in hospitals and organized in a multidisciplinary and interdisciplinary way. They have been described comprehensively (Campbell & Cole, 1987; Rubenstein, Rhee, & Kane, 1982) and evaluated for effectiveness (Rubenstein, Josephson, Weiland, English, Sayre, & Kane, 1984). In a randomly controlled prospective study (Rubenstein et al., 1984) frail aged with a high probability of being placed in a nursing home received an evaluation by the innovative geriatric evaluation unit, using an interdisciplinary team consisting of physicians, a physician's assistant, a social worker, and a group of nurses and nursing assistants. Consultants to the team included a clinical psychologist, dietician, occupational and physical therapists, a fellow in geriatric dentistry, an audiologist, and a public health nurse. Within 48 hours after admission to the acute-care hospital patients were randomly admitted to either a special inpatient unit to receive the services of the specialized interdisciplinary team, representing the treatment group, or to traditional inpatient services, representing the control group. The same consultative and specialized services were available to the control patients but were not organized as an interdisciplinary team. Both control and treatment patients were followed for 2 years with periodic assessments. At the end of 1 year, patients assigned to the specialized geriatric unit had lower mortality, were less likely to have been initially discharged to a nursing home, and were less likely to have spent any time in a nursing home during the follow-up period of 1 year. This group had fewer acute-hospital days, nursing-home days, and acute-care hospital readmissions. These patients also showed more improvement in functional status and higher morale than control patients. Moreover, direct costs for institutional care were lower in the treatment group. Lower cost, adjusted for survival, was due to fewer acute-hospital and, nursing-home days, and fewer acute-hospital readmissions in the patients managed by the interdisciplinary team.

In another study, in Monroe County, New York (Barker, Williams, Zimmer, Van Buren, Vincent, & Pickrel, 1985), aged patients were placed in more appropriate community facilities only after the introduction of a geriatric consultation team (consisting of a physician, nurse, and social worker) to six acute-care community hospitals. This ensured more appropriate and quicker placement of the aged hospitalized patients to appropriate community facilities, leading to lower costs to the patients and the community.

Teams have also been used in a home-care and nursing-home program as an alternative to expensive institutionalization with effectiveness and appropriateness of care (Master et al., 1980). In a randomized controlled study of a home-care team, consisting of a physician, social worker, and nurse practitioner, the team's patients had fewer hospitalizations, nursing-home admissions, and outpatient visits than controls (Zimmer, Groth, & McCusker, 1985), were more often able to die at home if this was their wish, used more in-home services than controls, and did not differ from controls in their functional abilities; finally, caretakers at home expressed higher satisfaction with the care the aged received.

Thus, recent experience suggests that an interdisciplinary approach to health care for the aged is effective and efficient and provides high-quality care. To introduce this approach in traditional settings, educational institutions must seek additional ways of educating health-care professionals in teamwork. Perhaps students can be exposed to the team model at some time in their professional development and have the opportunity of being a team member on an ongoing health-care team. It is clear that the team model works both at improving quality of care and decreasing the cost of that care. If the future of health care is to remain affordable and of high quality, we must look at ways of introducing the interdisciplinary team in all our communities and at some time in the education of all health-care providers.

## REFERENCES

Barker, W. H., Williams, F., Zimmer, J. G., Van Buren, C., Vincent, S. J., & Pickrel, S. G. (1985). Geriatric consultation teams in acute hospitals: Impact on back-up of elderly patients. *Journal of the American Geriatrics Society, 33,* 422.

Beckhard, R. (1972). Organizational issues in the team delivery of comprehensive health care. *Milbank Memorial Fund Quarterly 3*(50), 287.

Campbell, J. J., & Cole, K. D. (1987). Geriatric assessment teams. *Clinics in Geriatric Medicine, 3,* 99.

Ducanis, A. J., & Golin, A. K. (1979). *The interdisciplinary health care team.* Germantown, PA: Aspen.

Fisk, A. A. (1983). Comprehensive health care for the elderly. *JAMA, 249,* 230.

Harrison, R. (1973). Role negotiation: A tough-minded approach to team development. In W. Bennis et al. (Eds.), *Interpersonal dynamics* (3rd ed.), Homewood, IL: Dorsey Press.

Kane, R. L. (1975). *Interprofessional Teamwork, Manpower.* Monograph No. 8, Syracuse University School of Social Work, Syracuse, NY.

Kolb, D. A., Rubin, I. M., & McIntyre, J. A. (1971). *Organizational psychology: An experiential approach.* Englewood Cliffs, NJ: Prentice-Hall.

Likert, R. (1961). The nature of highly effective groups. In R. Likert (Ed.), *New patterns of management.* New York: McGraw-Hill.

Margotta, R. (1967). *The Story of Medicine.* New York: Golden Press.

Master, R. J., Feltin, M., Jainchill, J., Mark, R., Kavesh, W. N., Rabkin, M. T., Turner, B., Bachrach, S., & Lennox, S. A. (1980). A continuum of care for the inner city: Assessment of its benefits for Boston's elderly and high risk populations. *New England Journal of Medicine, 302,* 1434.

McKechnie, J. L. (Ed.). (1979). *Webster's Deluxe Unabridged Dictionary* (2nd ed., p. 1871). New York: Simon and Schuster.

Plovnick, M. S., Fry, R. E., & Rubin, I. M. (1978). *Managing health care delivery: A training program for primary care physicians.* Cambridge, MA: Ballinger.

Rubenstein, L. Z., Rhee, L., & Kane, R. L. (1982). The role of geriatric assessment units in caring for the elderly: An analytic review. *Journal of Gerontology, 37,* 513.

Rubenstein, L. Z., Josephson, K. R., Weiland, G. D., English, P. A., Sayre, J. A., & Kane, R. L. (1984). Effectiveness of a Geriatric Evaluation Unit, A Randomized Clinical Trial. *New England Journal of Medicine, 33,* 1664.

Rubin, I. M., & Beckhard, R. (1972). Factors influencing the effectiveness of health teams. *Milbank Memorial Fund Quarterly, 3*(50), 317.

Rubin, I. M., Plovnick, M., & Fry, R. (1975). Improving the coordination of care: A program for health team development. Cambridge, MA: Ballinger.

Rubin, I. M., Fry, R. E., & Plovnick, M. S. (1978). Managing human resources in health care organizations: An applied approach. Reston, VA: Reston.

Siegel, B. (1974). Organization of the primary care team. *Pediatric Clinics of North America, 21,* 341.

Silver, G. (1963). *Family medical care: A report on the family health maintenance demonstration.* Cambridge, MA: Harvard University Press.

Tichy, N. (1977). *Organization design for primary health care.* New York: Praeger.

Wise, H. (1972). The primary care health team. Archives of Internal Medicine, 130, 438.

Wise, H., Beckhard, R., Rubin, I., & Kyle, A. (1974). *Making health teams work.* Cambridge, MA: Ballinger.

Zimmer, J. G., Groth Juncker, A., & McCusker, J. (1985). A randomized controlled study of a home health care team. *American Journal of Public Health, 75,* 134.

# 16

## Attitudes, Values, and Ideologies as Influences on the Professional Education and Practice of Those Who Care for the Aged

Lisa Gurland

VARIATIONS IN CASE MANAGEMENT

The following case studies of Mr. James and Ms. Price demonstrate the differences in the way health-care clinicians understand and provide care to their clients.

### CASE 1

The staff in the coronary-care unit of an urban teaching hospital recently treated Mr. James, a man in his 80s who had suffered a myocardial infarction. Because of the diligent attention given to his physical condition and level of comfort, Mr. James's health status improved. Skilled-nursing care, monitoring of his medical condition by cardiologists through physical examination and appropriate use of diagnostic tests, and consultation with the departments of social work, pharmacology, dietetics, and physical therapy were used to provide Mr. James with the best health care the hospital had to offer. The staff focused on expediently diagnosing the medical illness and then set out to remediate the health problem as efficiently as possible. Getting as much done as quickly as possible without wasting either the patient's or the staff's time was seen as a high priority on the coronary-care unit. Discharge planning had begun upon admission and interventions were made with an eye toward the patient's being able to leave the hospital as soon as possible. In time, the staff was able to help Mr. James ambulate to the point where he was considered ready for discharge. After the taxi left him at the door to his home, it became apparent to Mr. James and his family that, however improved he might be, the climb to his apartment was more than he was capable of. With much commotion and distress, he and his family returned to the hospital and waited until an ambulance was available to take him home and bring him up the three flights of stairs on a stretcher. Though this man made a slow but full recovery, it was many months before he was vigorous enough to tackle the stairs.

## CASE 2

The home-care staff of a community health center has treated Ms. Price, a woman in her early 70s, in her home for the past 2 years. She suffers from hypertension, angina, difficulty in walking, confusion, and forgetfulness. The home-care staff, including a physician, nurse practitioner, and social worker, monitors her physical and mental status and has arranged for her to receive "meals on wheels" as well as homemaker and home health aide services. When her condition has required additional attention, a dentist, physical therapist, and podiatrist have provided her with treatment in her home. The home-care staff is prepared to provide comprehensive health-care services to Ms. Price on a long-term basis so that she might continue to live as comfortably as possible in her own home, where she has lived for 35 years. Because some of her symptoms have recently become more severe, a battery of diagnostic tests has been considered to possibly reveal a treatable condition. However, Ms. Price believes that medical intervention can sometimes "do more harm than good," and she has refused to undergo a brain scan or other diagnostic procedures that might shed light on her difficulties. The home health-care team has maintained a neutral position about diagnostic testing, and the staff does not think it impedes their ability to care for her adequately in her home.

How could the treatment of Mr. James and Ms. Price have evolved in a different way?

The organization of responsibility and control within an agency has implications for decision making and goal setting in patient care. The differences between the types of health-care settings affect ambulatory care and home care as follows:

| *Ambulatory Care* | *Home Care* |
| --- | --- |
| Focus on intrapersonal issues | Focus on person-in-environment issues |
| Focus of care oriented to the professional environment | Focus of care oriented to the home environment |
| Multidisciplinary professional relationships | Interdisciplinary professional relationships |
| Acute-care and crisis orientation | Long-term care orientation |
| Episodic client–clinician interaction | Continuous client–clinician interaction |

The case of Mr. James provides an opportunity to explore how professional roles in a hospital setting tend to be clearly delimited and each professional group tends to focus on the tasks and responsibilities specific to it jurisdiction. Because the demands of caring for a patient on a coronary-care unit are heavy, it is not unusual for no one staff person to have the "whole picture"; instead, as in the case of Mr. James, each practitioner manages a specific portion of the patient's total health-care needs. It is easy to see how the problem of the stairs might be overlooked because the hospital staff is intrapersonally oriented; that is, problem solving is focused on the dynamics that occur inside the individual instead of person-in-environment issues, whereby the individual patient is seen as one component of complicated problems and multifaceted solutions. Both the physical therapy department and the cardiology department found the patient to have the required physiological capacities to participate in the normal activities of daily living. Social services were not involved because Mr. James's finances were in order, he exhibited no unusual emotional or cognitive responses to his situation, and his family was attentive and supportive. The medical and nursing staff put their efforts into stabilizing his cardiac status and instituted a program of teaching the patient and his family how to keep him in the best health possible. This included following a strict dietary regime, participating in a regular exercise program, and scheduling follow-up visits to the medical center. Though all involved were interested in keeping Mr. James physically healthy at home, the hospital staff's perspective did not include an understanding of the home environment and the *home care* needed for him to function in it.

The goal of the professional staff in the coronary-care unit where Mr. James received care is the diagnosis and treatment of *acute* coronary disease. Meeting that goal includes judicious use of the medical center's resources in order to remedy a patient's cardiac difficulties. Various departments in the hospital provide either direct service to the client or consultation to the direct-care staff. For example, the medical staff examined Mr. James and ordered a series of diagnostic tests that monitored his physiological progress throughout his hospital stay. The pharmacist may have been consulted about the most appropriate medications for the client's condition, and the surgeon may have been asked to assess the need for an operative technique. Along with other professionals who helped to meet Mr. James's needs, the nursing, dietary, and rehabilitation departments provided a large portion of the daily care. The role of social services depended on the degree of financial, familial, and community support Mr. James had or needed. Direct service to patients and their families may be appropriate, or providing information to the nursing and medical staff regarding entitlement programs or rehabilitation centers may be the most beneficial use of social-service time. In some situations, social service is not used at all and in other instances the expertise of this department is relied on heavily.

In the hospital setting, the priorities and goals of health care necessitate carefully defined professional roles — that is, each discipline focuses on separate tasks coordinated to provide comprehensive health care to the clients. Hospital inpatient settings focus on short-term curative treatment and the goals include a timely discharge plan.

In addition to the distribution of professional duties, it is understood that the patient is *primarily* the responsibility of a particular physician, only secondarily is the patient the responsibility of the other staff of the coronary-care unit. In terms of professional role definition, the patient and the hospital staff think of Mr. James as Dr. Brown's patient, who was recently an inpatient on the coronary-care unit, who continued to be Dr. Brown's patient on a general medical floor, and who was then Dr. Brown's patient in a rehabilitation hospital.

Though most hospitals use a multidisciplinary approach to patient care, the physician is still viewed as the primary-care provider, and services from many departments can only be obtained through a physician's order. If the physician does not think that social services or physical therapies are necessary in a particular case, then the patient does not receive this care, regardless of how patient needs are viewed by other practitioners who actually may know the patient better than the physician.

Looking at another example of how health care differs between agencies, Ms. Price's health care might have been handled quite differently if she had been the patient of an ambulatory-care center of a general hospital instead of a home-care patient. In the outpatient department, care would have been centered on the resources of the hospital, not the home. The specialized and technically oriented staff might have strongly recommended that Ms. Price undergo an extensive evaluation for possible Alzheimer's disease, a brain tumor, and endocrine and other neurological or nutritional problems. A psychological assessment, including cognitive and projective tests, might have been used to rule out any underlying emotional illness contributing to her dysfunction. If the tests showed a treatable disease, medication, surgery, or other modes of intervention might have been instituted. Afterward, rehabilitation treatment might have been instituted to recoup any functional losses due both to the disease and the interventions that were meant to eradicate it. If the medical and psychological tests revealed a poor prognosis, then nursing-home placement might have been recommended for care and safety. In the nursing home, the emphasis on maintenance and safety for Ms. Price may have precluded more ambitious rehabilitative therapy.

Finally, the ambulatory-care staff would have had relatively few interactions with her (as compared to the long-term relationship of the home-care staff), and most of the interactions would have been task oriented (such as consultations with various specialty departments within the hospital). The end result of an ambulatory-care assessment could have been that, though a great deal of information was collected about Ms. Price, no one practitioner would have had a comprehensive view of the individual and how she functions in her home environment.

In contrast to the perspective of health-care delivery in both inpatient and outpatient hospital settings, home care per se presents a different view of the goals and treatment approaches to patient care. In the case of Mr. James, if the home health-care department of a community health center had to become involved, the discharge plan would have had a different focus. A careful assessment of the home environment and indigenous resources would have been the first priority. A home visit by the staff would have revealed the problem of the stairs and any other obvious circumstances that might impinge on a successful home transition. A meeting with the patient and key family members would have shed light on important cultural, religious, and social factors. These aspects of the patient's life would then have been integrated into the total health-care plan. Depending on the ability of the family to provide the daily health care, a schedule of visits by professional staff (nurse practitioners, physicians, social workers, physical therapists, etc.), home health aides, and homemakers might have been instituted. If, after the assessment, it had been clear that the family of Mr. James was not ready for discharge to the home, a period of time in a rehabilitation center could have been arranged for improving his functional level. The access the practitioners had to the important components of Mr. James's life, and the relevance and value they assign to them, affected the health care he received. Importantly, the focus of the coronary-care staff, which determines their approach to meeting the goals of treatment, differs in significant ways from the focus of the home health-care staff, which leads to quite a different approach.

In the case description of Ms. Price, the continuation of her present lifestyle depends both on her ability to maintain her level of functioning and on the support by the agency providing her health care. The home-care program is able to help keep her safe and comfortable in her own environment because its professional goals and priorities are similar to those of the patient. Because the philosophy of a community-based home-care program is not limited in its orientation to a strict medical model (i.e., the diagnosis and cure of self-contained disease), it is adaptable to the perspectives, values, and environments of patients in their home settings. The staff of the home-care program knows their patients over a long period of time (often years), and the treatment plan and health-care goals may change as the needs of the patient, family, and living situation change.

The professional roles of the home-care staff are neither rigidly defined nor permanently enforced (Gurland, 1985). In community-based, home-care programs, long-term care of patients in their individual homes requires more fluid boundaries between disciplines and a more generic view of task distribution. The primary practitioner for Ms. Price is likely to be the person on the staff most able to meet her needs, not a person designated by a predetermined hierarchy. For example, if the medical interventions needed by Ms. Price are minimal and the social-service needs are more complicated, then the social worker may be the professional in charge, though there will be direct care and consultation by the medical and nursing components of the program when needed. However, because Ms. Price is working with a program that understands her situation from a person-in-environment perspective as well as in terms of the intrapersonal issues in her life, the staff can take into consideration her personality, family, community, and health-care needs as well as her own wishes in making decisions about diagnostic tests and treatment.

It is important to note that individual staff members in an ambulatory-care department might be just as interested as the home-care staff in supporting Ms. Price's viewpoint, but because Ms. Price is well known to the home-care staff, they can weigh the pros and cons of diagnostic tests and treatment for this particular individual and are therefore able to support her desire to live out her life in a way that is meaningful to her.

These examples demonstrate some of the differences in the way practitioners and agencies perceive and treat the health problems of the aged. How practitioners and agencies understand clients and their problems determines their diagnostic and treatment procedures, extending from aggressive medical treatment to a less invasive psychosocial approach. Sometimes a combination of approaches is instituted; at other times one approach is rigidly adhered to.

What accounts for the variety of treatment approaches? One can understand the differences in care, in part, by looking at the attitudes, values, and ideologies (AVI) of practitioners and programs that treat the aged. AVI, though not the only determinant of health-care practice, exert an important influence on how practitioners conceptualize health status, problems, treatment, and goals.

## DEFINITIONS

*Values* are abstract ideals and principles of a group or society at large. A value is worthy of esteem or is desirable for its own sake; it is not simply a means to an end. For example, health is a positive social value in our society regardless of the circumstances or the individuals involved; conversely, illness is a negative value.

How do values originate? They are first learned in childhood through everyday life experiences. No one is born with a set of values; they are acquired as part of normal development through interactions with the environment. Just as other aspects of development take place through the assimilation of and accommodation to knowledge and experience throughout life, values also develop on a continuum. Though certainly the values learned early in life are the most ingrained, they can change through exposure to previously unexplored ideas, feelings, and situations. Values are integrated into the belief system of an individual, mediated through experience and relationships.

How does experience mediate values? Individuals' understanding of their environment is affected by relationships with other people who influence their thoughts and feelings. For example, if children are supported in their creative endeavors by their families and educators, then they will learn to value creativity. Later in life, relationships and experiences may support or undermine the value of creativity for these people.

*Attitudes* are likes and dislikes. They are our own affinities for and aversions to people, objects, and situations, including abstract ideals and social policies (Bem, 1970). It is important not to think of attitudes as static, for they exert a dynamic influence on people's responses to situations. Attitudes are the precursors of action; they create the impetus for much of human behavior. Using the example cited above, if people grow up valuing creativity, then their attitudes toward their own and others' creative endeavors will be positive. They will be likely to support creativity in their environments by using their positive attitudes toward creativity as the spark that fuels their activity in this realm.

Attitudes derive from values and provide the link in the relationship between belief and behavior: "Attitude is the intervening variable between conditions in the environmental context (stimulus input) [i.e., creativity as an internalized value] on one hand and behavioral activity in the other (output) [i.e., support of creative endeavors]" (McDavid & Harari 1968, p. 131). To understand the difference between an attitude and a value, consider the following example. Most medical personnel value good health achieved through the curing of disease. How a practitioner attempts to achieve a cure depends on the interaction of attitudes and values. Surgeons who want to use operative techniques and internists who want to prescribe medication for the same illness are sharing the same value (health through medical treatment) but are not sharing the same attitudes. In this situation, surgeons' values, which are acquired through a multitude of life experiences, including professional training, lead them to have a more positive attitude toward operative techniques and a less positive attitude toward medication in treating illness.

An *ideology* is a system of ideas reflecting the social needs and aspirations of an individual, group, class, or culture. Ideologies generally remain outside of our everyday awareness because alternative beliefs or conceptions of the world cannot be imagined. Bem (1970) uses the example of only unparochial and intellectual fish having the awareness of a wet environment. Fish usually have no understanding that it could be anything but wet.

Ideologies are the larger systems in which attitudes and values are embedded. An ideology is not an independent construct; it depends on attitudes and values for its definition (Eysenck & Wilson, 1978; Thouless, 1978). An ideology is formed through the interaction of values and attitudes, and it is through an ideological framework that attitudes and values are connected in an integral and meaningful way. However, usually ideologies remain unexamined, perhaps even unconscious.

For example, the attitude of community-based mental health treatment (a component of community mental health ideology) is based on the health-care value that mental health services are a right (not a privilege) and should be available to all people, regardless of ability to pay, in their own communities. The seeds of this ideology began to grow in the 1950s and 1960s, when a new, general definition of human equality became a value in this culture. With the integration of this new value into the mainstream of society, the attitudes toward long-term institutionalization of psychiatric patients in areas remote from their families and communities changed. With the change in attitudes came an opportunity for change in action. Thus the attitude of community-based care emerged as a component of community mental health ideology.

To gain a more complete understanding of any situation or experience, the *interaction* of attitudes, values, and ideologies must be explored. To investigate just one of these concepts is to miss a large piece of the picture. If one looks hard enough, under every action or attitude lies an ideology. Every independent decision made and every action taken presumes an attitudinal, valuative, and ideological base. Though not verbalized or even conscious, AVI operate together to create an idea, action, or emotional response.

## THE FUNCTION OF ATTITUDES, VALUES, AND IDEOLOGIES

AVI have three major functions for the health-care practitioner. According to Baker and Schulberg (1969, p. 433), "Ideological orientation must be considered a key variable since it very much reflects inner personality characteristics and choices in role definition." Thus, first, ideology is understood as a way of conceptualizing a self-definition (Bensman, 1967). It is the combination and interaction of attitudes, values, and ideologies that provide a framework for the tasks of a job, the reasons for decisions, and the way one feels about the work one does. In the case of Mr. James, the stairs to his third-floor apartment were not taken into consideration, in part because the health-care AVI of the coronary-care staff did not require specific information about his home as a necessary part of their professional practice to be included in discharge planning.

The second way AVI affect the clinician is by providing a link to a professional peer group. Ford (1980) states that clinicians want to feel good, and they identify with their peers by liking the same kind of clients, believing in the same treatment modalities, and so forth. According to Bensman (1967), the ideological base of one group protects itself through group solidarity against the ideological assaults of other groups. Groups provide the members with occupational pride, security, and motivation. If one does not share an AVI configuration with one's peers, then there is no place to recover when wounded, no place to seek shelter when things get overwhelming:

> What binds professionals together is not so much the facts we agree upon, or the knowledge we share, as the experiences we have all gone through, the way we understand them and fit them to the pattern of our values. (Fox, 1979, p. 77)

Finally, AVI provide a context for making decisions about client care. Health-care AVI influence treatment goals and methods. The qualities and ideas that clinicians think have intrinsic worth affect their clinical perspective: how they experience patients and perceive health-care needs. For example, if Ms. Price had gone to an ambulatory-care center, it is possible that a series of diagnostic tests might have been recommended by the professional staff. If a treatable condition were discovered, the staff might have encouraged her to use the resources of the medical center to undergo some form of medical intervention. It is the AVI configuration of the ambulatory-care staff that supports the idea of diagnosis and treatment of medical illnesses for Ms. Price. Likewise, it is the home-care staff's AVI that support Ms. Price in her decision not to undergo diagnostic tests and treatment but to maintain her daily activities.

These differences in AVI underlie differences in health-care practice. There is a relationship between AVI orientation and the way health-care programs are organized and the way practitioners function.

## THE DEVELOPMENT OF ATTITUDES, VALUES, AND IDEOLOGIES

What are the origins of AVI? Why do they differ from one person to the next?

We are all composites of our life experience. Our continual growth and development choreograph a complicated dance, with relationships, activities, and ideas as our partners. Though the lead may change hands depending on our circumstances, it is an undeniable fact that the partnership does not wither or die until we do. Throughout life, AVI development is influenced by relationships, environment, and one's ability to assimilate and accommodate oneself to new situations and experiences.

The influences of family, culture, physical environment, socioeconomic status, education, and professional training and experience are important in both the initial formation of AVI and in the ability to re-create personal belief systems based on experience and circumstances. If AVI are the trunk of the belief system, then AVI concerning the aged are a branch connected to that trunk, and health-care AVI concerning the aged are a twig stemming from the branch.

It seems pertinent to discuss first the development in early life of AVI toward the aged as a basis for understanding the development of the health-care AVI of clinicians who work with the aged. The fulcrum of family life allows for active inculcation of the individual's first set of AVI. Childhood years are impressionable, and many of the ideas and feelings assimilated during this period will be primary influences throughout life. Important and frequent exposure to grandparents or other older members of the community are forever embedded in one's accumulated experiences, conscious or unconscious, and provide a fertile soil from which AVI can bloom. If an aged person actually was a primary caretaker of a youngster, the influence is especially powerful, whether it be positive, negative, or ambivalent. How the adults in the family view their aged family members influences the children, who take their cue about how to think, feel, and act from their parents and other important adults. Adult responses such as joy, dread, condescension, and sadness in interactions with the aged affect the children's initial AVI toward them. If the aged are regular members of multigenerational households, then children have relationships with them as they would with any other person living in the family. With regular contact, children are able to learn in the context of a relationship about the positive and negative attributes of an *individual* who happens to be advanced in years. If visits with an aged person are rare, then there is a greater chance that the child will stereotype this person's characteristics and respond accordingly.

In terms of relationships with the aged outside of family life, the community's view of the aged population influences the children's developing AVI. If the aged are segregated through housing, social, and cultural activities, then children cannot help but experience the aged as different, handicapped, or stigmatized. If aged people in the community are employed, live in the neighborhood, and attend regular community activities, then the children have the opportunity to view them as functional members of society.

People interact with others according to their expectations of how those people are going to behave. No one discusses politics with a 3-year-old because they know the child's capabilities in this area are limited. Some people, however, because of exposure to poor role modeling or their own limited experience with children, are frightened of them or have very unrealistic expectations of age-appropriate child behavior. The same holds true for people's interactions with the aged. People who have had limited or no contact with the aged often find themselves frightened or without any knowledge of how to interact. As a consequence, the aged are often ignored, infantilized, or sent off to be with "other people like themselves." Children, who are quick to assimilate the AVI of their adult role models, interact with the aged according to their learned AVI configurations.

Issues of socioeconomic status affect the AVI children form about the aged. If children have contact with aged people who are thriving and functional, then the thought of reaching one's last decades may be viewed as a time of joy and independence. However, the aged make up a large proportion of the lower socioeconomic stratum in this country and are often unable to control their ability to provide for themselves in a safe and healthful manner. Because many of the aged are indigent, it is easy to understand why younger generations find the thought of aging frightening and unpleasant.

The media of mass communications have a tremendous impact on our view of the aging process. The aged are often depicted as frail in body, pitiful, annoying, silly, rigid in thought, and unable to understand and appreciate the aspects of life that the younger generations find indispensable. On television commercials, in magazine advertisements, and on the movie screen, the older person is usually presented as laughable or frightening — rarely sexy, wise, powerful, or heroic. An extension of the society they represent, the media often portray the aged in the same light as criminals, malformed infants, and an excess population of deer on public lands: "problems" for society to deal with expediently.

In recent years there has been some improvement in the depiction of the aged in the media. As the percentage of the aged in the population has increased, their visibility in the culture has also increased. Though certainly many aged live in poverty, each year the number who retire with financial means has risen. This group is now targeted by advertisers as potential consumers for a variety of products and services. In addition, there has been a recent upsurge in television and movie dramas that show the aged in a positive light. The mass media are a powerful force through which more realistic depictions of the aged will have a positive influence on society's AVI.

In addition to early life experience, the process of higher education, both general and professional, also influences AVI formation. College life is notoriously homogeneous. The student body generally consists of people within a narrow age group, and students tend to live in dorms or apartments with those of their own generation. Sometimes an aged professor will have direct contact with the student body, but many undergraduate courses are taught by young graduate students. Some universities encourage employees over 65 to retire to make room for the younger teachers who are trying to move up through the ranks.

Though facilities for the handicapped, by law, are becoming more a part of our experience, demonstrable illness or disability is not something that most college students have to acknowledge. College educators do not generally consider the concomitant effects of aging a learning priority for students.

In a liberal arts curriculum most universities offer few courses that address the issues of aging. Biology courses spend much more time on the formative aspects of life than on the processes of degeneration. In psychology courses much emphasis is placed on early life growth and developmental issues. Though developmental theories abound, there is a paucity of information and ideas on the later stages of life. Neither theoretical classroom discussions nor actual contact with the aged tend to exist as part of the educational experience. As an influence on AVI formation and modification, this message has far-reaching ramifications.

Besides contact in daily life, students learn about the aged through daily life and experience in practica and internships; through interaction with teachers who communicate knowledge, ideas, and feelings about the aged; and by reading the available literature on the issues of the aging process. Each of these arenas hopefully allows students to explore existing AVI (their own and others) toward the aged and to develop new AVI through the influences of their education. If a curriculum does not encourage learning in this manner, students are deprived of an important opportunity in their own educational growth and development. Without knowledge, experience, and support, students can easily be overwhelmed or turned off through the process of interacting with any group of people. Because of the ageist attitude prevalent in our society, the aged are particularly prone to stereotyping, prejudice, and ostracism.

## ATTITUDES, VALUES, AND IDEOLOGIES IN PROFESSIONAL EDUCATION

Because of the shaping of AVI by familial, educational, and societal influences, most students do not enter graduate education with the idea of specializing in geriatrics. However, some students do become interested in geriatrics while in professional training, and in recent years the number of geriatric/gerontological programs has increased. Others who may not have given much thought to the topic beforehand leave their graduate programs with an aversion to working with the aged population. What accounts for this difference in experience?

As discussed previously, AVI formation begins early in childhood and continues to be a developing process throughout life. By the time people enter professional training programs they often have well-established AVI concerning health care for the aged. How, then, is it possible for students to acquire new AVI configurations? Can they develop or modify their health-care AVI through education, or do professional schools only select students who share the AVI of the educators, institutions and professionals and thus only reinforce these AVI? There can be no definitive answers, since the response to these questions depends in part on the AVI of the author and readers of this chapter. However, the following discussion will take into consideration these salient issues.

In professional education programs, opportunities for reworking old beliefs and trying out new ones is an implicit part of students' curricula. The combination of the type of education offered by the institution and the ability of the student to make use of these opportunities promotes educational growth. If student training is effective, graduates emerge not only skilled in the theory and tasks of the profession but also with the ability to create personal and professional understanding of their work through the development of health-care AVI.

How does this process evolve? The culture of professions and specialties within them act as breeding grounds for new AVI toward the aged. This culture includes society's view of the different disciplines, the way they are viewed by other types of professionals and nonprofessionals, and their status and effect on health care in the community. Culture also refers to the ambiance of the educational institution, the teaching methods employed, the stigma or support inferred by the way a group of patients is discussed, the type of research that is acknowledged, and the range of employment opportunities graduates are encouraged to pursue. It is through the acculturation of students into the disciplines that health-care AVI are influenced by education. Once people have metamorphized from members of the general public to students of health care to full-fledged professionals, they have been exposed to numerous situations, which, upon careful analysis, promote the evolution of AVI.

The appropriate context for professional training involves a three-pronged process that integrates the *educational, psychological,* and *social* components of learning for the student with the professional needs and goals of the institution. The institution's *educational* goals are to impart the knowledge and skills appropriate to the general AVI of the profession within the context of the AVI specific to that particular institution. The students' *educational* goals complement those of the institution in that students assimilate the knowledge and skills they are exposed to by the institution. In addition, however, students must accommodate themselves to the AVI of the institution. In this context, accommodation refers to the integration of the institution's AVI into an already existing AVI configuration that each student brings to the professional training program.

The process of integrating students' AVI with the AVI, knowledge, and skills taught by the institution is influenced by *psychological* factors that affect learning. Students bring ideals and enthusiasm superimposed on a need for nurturance and support in an environment where the language, culture, and expectations are unfamiliar. Students are, by definition, at least somewhat uninformed and lacking in certain skills; however, at the same time they are also vulnerable to criticism and psychological injury. How does the student attain enough openness to learn in conjunction with enough healthy defensiveness to tolerate criticism for the normal ineptness of a student-in-training? How does the institution demand a level of competence in accordance with professional expectations while supplying the student with the encouragement and positive regard needed to assist in the transition from neophyte to professional?

The *social* component of professional training accounts for the integration of the educational goals and the psychological needs of both student and institution. By role-modeling appropriate standards of behavior, by requiring a level of expertise in knowledge and skill, and by providing opportunities to channel energy and enthusiasm, the institution fosters a social environment conducive to acquiring AVI consistent with the goals of the institution. Within an environment that supports the growth and development of the professional-in-training, the student is able to attain the knowledge and skills necessary to practice in the health-care field. Besides the theoretical and technical aspects of obtaining education, the identification with role models and the exposure to a wide range of health-care clinicians and settings will enhance the formation of AVI in a way that is meaningful for the student as a potential independent practitioner as well as a potential member of a professional group.

For example, suppose Ms. Price were to be evaluated in an ambulatory-care center by a professional team that included nursing and medical students. How would the other team members respond when the students wonder out loud if she is "too old" for a certain type of rehabilitation program? What would happen if the students expressed concern about the rigors of extensive diagnostic testing and its possible debilitating effect on Ms. Price? The response of the professional team members to the students' concerns and questions will affect the students' future interest in pursuing new ideas, raising different perspectives, continuing to ask questions about difficult subjects — and their views of the aged and readiness to work with them.

The way students experience new clinical situations also has an effect on their AVI. Nursing students are well informed about the advantages of diagnostic procedures as the first step in a process that will eradicate disease. If they are assigned to a clinical rotation in a home-care program, how do they make sense of the team's support of Ms. Price's unwillingness to accept this form of health care? Faced with what appears to be contradictory AVI, the students are forced either to reject this previously unexplored perspective as unethical or incompetent, or they must accommodate this new way of thinking about health care for the aged in their existing pattern of AVI. It is through the process of slowly and carefully integrating new ways of thinking about professional issues that AVI develop or are modified.

## ATTITUDES, VALUES, AND IDEOLOGIES IN PROFESSIONAL PRACTICE

### *Care of the Aged*

How do Health-care AVI affect the way in which the individual functions as a health-care professional? First of all, the general view of old age will have implications for the practitioner regardless of the type of work setting. Those who see old age as a *pathological* "condition" that needs to be treated will function differently from those with a *developmental* outlook, that is, the perspective that aging is a part of the normal life cycle.

The viewpoint of pathology looks at the aged person as being the sum total of component parts that may need to be fixed or cured. Using the example of Mr. James, each practitioner who treated this client on the coronary-care unit believed that he was healthy enough to go home. However, because the AVI of staff were narrow, a major impediment to a successful transition home was overlooked. Had Mr. James been assessed by a community-based home-care program or a rehabilitation center before discharge, the problem might have been recognized and a solution found. What is emphasized—the health-care goals of an inpatient setting—and deemphasized—the health-care goals of a home-care program)—in Mr. James's treatment reflects the AVI held by the health-care professionals treating him.

A developmental perspective of the aging process focuses less on pathology and cure through treatment and more on interventions that support the continued functioning and psychological growth of the patient. Psychological growth refers to the client's continuing need to function as independently as possible in the context of the best available lifestyle and interpersonal relationships. Regardless of age, human growth and development reflect a continual striving for an interesting and creative life. For Ms. Price, her way of creating a meaningful life did not include diagnostic tests. The home-care staff took a developmental view when they decided to support her wishes. Because of their orientation to health care, the home-care staff was able to see Ms. Price in her own environment, functioning day to day in a way that was meaningful to her.

Practitioners who see the aged as being hopeless because of their chronological age will offer a different view than those who find the life problems of the aged challenging. If the professionals who cared for Mr. James or Ms. Price had an AVI configuration that saw the aged as hopeless, then either patient might have received only custodial services at home, or perhaps a nursing-home referral would have been encouraged.

Thoughts and feelings about the *meaning of illness* affect the kind of care that is offered. Do health-care professionals believe that any change in ability to function is negative? Does being old and sick mean that a mistake was made in choice of lifestyle, nutritional intake, or some other controllable factor in the person's life? Is illness a punishment for serious indiscretions in thoughts or behavior? The implication is that if only one had behaved better, then all would have been well. Is illness seen as an enemy force to eradicate at all costs, or is it seen as distressing but a normal part of the life span with which to be coped? Do practitioners feel helpless or hopeless in the face of illness, or is it understood as a problem to solve within certain acceptable (to the patient) boundaries.

For example, a headache can be approached in a variety of ways: taking a pill, making an appointment with a neurologist for diagnostic tests, lying down with a cool cloth on the forehead, changing one's diet, praying to God, or ignoring the pain completely. The differences between these choices reflect differences in health-care AVI. Clinicians who believe in the medical model will assume that the headache is a response to the malfunctioning of a physiological system. Clinicians whose AVI are more holistic will look beyond the medical components to a larger range of possibilities. The practitioner who makes the decision to use extraordinary means to keep an aged person alive, regardless of the quality of life, has a different set of AVI from that of the practitioner who does not recommend any treatment for a particular problem because the client is "too old." It is the practitioner's AVI toward both the aged and health care that affect the decision-making process and treatment options for the aged.

### Relationships with Health-Care Institutions

Though it is certainly individuals who are ultimately responsible for treatment, no one functions in a vacuum. Usually practitioners are part of institutions that provide treatment. Consequently, the AVI configuration that practitioners bring to their work is modified by the already-existing AVI of the health- care agency. Of course, the individual has an effect on the agency, but unless the position a person holds is particularly powerful, major changes in the institution's set of AVI usually happen subtly over time, not with the addition of a single staff member.

Because agencies or departments within them have set AVI configurations (either stated or unstated), it is meaningful to look at the settings in which health-care professionals are employed. The economic needs of the practitioner and the staffing needs of the agency notwithstanding, the mutual attraction of employee and employer is related to a perceived concurrence of health-care AVI. The ability to function easily in a setting and the praise and support received from superiors and peers require a foundation of a mutually shared belief system. Conversely, dissatisfaction with the job role and clashes with the employer about role and function reflect a discrepancy in health-care AVI, at least in the way they are realized in that particular setting (see Chapter 15, Developing the Interdisciplinary Team).

In the example of Ms. Price, if a home health-care practitioner has AVI that support the idea that "where there is life there is hope," then going along with Ms. Price's wishes would be very uncomfortable for that practitioner within the AVI structure of that type of agency. That practitioner might be more comfortable with the health-care AVI and practices of an intensive-care unit in a medical center.

In the case of Mr. James, if the AVI of a staff member on the coronary-care unit supported the idea that the aged are "too old" for a cardiac rehabilitation program, then there may be a conflict between the AVI of the inpatient unit and the AVI of that staff person. Perhaps this particular person would be more in tune with the AVI of a nursing home or a non-rehabilitation-oriented medical unit.

### Relationships with other Disciplines

One of the ways that AVI manifest themselves in health-care practice is through the relationship of the practitioner with members of other disciplines. The vision of one's role both as a provider of service and as part of a health-care team, however limited the connection, is reflected in how one functions in a professional setting. For example, some practitioners find it important to be identified as the patient's primary caregiver, and some are more comfortable with the team approach of shared responsibility. Still others combine useful aspects of both approaches and identify themselves as primary practitioners within the context of an available team. The behavior of the practitioner in these circumstances is the consequence of AVI put into action.

Using the example of the coronary-care unit described, each practitioner is responsible for a particular part of the patient's health care. Individual providers often have no direct communication with each other and know of each other's existence only through progress notes or laboratory reports. For example, the physical therapist, one of the developers of the cardiac rehabilitation program, believes that a thorough, comprehensive program with an emphasis on instructing patients about their present limitations and teaching them safe methods of strengthening their cardiac muscle allows patients to leave the unit stronger and with the minimum of medication. The physician is not convinced of the benefits of the cardiac rehabilitation program and believes in the curative aspects of pharmacology. Therefore, many clients are discharged home on cardiac medication before receiving the full benefit of the inpatient rehabilitation program. Not only is the difference in opinions about treatment protocols influenced by health-care AVI, but the practitioners' AVI affect how they communicate their differences to each other. If both practitioners believe that interdisciplinary meetings are necessary, then the differing opinions can be addressed in this setting with an understanding of the areas of competence of the various disciplines and flexibility in disciplinary roles. If the practitioners believe that it is the role of the physician to take full responsibility for making treatment decisions, then the expectation of both staff members may be that no discussion is necessary because the physician will write the orders and the physical therapist will carry them out regardless of the professional judgment of the physical therapist. In this situation, the physical therapist may do a half-hearted job in providing treatment for Mr. James because the system (created by AVI) does not allow for action in accordance with the health-care AVI of this practitioner. The physical therapist confronts the ethical dilemma of being unable to act responsibly in light of professional judgment and personal values.

In part, variation in behavior in a health-care setting is related to the differences among professional groups. Through the process of education and acculturation into a particular health-care field, professionals have many ideas (conscious and unconscious) about their own identities, functions, and roles. How professional identity relates to the needs of the patient and the health-care team influences how the care is organized and delivered. Practitioners who believe that only health-care professionals are competent to make health-care plans would be appalled at the support the staff gives to Ms. Price in response to her treatment decisions. Practitioners who believe that treatment decisions are a team effort, and that the team includes the client, are more comfortable with the home health-care agency's interdisciplinary approach to decision making and would object to the narrow and dictatorial treatment of Mr. James.

Finances also affect the health-care practice of clinicians. The financial access to the different treatment options may influence the actual care a client receives, overriding the AVI of any practitioner or health-care team. If Medicaid benefits are the only available financial resources, then care will be dictated by what Medicaid covers. Here societal AVI affect the health care of individuals. Social values and policy determine taxation, funding of government programs (including medical assistance to the poor), and the health needs and services deemed worthy of support (see Chapter 12, Disability Trends and Community Long-Term Health Care for the Aged, and Chapter 13, The Economics of the Health-Care System).

In some health-care situations there is competition for financial resources among health-care agencies or departments within agencies. Government funds and private grant foundations are often available through a competitive proposal-writing and bidding process. Public health departments issue licenses based on an agency's ability to prove that a service is needed in a particular community. In these situations it is not always in the best interest of professionals to work collaboratively with other agencies. Practitioners stand to lose their jobs if programs in their agencies are not refunded or if budgets are cut. For example, there may be more than one agency capable of treating the homebound elderly in a given community. Because these agencies survive through the collection of third-party payments for services to these patients, each program is in competition with the others for patient contacts. Consequently, there can be animosity among the various professional groups which then compromises the working relationship and ultimately affects patient care.

Looking at the issue of finances from another perspective, the encouragement of additional patient services by other professional groups may be an exercise in futility if the services are not reimbursable. For example, if Mr. James's family is unable to participate in his care at home, nursing-home placement may be necessary for his physical well-being. If the staff at the nursing home believes that Mr. James (whose care is paid for by Medicaid) might benefit from attendance at the on-site adult day-care program, he will be unable to attend because Medicaid will not pay day-care fees for nursing-home residents. Here again the health care AVI of professionals and agencies are superseded by the AVI of government or society in determining the care of the aged. Because societal AVI are ageist and because the aged are the largest growing group falling below the poverty line, the aged are not seen as worthy of getting their needs met. Legislating the distribution of resources so that the aged get only a piece of what they need to function comfortably and safely is a clear statement about the nature of our society's health-care AVI.

## RECOMMENDATIONS FOR CHANGE

Because of society's various AVI toward the aging process, the aged are often discriminated against in terms of the availability of resources. AVI are reflected in the amount and quality of health-care resources available and the way care is offered and received. Limited reimbursable services, relatively few health-care practitioners who specialize in geriatrics, inadequate numbers of nursing-home beds, lack of affordable, safe housing for the aged; this is just a partial list of resources that have a low priority in the United States. If society changed its perspective toward the aged and took a more balanced view of the gains as well as the losses encountered at this stage of human development, then dramatic changes would be seen in the organization and delivery of health care. These changes could also affect the professional education of health-care clinicians, the availability of treatment resources, the practice of health care by professionals in a large variety of settings and, ultimately, the care and health of the aged.

### *Professional Education*

The process of education affects not only the patients cared for by students throughout their professional careers but also the care delivered by generations of future practitioners. In other words, the skills and knowledge imparted to one individual at one point in time is then passed on numerous times and in many different forms to students, colleagues, patients, families, health-care administrators, legislators, and others influenced by the AVI of one individual. Consequently, the way in which practitioners are educated has far-reaching effects on both the present and future health-care system.

One of the most important moments in a student's career is the first contact with actual patients. Even the most seasoned professional is able to recollect early experiences in patient care. It is not unusual to hear statements such as, "I remember my first patient when I was a nursing student. It was the first time I had ever seen a person who was that old and that frail," or "When I was an intern I had to tell this old man that he had cancer, so I went to my chief resident and she told me something that I never forgot."

Education is a powerful way we can effect changes in the health-care AVI of students and, ultimately, of clinical practice in health-care systems. The first clinical experiences of developing practitioners are often the most significant in that they force the integration of a new set of data (thoughts, feelings, and behavior) into an already-existing AVI configuration. A new experience — whether it be an actual interaction with a patient, a theory discussed in the classroom, or the observation of another practitioner carrying out a procedure — creates a window of opportunity by means of which one can access a previously unexplored way of understanding.

For example, how do students assigned to the coronary-care unit where Mr. James received treatment understand the problem of the stairs on the day of his discharge? What are the factors that will influence their AVI? Perhaps the most important influence is the observed reaction of other professionals on the health-care team. Was the problem seen as important enough to discuss in a team meeting, or was it shrugged off as an inconsequential piece of information? If a discussion did ensue, was one discipline blamed for "not doing its job," or did all practitioners present the issues from their unique professional perspectives? Was there an interdisciplinary process to modify the discharge planning procedures on the coronary-care unit in a way that avoids similar problems for future patients? The broader the array of professional opinions, the more likely it is that students will have a wide range of ideas and theories to integrate into their own understanding of what is important in discharge planning.

In the case of Ms. Price, it is important that students are exposed to a variety of opinions about the patient's wish to do without the benefit of diagnostic tests and treatment. To have just one viewpoint — that of the home-care staff — would be to deny students the opportunity to integrate new information rather than to simply accept or reject the AVI of the home-care staff as the determinant of care.

We have described how, when students are confronted with new situations, it is important to expose them to a variety of professional viewpoints as alternative perspectives to the same problem. One way to ensure a range of opinions is through interdisciplinary education (see Chapter 14, The Interdisciplinary, Integrated Approach to Professional Practice with the Aged). It is a mistake to continue the present trend, which follows a unidisciplinary approach — that is, nurses are trained almost exclusively by nurses, physicians by physicians, social workers by social workers, and so on. By creating a training program in which disciplines have the opportunity to teach and learn from each other, there is a greater chance that students will be better equipped to handle their relationships with patients, treatment options, and the expertise of other professional groups. Cooperative learning and teaching will dispel myths and stereotypes about the relative strengths and weaknesses of other disciplines that often grow up because students and teachers share little of the education of any group except their own. In the same way that exposure to the aged through everyday relationships reduces stereotyping and affects AVI toward the aged, interdisciplinary education reduces polarization of student groups and creates an environment in which AVI toward the aged can be broadened through everyday relationships with people who have an understanding of health care different from one's own. In addition, by sharing the learning process with a diverse group, students and educators have an opportunity to develop a more realistic appreciation of each other. A realistic view of other disciplines will affect the students' AVI toward other health-care practitioners and practices as well.

If professional education is to be considered more than just technical training, then education must go beyond the tasks and theories of any one particular discipline. For example, operating-room technicians can be trained in a number of months to do a safe, responsible job of completing tasks appropriate to a surgical setting. However, registered nurses who work in the operating room, through the process of professional education, understand not only the concepts and tasks pertinent to the surgical setting, but also learn about general health-care and nursing theory, political and social issues inherent in the hospital system, and ways in which nursing affects and is affected by the other professional groups involved in health-care delivery.

Besides the training students receive in the clinical setting, it is also important for students to learn about the lives of healthy and functional aged people. Since most people (especially the aged) who are seen in a clinical setting are ill or are having difficulty functioning, students naturally come to believe that aging is a purely debilitating process. Consequently, it is important for students to get to know aged people who experience the joys of their later years, the gains as well as the losses of aging. As part of students' curriculum, it would be useful for them to be acquainted with aged who live in and maintain their own homes and property, who are engaged in gainful employment, who live as functional members of multigenerational families, and who enjoy and contribute to the mainstream of cultural and social events in their communities. Knowing the range of functions possible for the aged would broaden the concept of treatment goals and methods of health-care practitioners. It is by knowing what is desirable and also possible for the aged that practitioners are able to make treatment recommendations that include the broadest range of alternatives for their patients. If practitioners have the most complete perspective possible of client needs both in illness and in health, they can be more competent and flexible in providing information, support, and services. Also, though it may not be reasonable to expect all professionals to have the same expertise, a broad base of clinical knowledge and experience will encourage the provision of better, more comprehensive care.

For example, if the team leader or primary practitioner is limited in knowledge, experience, or accessible options, then the treatment plan created will also be limited. Health-care providers, if they have a strictly medical orientation, can easily overlook social needs, and vice versa. Consequently, through narrowness, important health-care needs can be easily overlooked or underestimated. Conversely, if different professionals in a given case prioritize differently what is important, it is possible that the overall care of the patient may be fragmented or inconsistent. One way to ensure a broad base of knowledge and understanding is through a team approach to health-care education and practice, using professional skills from a variety of disciplines. If clinicians of different disciplines share treatment planning responsibilities, then health care can be organized in a way that meets clients' needs in the most suitable and efficient manner possible. In the process the differing priorities of the involved disciplines might then be coordinated.

Patient care suffers when clinicians are expected to make decisions without the proper expertise. Though no one practitioner (or discipline) can be expected to have all the knowledge and skills needed to care for every patient, each clinician must have enough ability at least to identify the problems and know the sources of appropriate care. This can come from pooling resources through a team-oriented case-management approach. A broad health-care perspective is achieved not only through the organization of the health-care team, but also through the training of professionals. Through the educational process, students can be exposed to a variety of professionals and, with proper training, can understand the similarities and differences of disciplinary roles. The health-care AVI of professionals can be influenced through interdisciplinary training and experiences and an organized team approach to health care.

### Staff Selection

The health-care AVI of practitioners have implications for the selection of staff who work with the aged. It is beneficial for health-care agencies to seek out practitioners whose customary approach to patient care matches the role expectations of that particular institution. Conversely, practitioners who choose to look at institutional AVI when considering employment make professional choices appropriate to their needs and interests.

Though aspects of institutional AVI are often clear to health-care professionals, either through exposure or hearsay, there is little direct communication from the institution to the staff, explicitly outlining (1) the rationale behind the organizational hierarchy, (2) the reasons for the unequal dispersion of resources among departments, and (3) perhaps most importantly for the staff, how the various disciplines interact and communicate — whether it be through a unidisciplinary, multidisciplinary, or interdisciplinary mode.

Conflicts between professional peers, distrust between supervisors and staff members, and antagonism between employees and agencies are often the result of clashes of health-care AVI. For example, consider the nurse who spends an hour each week talking with the family of a newly admitted patient. In this meeting, the nurse includes some information on the patient's condition, prognosis, and future health-care needs. The family uses the time to vent feelings of grief, fear, and anger. The nurse thinks it prudent to invest time in building an alliance between staff and family so that decisions about patient care are made cooperatively with the support of all parties concerned. Interestingly, depending on the AVI of the agency, the amount of staff time involved (1 hour per week) may be considered inappropriately large or small for the tasks described.

In a home-care program, the supervisor may encourage the nurse to spend more than an hour a week with the family in this initial period so that a successful treatment plan can be organized and implemented. The nurse may be encouraged to visit the home and meet with the family members at their place of business. If the nurse agrees with this concept, then the staff member and supervisor (as an agent of the institution) have congruent AVI and care will be provided with mutual satisfaction. If the nurse disagrees with the supervisor and does not want to spend additional time with the family but instead wants to do more bedside nursing of the patient, then a discordant relationship between practitioner and agency emerges.

In a hospital setting, however, the supervisor might consider an hour each week to be an inordinate amount of time for the nurse to spend with the family because it takes time away from bedside care, the designated role of the nurse in that institution. If the practitioner does not share this understanding of health-care AVI, then an inappropriate staff-employer match results in dissatisfied, frustrated practitioners and angry employers. This, in turn, leads to increased turnover in employment and, ultimately, less than optimum care for the client.

Moving away from specific client care issues, the differences in role definition among professionals is affected by institutional AVI (Gurland, 1985). How the health-care AVI of an individual as part of a particular professional discipline relates to the AVI of the workplace has implications for the selection of staff in any type of agency. For example, people interested in sharply defined professional roles and clear functional expectations may find working in large medical centers (in both inpatient and outpatient departments) most congruent with their configuration of health-care AVI. Those same clinicians may not be suited to employment in smaller community-based programs because of the limited number of specialized services and the overlapping of professional functions. In contrast, clinicians who resist role definition and are comfortable with unstructured and less traditional resources are likely to be well suited to work in small community agencies. These same clinicians might feel restricted by the clearly defined professional roles and strict treatment protocols of larger, more compartmentalized institutions.

Though there is no clear formula for making perfect choices, the issues inherent in the selection process of both agencies and staff are worth careful consideration. How practitioners understand and feel about the work they do relates to the way agencies function, affects the level of professional satisfaction, and most certainly influences the type and quality of patient care.

### Client Referral

As patients, families, and health-care professionals assess health-care problems and needs, consideration must be given to the appropriate choice of practitioner and institution for evaluation, diagnosis, and treatment. When confronted with a request for the name of a practitioner or health-care institution, most people — health-care professionals as well as non-health-care professionals — will send the patient to a person or place the referring person believes to be of high quality. This is done without asking questions about or giving much thought to what the particular patient might need. It is not uncommon to hear statements such as, "Dr. Brown is the only doctor I would trust," or "Ace Hospital is the best, go there for your surgery." Usually these well-meaning referrals are not based on any understanding of the need to identify the health-care AVI of the patient, practitioner, or institution. In addition, little thought is given to how the relationship among these AVI will actually influence the health care of the patient.

In the case of Ms. Price, her health-care AVI affect not only the kind of treatment she will be open to but also how she will relate to the health-care providers who offer her care. The particular way that Ms. Price's AVI interact with those of her practitioners influences her ability to receive the optimal care *best suited to her own needs and wishes* and affects the practitioners' ability to provide her with treatment that does not compromise their own health-care AVI. The best care is given and received when the AVI of practitioners and patients are similar enough to allow for communication, trust, and the development of a treatment plan that meets the needs and abilities of all concerned.

In the case of most referrals, little thought is given to how the medical condition, understanding and beliefs about health and disease, and life situation (family support, community resources, finances, religion, etc.) of the patient will interact with the health-care AVI of the practitioners. If the patient is refusing to consider hospitalization as an option, then it is probably a waste of time to refer the patient to a practitioner who works primarily in an inpatient setting. Conversely, a client who is anxiously anticipating the possibility of surgery for a malignant lump may initially be referred to a surgeon and later referred to an agency that provides long-term follow-up care. The word "best" or "good" when applied to health care or an institution only has meaning in the context of individualized, appropriate health care.

In the case of Mr. James, it would not be unusual for the physician to rely on Mr. James's wife to make decisions or contemplate treatment options during periods when the patient was not able to do so himself. However, because of the background and inter-personal dynamics of this family, the oldest son, not Ms. James, was considered to be the head of the household during his father's illness and, consequently, the one expected to make decisions about Mr. James's health care. Whenever the oldest son tried to contact the physician, the physician referred him to his mother, Ms. James, because *she was the head of the household from the physician's perspective.* After must discomfort and anger on the part of the family, the physician was finally able to meet the family's need by communicating directly with the oldest son. If the physician had known more about the family's AVI, then communication could have resulted in a smoother hospital stay for the client and less disruption and disharmony for Mr. James's loved ones.

An appropriate referral is one whereby attention is paid to the integration of the individual needs of patients and the health-care AVI of the institutions and practitioners available to provide treatment. In addition, the health-care professionals must be willing to learn about the patients' AVI and adjust their own accordingly so that the care is given in the best interest of the patient, not for the convenience of the staff and institution.

Unfortunately, in both the health-care community and in the general population, it is apparent that some health-care AVI are believed to be universal. For example, one common belief is that disease should be treated by the latest medical technology and this way of managing illness is considered to be the best alternative for everyone. However, another way to understand medical technology is to think of it as *one* intervention that lies on a continuum of possible treatment options. For example, in the usual mode of making a referral, if Dr. Brown is considered to be a "good" doctor, then Dr. Brown is the physician of choice to treat whatever medical problem exists. If Ace hospital has the latest and most extensive diagnostic and treatment equipment, then it is believed to be the "best" hospital in the area. This is a common misconception that can lead to poor care despite the supposed worth of the individual practitioner or institution.

In a more general sense, the health-care AVI of patients have ramifications for both the choice of medical treatment and the patients' ability to use the care to the best advantage. With patients' knowledge and consent, diseases and problems that require complicated medical technology are best treated in the specialized departments of well-equipped medical centers. In addition, if health-care treatment can be accomplished by health-care clinicians alone (e.g., treatment of a discrete disease entity within the individual), then large medical centers have the professional resources needed to handle these problems.

However, if patients have needs that involve interrelated problems (e.g., chronic physical disabilities that require assistance in the activities of daily living and therefore social services), then the referral may be most appropriately made to a local community agency. These agencies are limited in the realm of immediately available medical technology but are equipped to organize the nonmedical community resources that allow for coordination of care with minimal disruption to the client life at home. Sometimes, a combination of specialized services in a large institution can be combined with the long-term care of a community-based program.

Ultimately, it is the concomitants of the health-care problem combined with the health-care AVI of the patient, the family, and involved professionals that determine the setting of choice to meet the treatment goals. These factors, in combination with knowledge of the different services available in the different agencies, increase the likelihood of making an informed decision about optimal health-care programs for individual clients.

## REFERENCES

Allport, G. W. (1967). Attitudes. In C. Murshison (Ed.), *A handbook of social psychology.* New York: Russell & Russell.

Amor, D., & Klerman, G. L. (1968). Psychiatric treatment orientation and professional ideology. *Community Mental Health Journal, 9,* 243–255.

Baker, F., & Schulberg, H. (1967a). *CMHI scale.* New York: Behavioral Publications.

Baker, F., & Schulberg, H. (1967b). The development of a community mental health and ideology scale. *Community Mental Health Journal, 3*(3), 216–255.

Baker, F., & Schulberg, H. (1969). Community mental health ideology: Dogmatism and political-economic conservatism. *Community Mental Health Journal, 5*(8), 433–466.

Bem, D. J. (1970). *Beliefs, attitudes and human affairs.* Belmont, CA: Brooks/Cole.

Bensman, J. (1967). *Ideology, ethics and the meaning of work in profit and non-profit organizations.* New York: Macmillan.

Birnbaum, N. (1960). The sociological study of ideology. *Current Sociology, 9*(2), 91–117.

Brauer, L. D., Gilman, E. D., & Klerman, G. L. (1975). Psychiatric treatment of ideologies among university faculty. *Psychiatric Opinion, 10*(1), 25–35.

Cranston, M. (1974). *Ideology.* London: Encyclopedia Brittanica.

Curtin, S. (1972). *Nobody ever died of old age.* (p. 16). New York: Atlantic Monthly Press.

Dekadt, E. (1982). Ideology, social policy, health and health services—A field of complex interactions. *Social Science Medicine, 16*(6), 741–745.

Destuff de Tracy, S. L. C. (1978). Elemens d'Ideologie. In H. J. Eysenck & G. D. Wilson (Eds.), *The psychological basis of ideology.* Baltimore, MD: University Park Press. (First published in Paris in 1817)

Eysenck, H. J., & Wilson, G. D. (Eds.). (1978). *The psychological basis of ideology.* Baltimore, MD: University Park Press.

Festinger, L. (1959). *The theory of cognitive dissonance.* Stanford, CA: Stanford University Press.

Fishbein, M., & Ajzen, I. (1981). Formation of intentions. In M. Fishbein & I. Ajzen (Eds.), *Belief, attitude, intention, and behavior* (pp. 21–52). Reading, MA: Addison-Wesley.

Ford, C. V. (1980). Attitudes of psychiatrists toward elderly patients. *American Journal of Psychiatry, 137,* 571–575.

Fox, R. (1979). *Essays in medical sociology.* New York: Wiley.

Gastorf, J. W., Anderson, R. L., Gaskins, S. E., & DeShazo, W. F. (1982). Attitude change as a result of role defining conferences. *Family Practice Research Journal, 1*(3), 172–176.

Gilbert, D. C., & Levinson, D. J. (1957). Custodialism and humanism in mental hospital structure and in staff ideology. In M. Greenblatt (Ed.), *The patient in the mental hospital.* Glencoe, IL: The Free Press of Glencoe.

Gurland, L. (1985). *Who you are is what you do: A study of the health care attitudes, values, and ideologies of clinicians who work with the elderly.* Unpublished doctoral dissertation, Massachusetts School of Professional Psychology, Boston, MA.

Katz, D. (1960). The functional approach to the study of attitude change. *Public Opinion Quarterly, 24,* 164–204.

Kestenbaum, V. (1982). *The humanity of the ill.* Knoxville: University of Tennessee Press.

Krishef, C. H. (1982). Who works with the elderly? A study of personnel in gerontological settings. *Education Gerontology, 8*(3), 259–268.

McDavid, J. W., & Harari, H. (1974). Attitudes, development and change. In McDavid and Harari (Eds.), *Psychology and social behavior* (pp. 84–106). New York: Harper and Row.

McDavid, J. W., & Harari, H. (1968). *Social psychology — Individuals, groups, societies.* New York: Harper and Row.

Parson, T. (1958). Definitions of health and illness in the light of American values and social structure. In E. G. Jaco (Ed.), *Patients, physicians and illness.* Glencoe, IL: The Free Press of Glencoe.

Ryden, M. B. (1978). An approach to ethical decision making. *Nursing outlook. 26*(11), 705–706.

Schulberg, H., & Baker, F. (1969). Community mental health: The belief system of the 1960's. *Psychiatric Opinion, 6,* 14–26.

Sharaf, M. R., & Levinson, D. (1957). Patterns of ideology and role definition among psychiatric residents. In M. Greenblatt (Ed.), *The patient and the mental hospital.* Glencoe, IL: The Free Press of Glencoe.

Strauss, A. (Ed.). (1964). The questionnaire study. In *Psychiatric ideologies and institutions.* Glencoe, IL: The Free Press of Glencoe.

Taylor, H., Hirschboeck, J., Westberg, G., & Smith, J. (1960). What are the effects of the physician's view of human nature upon his patients? In *The place of value systems in medical education.* Fourth Academy Symposium of the Academy of Religion and Mental Health, with Josiah Macy, Jr., Foundation (pp. 105–160), New York.

Thouless, R. H. (1978). The tendency to certainty in religious beliefs. In H. J. Eysenck & G. D. Wilson (Eds.), *The psychological basis of ideology.* Baltimore, MD: University Park Press. (First published 1935 in *British Journal of Psychology, 26,* 16–31)

Zimbardo, P. G., Ebbeson, E. E., & Maslach, C. (1977). *Influencing attitudes and changing behavior.* Reading, MA: Addison-Wesley.

# IV

# The Interdisciplinary Care of Aged Persons—An Integration of the Issues

Part IV of the text presents a concrete example of the interdisciplinary team at work in evaluating and planning the clinical treatment of an aged person, Mrs. Steinfeld. In Chapter 17, An Interdisciplinary Case Conference, the various health care professionals demonstrate both the technical expertise their disciplines contribute and the perspectives (attitudes, values, and ideologies) they hold. Thus, a vigorous debate arises about the nature of health problems, the goals to be desired, the types of helping intervention to be applied, and the settings in which treatment should take place. The interdisciplinary process consists not only of various contributions but also of mutual understanding and respect among colleagues, and the pursuit of common goals and complementary efforts. Especially interesting is the discussion of both team functioning and the interdisciplinary working relationship that is an ongoing part of the team's work.

As part of the commentary on the interdisciplinary care of aged persons, David Satin, a psychiatrist, notes that several fundamental questions relevant to the interdisciplinary clinical care of the aged are raised in this illustration of the interdisciplinary case conference: Who appreciates the importance of the insight and skill with which helping interventions and the use of resources are understood, taught, and practiced, and how these impact on clinical care? Who recognizes the health implications of the social context in which people function or fail to function? How are clinical issues for individuals related to interpersonal and societal issues? And who finally integrates all these factors? Ideally, the clinician – or a good interdisciplinary team – does this, and practicing clinicians should incorporate into their work an understanding of team development; interdisciplinary practice; and appropriate attitudes, values, and ideologies. However, in practice it is often those seeking care – aged people, their families, and informal caregivers – who are left trying to understand what is needed, find what is available, and wring practical, caring help out of real-world settings. This highlights a dilemma about who controls clinical care. One approach puts the aged and their families at the hub of the caregiving team and policy-making group. In this model it is paradoxical that, in practice, they are almost always left out of formal evaluation and planning. The other approach makes health care professionals responsible. In this model it is inappropriate that professionals are often too narrowly focused to plan and deliver comprehensive care, and the aged and their loved ones – the least sophisticated and least powerful participants in this interaction – are left to make the best of the scattered and arcane helping interventions they encounter. In nature, the various components of an ecosystem reach a balance. When people intervene, they must take responsibility for understanding the significance and consequences of their interventions. In health care delivery, intervening professionals know more about specific caregiving techniques than about the whole pattern of care, which involves patients, clinicians, caregiving institutions, and the larger community and society.

As a nurse, Barbara Blakeney notes that we have suggested throughout this volume that an interdisciplinary training program and practice makes it possible to integrate the knowledge and perspectives of all the professions that interact in the clinical setting. The strength of this approach is that these perspectives can be synergistic. Our goal is for all of us together—clinicians, patients, and their families—to make something happen that each of us individually cannot achieve, even with all our knowledge, skill, and technology. Jennifer Bottomley, physical therapist, finds all patients so different that the expertise of all disciplines are needed to deal with the physical, emotional, and socioeconomic areas important in an individual's life. The interdisciplinary team provides the many areas of expertise as well as the flexibility that allow individual disciplines to come to the fore when necessary to help the team meet individual patients' needs.

Indeed, Satin notes, health care is a continuously creative endeavor. Caregivers must be flexible and must be able to adapt to the needs of specific persons, situations, and resources. We are all seeking, struggling, and experimenting to help our patients. We need to continue to struggle, to find better ways, to find a more comprehensive understanding of all these factors, to tune and shape our efforts so that the individual, society, and theory fit together in a beneficial relationship.

The case conference, which epitomizes and synthesizes the subject matter of this book, puts our theory into practice, according to Blakeney. Each discipline contributes its perspective and expertise to the process of finding out how to address Mrs. Steinfeld's needs and help her to realize a life that is more meaningful, healthy, and consistent with her wishes. The issues of goals, roles, and procedures, presented in Chapter 15, Developing the Interdisciplinary Team, come especially to the fore: Who will do what and when? The conference illustrates how a team raises and addresses crucial issues. We encourage readers to apply the theoretical principles presented in this book to the example of the case-conference team's work—and to their own work.

# 17

## An Interdisciplinary Case Conference

David G. Satin (ed.)

ROSE STEINFELD: A CASE STUDY IN GERIATRIC HEALTH CARE

Rose Bloomberg was born in the United States 77 years ago to a Jewish family that had immigrated from Russia seeking economic opportunity and religious tolerance. They settled in a small city (part of a major metropolitan area), at that time populated largely by Eastern European Jews and Mediterranean immigrants who worked as artisans, factory workers, and small merchants. Both parents (and the children, when they were old enough) worked long hours in a small family grocery and lived a meagre existence. Nevertheless, the parents encouraged their children to seek education, culture, and a higher socioeconomic status. They were all regular members of an orthodox synagogue, but not preoccupied with religion.

Rose completed high school and a 2-year business school, and then worked as a secretary while living with her parents. She married Joseph Steinfeld and helped him build a successful retail jewelry business in the same city. They lived comfortably but modestly, bought a house, and raised a son and two daughters. Although they "modernized" and dropped some of the ritual practices, Mrs. Steinfeld and her family retained their religious and cultural identity, and the congregation was an important part of their social network. She was an intelligent, vigorous, healthy, warm woman with broad cultural interests and social involvements. Her two sisters and their families also settled in the same city, and her brother in a nearby suburb. They were in touch with one another often and looked after their parents — largely in the parents' home — in their old age and last illnesses. The brother and one sister have died; the other sister, who is physically disabled and mentally impaired, lives in a nursing home.

Mrs. Steinfeld's children all attended college, married, and moved away — her son to an upper-middle-class suburb 12 miles away, one daughter to a neighboring state, and the other daughter thousands of miles away. Mrs. Steinfeld began to develop osteoarthritis of her fingers and knees. Her husband developed coronary artery disease with angina and had a mild heart attack. They were cared for by their local family physician, with whom they had had a long relationship, with occasional visits to a nearby teaching hospital for specialty procedures. Their local pharmacist, a former schoolmate who owned and operated a small drug and candy store two blocks from their home, regularly filled their prescriptions and was both a friend and medical counselor.

The population of the city changed: The first-generation immigrants died, their children moved to more distant suburbs or other parts of the country, and a new wave of working-class immigrants — first Hispanic, then Caribbean, and later East Asian — moved in. A general atmosphere of discomfort and tension developed between the "old-timers" and the "newcomers," with occasional personal or political conflicts, though warm relationships between individuals also existed. At the same time, the small factories, warehouses, and retail businesses on which the city's economy had been based were replaced by larger manufacturing and chemical industries, a change that brought with it economic depression, increased pollution, and overcrowding.

After struggling to continue business as usual, Joseph Steinfeld finally closed his jewelry business for economic and health reasons and moved some of its contents into the attic of his home. The house was subdivided into two apartments, the Steinfelds living on the second floor and the first-floor apartment rented out to increase their income. Mr. Steinfeld's heart disease, prostatic hypertrophy, and osteoarthritis increased, and Mrs. Steinfeld developed otosclerosis with moderate hearing impairment in addition to worsening osteoarthritis. As their health deteriorated, contemporaries died or moved away, and the local population changed, the Steinfelds' social activities became more restricted. Their involvement with their religious congregation — a shrinking remnant of aging couples and individuals — became more important in their social lives, and religious beliefs became more important to their sense of meaning in life. The rabbi, whom they had known for decades, visited congregants at home with ritual on ceremonial occasions, with authority when they had problems, and with comfort in time of pain.

Five years ago Mr. Steinfeld died of a heart attack. Mrs. Steinfeld continues to live in the second-floor apartment on income from Social Security Old Age Assistance and Survivors' Benefits, with slight supplementation from a dwindling inheritance from her husband. Her children occasionally buy her a household appliance or article of clothing but make no regular monetary contribution to her support. The pharmacist friend has died and his family moved away. Mrs. Steinfeld must now go or send someone for her medications to a chain discount drug store 2 miles away. Her family physician retired 2 years ago. A dwindling number of aging physicians remain in the community, and health clinics and nearby teaching hospitals have varying interest in and resources for serving this community. Mrs. Steinfeld has not developed a relationship with another physician or clinic, receiving only sporadic medical care from a variety of sources. The rabbi at her synagogue died 8 years ago and has been succeeded by a series of younger, part-time men who have not gotten to know the congregation. Mrs. Steinfeld has not been to her synagogue in 2 years. Her physical disabilities, discomfort with the strange customs and language of the current community residents, and fear of the crime in the area have increasingly confined her to her apartment and made her feel socially isolated and lonely. Occasionally old friends phone but rarely visit, since they, too, are old, disabled, and fearful. She misses her husband, cries often, sleeps poorly, and sometimes wishes God would "take me." She telephones her son more and more often to talk and ask him to visit. He is concerned about her, but his responsibility to his family and work do not permit him to visit more often than every 2 to 4 weeks.

In the past 2 years Mrs. Steinfeld developed hypertension and hypertensive heart disease, which make it hard to climb stairs. Her medications are digoxin for her heart disease, methyldopa (Aldomet) for her hypertension, occasional injections of hydrocortisone for her arthritis, and occasional prescriptions for diazepam (Valium) for depression and insomnia.

In the past 8 months Mrs. Steinfeld has become increasingly forgetful, anxious, and confused. She has begun to suspect that her tenants are not caring for their apartment well or paying their rent on time, and knocks on their door at odd hours of the day and night to complain and threaten eviction. She has begun to fear that neighbors have learned that there is a stock of her husband's jewelry hidden in the attic and might break in to steal it. For the past 4 months she has been calling her son and the police to report that her tenants' teenage nephew is breaking into the house at night through the attic window to burglarize the attic and her apartment. She has heard and seen him at night and has found some of her posessions missing. Her son nailed boards over the attic window, but Mrs. Steinfeld now claims that the boy comes in through a hole he has made in the roof. The police no longer take her calls seriously. The tenants, sympathetic but annoyed, are thinking of moving out. Her children are worried and exasperated, and do not know what to do with her. They have suggested nursing home placement, but Mrs. Steinfeld is violently opposed to being "put in that graveyard for the living" where children get rid of their unwanted parents. She reminds her children that she and her siblings cared for their parents at home no matter what their needs.

On examination, Mrs. Steinfeld is neatly and attractively dressed and groomed, though her clothes are slightly untidy and stained. Her apartment is neat and clean, but the furnishings are worn. She is a thin, frail-looking woman. Her hands are deformed and have swollen joints, she has difficulty holding and manipulating objects (such as buttons and bottle caps), her gait is hobbling, and her balance is unsteady. In embarrassment, she tries to hide and minimize all these disabilities. She is warm and polite, and welcomes visitors into her home even when they are strangers. She readily describes her life, health, and worries realistically and easily shows her sadness and loneliness. She talks about her earlier life in great detail and with much feeling but cannot remember or is confused about recent happenings and knows little about current events. Her thinking and speech are clear and logical except that she describes clearly and convincingly her fears and beliefs about the invasion of her home by the neighborhood teenager. She is uncertain about what help or changes in her life she wants except to be protected from the danger she fears and to be less lonely.

## INTERDISCIPLINARY CASE CONFERENCE

A list of conference participants, the authors of this volume, follows. The discipline of the participant is provided along with an abbreviation of this discipline, which will be used for reference purposes in the pages that follow.

David Barnard: Ethics (ET)
Barbara A. Blakeney: Nursing (NS)
Johanna T. Dwyer: Nutrition (NT)

Marjorie Glassman: Social Worker (SW)
Lisa Gurland: Attitudes, Values, and Ideologies (AVI)
Margot C. Howe: Occupational Therapy (OT)
Glenn S. Koocher: Economics (EC)
Thomas F. O'Hare: Law (LW)
Terrence A. O'Malley: Internal Medicine (IM)
Athena S. Papas: Dentistry, Nutrition (DT)
Diane S. Piktialis: Economics (EC)
David G. Satin: Psychiatry (PS)
Joseph M. Scavone: Pharmacy (PH)
Benjamin S. Siegel: Teamwork (TM)
Helen D. Smith: Occupational Therapy (OT)

## First Team Meeting: Planning the Evaluation

SATIN (PS): This team has been organized at the request of the Visiting Nurse Association and family to provide consultation to them about Mrs. Rose Steinfeld, and perhaps to provide services to her and them.

Speaking as a psychiatrist, I think Mrs. Steinfeld is dealing with many obvious cognitive and emotional problems and needs help with them. The first that comes to mind is that she's sad and lonely. She is dealing with an existential condition— something real—that makes her sad and lonely: not only the loss of her husband and other important people in her life but her whole life style and context. I'm not comfortable talking about this as an individual's intrapsychic pathology, but rather as a life crisis (as Dr. Erich Lindemann would have put it). It produces normal emotional reactions that need clinical intervention in order to help Mrs. Steinfeld deal with her predicament in an adaptive rather than maladaptive way.

Another concern is what I would call her delusions about the boy breaking into her house. I think the evidence is fairly strong that this is not reality but her belief and her way of handling her predicament. I don't know at this point what the cause of the delusion is or whether it is reversible: whether it's her way of handling her loneliness and forgetfulness, a reversible toxic reaction or some kind of permanent brain dysfunction.

Finally, there is her forgetfulness itself, which is a grave symptom. I wonder whether this will turn out to be a permanent disability for her.

I think that evaluations of the physical, nutritional, and social aspects of her condition would shed light on her mental state.

BLAKENEY (NS): I think one of the things we're missing is a current data base in general. We don't really know Mrs. Steinfeld's current physical health status, including her cardiac status. I agree that we don't know why she has an altered mental status. A good physical evaluation will help answer these questions and suggest a plan of care. We probably should arrange this quickly.

HOWE (OT): I think we need to evaluate her level of physical health first and then apply the results to her psychosocial and behavior problems.

O'MALLEY (IM): I echo that as well, and would add a few things. It's important to have the data base as complete as possible so that we can set our priorities for intervention. There are quite a number of medical issues that are not clear, such as the cause of Mrs. Steinfeld's hypertension, the extent of her hypertensive cardiovascular disease, and whether her current treatment is contributing to her depression or cognitive disorder. Our team pharmacist can comment about the well-known effect on cognitive function of digoxin in toxic doses and alpha-methyldopa in therapeutic doses. We certainly would want to clarify that as part of our initial evaluation.

The problem list we have on the basis of the history suggests that this woman's long-term ability to remain at home depends more on her cognitive state than her physical state. I for one would direct more attention to her cognitive disorders than her degenerative arthritis or hypertension.

SATIN (PS): But don't her physical disabilities limit her ability to survive outside an institution? If she can't get up and down the stairs, whether because of her cardiovascular impairment or her arthritis, isn't she disabled? People end up in nursing homes because of physical problems, too.

O'MALLEY (IM): Physical impairments certainly can cause limitations, but on the list of priorities we should rate more highly those things that are going to impair her function most. I think her mental status is probably going to be more disabling than her physical problems, or at least so it appears by history. Her arthritis and hypertension are relatively simple problems compared to the difficulties resulting from her changes in judgement and questionable ability to take care of herself because of her mental status. Also, it's problably easier to overcome her physical limitations by making alterations in her environment, such as adaptive devices and a move to a first-floor apartment. These simple changes would avoid the need to relocate her from the house.

PAPAS (DT): She seems to have a neat apartment; she's a neat person, but she's frail. Maybe she has some nutritional problems. Her cognitive impairment might be because her medication is incorrect or it could be nutritional. Perhaps these factors can be addressed and reversed.

She seems isolated. People who eat alone tend to have more nutritional problems because they sometimes develop very strange diets. We have taken histories and discovered people who have tea and toast in the morning, canned pasta for lunch, and tea and toast for dinner. The nutritional content of that diet is not very good. We would want to assess whether she is still able to cook, how she shops, and the kinds of food she buys. If Mrs. Steinfeld is having trouble going out into her community, she's probably not shopping. If she is not getting a lot of green, leafy vegetables, salads, and so forth; is not eating a lot of fruit; has a pretty low-protein and high-carbohydrate intake; and doesn't have enough vitamin in her diet, she is in nutritional trouble.

The medications she's taking may be causing her to lose nutrients like potassium. Also, people who don't have roughage in their diets frequently get constipated and then turn to remedies such as mineral oil, which cause them to lose even more nutrients. She may be thin and frail-looking for these reasons.

Changing hats and speaking as a dentist, Mrs. Steinfeld needs a dental evaluation in addition to a medical evaluation. Frequently, chronic problems lead to poor eating. People may have several teeth that are loose and abscessed. They'll flare up for a few days, a fistula will drain it, and then the problem will subside and show up again 2 months later. Such problems don't necessarily disable people completely, but they degrade the general quality of life and cause enough discomfort that people avoid the kinds of foods that get them into trouble and move toward a softer diet. These sorts of situations may cause a fever of unknown origin and can contribute to confusional states like Mrs. Steinfeld's.

So she needs to have a dental workup. Once her dental status is determined, she needs dental work done that she can handle. Her ability to take care of her dental needs should be assessed, and she needs help in learning how to maintain her oral health as well. Her arthritis may be giving her problems in brushing her teeth. If so, we can also adapt a toothbrush. If she has dentures, we can set up a little scrub brush on the sink with suction cups for her to use. If she has trouble with one hand, she can use her good hand to clean the dentures. Little things like that can make life easier and help her to function.

It's hard to take an older person completely out of her environment It would be better if she could remain and function well in her familiar environment.

SATIN (PS): You raise an issue of real psychiatric concern. Taking this person out of her environment, especially if she has trouble learning and adapting because of even a slight degree of dementia, would add so much to the problems of her dementia itself! Confronting her with evidence of her incapacity may make her anxious, depressed, or precipitate some other reaction. One is sometimes very torn in deciding which course of action would do her more good: caring better for her physical condition by getting her into a safe setting or maintaining her mental functioning by keeping her in a familiar setting.

BLAKENEY (NS): A couple of things come to mind from a nursing perspective. First, it seems to me that Mrs. Steinfeld is profoundly isolated physically, emotionally, and spiritually. She has no dependable support system in any of these areas, and that puts her at great risk of having to either alter her life style or having it altered for her by concerned family or because of her behavior and inability to function.

From the history it strikes me that she might have a very poor self-image. She hides her hands deformed by arthritis, and that adds to the isolation. Her activities of daily living may be profoundly affected by her physical limitations. Can she see well enough to know that the gas is on in the cooking stove and otherwise avoid injury in the kitchen? The history indicates that the house is clean, telling us that she is able to do some basic activities of daily living, but there are others that we don't know about. In addition, she's got a sleep disturbance for which she may be treating herself with *exactly* the wrong medications.

A variety of support services could be built into her daily life to help with physical tasks such as shopping and cooking. Perhaps even more importantly they could help her break out of her social isolation and build a support network of people who interact with her and give her access to outside activites and resources. This is vital in making it possible for her to remain in her home. I am concerned even about moving her downstairs, because if she's worried about people breaking into her house, the ground floor might be more frightening because it is much more accessible. I'd prefer to do everything we can to make her life in her current environment successful. Only if we find that we're unable to do that, would I consider environmental change.

SCAVONE (PH): One of our goals should be to straighten out Mrs. Steinfeld's medical problems. It seems that she hasn't had any coherent medical help in 2 years. She's been getting prescriptions from who-knows-where, and then getting them refilled. As a pharmacist, I think we need to consider these medications and their side effects, because they could either be causing her medical problems or magnifying them. For example, consider digoxin: some possible side effects are delirium, visual and auditory hallucinations, delusions, changes in appetite, nausea, vomiting, and disruption in the way a person thinks of eating or perceives food. Methyldopa can produce side effects such as depression, nightmares and other sleep disorders, drowsiness, and dizziness. Diazepam toxicity can produce delusions, depression, disorganization of thought, incomprehensible remarks, incomplete statements, and problems with recall.

We need a review of her medications either by meeting with her or with her family. I think her medical situation needs straightening out before we proceed.

O'MALLEY (IM): I'd like to suggest that we develop a problem list of sorts. To begin with, I would like to raise the issue of whose problems we are trying to solve here, what we are trying to accomplish, and under whose auspices. Are we intervening in this woman's life because of *her* request, because something has gone wrong and *she* wants a change? Are we intervening because the *family* is concerned or can't take the situation any longer and wants something done? Are we intervening because the *neighbors* are tired of being harrassed? Or have the *police* or some other *social agency* been contacted and asked for intervention?

I think that it's important to answer that question for a couple of reasons. One, it helps focus the team on concrete goals rather than trying to accomplish everything in this situation. Two, it raises profound ethical and rather tricky legal issues about just whose rights we are respecting or violating in this situation.

BARNARD (ET): The question of who has requested help from the team is very important. It is easy for the family to emerge as the most vocal party and for the team to be misled into thinking the *family's* needs determine the focus of attention. It will be crucial to arrive at a mutual understanding (perhaps we could call it a contract) between the team and Mrs. Steinfeld based on her statement of the help *she* desires. She has articulated desires to be less lonely and less vulnerable. Presumably she also needs to have medication provided, her hypertension monitored, and so forth. These are the beginnings of contract development. We need more explicit expressions of what she is prepared to do for herself, what she will allow done for her, her expectations of the team, and so on.

SIEGEL (TM): From a team process point of view let me make an observation at this point. The providers have raised many questions about the need for data and the task of developing a problem list and set of care plans to meet the patient's needs. There have been many suggestions about what ought to be done but it wasn't until Terry O'Malley raised some questions about fundamental goals that the team process became crystalized. Team effectiveness is determined by the team's goals.

Until the goals are defined, the team cannot go on to the next step of assigning team roles: who does what, about what problem, and how we're going to evaluate effectiveness.

KOOCHER (EC): It appears that she has a great number of medical and social problems. Her problems with medications may be indicative of the fact that she hasn't had a primary-care physician for some time and may be shopping around and receiving uncoordinated, duplicated medical care. These problems are not going to be met by a single agency or a group of individuals or agencies. She needs to be close to a comprehensive treatment source with a single entry point and a coordination mechanism that will direct her through the various services she will need. These are the reasons this interdisciplinary team has been assembled: so that we can evaluate her needs and direct her to the entry point of an appropriate, coordinated treatment system.

SATIN (PS): In trying to decide what treatment system to refer Mrs. Steinfeld to, we've talked about her physical and mental health needs, and we've at least alluded to her ethical and legal needs. Another consideration is what health care facilities are available to her.

KOOCHER (EC): This requires careful consideration. Since Mrs. Steinfeld lives in a metropolitan area rich in health care resources, a large array of social, medical, and institutional services are available. If she lived in a small population area with sparse health care resources, she'd be in a totally different health care environment, better and worse in various ways.

SATIN (PS): But even in a metropolitan area rich in resources, realistically one of the first questions caregivers are going to ask is, "Is she on Medicaid or Medicare, or is she 'private pay'?" And that's going to influence the services she has access to. There are some places where she is not going to be welcome.

KOOCHER (EC): The effect of these factors on medical services will depend on the political, social, economic, and other pressures placed on the provider community.

SATIN (PS): Realistically we know that lots of pressures are placed on the provider community, and good social workers who think about getting access to community resources for people such as this are going to ask themselves, "How are these services going to be paid for and what facilities are going to accept these sources of funding?"

KOOCHER (EC): It appears from her income information — her reliance on Social Security Old Age and Survivors' Benefits and some savings — that she is probably not eligible for much subsidized service. She's not getting a whole lot of money, and it looks like she relies primarily on Medicare, possibly with the addition of a form of Medicare-supplement insurance, to pay her bills. She probably does not have Medicaid, based on the income information we have. That's still going to leave some portion of her income for her use after basic living expenses. I would think her access to medical care will not be limited. Mrs. Steinfeld will have to be willing to spend money, at least with regard to dental care, because if she has dental problems, as most of the other thousands of Mrs. Steinfelds have, she's going to be paying for those almost entirely on her own. In this sense she has as much medical coverage as many other older persons.

PAPAS (DT): That's why we have the Geriatric Dentistry Clinic, where the fees are half-price. Also, we try to have a nice environment — a penthouse with a little courtyard.

KOOCHER (EC): If she's fortunate enough to be near that type of facility. A geographic inventory of health care resources would tell us.

PAPAS (DT): That's why we have transportation as another service.

KOOCHER (EC): If that clinic is close to other focal points of service, that would be very valuable to her.

O'MALLEY (IM): She may not have access to homemaker or home health aide services except by paying for them out of her own pocket.

KOOCHER (EC): That's clear, but her access to medical services should not be limited.

PAPAS (DT): Her medical fees would probably have to be set on a sliding scale.

KOOCHER (EC): Her access to superior medical services, as opposed to just whatever medical services might accept her funding sources, is an issue. That is, her limited finances might enhance her access to an outstanding specialist rather than restrict her to seeing a local physician who may not be as skilled or as willing to refer her to expert consultants.

PAPAS (DT): I would hope her children would become involved at that point. They've been willing to buy major appliances and things like that; if it came to a major health need, they might help pay some of the medical bills.

SATIN (PS): I wish the social worker would comment on the issue of individual priorities. We have talked about Mrs. Steinfeld's need to spend money so that she has access to health care, or having her family contribute to her care. In doing so, we are talking not only about economics but psychology and social relations as well. Will she want to spend money on her medical care, which does not have any very immediate reality to her, or would she rather economize for the sake of saving her money so she doesn't starve in the future, which may be something she learned in childhood? If her family members are asked to contribute to her support, what kinds of family relationships — rejection or responsibility — is this going to stir up? Such old issues may make them decide, for instance, that they don't want to or they wish they hadn't been asked. These are not simple questions.

KOOCHER (EC): With the exception of the son, who may be fed up with his mother's belief that someone is breaking into the house, we haven't heard from the children.

Financial issues aside, if, at some point, this woman faces a catastrophic illness or even a serious illness requiring some hospitalization, are the clinicians making decisions about her care going to consult with the children without consulting Mrs. Steinfeld? Are they going to make decisions on her behalf without her input? A whole range of self-determination ethical issues are raised.

BARNARD (ET): Now is the time to have serious discussions with Mrs. Steinfeld concerning how decisions should be made regarding medical care. Her preferences regarding critical care, limitations to treatment (such as cardiopulmonary resuscitation), and other matters should be documented in the medical record. She is still competent and can express herself articulately. Even if her family expresses contrary wishes, hers take precedence. All of this is easier said than done, of course. I would suggest that these issues gradually be worked on in the course of establishing a trusting, open relationship. Many of the serious legal and ethical problems in decision making for incompetent patients can be minimized with this sort of advance discussion.

O'HARE (LW): I hope that clinicians aren't going to be making decisions on her behalf without consulting her, or imposing diagnostic or treatment procedures on her simply by talking with her children and getting their permission. They simply do not have legal authority in this situation. To minimize exposure to legal risk I would advise clinicians not to involve themselves in that kind of action.

SATIN (PS): But don't clinicians usually do just that as a matter of course?

O'HARE (LW): Many people don't take my advice.

SATIN (PS): In what percentage of cases are such actions ever challenged? How many people get into trouble for not taking your advice?

O'HARE (LW): Realistically, liability only becomes an issue when something goes wrong or when someone is unhappy about the outcome. The complex medical, social, and psychological issues involved in the treatment of elderly persons means that the possibility of a "bad outcome" is greater than it is in the treatment of younger, more resilient persons. As a result, the liability exposure is also increased in working with the elderly. I'm simply saying that legally there is no authority to impose treatment on this lady without her consent.

PAPAS (DT): What if she is adamantly opposed to being placed in a nursing home, as has been reported, and her son has had it with her and decides he's going to put her in a nursing home? What then?

O'HARE (LW): Legally, the first issue that must be resolved is that of the person's competence. As a consultant, I would ask the clinical people who have directly observed her for their impressions of her competence to direct her own affairs. I see some mildly delusional behavior, but it does not appear to grossly impair her judgment. I don't see anything in the case report that tells me that she's incompetent: that she doesn't understand the consequences of her behavior or decisions. That is a basic test of competence.

SATIN (PS): My understanding is that clinicians cannot determine competence. This lady is competent — she is legally in charge of herself — until a competent authority says she is not. She can be as bizarre as can be, but until a court says that she is no longer going to make her own decisions, she is in charge.

O'HARE (LW): That's quite true. I'm asking whether there appears to be sufficient evidence to bring the issue before a court with the likelihood of having a guardianship or conservatorship imposed.

SATIN (PS): Will a court condone overriding her preferences retroactively? If she says, "I don't want to go to a nursing home," and somebody says, "You're going to burn yourself up in this apartment," and carries her off to a nursing home, and she sues, and a petition for guardianship is brought to the court, and the court says she is not competent and she was not competent last month either, is the person who carried her off to the nursing home off the hook?

O'HARE (LW): Probably. First, it is unlikely that a nursing home would admit her if she actively resisted the admission and declined to sign herself in as a resident. And the persons accompanying her would have no legal authority to sign for her. I would hope that most long-term care facilities are sensitive enough to their own liability exposure to know this.

Realistically, however, any court would have to look to the bottom line, which is damages. If the individual was not damaged in any meaningful way by the action, the only liability would be for violation of Mrs. Steinfeld's civil rights. If the violation was committed by an individual not acting for the state and the motivation for the action was humanitarian, it is not likely that damages would be imposed. If they were imposed, they would be nominal. Still, it is entirely possible that a court might wish to "send a message" regarding the rights of the elderly and find that a serious invasion of Mrs. Steinfeld's civil rights had occurred. There might be penalties imposed for this.

Regardless of the likelihood that monetary damages would be awarded, it seems to me that a desirable approach in working with the elderly is to respect the integrity and autonomy of the individual. I think we should accept that this woman appears to be legally competent to make her own decisions and that if those decisions are contrary to her best medical or social interests, we must persuade rather than coerce her.

O'MALLEY (IM): Let me try to put Mrs. Steinfeld's case into a different perspective. First, she does not appear to be in a crisis or at risk of imminent harm to herself or others in the household: she's not leaving the stove on, she's not lighting fires in hallways. She appears to be functioning at an appropriate level.

SATIN (PS): As a psychiatrist, I'm not entirely comfortable that there's no emergency. She's not going to drop dead immediately, but she is at risk of embedding her delusional system — her maladaptation to her crisis. The longer she practices this delusion, especially if she's got some degree of dementia and is therefore inflexible, the more it's going to be set in place and the harder its going to be to get it out. So I think we need to do something about it with all deliberate speed.

I'm also sympathetic to the need to avoid overwhelming her. We don't want to brutalize her and harm her in that way. But I don't want to delay action any longer than necessary.

HOWE (OT): That's a good point. I agree.

O'MALLEY (IM): The degree of urgency of the problems determines the speed with which any interdisciplinary group must arrive at either recommendations or interventions. This situation allows us some time — not available in all cases — to systematically develop the data base. We can get the information we need in a way that doesn't irreparably interfere with the establishment of a good, close, therapeutic alliance with Mrs. Steinfeld over time. For example, we needn't go in there like gangbusters — 90% of this group knocking on her door some day to assess her mental, medical, social, environmental, nutritional, and dental health.

What we need instead is probably an approach that brings as few people as possible into her home — with her permission — to begin two simultaneous tasks. One is to establish a close relationship upon which further interventions would be based. The second is to begin to gather data and establish the priorities of issues requiring intervention. Our priorities would be established, in large part, by listening to what Mrs. Steinfeld tells us her priorities are.

SIEGEL (TM): Let me make a comment on team dynamics. Terry O'Malley has just performed an important function of leadership. He has summarized the approaches of the various team members and tried to outline a set of goals for the team to address.

At this point, it's up to the team to decide whether it makes sense to define emergent versus nonemergent problems for the patient or whether there are other goals to be addressed.

In setting goals, the team must make a series of decisions. For instance, what kind of assessment is needed? The providers have questioned whether Mrs. Steinfeld should be in a nursing home, but it doesn't sound like that can be decided until more information is gathered. So one of the major goal issues is to get more information about the patient and her social, psychological, and medical status.

The next question is: Are there other goals that need to be identified besides gathering more information?

O'MALLEY (IM): One important issue to raise now is how we get her into medical care? Are we prepared to make that an involuntary step? Can we do that? I think it has to be her choice.

SCAVONE (PH): I agree there would be problems with involuntary treatment, but her reluctance has really not been established. We know that her son is starting to get fed up. If he's convinced that her behavior might be influenced by her medical condition, he might help convince her to get a checkup after having none in 2 years.

BLAKENEY (NS): People whom patients know, whom they feel more comfortable with for whatever reason, can establish trusting relationships. Those relationships then open the door to trusting others, to coming into health care systems that are frequently very large, confusing, and difficult for patients not used to them. So having advocates and people they can trust helps caregivers establish treatment programs. We hope that then leads to evaluations and ongoing positive relationships.

For these reasons, our first task is to get a person into Mrs. Steinfeld's home on an ongoing basis, with the goal of arranging a comprehensive evaluation when she's ready. Because there's no immediately danger, we have time to establish such a relationship.

SATIN (PS): I agree there is evidence that she would accept help. She let evaluators in to see her without objecting, treating them as old friends — she was probably too trusting of them — and was perfectly willing to talk about her problems.

As a team member, not as a psychiatrist, I am sympathetic with Ben Siegel's gentle but persistent observations that episodically we experience team leadership efforts, but we keep going on to something else. When Terry O'Malley suggests that we ought to get this project together into some structured form I, as a team member, feel the need for some kind of leadership. We need somebody to help us organize our plans and put all these interesting ideas into some form of action. As a physician — that is, as a medical engineer — I am used to getting something done, rather than continuing to talk about it.

SIEGEL (TM): Now you have just taken on a leadership function. It is important to realize that anybody can perform leadership functions within a team. The question for the team at this point is, Does the team want to select a leader or continue in this leaderless form? It is not essential to make the decision just now.

Even before addressing the question of leadership, the team really has to agree on what its goals are. It is very important to define what it is that you think ought to happen next and then get consensus on it. This is the team function of *decision making.* Terry O'Malley and David Satin have been exercizing some leadership by trying to get people back to focusing on what the essential problem is. The team cannot function unless you have shared lots of information first and have begun the process of involving all members in defining their priorities and care plans. This you've done. Now it's appropriate for someone to take responsibility for helping the team define its goals and priorities.

BLAKENEY (NS): There are three spheres of leadership. One is the establishment of trust and coordination of access. The second is clinical evaluation — finding out if there are physical problems that would account for altered mental status and other disabilities. Finally, there's leadership in treatment once those issues are clarified, which involves including the patient in establishing a treatment plan. This plan may be to help her maintain herself in her home environment or, alternativley, in an environment that's comfortable, supportive, and acceptable to her if that's her desire. Her wishes and participation in evaluation and treatment are especially important if no physical causes of the delusions are found.

So I think leadership must be built into the clinical care system, into identifying, defining, treating, and long-term managing of the problems. The ultimate goal is to help Mrs. Steinfeld to function safely and productively in the environment that makes most sense for her today.

SIEGEL (TM): There are different kinds of leadership currently being exercised. One is team leadership in deciding what the team's goals are, summarizing, pulling together various opinions, and so forth. Terry O'Malley and David Satin each started to do it. Another addresses clinical issues of defining which health care problems have high priority. Yet another addresses the choice of the professionals who will gather the data, manage the problems, and assess the effectiveness of the team interventions. Barbara Blakeney is really talking about clinical leadership about case services. Still another form of team leadership concerns team process: How does the team make decisions about who will do what (roles) and how the team functions (process, or team procedures)? There may also be team members who are not directly involved in the case but must be informed about team plans.

SCAVONE (PH): I think Barbara Blakeney was also talking again about defining goals, prioritizing them, and then developing leadership in addressing them.

SIEGEL (TM): Okay, but you really can't do anything until you've clearly defined what the goals are. The team has already defined broad goals: getting Mrs. Steinfeld appropriate evaluations and comprehensive care; determining the variety of people who should be involved; consulting someone in economics to help consider the various resources available; and examining the legal issues related to getting her informed consent before doing anything, since she is a competent person.

Now, team, we've got to define some interim goals. You might want to make one goal statement very concretely, such as, "We need to get more information, and it probably ought to be done by one person." The team has to decide whether that's an appropriate initial goal at this point.

SATIN (PS): But don't we need a team leader or a team administrator to define goals? To move us beyond throwing out interesting and useful ideas?

SIEGEL (TM): I don't know that you need a specific person, but you do need that function.

So, does anybody want to get the team together to define what it is you want to do? It could be anybody.

SATIN (PS): Nobody is volunteering and nobody is being drafted. Terry O'Malley has tried to do this twice. He's asked us to pull our ideas together. Since he seems to be thinking things out in an orderly and planned way, it seems to me that we ought to invite him to continue organizing our work.

O'MALLEY (IM): Well, okay, thank you. Having been drafted, I suggest we go about establishing an agenda of immediate activities that we can undertake to further the team's long-term goal of assisting Mrs. Steinfeld to function at the highest level possible in circumstances she finds most appropriate and acceptable. I think we discussed before the need to gather further information, so that is one important goal. When we gather the information, we'll move on to other goals, with team members reassigned to tasks of gathering additional information, intervening helpfully in ways we all determine to be appropriate, and so forth.

At this point, I suggest we talk about how we should gather information. By that, I mean defining the areas of information we want gathered and who we think should do it. What do we do with that information is a second step in decision making.

SIEGEL (TM): Before we get to that, you, as leader, might want to check out whether everyone is in agreement. Is there consensus? Is there any major disagreement?

O'MALLEY (IM): Certainly.

SATIN (PS): I agree that we ought to go about it in this way. I'm willing to start off with what information I would like to see gathered from a psychiatric point of view. For one thing, I would like to have somebody do a more extensive evaluation of Mrs. Steinfeld's mental status. We have some interesting observations about it, but somebody should complete the evaluation in an orderly fashion. It need not be a psychiatrist; it could be a psychologist, a nurse, an occupational therapist. Anybody who would look carefully at her cognitive, emotional, and behavioral status would be helpful. Second, I would like to get some history about her emotional function and social relations. This could come from her family and from other third parties to let us know how she is with them and how they relate to her. Third, I would like to get some medical, nutritional, and pharmacological data about factors other than psychosocial dynamics that might help account for her thinking and behavior. That body of information would help me to figure out what to do about her emotional and cognitive condition.

O'MALLEY (IM): And, Barbara Blakeney, would you want some Activities of Daily Living (ADL) data?

BLAKENEY (NS): Yes, I think we need to look at her ADL skills and her support systems. We are interested in the physical support system in terms of her ability to accomplish activities of daily living and how she gets help doing the things she can't do. It's also important to look into her social support system in term of sources of support she might most easily accept. Her past history tells something about where that support might come from, and we should use our knowledge of community resources to determine where supplemental care might come from.

The basic goal is for Mrs. Steinfeld to function at the maximum level she is capable of and interested in. We should use the data we gather — our interim goal — to achieve this overriding goal.

GURLAND (AVI): One thing I was thinking of is who should do these kinds of evaluations. Mrs. Steinfeld lives in an urban area, so we can assume there is a variety of health care available. The decision about whether the evaluations should be done in a large urban teaching hospital, by a private internist whom she may know, or by a home care program has important implications in terms of the goals of these clinicians, and how these goals influence the nature of the evaluations done and the health care outcomes that will result. In other words, outcome goals should determine who does the evaluations and treatment.

SATIN (PS): Would you expand on how the health care goals determine who should do evaluation and treatment, and what the consequences are of the evaluation taking place in these different institutional settings? Couldn't one choose whichever institution is most famous or closest?

GURLAND (AVI): The nature of the health care institution or the discipline of the clinician may have implications in terms of the attitudes, values, and ideologies of the people who gather these data. They should represent the widest ideological base possible. Often professionals go into situations like this with their own agendas. They may have preconceived notions about what the clients are like and what they want and how demented they are. Or, because of their funding sources, they want to plug the clients into their parent systems because that's what they can get paid for instead of considering what the clients might need.

One of the things that was mentioned in regard to Mrs. Steinfeld was the consequences of dealing with her only as a physical entity with a variety of problems; that taking care of physical needs by doing some traumatic diagnostic or therapeutic things might interfere with her cognitive abilities. One must strike a balance among what she wants, what she is capable of, and what agencies are capable of meeting her needs. To some extent that is determined by the caregivers' values. If their values indicate that it's more important for her to stay home, then they will accept her not getting all the tests she needs and a medical workup in as much depth as they might like because these losses are outweighed by the benefit of having her home, comfortable, and maintaining more functional capacity.

So not only is it important to gather the data but to make sure it is done by appropriate professionals from appropriate agencies. The options are a home care program, the visiting nurse association (which is different from home care), or a medical center of some kind. Only after we decide on the kind of agency that might be best suited — might have the best resources for Mrs. Steinfeld — can we decide which discipline or particular person might have the most expertise for this task.

O'MALLEY (IM): I think quite often the choice of agency or professional is determined by what is available. If you're in Boston, then you have many options to choose from and, yes, you can go about deciding whether you're going to hook up with a tertiary care hospital with a geriatrics program or use a small home care agency. But I wonder if the prior issue still isn't which one or two people are available to gather this data base, at least preliminarily, and then we can reach out to the various more specialized people. I may be wrong, but the choice of an agency seems not as much of a problem as the identification of the kind of person you want.

SATIN (PS): Some of Lisa Gurland's research has indicated that the kind of agency you ask for will determine the kind of data you get. The social worker from a tertiary care hospital is going to get different data than a social worker from a home care program, just because these professionals emphasize different things, value different kinds of data, and will see different implications in them. You're not going to get a recorded transcript of what the patient does. You're going to get an interpretation, and different clinicians are going to interpret the same data differently. So, in a way you decide what kind of intervention and outcome you would like to see recommended, and then you pick the kind of agency that is likely to give you those results. If you want to see Mrs. Steinfeld stay at home, you are better advised to ask a home care agency to send a social worker than to ask a tertiary care center to send a geriatric fellow.

Since we have generally agreed that we want to help Mrs. Steinfeld stay as functional as possible and as close as possible to her natural environment, I would pick a home health agency to do the evaluation. This is a way of building our prejudice into the evaluation process by choosing evaluators who are prejudiced in favor of evaluating her at home and evaluating home as a viable setting for her services.

KOOCHER (EC): Is that true, though? Won't a tertiary care center want a new outpatient? Wouldn't the home-care unit of a tertiary care center provide you with an objective, high-quality assessment that would equal that of a home health agency or a community social service agency? The tertiary care center would provide comprehensive home care sevices and a liaison to the social service deparment as well as access to good medical and related clinical specialties and subspecialties.

GURLAND (AVI): On the contrary, as far as I know in this area, there is only one real home care program connected with a tertiary care hospital. The other such hospitals don't have the same kind of primary care services.

BLAKENEY (NS): The city hospital has a small program at this time.

SATIN (PS): I'm not sure how well even that one tertiary care hospital's home care program compares to a free-standing home care program in terms of commitment to home care and range of services. Tertiary care facilities are really not used to looking at home care as a valued option. They look at tertiary care as the important option. For those patients who are so disabled that they are not going to be cured quickly at tertiary care hospitals, the alternative is some kind of chronic institutional placement.

KOOCHER (EC): The tertiary care hospital makes a referral for assessment outside their facility. That might be a social service agency, such as Margery Glassman's, or a home health agency such as the Visiting Nurse Association, or a range of others. The VNA might not have the same perspective on homemaker chore assistance, laundry assistance, or transportation services that a home care or home social service agency would have. The home social service agency would probably have less breadth of expertise in terms of all the medical issues involved.

This raises a major social policy issue: the institutionalized separation of health and social services for older people. This creates a problem for anyone trying to help Mrs. Steinfeld.

GURLAND (AVI): There are some agencies that do both health and social service care well. Maybe they are not found in every community in the United States, but certainly in larger urban areas.

SATIN (PS): A related issue I was thinking of was financial. As Lisa Gurland mentioned, people and agencies are going to do what they are going to get paid for, and they're not going to spend a lot of time doing something they're not going to get paid for, such as completing an evaluation so that the patient will be cared for by somebody else. Nor will they want to lose business by sending a customer someplace else. So clinicians are going to recommend services that they perform and will be paid for.

KOOCHER (EC): As the self-proclaimed resident cynic, I agree. We must continue to be mindful of the fact that people's financial interests may govern their perspectives on this case. Anything — medical, social, or any other of a wide range of services — will be influenced by economic advantage. Someone will have to be looking out for Mrs. Steinfeld in this regard. It could be a social worker or maybe some other discipline.

O'MALLEY (IM): Actually, agencies perform services and assign disciplines they will get paid for but lie and do other things under the guise of the things they are reimbursed for. If the agencies get paid for a nursing visit but not a social worker visit, then the nurses end up doing most of the social service.

BLAKENEY (NS): It's called creative record-keeping. Based on the information we have on Mrs. Steinfeld now, if we were to say to a visiting nurse agency, "Go and provide her care," there is nothing we know of that they would be reimbursed for. There is no dressing change, there is no clear need for much of any hands-on nursing service.

KOOCHER (EC): Plus she can leave the house.

O'MALLEY (IM): Her cardiovascular status would probably come under the standards for home nursing.

SATIN (PS): If you, as the attending physician, say so, it is so.

KOOCHER (EC): What that means is that any physician who does a full physical on her is going to bill that to Medicare as the diagnosis and treatment of a medical problem, and Medicare pays for that. But in terms of home health care, as long as she can leave the house on her own two feet she is not covered by Medicare without other justification.

BLAKENEY (NS): Do you know how many slips have been signed and sworn to in a primary care center attesting to the fact that somebody is homebound?

KOOCHER (EC): I understand that, but I'm not sure students of gerontology should be encouraged to find ways of having needed services fall under reimbursement guidelines.

O'MALLEY (IM): They *should* be encouraged.

PAPAS (DT): That's a very important issue. There was once a grant to treat homebound dental patients. The agency required clinicians to attest that the people were homebound, so a visiting nurse or somebody else had to attest that the people were homebound before they could be visited. And very weird situations would occur when the clinicians arrived at the homes of these "homebound" people just as they were on their way out the door.

KOOCHER (EC): The fact is that clinicians and clinical care agencies recognize that it may be important to get a little creative with reporting in order to deliver the services patients may need.

GURLAND (AVI): A sad fact is that being truly homebound is not enough to assure Medicare coverage. If Mrs. Steinfeld couldn't walk, it does not necessarily mean she would be able to get very many homebound services, certainly not professional care.

BLAKENEY (NS): The agencies that do well in getting reimbursment know what they can get reimbursed for and focus their record-keeping system to document that clearly, and that allows them then to do the things for which they cannot be reimbursed but which are vital in making it possible for patients to stay at home.

So the nurse who goes into the home and takes one minute to check Mrs. Steinfeld's blood pressure and write it down and comment on it, and then spends the next half hour working with her on another issue that is vitally important, gets reimbursed for that half-hour visit. She is reimbursed because she took the blood pressure, not because she did any skilled intervention using cognitive processing, intervening with another person's ways of thinking, teaching Mrs. Steinfeld, or somehow addressing issues that allow her to live more successfully.

The blood pressure is a vehicle. It's important to take action if the blood pressure is erratic, but blood pressures may be ordered every 2 weeks on patients whose blood pressures have not varied more than 10 points, because clinicians know how vital it is for the interaction and monitoring to occur. The reimbursement system makes clinicians circumvent the rules because it does not value care modalities that are necessary to keep people at home. It values technical procedures, and yet what we're about is much more than technical procedures.

PAPAS (DT): Some method of reimbursement is needed in situations not covered by Medicare. I have cancer patients who will lose their jobs and possibly their lives because they need dental care. They've had radiation that necrotizes bone and compromises the immune system. They could develop abscesses that involve the whole jaw, and lose the jaw. I tell Medicare this and they say, "We realize that. It's too bad." And I say, "Well, what happens when you get this person with an osteoradionecrosis in the hospital for 3 months and the person dies? How much are you going to have to pay for that?" They don't want to pay $50 for a visit to the dentist for an initial evaluation and $25 for a follow-up—we're not talking about huge sums. But they won't pay even for medically indicated dental interventions. Day-to-day dentistry just doesn't exist under Medicare. So we have to charge the patient. Unless we have a grant, we have to charge homebound patients $50 extra to transport us there physically. That's quite a hardship for someone who has very limited means.

BLAKENEY (NS): Health education will be another important service for Mrs. Steinfeld. It's important to know what she understands about her medications and her illnesses. Getting information about this allows us to plan to help her become more knowledgeable. The more knowledgeable she is, the more able she'll be to participate actively and have meaningful input into the ultimate plan.

O'MALLEY (IM): We also want to get a data base on her physical health in addition to any other information.

HOWE (OT): We need a complete history to understand her former level of function, her values and beliefs, and her interests, as well as present skills and supports.

O'MALLEY (IM): I can summarize the data base that we have; chime in if you have things to add: a deeper and more exact mental status evaluation, history of her past and present social support system — who and where she might accept help from, her medications, her ADL skills, what she knows about her illnesses, medical evaluation, and dental evaluation.

KOOCHER (EC): The social assessment should include a financial assessment including an analysis of her health insurance coverage.

BARNARD (ET): In discussing the data to be gathered, let me repeat the importance of a "values history" that I discussed in the chapter "Ethical Issues at the End of Life." We need to know her attitudes toward independence and dependence, medical care, life support, and so forth. How were things handled when her husband died? What impression has she formed of emergency care, hospitals, and other forms of treatment? What does she envision and desire for herself? Again, I assume this will be done with tact.

SATIN (PS): Nutritional and pharmacological evaluations should be included in the list.

KOOCHER (EC): Also religious considerations.

O'MALLEY (IM): They should have been in there if they weren't.

PAPAS (DT): Mrs. Steinfeld seems to have a lot of problems with ambulation and other physical tasks. Maybe a physical therapist could be brought in to help her with her arthritis and see if exercize tolerance can be improved. She's also at high risk for osteoporosis.

O'MALLEY (IM): That may be appropriate, but we have yet to identify specific needs. What we have to do is reassess all her activities of daily living.

PAPAS (DT): Yes, activities of daily living will tell us whether she needs physical therapy intervention.

O'MALLEY (IM): We may also have the social worker contact the family and begin getting parallel information about them, their perceptions of what's going on, and their ability to provide supports in the future.

PAPAS (DT): It might also be good to get the family involved in the decision making. My experience has been that if you make decisions with the patient alone, the family can reverse them all. That's why I think it's very important to achieve consensus early on.

BLAKENEY (NS): I think you all are absolutely right in your concern about whether the family feels they're participants and partners in whatever happens. One of the most frustrating experiences is to develop a plan that the client wants and that fits well with our own perspectives, and to have the people who are expected to implement parts of that plan and be affected by it create situations where you can't implement it because they haven't participated in the planning. Then everybody is angry and upset with everybody else.

SATIN (PS): I would expand that to include all care-givers.

BLAKENEY (NS): I agree.

BARNARD (ET): Getting the family involved is a very good idea, but to say they will reverse plans they disagree with leaves out the important role the team (or whichever member is carrying the ball) can play as an advocate for Mrs. Steinfeld's interests if conflict does exist. In a supportive way, which may include sympathetic attention to the son's feeling about his mother, the family needs to be reminded that Mrs. Steinfeld's needs and interests are primary here. Perhaps if the son hears this message in concert with empathy for his own perceptions and feelings, serious conflict can be minimized even if choices are made that he disagrees with.

SIEGEL (TM): Then everyone is agreed and there are no conflicts about the interim goals and broad issues. The next question for the team is who is going to do what—a role issue.

O'MALLEY (IM): We can now go about deciding who is going to collect the information. I think there are a couple of ways we can approach that. There are certain parts of the data base that are only going to be available through subspecialty practitioners. The dental evaluation is probably going to require a dentist if it is to be more than just the initial quick look in the mouth to see if dentition is adequate.

PAPAS (DT): Actually, we're trying to teach nurses how to do that too.

SATIN (PS): Maybe somewhere along the line we could do some in-service training within our team so that we broaden skills for all of us in this and other areas.

O'MALLEY (IM): We need information in medical, dental, nursing, psychiatry, and social work spheres. We should look to see if there's any one person among us who can bridge all these areas for an initial evaluation. The traditional choice of the intital responder is often someone in social service or nursing.

PAPAS (DT): A nurse could visit Mrs. Steinfeld, establish trust, introduce her to the team, and get the necessary medical evaluations.

SATIN (PS): We seem to be looking for one person who could do all the evaluation. I wonder if we couldn't get more than one person to do these things, perhaps serially, so that a wider array of expertise could be brought to bear. We don't want to overload this woman, but couldn't she meet two or three or four people for various purposes if they are all identified with one gate-keeper? There are even times when more than one person could come at the same time. I wonder if two or three people couldn't collaborate well enough to do a combined evaluation.

O'MALLEY (IM): I think your suggestion raises the problem of overwhelming this woman with a cast of thousands coming into her home. One or two people I'm sure would be no problem.

PAPAS (DT): I think she might enjoy a cast of thousands. She's been isolated. Our major problem is to get *out* the door once we're in!

HOWE (OT): Perhaps we need to consult with Mrs. Steinfeld to get her ideas and attitudes regarding the type of health care program she wants and past experiences with health care personnel. She may have definite preferences.

KOOCHER (EC): I think a home health agency is the wisest course. It seems to me that their intake person, which is a nurse, should and would collaborate with a home care caseworker.

SIEGEL (TM): As soon as you start dealing with other agencies there are issues of collaboration, communication, and how you and the other agency relate. There are also questions of data sharing, the other team accepting your data as valid, and not knowing the attitudes, values, and ideologies of the people who are generating the data. So the more complex the institutional relationships, the more fragmented the work may become.

Is there anybody on our team who could do this evaluation?

SATIN (PS): We have a nurse on the team.

BLAKENEY (NS): Mrs. Steinfeld's case is wonderful from a nursing perspective. There are so many issues and nuances to be explored and dealt with. Several of the disciplines around this table can be active in collecting and analyzing essential information. Assuming we have a financial limitation, we can be reimbursed for an initial visit to gather some data and establish priorities. It makes the most sense to have one person develop the data base so that we know what we're about and then introduce services in a way that's going to benefit her physically and emotionally. Eventually a cast of thousands for socialization purposes might be exactly what we need.

SATIN (PS): At some point the nurse might introduce Mrs. Steinfeld to her friend the occupational therapist to evaluate her ADLs.

BLAKENEY (NS): It makes sense to establish a relationship, do an initial assessment of physical, mental, and social health status and support resources in the home community. With that, the team will have much more data vital for setting priorities among the needs to be met. This task is also the vehicle for establishing a good relationship. Then we can proceed to get her into the ambulatory-care center or admitted to the hospital or whatever else is necessary for further evaluation and treatment. The data base is vital in order to prioritize needs before we begin management.

SATIN (PS): Since the hour is growing late, would it be appropriate for our team administrator to summarize where we are and what we do next?

SIEGEL (TM): Or whoever feels moved. Anybody can do that.

O'MALLEY (IM): Who wants to summarize?

BLAKENEY (NS): I can meet Mrs. Steinfeld within the next couple of days to gather the data that we've talked about and establish a working relationship with her. I will bring that data back to the team within a day or two of the visit. Perhaps we could have a follow-up conference at which I will present the information we have so far. Then, based on the data, we can plan our next actions.

SIEGEL (TM): Before we end the team meeting, is there general consensus around the next step? Does silence mean consent?

O'MALLEY (IM): Silence means consensus. Let's adjourn until the next meeting.

### Second Team Meeting: Review of Evaluation and Planning Treatment

BLAKENEY (NS): Since our last meeting I visited Mrs. Steinfeld on three occasions over a 10-day period. In light of our discussion, I attempted to visit her at different times of the day to get a sense of what she and her life are like in the morning, afternoon, and early evening.

First, some basic information with regard to these visits: I visited her at 10:00 A.M., 1:00 P.M., and 5:30 P.M., and spent about an hour and a half with her on each visit. Generally, Mrs. Steinfeld is a delightful person, very friendly, very sociable, very happy to have company, very eager to talk and share experiences. She had to come down the stairs to let me in on all three occasions and had considerable difficulty physically negotiating the stairs. She also developed shortness of breath, especially when going up the stairs. Her living room and dining room are both very neat and clean, but I found that most of her activity occurs in the bedroom, kitchen, and bathroom, which are less neat and clean. She has considerable difficulty maintaining basic cleanliness because of her physical limitations, which I'll discuss in a few minutes.

Mrs. Steinfeld's blood pressure ranged from 160/94 to 172/100, and pulse 88 to 94. After going up and down the stairs, respiration increased to 25 to 30 breaths per minute with considerable shortness of breath. Physical examination revealed a woman with moderately severe deformities in her hands, making fine motor coordination, such as buttoning things and handling cups and saucers, difficult. She also had considerable enlargement of both knees, with limitation in range of motion. She had considerable pain in both her hands and knees, worse in the morning but improving during the day. She is unsteady on her feet. Early in the morning she has considerable difficulty getting around, but this improves during the day.

Cardiovascular status includes an $S_4$ heart sound. Her lungs show mild râles in both lower lobes, and, as I mentioned before, she has considerable dyspnea after climbing one flight of stairs. She has 1+ pitting edema in both ankles. Pulses in both legs and feet are strong.

The rest of her physical examination was within normal limits given the level of examination possible in her house.

Mrs. Steinfeld keeps all her medications on her kitchen table. These include digitalis and methyldopa. She uses diazepam occasionally. She is somewhat unreliable in remembering to take her medications, and I'm not convinced that she takes them regularly.

Food supply in the kitchen consists mostly of tea, coffee, bread, and some canned goods. There is not much food in the freezer, and this is prepared foods like frozen complete meals and entrees. She does not get out to shop very often but depends mostly on neighbors, whom she pays for this.

Mrs. Steinfeld is very anxious about her life: what's going on presently and what's going to happen to her in the future. She's very sad and continues to grieve over the loss of her husband. I am worried about a pathological grief reaction, given the length of time since her husband's death and the level of sadness she continues to manifest. Short-term memory is impaired. She tends to cope by hiding it, giggling, or making a joke about it, but becomes anxious when it becomes obvious. Long-term memory is excellent.

Mrs. Steinfeld is very convinced about the young man breaking into the house. It is significant that when she and her husband were running their store, they suffered a couple of robberies and break-ins, and she may be drawing on that past experience.

Mrs. Steinfeld's social network is extremely limited. She hasn't been out of her house in the last 6 months, and the idea of doing so raises considerable anxiety. Frequently several days pass without her receiving or making a phone call. This concerns her, and she says, "What if something happens to me? Nobody would know!"

My overall impression of her physical condition is that her hypertension and congestive heart failure are not well controlled either by diet or medication. We drew a blood sample for a digitalis level on the last visit and are waiting for the results. I am also very concerned that her arthritis causes problems both with self-image and mobility. Her ataxic gait is, I think, in part due to arthritis, but may reflect other pathology.

In terms of mental status, Mrs. Steinfeld's short-term memory is impaired. She's anxious and concerned about that. She appears to be deluded in that she continues to believe strongly that someone is breaking into her house although there is no evidence to support that. She continues to actively grieve her husband's death.

This woman has a limited to nonexistent social network except for the rare visits from her son, and she's very lonely. She's very outgoing and responsive with visitors. On my second visit she made a special effort to get dressed up for the occasion, had the table set, and served tea to make it a little social event. So she looks forward to visits and wants more company.

My sense is that once we understand her needs, she will be responsive to active treatment and attempts to increase her social involvement.

O'MALLEY (IM): Unless someone else wants to, I will take administrative charge of the team to make efficient use of our time.

First of all, Barbara Blakeney's presentation was excellent. I think it really filled in a large number of gaps that we all recognized prior to her evaluation. I would suggest the following tasks for the group, and we can discuss whether or not we think we can complete them in the limited time we have.

The first is for us all to address the data Barbara Blakeney has brought from the perspectives of our own disciplines to see if she can fill in any gaps or whether we feel further assessment is required. The second task is to determine the priorities of therapeutic interventions. This means priorities within the various disciplines, and also combined priorities for the immediate future. The third task is to delegate specific jobs to team members to fill in information gaps and pursue therapeutic interventions. I thought this might be the way to approach this woman.

If there are no comments or additions, I'd like to ask Barbara Blakeney some medical questions about the problem areas we identified in our first team meeting. The first I'd like to tackle is Mrs. Steinfeld's cardiovascular status, to give us a line on the etiology of what sounds like her congestive heart failure. From the exam she certainly has that until we prove otherwise. Apparently we don't have very good history about whether she's had myocardial infarctions. Our treatment would be different if she has hypertensive cardiovascular disease with heart failure rather than valvular heart disease or a large loss of myocardium from heart attacks.

We also ought to know if she is currently under treatment, where she is getting her medicine from, who her physician is, and whether we can get more data from her source of treatment.

BLAKENEY (NS): In answer to these questions, the medication prescriptions are dated almost a year ago. Dr. Bertinelli, the physician whose name is on the medication bottles, was a nice young man Mrs. Steinfeld saw then in the walk-in clinic at a local teaching hospital. She's not been back to see him since because she doesn't want to bother people with her problems. I think also travelling to the hospital is difficult for her in her current condition. She seems very, very anxious about leaving home.

This woman's medical care is extremely sporadic. Given her cardiac status, the lack of clarity as to her perfusion, and the uncertainty about her digitalis compliance, I'm anxious to have a very complete evaluation of her cardiovascular status. This would shed light both on her heart and dementia.

O'MALLEY (IM): A few more questions about Mrs. Steinfeld's mental status. Did you do a formal mental state evaluation? If so, I'd love to hear the results. That will help determine the underlying cause of her cognitive impairment. Several diagnostic alternatives come to mind: Is this a true dementia, a dementia-like illness due to her drugs or other reversible causes, or is it a pseudodementia resulting from her depression and isolation? If we can get a handle on that issue it will help us tremendously in predicting Mrs. Steinfeld's ability to stay at home and in selecting services to introduce. If the answer is unclear or she appears to have a true dementia, we need to do a formal dementia evaluation to rule out reversible causes. You mention an ataxic gait. If she's incontinent in addition to ataxic and demented, we ought to think of normal pressure hydrocephalus, a potentially reversible cause of dementia.

If her digoxin level proves elevated, that can contribute to confusion. We should probably also discontinue her methyldopa.

SATIN (PS): From the point of view of psychiatry, I think that Barbara Blakeney gave all the evidence that she has. More data must come from some special interventions, such as neuropsychological testing and brain imaging. The fact that Mrs. Steinfeld is able to function as well as she does and can rise to new tasks makes me hope that she has little permanent neurological and emotional impairment and a lot of reserve capacity that can be brought up to better function.

In the social area she's very isolated and lonely and is, in a sense, suffering sensory deprivation. This woman needs to reestablish a relationship with some stable person or small group of people both for her current well-being and as a bridge to reintegration into life and society. I would like to see her more active. If these activities are health evaluation or treatment procedures she can get some company and interaction from that. One or more members of the interdisciplinary health team can collect health data, develop a therapeutic relationship, and act as the bridge to other social groups and activities in the community. Maybe we can turn to social work to identify those resources and how appropriate they are for her.

She has real grieving to do. I'm not inclined to approach that through formal psychotherapy, but rather again social interaction and enriching her environment to recreate the social network that was dependent on her husband's presence. This would be more effective than abstract insight work about her feelings and her associations to the loss of her husband.

In terms of her cognitive functioning, I suspect that we're not going to know what her maximum capacity is until we alleviate several of the stresses that are impairing it and find out what defects remain. A good medical evaluation and correction of her congestive heart failure, hypertension, and so forth, have to be accomplished before we can tell how much these contribute to her cognitive state. I would also look to a nutrition evaluation to determine what nutritional deficiencies are contributing to her physical and mental impairments.

I know that the diazepam is not good for her. It does not help depression as was intended, and it carries great risk of impairing her mental functioning through cumulative toxicity and adding to depression. I would stop that forthwith and not replace it with any psychotropic medications until we have good evidence that other, less risky approaches won't work better for her. I would turn to pharmacy for some advice on the rest of her medications, including the ways she takes them as well as their chemical effects. How much are they are contributing to her depression, delusions, and cognitive impairments?

In summary, the first step I would take is to remedy the various things that are impairing her functioning. Secondly, I would take the positive approach of social interventions: enriching her life with people and activities and meaning.

BLAKENEY (NS): I deliberately visited Mrs. Steinfeld at three different times of day to evaluate variations in physical ability and stamina as well as mental function. Her Mini-Mental Status Exam score was eight, and we repeated the exam on the third visit with the same result; this suggests true dementia. Ability to recall information given a few moments before, ability to recall what she had eaten, and ability to recall activity of that morning were all somewhat impaired. However, what was very interesting was her ability to keep quite straight the plots in the TV soap operas she watches every day. I'm not sure what this means.

In terms of drugs, on our last visit I gave her a pill organizer and pill-taking schedule to cover 7 days. When I return to reevaluate her, I'll have a better idea whether she's taking her medications properly and how her function changes with proper medication.

In light of the way that she's eating and the amount of food in the house, I'm very worried that her cognitive impairment may be a result of malnutrition and would really like to see the nutritionist explore that more fully.

SATIN (PS): One further comment on Mrs. Steinfeld's mental status: I feel strongly that you cannot do a dementia evaluation anytime you want to and obtain valid results. Some factors contributing to dementia can be tested no matter what else is going on in the individual's life. For instance, you can do a CT scan of the head and find out whether she's got a subdural hematoma, a tumor, cerebral infarcts, or cerebral atrophy. If she's got normal pressure hydrocephalus, it will show up now and we ought to do something about it now.

Other factors are so responsive to environmental conditions that you cannot get an accurate measure until you clear up environmental problems. For instance, I would not do detailed neuropsychological testing of Mrs. Steinfeld now because we won't be able to tell whether deficits in her functioning are coming from nutritional, psychological, or neurological sources. I would put off this evaluation until her nutritional status is improved, her medications are adjusted, and she is less sensorily and socially deprived.

DWYER (NT): What is in the attic? Is Mrs. Steinfeld's concern in fact a delusion? It may be a delusion that somebody is coming to get what's there, but if there's something up there that could be removed perhaps that would solve the problem. In some sections of the city, if there are jewels in the attic I can tell you she does have a problem because somebody will come and get it sooner or later.

BLAKENEY (NS): Frankly, I don't know what's in the attic as yet, but I assure you I will try to find out. I'm going to go to the attic!

SCAVONE (PH): I have two questions. One relates to compliance. Did Mrs. Steinfeld mention how she takes her medicines? If she does not take them regularly does she take them when she feels symptomatic? Second, does she take an analgesic when she has pain and stiffening?

BLAKENEY (NS): I honestly don't think that she knows how often she takes the digitalis and methyldopa. She is confused, and I don't have confidence that she's taking medications on a regular basis or fully benefiting from them. Pulses of 88 to 94 would indicate that she's probably not taking her digitalis regularly, which is a problem. We've set up a 7-day pill organizer for her with large signs to remind her what day it is. We'll see how well she does with that.

     She tends not to take her analgesic but just to wait it out and move around. She knows that after a couple of hours she'll start to feel better.

PAPAS (DT): Did you have any estimate as to what her dental status is? Did she have teeth? Dentures? Were they clacking?

BLAKENEY (NS): She has a full set of dentures.

PAPAS (DT): Could you tell whether there was a problem with them, whether she was having trouble manipulating them or keeping her mouth closed? One of the things we've found is that the aged who have trouble with their dentures have deficient food intake. That may be one of her problems.

BLAKENEY (NS): She said she had no problem and none was obvious.

DWYER (NT): From a nutritional point of view I would like to know first of all what this woman weighs, what her height is, and if she's had any changes in weight over the past 6 months or year. I was interested that she seemed more alert at one time of day than another. Were you able to watch her preparing food, eating, or anything else relating to nutrition? Does she have problems in this area?

BLAKENEY (NS): Her height is 5 feet 4 inches, and her current weight is 112 pounds. I have no clear idea what her weight was in the past, but I can say that her clothes hung somewhat loosely. As far as activity during the day goes, in the morning her energy level is high but her mobility is decreased because she is stiff and sore. In the late afternoon and early evening, mobility is better but her energy level is decreased and she tires more easily, becomes a bit more confused, and has more difficulty following a conversation for long. Also, her dyspnea on exertion increases at the end of the day.

PAPAS (DT): Mrs. Steinfeld may not be getting sufficient quantities of essential nutrients because of physical disability and isolation. To remedy this, foods that are familiar to her must be reintroduced so that her diet is healthy. We want to avoid changing her diet so drastically that she won't accept what we give her. We would want to stay within her Kosher diet and reintroduce nutritious things that she once ate. We can try such approaches as, "Mrs. Steinfeld, you're eating A, B, and C. You need that C with a little bit of D and F in it. Try to put a little of this into your diet. For instance, if you don't like drinking milk, have you considered eating cheese?" Trying to give dietary supplements in this age group frequently fails; making minor modifications to the diet is much more successful.

In addition, we might try to have someone help her with the shopping. A home health aide could come to stock her cabinets and set up meal plans so that she can cook simple, healthy meals. In regard to her arthritis, assistive devices such as special plates with broad rims and mugs with big handles would make it easier for her to eat the food.

We might also try to get her to a nutrition site where other people to socialize with would increase her interest in eating. Perhaps she should move to a different setting, such as a geriatric housing complex, where she can be better cared for.

These are all reasons why we need a complete nutritional assessment as well as assessment in other areas.

SMITH (OT): I would be interested in knowing if Mrs. Steinfeld herself identified any specific problems with self-care or homemaking activities. Your description of her hand deformities and function suggests that she has difficulty manipulating and grasping objects, as well as reaching items in high or low places. Thus dressing, bathing, and eating as well as homemaking activities would probably be affected. Also I would imagine that her arthritis, in particular her gait problem, would limit her endurance for daily activities and possibly pose a safety hazard.

In addition, I would like to know how she fills her time each day. Did you see any indication that she is involved in any activities such as reading, sewing, or watching television?

From what we have heard it would seem that Mrs. Steinfeld would benefit from an activity evaluation as well as an analysis of how she uses her time each day. This would give the team specific information on how functional she actually is.

BLAKENEY (NS): This area of her life is interesting. She has coped in terms of feeding by using a lot of prepared, frozen foods. Verbally she covers over her limitations quite well by saying such things as "I manage" or "It's not important anyway." As I mentioned, the clothing I saw her wear was loose-fitting and either pull-over-the-head or zippered. I suspect she has some difficulty managing the zippers, as some of them were not completely closed.

I didn't get the sense that she reads very much, but at one o'clock in the afternoon we had the television soaps on throughout my visit, and she knew what was going on in each soap. My sense is that her afternoons are filled with television.

In terms of care of her environment, she's managed some basic activities in a minimal way, but the rooms that she lives in are somewhat cluttered and dirty. There's clear evidence that she has trouble making the bed and changing the bed linen. Instead of fitted sheets she uses the old open sheets: my sense is it's just too difficult for her to pull that last corner of the sheet down taut. Such activities seem extremely difficult for her, and it takes her a long time to accomplish basic activities of daily living.

At this point, she has adapted in most instances through avoidance, and done it quite skillfully. I see evidence that she would benefit from adaptive equipment throughout the house and training in its use. She was very open to my suggestions and made some changes in the bedroom so that it's now a bit safer physically than it was when I arrived.

PIKTIALIS (EC): I'm wondering if there was any discussion with Mrs. Steinfeld about what kind of health insurance or other health coverage she has or anything about her financial situation. Some of the things you're suggesting could be done free, at least initially. Others would require some kind of reimbursement. Clearly, if she's been taking so many drugs she must either have some money and is paying out of pocket, or she has health insurance coverage. It is likely that she has Medicare coverage, but we should confirm that. We should determine if she has any Medicare supplement insurance. In any case, it would be very helpful to get financial assistance. We need to look at her finances to see if she is Medicaid-eligible now. If not she may become Medicaid-eligible after a lot of the medical interventions and other services we suggest are paid for.

I think it would be very important to get a social worker or case manager to sit down and to talk to her about how she's been paying for health care bills if this information is not otherwise available. If this lady is too confused or fearful or reticent about exploring her financial situation, her children may have to be contacted in order to get some better information.

I think data on her finances are going to be very important in pursuing an interdisciplinary plan of care.

BLAKENEY (NS): Mrs. Steinfeld believes that she's got Medicare and referred me to her son for other information. Her son pays most of her bills by check. He comes once or twice a month, picks up the bills, and "handles all those things." My sense is that she does not have much information about her finances and depends heavily on her son to handle them. Phone calls to her son have not yet been returned, so I don't have more answers.

GLASSMAN (SW): I still don't quite get a picture of what Mrs. Steinfeld wants and what her goals are. It's a mystery to me how she remains in her current situation. Has she no knowledge of resources, or does she wish to remain as she is? You say that she's a very sociable person. Would she like to go out into the community? In her community there are Jewish community centers, day-care programs, and housing for the Jewish elderly.

BLAKENEY (NS): I think she wants to remain where she is. She's lived in that house for many years. She knows where everything is and she's quite comfortable there. She feels very safe except for her conviction that this young man breaks into her apartment periodically and steals things from the attic.

My sense is that she wants very much to have a social network but either doesn't know how to go about getting it or is fearful because of her physical problems and because of the ethnic change in the neighborhood. If we could provide her with support, for example somebody who would pick her up and bring her to an activity or to visit an old friend who lives several blocks away, that would begin to build her social contacts.

Once we are clear about her physical health problems and stabilize them, we can begin to either move people and stimuli into her life or move her out into a more socially stimulating environment. This must be done gradually because her anxiety and confusion increase when she's bombarded with stimuli, but I think generally she'd respond positively. The challenge is for us to find a way for her to get that kind of support and interaction.

GURLAND (AVI): It sounds like Barbara Blakeney did a very thorough evaluation from a very nonbiased perspective. Also, I think that people have been raising a lot of well-founded questions. We need to find the answers to those questions in order to provide for Mrs. Steinfeld's care.

I'm concerned about delivering services without having a lengthier discussion with her about her feelings about health care. What are her feelings about death? What does she see as her future? Would she like to end up in a nursing home or an elderly housing development with people of her faith, or does she want to die at home in that apartment no matter what? What kinds of medical interventions does she see as being important?

This woman probably won't be able to answer some of these questions because she probably hasn't thought much about them. However, I think that before we decide what kind of agency and what kind of professionals we're going to bring in even to do evaluations, we need to have some idea about her beliefs about life and death and who she is.

BLAKENEY (NS): Clearly those questions have to be explored. However, after only three visits I didn't feel we'd established enough rapport to get into that. I do know that when I asked how she felt about continuing to live in that apartment, her anxiety level rose so that I was afraid I'd scare her beyond what was useful if I pursued that avenue without first establishing a more trusting relationship. My sense is that spending more time with her, dealing with immediate issues, and helping her to function better in certain areas will bring us to the point where we can begin to explore these basic questions.

GLASSMAN (SW): I think we are missing a meeting with the family and getting the data they can give about what this woman was like before her current problems. I also feel that it's very important to include her children and her in the planning process. I hear about all the things that are going to be done for her, but I don't have a clear idea about her own goals. This does not have to await a number of visits.

PIKTIALIS (EC): My comments aren't related to economics but with some other work I'm involved in. I disagree a bit with Marjorie Glassman. Given the history we have about the family, it sounds to me as if the children have not been particularly involved with Mrs. Steinfeld other than showing up once a month to pay bills. Oftentimes getting family members together with the older person must be preceded by getting the family members together among themselves. As David Satin mentioned in the last team meeting, the family needs to talk about the history of their communication, what roles they are currently playing, and what roles they are willing to play in the future. Only when that kind of family meeting is held without the older person do I think the family is ready to come together with the older person, particularly when there's evidence that the family has not been working together.

GLASSMAN (SW): I would certainly agree with you in that. Still, from where I stand you ultimately have to involve both families and the elders in any kind of treatment planning. We certainly will talk with the family before we bring them together with the older person, but the woman and her family need to have an active role in planning. Too often I hear clinicians making plans for elderly people as we have for Mrs. Steinfeld. But the team's goals need to be the goals of the patients and their families, and the priorities need to be the priorities that the recipients of care have set. Sometimes clients don't set the kind of priorities that we as a team would set.

If we're going to get cooperation, I think we really need to pay attention to the elders and their informal caregivers. One of the roots of noncompliance — and we see many noncompliant older people — is that our priorities are not the same as their priorities. Sometimes we see a family being subversive to the plan we set up because we haven't worked very closely with them.

BARNARD (ET): My comments in the last team meeting also apply here. The involvement with the family, especially the son, may well have to address emotional reactions of sadness, guilt, or whatever other feelings he has as the son contemplates his mother's situation and his own involvement with her (or lack of same). The same may well apply to other family members who live even farther away. It will be important to minimize the impact of unacknowledged feelings that might prompt the children to advocate or resist plans for their mother based on those feelings rather than on a fair assessment of Mrs. Steinfeld's needs.

O'HARE (LW): I'll make one suggestion to both Diane Piktialis and Margery Glassman. When we talk about involving family (family, I take it, is only the son who's in the immediate area here), I would want to take a long look at what his participation in the finances has been and is going to be in the future, and how his financial self-interest may color his input into what treatments may be offered and what placement might be decided upon. Presumably the house is paid off and there's been an income from the tenant all these years. I don't know what Mrs. Steinfeld's expenses have been, but if the son's been paying them out of her income it would be important to understand how his financial self-interest affects his advice about expenditures for her care. Next to "*Cherchez la femme*," "Keep an eye on the family's financial interests" is a very operative phrase in family law.

SIEGEL (TM): I want to reflect on where the team has been. It's very clear that this team works together very well because there seems to have been general consensus without very much conflict concerning team goals. Specifically, the team decided to send the nurse to gather information. The physician took a leadership role in outlining how the information can be used, what goals can be established, what priorities need to be set, and what tasks need to be accomplished.

It's clear that, although solutions have been suggested, the team members agreed that particular tasks and solutions can't be decided until as much information as possible is available and the team has set priorities for problems and issues. You established a number of potential tasks and goals.

The team has done well in its first phase of team functioning as defined by the team leaders: gathering information, defining the problems and issues, and beginning the task of setting priorities and deciding the next steps.

O'MALLEY (IM): I think that's an excellent lead-in to the next phase of the team's work, which is to organize our priorities in two groups: We need to list those issues which require early intervention, and then we need to establish priorities among those issues that must be resolved in the longer term. If I may, I'll summarize very briefly, then we'll go around the team and address issues that I overlooked.

There seems to be general agreement that we need a very detailed physical evaluation of this woman, which includes both a close look at her cardiovascular system and also further evaluation of what appears to be a dementia. At a minimum this will include a CT scan or MRI of the brain, chest X ray, EKG, blood work (complete blood count, sedimentation rate, electrolytes, BUN, creatinine, blood sugar, thyroid functions, liver functions, vitamin $B_{12}$ level, folate, serology, and digitoxin level), and a good neurological exam. This will supplement a good general physical exam and be particularly attuned to her cardiovascular system.

Having done those things, we should begin to treat her appropriately, based on what we find. We aim at correcting treatable causes of dementia and managing her hypertension with medication that will neither exacerbate her dementia nor create great compliance problems because of side effects or complexity of regimen.

Two other issues are a little less clear to me. One is the assessment of her priorities and of her family's ability to be engaged in her care. I would also propose that we explore alterations in her situation and environment that will make life easier for her and that she might find helpful, such as the suggestions that occupational therapy has made about changes in adaptive devices, help with the way her apartment is organized, and homemaker and home health aide services. I would add a financial assessment of the patient.

Let's discuss these priorities, add to them, or change them.

SIEGEL (TM): Before a team decides what it's going to do, it's important to get some consensus about what the problems are, because if there's conflict concerning goals, you can't decide who's going to do what (roles).

O'MALLEY (IM): Thank you. Let's find out if everyone agrees with the list of goals that I outlined: that it's complete and that everyone feels that these are the proper priorities.

PIKTIALIS (EC): Where would you fit the evaluation of her drugs and nutritional needs and deficits? Did you encompass them in the physical evaluation?

O'MALLEY (IM): Yes, although I didn't make that explicit. Those are certainly important parts of her physical evaluation.

GLASSMAN (SW): I think we also need to evaluate the kind of social resources that are available to her. We need to find out about transportation, home care, and day care. There are a number of social services that she probably is eligible for and that may reduce her isolation.

PAPAS (DT): Although her physical and mental needs may come first, I think we also have to do a dental evaluation. Problems with eating and pain may contribute to her nutritional status and overall health. One of the things we find with homebound elders is that they have a lot of dental problems they are resigned to and deal with by making modifications in their diets which, in turn, lead to nutritional and other problems.

SATIN (PS): I agree with Terry O'Malley's formulation of tasks and priorities in general. One thing I would remind the team to add high on the list, though, is to form a task force of people who will develop a working relationship with this woman. Without her sense that she has a relationship with those identified people, and without the workers' sense that they have a responsibility for her and the coordination and facilitation of her care, the tasks won't be done no matter how high their priorities. I think the method—the vehicle—for doing these things needs to be put in place.

From an interdisciplinary point of view we'll certainly have to decide what combination of disciplines will do what. My suggestion is that the task force consist of nursing, social work, and occupational therapy. These seem appropriate to me partly because nursing already has established a relationship with Mrs. Steinfeld and has been well received. Another consideration is that these are some of the more pragmatic, action-oriented disciplines, and they will have more face validity and bring more immediate helping results for this woman. Other disciplines, such as medicine, psychiatry, nutrition, and the rest of us on the team, can act as consultants and provide technical services to back up this task force of people providing primary care to this woman.

GURLAND (AVI): Let's not forget to clarify attitudes, values, and ideologies of the team as a whole and of the clinicians in the task force who are going out to do the assessment and interventions. For example, if the occupational therapist feels that this person really should be in a nursing home but forces herself to go out and do what she can, that's very different from an occupational therapist who is very committed to home care and feels very comfortable with putting a lot of adaptive devices into the home.

I think we as a team we need to talk about this before we send any individuals out.

DWYER (NT): I'm concerned that we've assumed a hierarchical relationship whose goals are provider-oriented. My experience as a nutritionist teaches me that we should find out what Mrs. Steinfeld herself really wants before we go through a $2,000 medical workup.

GLASSMAN (SW): I think the very highest value that we have to look at in this situation and in working with older people in general is self-determination. It's extremely important if you're going to get this woman's trust and cooperation.

SATIN (PS): I have a question of law. I'm beginning to have some concern about the potential conflict between this woman's right to choose what kinds of evaluations and treatments she wants and our responsibility, both legally and in terms of public opinion, to care adequately for the welfare of an elderly person. If the patient refuses to be a patient, to accept some of our recommendations and care, and there's some terrible outcome from her refusal, are we liable for neglect or some kind of abuse for not having seen to it that she gets good care?

O'HARE (LW): The short answer is no, you are not liable if the patient refuses to become a patient or continue as a patient so long as the refusal is a knowing one and the obverse of informed consent—informed refusal. The patient certainly has the right to choose what kinds of evaluations and treatments she wants to participate in.

At the same time, I think we have obligations to educate her as to what treatments and evaluations are available and what the risks and benefits are. The informed consent process isn't a one-way street where we sit back and wait for patients to ask the right questions of us. We have a positive obligation to provide information to patients or prospective patients, as in this case. So I think it's as much an education process — a real *process* with her — soliciting consent to a particular evaluation or treatment, as it is avoiding forcing unwanted care on her.

BARNARD (ET): I agree with the thrust of the legal comments on informed consent. I would reemphasize that the informed consent process is not simply the act of getting patients' permissions to do things. It is an *opportunity* to learn people's values, to help them envision the goals they have for themselves. The *legal* requirement is the occasion for a more profound *social* and *spiritual* exploration.

Remember, too, that if people reject your professional advice, no matter how much *you* think it is in their best interests, the refusal itself is not necessarily evidence of incompetence. The key is what kinds of reasons the people put forward. Competency evaluations should not be used as threats or bludgeons to get people to do things *we* think they should do if their refusals are based on an understanding of the consequences of their refusals and on expressions of their own values and preferences.

O'MALLEY (IM): Let me respond to that. I think that's an absolutely essential point. Perhaps we should move the issue of defining her priorities higher on the list and use that as the branch point to determine who does what for this woman.

I would make the argument that she really does need physical and mental status evaluations at this point almost regardless of what her priorities are. I see the legal consultant stirring over there, but I'm not saying that we usurp her prerogatives as an independent individual. I think we can easily gain her acquiescence to proceed with an evaluation. We should certainly attempt to do so, and, if she says yes, go ahead.

SIEGEL (TM): It is costly to bring you together as a team, and thus you want to use your time efficiently.

What you've done in these team meetings is very important. You have struggled through a process of defining all the problems (goals) and negotiating those explicitly and openly. You need to do that so that each member of the team has a sense of what each other member can contribute and how each analyzes the case. It's very important for the team to synthesize and analyze all the data in order to define the priorities from the various professional perspectives and decide what can be offered to the patient. As a result, the team itself or a subcomponent of the team will understand what the general consensus of the team is in terms of the care plan. This initial process of goal-setting or problem list-definition is important even before you assess what the patient wants, though that, too, needs to be integrated into the care plan. When the team has worked extensively together, each team member will know what each other member's role is and what contributions each team member can make.

O'MALLEY (IM): We have 10 minutes left in our discussion. Let's reset the priorities for our intervention. I certainly would agree that we put defining Mrs. Steinfeld's priorities high on the list and that we be sure to find those out on our next home visit.

As a procedural issue, I would suggest that we prepare the next set of actions to take when she agrees to let us do our evaluations. If we're all in agreement about the issues that we've listed, let's divide the next set of tasks up and be prepared to undertake interventions when we get her acquiescence.

BLAKENEY (NS): I think I share with Terry O'Malley the concern that at some point it is going to be important to get the basic physical health data and history, both from the patient and the family, regardless of what she wants in terms of the outcomes of where she lives and how she lives. She doesn't have an ongoing care provider. She needs to have that regardless of what else happens.

We did three things together at the end of our last meeting, and she has agreed to them. We have initiated a homemaker to help her with the daily cleaning of the house, and a home health aide for personal care. She has agreed to having hot meals delivered to her home, which will begin next week. She also has agreed to, and felt very positive about, getting an emergency call system, which will give her some personal security in case she falls or has some other urgent need. Her response to these suggestions is very positive and enthusiastic.

My sense is that once we're ready to work with her on the next issues, such as a better physical exam and perhaps coming to the hospital for complex evaluation, she's going to have a positive response. I don't have the sense that she's negative about wanting to feel better.

It is our problem to decide what course of action to propose to her.

O'MALLEY (IM): It sounds like this might be the appropriate time to designate that small group of individuals who will form the core team for the next stage of intervention. David Satin's suggestion that it be nursing, social service, and OT sounds good to me. If everyone else agrees with that, we should assign that group to go ahead and begin the intervention with the priorities we've set.

If there are no more suggestions, we'll meet again to review progress and extend our plans. It is now the end of our scheduled meeting.


*Commentary*

SATIN (PS): Maybe it would be appropriate to follow up our team meeting with some feedback from our team consultant about what we are doing.

SIEGEL (TM): I think that the team did a terrific job, considering that it was working together for the first time. If you had worked more and solved a lot more problems together, you would have known each other better and been even more efficient.

All of you shared your different perspectives about what you thought the needs were. You also defined a set of problems that needed to be addressed, and then you engaged in setting goals. You didn't do more formal setting of priorities because, by consensus decision making, you agreed that the most important goal was to get more information. It was deemed more efficient to say that we need to get more data before we jump in and make such statements as, "She obviously needs to be hospitalized," or "She needs to be in a nursing home."

There was then the role issue of who does what, a sorting out of the alternatives using a problem-solving model, and then coming up with a decision to designate a team person to carry out the goal of gathering more information. Each of the team members then consulted with the provider who would be making the home visit to ensure collection of the data important to the next step of identifying the needed interventions.

Communication was clear, with very little interruption. There was consensus with little conflict. What conflict did exist was openly discussed and managed.

In terms of team functioning, not only one team member but a number of people took on leadership roles as well as process functions. Three or four people took leadership in terms of summarizing, defining the problems, and getting the team back to the task of defining the goals and achieving them.

This process ended with a general consensus that everyone can live with. It's really important, once you define your goals and roles, that people agree to carry them out because sabotage or other impediments to team function can occur if people really aren't committed to the team plans.

So, congratulations on good team functioning!

SATIN (PS): From an interdisciplinary point of view I was impressed that people spoke clearly from the perspectives of their own disciplines but also felt free to discuss in a nondisciplinary fashion issues that were generic or were outside their disciplinary expertise. For example, there was a lot of discussion about economic issues, value issues, and helping Mrs. Steinfeld remain functional, during which it was probably not possible to identify people's disciplines because they were using a more shared background. There is a lot of respect among us that allowed us to learn and overlap with another.

Good job!

# Index

"Accidental immobilization," 239–40
ACE inhibitors, 179
Achlorhydria, 119–20
Active-assistive range of motion, 249
Active, voluntary euthanasia, 324–26
Activities of daily living: assessment, 232–33; disability trends, 349–50; and nutritional state, 200; Performance Activities of Daily Living, 235–36. *See also* Basic activities of daily living; Instrumental activities of daily living
Activity level, 239–50
Activity theory, 294
Acute care: health insurance, 381; and professional roles, 428
Acute confusional state, 74–75, 81
Acute myocardial infarction, 55–56
Acute pain, 258
Acute renal failure, 47
Adaptational approach, 70–71
"Add-on" effect, 354
Adjusted average per capita cost, 383
Advance directives, 321
Advocacy, 319
Against medical advice decisions, 340
Ageism: definition, 63–64; formation of, 434–35
Agitated depression, 71
Albumin, drug binding, 150–51
Alcohol intake, 208
Alcoholism, 77–78; treatment, 77–78; vulnerability in the aged, 208
Allocation of health care, 105
"Allowable" charges, Medicare, 372
Alpha$_1$ acid glycoprotein, 150–51
Alpha$_1$ antagonists, 180
Alpha$_2$ agonists, 180
Alprazolam, 174
Alveolar bone, 110–11; anatomy, 110–11; and Cushing's disease, 123; osteoporosis effects, 119
Alzheimer's disease, 81–82; clinical issues, 36–37, 81–82; family effects, 85–86; financial impact, 380–82; health care team role, 36–37; rehabilitation therapies, 256, 261; treatment, 84–86
Ambulation, fall prevention, 271
Ambulatory care. *See* Outpatient care
Aminoglycosides, 184
Amitriptyline, 176
Amoxapine, 177
Amputation: in peripheral vascular disease, 58–59; rehabilitation therapies, 255
Anemia, 210; microcytic hypochromic, 210
Anger, in dying patients, 96
Angioplasty, 56
Angiotensin-converting enzyme inhibitors, 179

"Antabuse," 77
Antacids, 183
Anterograde amnesia, and triazolam, 172
Antianxiety drugs, 173–75; in dying patients, 96; in long-term care, 89; short- versus long-acting, 174
Antiarrhythmic drugs, 181–82
Antibacterial agents, 183–84
Anticholinergic drugs: in Parkinson's disease, 39–40; in sleep disorders, 167–68
Anticoagulants, 182
Antidepressant medication, 73, 90, 175–77; adverse effect profiles, 175–76; in dementia, 85; dosage, 175; in long-term care, 90
Antidiuretic hormone, 53
Antihistamines, 167–68
Antihypertensive agents, 178–80
Antipsychotic medication, 177–78; in dementia, 85; dying patients, 96; indications, 177–78; in long-term care, 90; in paranoia, 76; in physical illness reactions, 88; right to refuse treatment, 334; side effects, 178
Anxiety: clinical presentation, 74; drug therapy, 173–75; and dying patients, 95–96; rehabilitation component, 253
Aortic valve disease, 57–58
Apathetic depression, 71
Apathy, in dying patients, 97–98
Aphthous ulcer, 128
Area Agencies on Aging, 377–78
Arthritis, 43–45; clinical issues, 43–45; rehabilitation therapies, 255
Articular cartilage, 248
Aspirin; burn, 127; coronary disease treatment, 55
Assignment billing, 368–69
Assistive devices, 259–60; in fall prevention, 266–67
Asthma, 49
Atherosclerosis, 198, 204–5
Atrial fibrillation, 57
Atrophic gastritis, 60
Attitudes, values, and ideologies, 426–47; and ageism, 434–35; definitions, 430–32; development of, 433–35; function of, 432–33; and interdisciplinary practice, 440; in professional education, 435–37, 441–44; in professional practice, 437–41; in team-patient relationship, 408
Auditory system. *See* Hearing
Authoritarian decision making, 94
Autonomy: and active euthanasia decisions, 325–26; health care financing effect, 385; living environment principle, 303–4; and rehabilitation, 252; stroke patients, 38–39

Baccus Amendment, 370
Bacterial endocarditis, 58
Balance: and fall prevention, 270–71; inactivity effects, 241–42; sensory conditions, 270–71; therapeutic exercises, 270–71
Balance billing, 368–69
Barbiturates, 165–66
Barthel Index, 234
Basal-cell carcinoma, 50
Basic activities of daily living: assessment, 332–33; and disability trends, 350. *See also* Activities of daily living; Instrumental activities of daily living
Bedrest: cardiovascular consequences, 242–43; deconditioning effect, 240; metabolic effects, 249; nervous system effects, 241; sensory deprivation comparison, 241; skeletomuscular effects, 244–46
Beliefs, 253. *See also* Attitudes, values, and ideologies
"Benefit ratios," 374
Benign familial tremor, 39
Benzodiazepines: adverse effects, 174; in anxiety disorders, 173–74; half-life implications, 169, 174; hepatic clearance, 158–59; sleep disorders treatment, 168–73
Best-interests standard, 322
Beta-blockers: in anxiety, 175; in hypertension, 179
Biliary tract disease, 60–61
Bioavailability of drugs, 143–46
Biotransformation of drugs, 157–59
Black aged women, 288–89
Blood levels of drugs, 152–53
Blood pressure, 215–16, 243
Blood volume, inactivity effects, 246
Body fat, and drug distribution, 149
Body weight: desirable levels, 202–3; and energy intake, 201–2; surveys, 201
Bone health: age-related changes, 42, 118–19; and calcium nutrition, 211–14; and inactivity, 245–46
Bone loss, 245–46
Bone meal, 218–19
Bone structure: age-related changes, 42, 118–19; and oral health, 118–19
Bradycardia, 56–57
Brain mass, 261
Bromocriptine, 39
Bronchitis: chronic, 49
Bruxing, 126
Buccal drug dosage, 145–46
"Buddy system," 268
Bupropion, 177
Buspirone, in anxiety, 174–75

Caffeine, and calcium loss, 212
Calcium balance, and osteoporosis, 42
Calcium channel antagonists, 180
Calcium losses, and bedrest, 249

Calcium nutrition, 211–15; absorption, 211; bone health role, 211–14; clinical implications, 211–15; hypertension effects, 214–15; and osteoporosis, 211–14; protein interactions, 212; recommended dietary allowance, 211; requirements, 213; supplements, 218–19
Calcium supplements, 218–19
Calories: recommended dietary allowance, 200; needs in the aged, 200–3
Canadian health care system, 18–20
Cancer: emotional factors in survival, 93; oral complications, 125
Candidiasis, 127
Capitated payment, 388
Capsule drug dosage form, 143
Carbohydrate intake: clinical implications, 205–8; and dental health, 116, 205; diabetes mellitus implications, 205–8; recommended diet, 205
Cardiac catheterization, 56
Cardiac conduction system, 56–57
Cardiac disease. *See* Cardiovascular disease
Cardiomyopathy, 54–55; hypertrophic, 55
Cardiopulmonary resuscitation, 319–20
Cardiovascular disease, 54–59; clinical issues, 54–59; dietary fat recommendations, 204–5; and oral health, 123; rehabilitative therapies, 255–56
Cardiovascular system, inactivity effects, 242–44
Caregivers: burden on, 291; and dementia patients, 37; and disclosure, 316; environmental considerations, 272; family role, 289–91; and female responsibility, 290; financial impact, 380–82; functional abilities, 233, 236–37; and public policy, 292
Caries, dental. *See* Dental caries
Cartilage, inactivity effects, 248–49
Case management: in channeling programs, 355–57; cost offset failures, 357; dementia patients, 37; in Medicare waiver programs, 354–55
Cataracts, 33
Catastrophic costs, 383
Central nervous system: diseases, 39–41; normal aging, 31–34
Cerebrovascular diseases: clinical issues, 37–38; oral health effects, 123; rehabilitation, 38–39, 254
Cervical spondylosis, 40
Channeling programs, 355–57
Cheek biting, 127
"Chemical restraint," 334
Chemotherapy, oral complications, 125
Chinese families, 92
Chloral hydrate, 165
Chlorpromazine, 178
Cholecystectomy, 61
Cholelithiasis, 60–61
Cholesterol: high-density lipoprotein, 204
Cholesterol level: dietary recommendations, 198, 204; as risk factor, 203–5

Chronic care. *See* Long-term care
Chronic inactivity: cardiovascular consequences, 243–44. *See also* Sedentary life style
Chronic obstructive lung disease, 49
Chronic renal failure, 47
Cimetidine, 183
Clonidine, 180
Coercion, and informed consent, 332
Cognition, 62–107; functional variability, 238–29; and normal aging, 67–60; and physical illness, 86–88
Cognitive disorders, 79–86; dying patients, 95–98; and organic brain syndromes, 34–37; overview, 79–86
Coinsurance charges, and Medicare, 369
Collagen fibers, 262, 247–48
Colon cancer, 60; and dietary fiber, 209
Color contrasts, 273–74
Color vision, 33, 273–74
Commission on Chronic Illness, 232
Communication: environmental facilitation, 273; on health care teams, 418
Community care, 346–61; cost offsets failure, 357, 359–60; demonstration programs, 354–59; professional roles in, 427–31. *See also* Home care
Compensatory intervention, 306
Competence: ethical issues, 318–23; and extent of care decisions, 2, 341–42; fluctuations in, 330–31; informed consent condition, 332–33; legal issues, 329–31; and refusal of treatment, 318–19; values in, 318–19
Complex carbohydrates, 205–7
Conflict management, teams, 412–13, 418, 444
Confusional states, 34–35; in dying patients, 96–97
Congestive heart failure: clinical issues, 55; dietary recommendations, 198
Conjugation reactions, drugs, 157–58
Consensus decision making, teams, 415–16
Consequentialist ethic, 312–13
Conservatorship, 336
Constipation: clinical issues, 60; dietary fiber benefits, 209; and inactivity, 249
Continuing-care retirement communities, 384
Coordinated care, 357–59
Coordination: aging effects, 262; inactivity effects, 241–42
Coronary artery disease: clinical issues, 55–56; dietary recommendations, 198, 204–5
Coronary bypass grafts, 56
Corticosteroid disorders, 80, 123
Cost-containment programs, 371–73
Cost factors: community care programs, 357, 359–60; and life-sustaining treatment decisions, 322–23; in long-term care, 323, 376–82; medications, 163–64; and professional practice, 438–39
Cost offsets, 357, 359–60

"Cost shifting," 364
Coumadin, 123
Creatinine clearance, 153, 160–61
Crown (tooth anatomy), 109
Cushing's disease, 80; dental complications, 123

Dancing, 271
Death, 92–100: attitudes toward, 92–93; emotional and cognitive issues, 92–100; ethical issues, 311–28; family issues, 94, 98–99; and health professionals, 99–100; legal issues, 340–42; and life-sustaining decisions, 316–23; perspective of the elderly, 20–21; religion role, 95. *See also* Terminal care
Decision charting, 416
Decision making: of dying patients, 94, 319; and extent of care, 28–30; in health care teams, 415–16
Deconditioning: definition, 240; and functional capability, 240–51
Decubitus ulcers, 51. *See also* Inactivity
Degenerative joint disease, 43–45
Dehydration: bodily effects, 120; renal effects, 46
Delirium, 34–35, 79–81; clinical issues, 34–35; in dying patients, 96–97; sources of, 79–81; treatment, 81
Delusions, 97
Dementia, 81–86; causes, 81–84; clinical issues, 35–36, 81–84; family effects, 85–86; health care team role, 36–37; health professional reactions, 86; treatment, 84–86. *See also* Alzheimer's disease
Demographics, 346–48
Demonstration programs: community long-term care, 354–59; cost offsets, 357; hospital-based, 357–59
Dental care, 108–36; progress in, 129–30; protocol for, 133–36; utilization by aged, 128–29
Dental caries, 111–12; and carbohydrates, 116, 205; cheese and dairy products as protection against, 117; coronal caries, 112, 116; food-related factors, 115–16, 205; prevalence, 114; root caries, 116–17; and starch, 116; and sugar intake, 116; treatment, 129–30
Dental implants, 129–30
Dental Longitudinal Study, 115
Dentin, 110, 117, 119
Dentures: dyspepsia link, 120; and food intake, 115; protocol for inspection, 136
Dependence, and self-worth, 304–5
Depression, 71–74; clinical forms, 71–73; drug therapy, 175–76; in dying patients, 97–98; and extent of care decisions, 28–29; institutionalization reaction, 89–90; treatment, 73–74, 175–76
Depressive personality, 72
Desalkylflurazepam, 169–70
Desipramine, 176
Developmental perspective: and care of the aged, 437–38; on emotional problems, 70–71

Diabetes mellitus: carbohydrate intake, 205–8; control of, 206–7; dental complications, 123; dietary modification, 207–8; and glucose metabolism, 53

"Diabetic diet," 207

Diabetic neuropathy, 41

Diagnosis Related Group program: and hospital discharge, 351; impact, 371–73; outlier limit, 372

Diastolic blood pressure, 215–16

Diastolic dysfunction, 55

Diazepam, 174

Dictatorial decision making, 415–16

Diet: and dentate status, 115–17; drug interactions, 195

Dietary fat: clinical implications, 204–5; heart disease recommendations, 198; as risk factor, 203–4

Dietary Guidelines for Americans, 199

Diffusion (pulmonary function), 246–47

Digestive system, 119–20

Digoxin, 181

Dilantin, gingival effects, 125

Diltiazem, 180

Disability: community long-term care, 350–61; definition, 230–31; demographics, 231–32, 346; demonstration programs, 354–59; trends in, 349–50

Disability Insurance Trust, 366

Discharge planning, 340. *See also* Hospital discharge

Disclosure, 312–16; communication skills, 315–16; informed consent condition, 314–15, 332; psychological effects question, 312–13; truth in, 314–15

Disengagement theory, 294

Disopyramide, 182

Disulfiram, 77

Diuretics, 179

Diverticular disease, 209

Divorce, 289

Do Not Resuscitate order: court decisions, 341; ethical issues, 320

Dolomite preparations, 218

Doral (quazepam), 170

Doxylamine, 167

Dread-disease insurance, 374

Drug absorption: in the aged, 147; basic concepts, 143–44; gastrointestinal tract, 144–47

Drug abuse: "maturing out" concept, 41; treatment, 78–79

Drug clearance: and clinical practice, 153–54; and drug sensitivity, 140; elimination half-life relationship, 155–56; general principles, 153–54, 160–61

Drug compliance, 185–86

Drug distribution, 147–53; and aging, 149, 163; drug choice relevance, 147–48; gender-related differences, 149; protein binding effect, 150–53

Drug dosage forms, 143

Drug interactions: drug selection factor, 163; and protein binding, 152

Drug intoxication, 46–47

Drug metabolism, 157–59

Drug sensitivity: and aging, 161–62; basic mechanisms, 140–41, 161–62

Drug therapy, 137–92; anxiety, 173–75; depression, 175–77; diet interactions, 195; general concepts, 138–62; hypertension, 178–80; sleep disorders, 164–73

Dry mouth, 121–22

Durable power of attorney, 342–43

Duty to save, 325

Dysnomia, 82

Dyspepsia, 120

Dysphagia, 59

"Dysphasia team," 265

Dyspnea, 49

Early retirement, 298

Economics, 362–86: and availability of health care, 105; long-term care aspects, 376–82; and managed care, 382–84; Medicare and Medigap, 364–74; professional practice effects, 438–39; quality of care issues, 384–85. *See also* Cost factors

Education, 435–37, 441–44

"Ejection" chairs, 260

Elastic cartilage, 248

Elastin fibers, 247

Electroconvulsive therapy, 73–74

Electroencephalogram, and bed rest, 241

Elimination half-life, 154–57; benzodiazepines, 169, 174; clinical implications, 156–57, 169; drug selection factor, 162–63; general principles, 154–56

Emergencies, and right to refuse treatment, 334

Emotions, 62–107; dying patients, 92–100; and long-term care settings, 88–92; and normal aging, 67–70; in physical illness, 86–88; and professional practice, 65–67

Emphysema, 49

Employer At Risk program, 384

Enamel (tooth anatomy), 119, 126

Endocarditis, 58

Endocrine disease, 51–54, 123

Energy intake, 200–203; and body weight, 201–2; declines in the aged, 201; and diabetes, 207. *See also* Calories

Enophthalmos, 33

Enteric-coated tablets, 145

Entropion, 33

Environmental factors: in geriatric rehabilitation, 271–74; and self-esteem, 303–4

Epilepsy, and oral health, 125

Estate planning, 342–43

Estrogen replacement therapy: and calcium nutrition, 213–14; in postmenopausal osteoporosis, 214

Ethchlorvynol, 167
Ethical issues, 311–28; and disclosure, 312–16; and euthanasia, 324–26; in life-sustaining decisions, 316–23
Euthanasia, 324–26
Exercise: balance improvement, 270; benefits, 253–57, 268–70; fall prevention benefits, 268–70; precautions, 270; as primary rehabilitation modality, 240, 253–57; theories of, 240
Existential depression, 71–72
Extended families, 288
Extent of care, 28–30
Extropion, 33

Falls, 266–71; balance exercises, 270–71; home assessment in, 268–69; preventive measures, 266–71; safety education, 268–69
Family care: burden of, 291; cost impact, 380–82; long-term conditions, 91–92, 351, 353; and mourning, 290–91; perspective of the aged, 11–14; public policy, 292; terminally ill, 94, 98–99; values in, 289–90
Family conflicts, 286–87
Family education, 91–92
Family relationships, 285–93; dementia effect, 85–86; perspective of the aged, 11–14; shifts in old age, 69–70, 285–87
Family structure, 287–89
Family visits, 288
Famotidine, 183
Fast muscle fibers, 244
Fat. *See* Dietary fat
Fat-soluble drugs, 147–49, 163
Fatigue, 264
Fear of death, physicians, 100, 313
Fear of falling, 266
Federal employees, insurance, 371
Federal food assistance programs, 220
Federal Health Employee Benefit Program, 371
Federal Insurance Contribution Act, 366
"Fee-for-service" system, 372, 382
Feeding programs, 265
Feeding tubes. *See* Tube feeding
Fermentable carbohydrates, 116
Fertility rates, 347
Fetal tissue transplantation, 40
Fiber intake, 208–9; clinical implications, 209; colon-rectal cancer decreases, 209; and diabetes mellitus, 205–7; recommendations, 208
Fibrin, 248
Fibrinogen, 248
Fibroblasts, 247
"Fiduciary" capacity, 339
Finances. *See* Economics
Fissured tongue, 126
Flow charts, 416
Flow experiences, 303
Fluid intake, recommendations, 218
Fluoride treatment: dental caries prevention, 129–30; dry mouth patients, 122

Fluoxetine, 177
Fluphenazine, 178
Flurazepam, 169–70
Folic acid deficiency, 210–11
Food stamps, 220
Foot pain, 258
Fordyce granules, 126
Free drug fraction, 150–53
Functional assessment, 232–36
Functional capacity: levels of, assessment, 233; and nutrition, 264–65; old age definition, 63
Functional Health of Institutionalized Elders, 235
Functional Health Scale, 236
Functional variability, 237–39
Functioning for Independent Living, 236

Gait changes: evaluation, 266; and fall prevention, 266; and rehabilitation, 262–63
Gait patterns, 263, 266
Gallstone disease, 60–61
Gastric cancer, 60
Gastrocsoleus muscle, 244–45
Gastrointestinal disease, 59–61
Gastrointestinal tract, 59–61; drug absorption, 144–47
Generic drugs, 163–64
Geographic tongue, 126
"Geri-chairs," 260
Geriatric evaluation units, 423–24
Geriatric psychiatry, 63–65
Geriatric rehabilitation. *See* Rehabilitation
Geriatrics: legitimacy, 63–65; as pandiscipline, 399; professional education, 435–37
Giant-cell arteritis, 44
Gingiva, 110–11
Gingival disease, 112–13, 123
Glare, 273
Glucose intolerance, 206
Glucose metabolism, 53
Glucose tolerance test, 206
Glutethimide, 166–67
Goal setting, in teams, 412–13
Gout, 44
Government employees, insurance, 374
Graduate education, 435–37, 441–44
Graves disease, 80
GRPI model, 411–19
*Guardian ad litem*, 338
Guardianship, 336–40; temporary, 339

Hairy tongue, 126
Halcion. *See* Triazolam
Half-life. *See* Elimination half-life
Hallucinations, 97
Haloperidol, 178
Handicaps, definition, 231
Harvard University Medicare Project, 380
Health-care institutions. *See* Institutional care
Health-care proxies, 342
Health-care team. *See* Interdisciplinary team

Health maintenance organizations, 382–84
Health professionals: attitudes, values, and ideology, 437–41; education, 435–37, 441–44; emotional and cognitive issues, 100–102; roles of, 413–15, 427–31, 444–45; and terminal care, 94–95, 99–100
Health status perceptions, 252–53
Hearing: evaluation of, 105; geriatric rehabilitation consideration, 261; normal aging, 32
Heart disease. *See* Cardiovascular disease
Heart rate: age-related changes, 264; bedrest effects, 242–43
Heparin, 182
Hepatic blood flow, 159
Hepatic clearance, 157–59
Hepatic function, and drug selection, 163
Herpangina, 128
Herpes zoster: clinical issues, 50–51; oral effects, 127–28
Hip fracture: incidence in the aged, 231; rehabilitation therapies, 256; Year 2000 goals, 221
Histamine$_2$ antagonists, 182–83
Home care: and caretaker abilities, 233, 236–37; cost-containment impact, 375; environmental considerations, 272–73; interdisciplinary team use, 424; Medicare coverage, 370; out-of-pocket expenses, 379; professional roles in, 427–31, 444–45
Home-delivered meals, 220
Hope, 316
Hospice care, 99–100; Medicare coverage, 367
Hospital-based demonstration programs, 351–59
Hospital care. *See* Inpatient care
Hospital discharge: cost-containment impact, 372; planning of, 340; and prospective payment system, 351, 372
Hospital insurance. *See* Medicare Part A
Hospital Insurance Trust, 366
Hyaline cartilage, 248
Hydralazine, 180
Hydrochlorothiazide, 179
Hydrophilic drugs. *See* Water-soluble drugs
Hyperalimentation, 221
Hyperglycemia, 53, 206–7
Hyperkalemia, 46
Hypernatremia, 215
Hyperosmolar nonketotic coma, 207
Hyperparathyroidism, 54
Hypertension: calcium nutrition, 214–15; clinical issues, 58; drug therapy, 178–80; nonpharmacologic therapies, 178; sodium nutrition, 215–16
Hyperthyroidism, 52
Hypnotic drugs, 164–73
Hypokinetics: definition, 240; and functional capability, 240–51. *See also* Inactivity
Hyponatremia, 215
Hypoparathyroidism, 54
Hypothyroidism, 52

Iatrogenic effects, 103–4
Ideology: definition, 431–32. *See also* Attitudes, values, and ideologies
Immobility: functional capability losses, 239–50; nervous system effects, 241–42
Impairment, definition, 231
Inactivity: and functional capabilities, 239–50; health interactions, 240
Income, 296
Incompetent patients, 320–23; ethical issues, 320–23; extent of care decisions, 29, 320–22, 341–42; guardianship proceedings, 338–39; legal issues, 329–31; right to refuse treatment legalities, 333–34
Indemnity insurance plans, 371
Independent living, 305–6. *See also* Autonomy
Individual medical accounts, 384
Information sharing, terminal patients, 93–94
Informed consent: conditions for, 332–33; legal issues, 331–36; patients' rights, 313–14; and treatment refusal 318–19, 333; truthful disclosure in, 314–15, 332
Inpatient care: cost-containment impact, 372–73; professional role perspective, 428, 444–45
Insomnia, drug therapy, 164–73
Institutional care: adjustment to, 88–91; emotional/cognitive aspects, 88–92; family issues, 91–92; iatrogenic effects, 103–4; patients' functional needs, 102–3; viewpoint of the aged, 17
Institutional environment, 303–4
Institutional ethics committee, 323
Instrumental activities of daily living: assessment, 233; and disability trends, 350. *See also* Activities of daily living; Basic activities of daily living
Insulin, 185
Insulin-dependent diabetes, 207
Insulin dosage, 207
Insurance. *See* Federal employees; Indemnity insurance plans; Medicaid; Medicare; Medigap; Private insurance; Public employees; State employees
Intelligence, functional variability, 239
Intentional killing, 325
Interdisciplinary education, 442–43
Interdisciplinary team, 391–424; administrative support, 419–23; advantages, 399–400; complexity of, 406–7; conceptual framework, 392–93; conflict resolution in, 418; decision making, 415–16; dementia intervention, 36–37; development issues, 404–24; difficulties in, 400–401; dynamics of, 411–19; effectiveness, 423–24; and extent of care, 28–31; goals, 411; in independent living assessment, 305–9; interpersonal issues, 418–19; leadership issues, 417–18; liability issues, 344; matrix organizational support, 419–23; model of, 396–97; versus multidisciplinary approach,

405–6; patient relationship, 408; primary care structure, 407; professional identity in, 399–402, 440; and professional practice, 440; roles in, 413–15, 440; size and composition, 407–8; spectrum of models, 393–402; spheres of competence, 392–93
International Medical Centers, 383
Interpersonal issues, in teams, 418–19
Involuntary commitment, 333–34
Involuntary treatments, 334
Iron absorption, 209–10
Iron deficiency anemia, 210–11
Ischemic heart disease, 55–56
Isometric exercise, 270
Italian families, 92

Joints, degenerative changes, 43–45

Katz ADL instrument, 234
Kenny Self-care scale, 234
Ketosis, 207
Kidney failure, 47
Kidney function. *See* Renal function

Lactose intolerance, 120
Laxation, dietary fiber benefit, 209
Laxatives, 183
L-dopa, 39–40
Leadership, in health care teams, 417–18
Lean body mass, 244, 263
Learned helplessness, 304
Legal issues, 329–45; and allied health professionals, 344; competency decisions, 329–31; guardianship, 336–40; and informed consent, 331–34
Leisure activities, 295, 302
Lesbians, 288, 291
Lichen planus, 127
Lidocaine toxicity, 181
Life expectancy: improvements in, 346–49; Year 2000 goals, 221
"Life-line," 268
Life satisfaction: postretirement factors, 299, 302–5; and productive activity, 295
Life-sustaining decisions: cost factors, 322–23; ethical issues, 316–23; legal issues, 341–42; and quality of life, 322–23
Lipid-soluble drugs. *See* Fat-soluble drugs
Lithium, 178
Living will, 341–42
Long half-life drugs: advantages and disadvantages, 157, 169; benzodiazepines, 169, 174; and drug selection, 162–63
Long-term care: adjustment to, 88–91; community demonstration programs, 354–59; costs, 323; definition, 351; family issues, 91–92, 351–52; financing of, 376–82; formal and informal services, 351, 353; fragmentation, 353–54; insurance system limitation, 353–54, 370, 376; pro-

fessional role perspective, 427–30; societal lack of support, 353–54
Long-Term Care Project of North San Diego County, 354–55
Longevity: trends, 346–47; Venice, California study, 304
Lorazepam, 174
Low back pain, 256
Low-calorie diets, 203
Low-density lipoprotein cholesterol, 204
Low-sodium diets, 198
L-tryptophan, 168
Lumbar spine, 43
Lung function. *See* Pulmonary function

Majority rule, in teams, 415–16
Malignant melanoma, 50
Malnutrition. *See* Nutritional deficiencies
Managed care, 382–84
Managed teams, 409
Maprotiline, 177
Maslow's theory, 303–4
Mass media influences, 434
Matrix organization, 409, 419–23
"Meals on Wheels" program, 220
Media influences, 434
Medicaid, 373–74; benefits, 374, 376–77; eligibility, 373–74; legal issues, 343; long-term care limitations, 353, 376–77; "spending down" process, 376–77; and transfer of assets, 343
Medical expertise, 313
Medical model: definition, 70–71; effect on professional practice, 437–38
Medicare, 364–74; balance billing in, 368–69; benefits and coverage, 366–70; cost-containment impact, 372–73; eligibility, 366; financing and structure, 365–66; history, 364–65; HMO programs, 382–83; long-term care limitations, 353, 376, 381; non-covered services, 370, 375–76; Part A, 365–70; Part B, 365–70; rationale for, demographics, 347–48; viewpoint of the aged, 18–20
Medicare Catastrophic Coverage Act of 1988, 382
Medicare waiver demonstration programs, 354–55
Medication compliance, 185–86
Medigap insurance, 370–73, 375
Megaloblastic anemias, 210
Melanomas, 50
Menopausal women, 212–14
Mental ability, 238–39
Mental health services, insurance, 367–68
Mental hospital care, Medicare, 367
Metabolic brain syndromes, 34–35
Methyldopa, 180
Midazolam, 148
Mineral supplements, 218–19
Minerals, recommended allowances, 199
Mitral valve disease, 57
Mobility: disability trends, 349–50; in functional

assessment, 233; and functional capabilities, 239–50
Monoamine oxidase inhibitors, 176
Monroe County, New York study, 424
Morale, and retirement, 298–99
Mortality rates, 348–49
Motivation: living environment role, 303–4; rehabilitation component, 253
Motor coordination. *See* Coordination
Mourning, in caregivers, 290–91
Multidisciplinary working relationships, 395–96, 398–99,; 405–6
Multigenerational family, 286
Multi-infarct dementia, 36, 82
Multiple sclerosis, 124
Muscle: and geriatric rehabilitation, 262–63; inactivity effects, 244–46; normal aging effects, 41, 118, 262–63; oral health role, 118
Muscle mass: aging effect, 262–63; and inactivity, 244
Muscular dystrophy, 124
Musculoskeletal system: inactivity effects, 244–46; in normal aging and disease, 41–45; and rehabilitation, 262
Myocardial infarction, 55–56
Myopathy, 41–42
Myositis, 41–42
"Myxedema madness," 80

Narcotic analgesics, 184
Nasogastric tube feeding. *See* Tube feeding
National Health Interview Survey, 349–50
Nerve conduction velocity, 262
Neuronal loss, 261
New York City Home Care Project, 354
NHANES I/NHANES II, 201
Nifedipine, 180
Nizatidine, 183
"Nonaccumulating" drugs, 156
Noncompliance, 185–86
Non-insulin-dependent diabetes mellitus, 207
Non-ketotic hyperosmolar coma, 53
Nonsteroidal anti-inflammatory drugs, 145
"Nonsusceptible" metabolic pathway, 158
Normal-pressure hydrocephalus: and dementia, 83; general features, 40
Norms, and health care teams, 418
Nortriptyline, 176
Nurse's role, 444; historical perspective, 405; medicalization of, 101
Nursing homes: adjustment to, 88–91; extent of care guideposts, 29–30; financing, 376–82; lack of Medicare coverage, 370, 379; out-of-pocket expenses, 379; patients' emotional/functional needs, 102–3; reimbursement limitations, 353
Nutrition, 193–229
Nutritional Status Survey, 115

Oars assessment, 235
Oars II assessment, 236
Obstructive lung disease, 49
Occupational role, and self-esteem, 297
Occupational therapists, 305–9
Old Age Survivors Trust, 366
Old-old group, 231, 349–50
Older Americans Act, 220
Olfaction, 33–34
OnLok Community Care Organization for Dependent Adults, 355
Opiate analgesics, 184
Oppositionalism, in dying patients, 96
Optimal health, 250
Oral cancers, 125
Oral cavity: age-related changes, 118–22; anatomy, 109–11
Oral diseases, 110–15, 126–30; and nutrient quality, 115–17; treatment, 129–30
Oral health, 108–36
Organic brain syndromes, 34–37. *See also* Alzheimer's disease; Delirium; Dementia
Orthostatic hypotension, 243
Osteoarthritis, 43, 249, 252
Osteoclasts, 245
Osteomalacia, 42–43, 119, 216–17, 219
Osteons, 245–46
Osteoporosis, 42–43; and calcium nutrition, 211–14; clinical issues, 42–43; and dental problems, 119; inactivity role, 245; mineral supplements, 219; postmenopausal women, 212–14; prevalence, 118–19; and rehabilitation, 263
Out-of-country care, 370
Out-of-pocket expenses: cost-control impact, 371–73; Medicap premiums, 375–76; and Medicare, 369
"Outlier" limit, 372
Outpatient care: cost-containment impact, 372; and goal setting, 427–30
Over-the-counter medications, 137–38
Oxidation reactions, 157–58
Oxygen uptake, and bed rest, 243

Pace II, 235–36
Pain: chronic, 258; management of, 258
Pandisciplinary model, 397–99
Panic, 74
Papillary hyperplasia, 118
Paradisciplinary model, 394–95
Paraneoplastic syndrome, 80
Paranoid depression, 71
Paranoid state, 75–76
Paraphrenia, 75
Parathyroid disease, 54
Parent-child relationship, 69–70
Parkinson's disease, 39–40; clinical issues, 39–40; and dementia, 83; drug treatment, 39–40; oral complications, 124; physical therapy, 40; rehabilitation therapies, 40, 254–55
Parkinson's syndrome, 39
Passive range of motion, 249
Pathology model, 437–38

Patient classification index, 235
Patient Self-Determination Act, 321
Peak plasma drug concentration, 143–44
Peer review organizations, 375
Pemphigus, 127
Pepsin, 120
Peptic ulcer, drug therapy, 182–83
Perception of health, 252–53
Performance goals, teams, 412
Periodontal disease, 110, 113–14
Periodontal ligament, 110
Periodontitis, 114
Peripheral neuropathy, 41–42
Peripheral vascular disease, 58–59
Pernicious anemia, 60
Personality: and adjustment, 294–95; continuity
    of, 68
Personality conflicts, team members, 419
Perturbation response, 270
*p*H level, 116–17
Pharmacodynamics: aging effects, 161–62; defini-
    tion, 142–43
Pharmacokinetics, 141–42. *See also* Drug clear-
    ance; Drug distribution; Elimination half-life
Phase I/Phase II biotransformation, 157–58
Phenomenological perspective, 71
Phenytoin, 184
Philadelphia Geriatric Center Scale II, 236
Physical activity: benefits of increased levels, 202;
    and calorie intake recommendations, 201;
    rehabilitation benefits, 253–54, 257. *See also*
    Exercise
Physical strength, 238
Physical therapy: Medicare B coverage, 368;
    stroke patients, 38–39
Physician-patient relationship: economic factors,
    384–85; and informed consent, 313–14;
    respect for patient's autonomy, 313–14
Physicians: and disclosure, 312–13, 332; fear of
    death, 100, 313; health care team role, 410; lia-
    bility issues, 344; professional role, hospital
    setting, 428
"Piggy-backing" claim process, 372
Plasma drug concentrations, 152–53
"Plop effect," 415–16
Pneumonia, 48
Polymyalgia rheumatica, 44
Positive reinforcement, 253
Postherpetic neuralgia, 51
Postmenopausal women, calcium nutrition,
    212–14
Postural hypotension, 268
Postural sway, 262
Posture: and fall prevention, 270–71; and feeding,
    265; and rehabilitation, 263; therapeutic exer-
    cise, 270–71
Potassium balance, 46
Potassium depletion, 208
Potassium supplements, 208
Prazosin, 180
Preferred-provider organizations, 384

Prepaid health insurance plans, 382–84
Preretirement groups, 299
Presbycusis, 32
Presbyopia, 33
Prescription drugs: Medicare coverage, 368; use
    by the aged, 137
Pressure sores, 51
Prevention; of nutritional deficiencies, 195, 197;
    and optimal health, 250–51
Private insurance: in catastrophic care, 380–81.
    *See also* Medigap insurance
Procainamide, 181
"Process consultant," 419
Process issues, teams, 410–19
Productivity, 299–302; aging process effects,
    300–301; definition, 299–300; disuse versus
    aging issue, 301; as identity criterion, 69; and
    leisure activities, 302; and worth, 69,
    294–309
Professional education, 435–37, 441–44
Professional identity, 399–400, 440
Professional roles: ambulatory versus home care
    settings, 427–31; hospital settings, 444–45; in
    interdisciplinary teams, 413–15
Professional standards review organizations, 372
Project OPEN, 354–55
Prolongation of life. *See* Life-sustaining decisions
Proprioceptive neuromuscular facilitation, 257
Prospective payment system: hospital discharge
    effects, 351; impact, 371–73
Protein, recommended intake, 203
Protein binding, drugs, 150–53
Protriptyline, 176
Proxies, health care, 342
Pseudodementia, 83–84
Psychotherapy: dementia patients, 84; dying
    patients, 96
Psychotropic medications, 168–78; in dying
    patients, 96–98; in physically ill, 88
Ptosis, 33
Ptyalin, 120
Public employees, insurance, 371
Pulmonary edema, 55
Pulmonary function, 47–48; age-related changes,
    264; clinical issues, 47–48; inactivity effects,
    246–47; rehabilitation therapies, 256
Pulp (tooth anatomy), 110, 119
Pyrilamine, 167

Qualified Medicare Beneficiary program, 368
Quality of care, 384–85
Quality of life, 322–23
Quazepam, 170
Quinidine, 181–82

Radiation therapy, oral complications, 125
Range of Motion scale, 234–35
Ranitidine, 183
Rapid Disability Rating, 234
Rate-of-living theory, 240
Reaction time: age-related changes, 262; exercise

benefits, 254; functional variability, 238; sedentary life style effects, 242
Reality orientation, 97
Rebound insomnia, 169, 172
Receptor sensitivity: aging effects, 161–62; and drug reactions, 140–41, 161–62
Recommended dietary allowances, 198–99
Rectal cancer, 209
Red blood cells, and inactivity, 246
Reducing diets, 203
Referral, 445–47
Refusal of treatment, 318
Rehabilitation, 230–79; environmental factors, 271–74; functional assessment in, 232–33; nutritional considerations, 264–65; pain management, 258; principles of, 237–51; and safety, 257–58; and "threshold" physiologic values, 240
Relief of suffering argument, 324
Religion: and dying patients, 95; perspective of the aged, 14–16
REM rebound, and barbiturates, 166
REM sleep, bedrest effects, 241
Remedial intervention, 306
Renal disease: clinical issues, 45–47; nutritional considerations, 197–98
Renal failure, 47
Renal function, 45–47; and drug selection, 163; and protein overnutrition, 198
Respiratory disease, 47–49
Respiratory function. *See* Pulmonary function
Response to perturbation, 270
Resting metabolic rate, 201;
Restraints, in dementia, 85
Resuscitation decisions, ethics, 319–20
Retirement: adjustment to, 294–95, 298–99; compulsory, 298; and identity, 69; life satisfaction factors, 299; regrets, 298; self-worth factors, 302–5
Rheumatic valvular disease, 57
Rheumatoid arthritis, 43–44
"Right to die," 341
Right to refuse treatment, 333–34; antipsychotic medications, 334; in emergency conditions, 334; ethics, 318; in incompetent patients, 333–34
Right to treatment, 334–36
Robert Wood Johnson Foundation, 357
"Role contracts," 414
"Role reversal" theory, 69
Roles. *See* Professional roles

Safety measures: fall prevention, 268; in rehabilitation, 257–58
Saliva, function of, 121–22
Saturated fat, 203–5
Sedatives, in dying patients, 96
Sedentary lifestyle: deconditioning effect, 240; neuropsychological consequences, 242
Seizure disorders, 125
Self-esteem: and retirement, 298–99, 302–5; as work function, 297

Self-image, 70
Senile extropion, 33
Senior centers, 304
Senses, and normal aging, 32–34
Sensory deprivation, 241
Sensory integration techniques, 257
Serum creatinine, 160–61
Serum drug concentrations, 152–53
Shingles, 128
Short-acting drugs: advantages and disadvantages, 156–57, 169; benzodiazepines, 169, 174; and drug selection, 162–63; in dying patients, 96
Single older women, 288–89
Sjögrens syndrome, 122
Skilled-nursing facility: cost-containment impact, 372; Medicare coverage, 367
"Skimming," 383
Skin disease, 49–51
Sleep disorders, drug therapy, 164–73
Smell, in normal aging, 33–34
Social/health maintenance organizations, 384
Social isolation, 103
Social relationships, and work, 297
Social Security, 365
Social status, as work factor, 297
Social support, 11–14
Social withdrawal, dying patients, 97–98
Social worker's role, 405
Socialized medicine, 18–19
Societal issues, 104–5
Sodium balance, 45–46
Sodium nutrition, 215–16
Somaticizing depression, 71
South Carolina Community Long-Term Care Project, 354–55
"Spending down" process, 376–77
Squamous-cell carcinomas, 50
Starvation, 201–2
State employees, insurance, 371
Steady-state drug concentrations, 153–54, 156
Stomach cancer, 60
Stomatitis, 125
Stress reactions, 74–75
Stroke. *See* Cerebrovascular diseases
Stroke volume: age-related changes, 264; inactivity effects, 243
Sublingual drug administration, 145–46
Substance abuse, 77–79
Substituted judgment: ethical issues, 321; legal issues, 333
Sucralfate, 183
Sucrose, 116
Sugar intake: and dental caries, 116; diabetes mellitus implications, 205–7
Suicide, 72–73; assisted, 324–26; rate, 72
Supplemental medical insurance, 365–66, 370–73
Supplemental Security Income program, 373
Support system, 37, 106
Surrogate decision makers. *See* Substituted judgment

Survival, 93
"Susceptible" metabolic pathway, 158
Sustained-release tablets, 145, 162
Syndrome of inappropriate antidiuretic hormone, 45, 53
Synovial membranes, 43
Systolic blood pressure: age-related changes, 215; inactivity consequences, 243; and sodium nutrition, 215–16

Tablet drug administration, 143, 145
Tachycardia, 56–57
Tactile sense, 261–62
Tardive dyskinesia, 178
Taste, in normal aging, 34
Tax Equity and Fiscal Responsibility Act, 383
Team treatment. *See* Interdisciplinary team
Tear production, 33
Teeth: anatomy, 109–11. *See also* Dental care; Dental caries
Teeth loss, 114–15
TEFRA, PL 97–248, 383
Television depictions, 434
Temazepam: dosage forms, absorption, 143–44, 171; elimination half-life, 171; hard- versus soft-gelatin capsule, 171; in sleep disorders, 170–71
Temporal arteritis, 44
Temporomandibular joint disease, 127
Terazosin, 180
Terminal care: family issues, 94, 98–99; information sharing in, 93–94; in normal dying experience, 93–95. *See also* Death
Testamentary capacity, 331
Theophylline, 185
Therapeutic range, 138–39
Thermogenesis, 201
Thermoregulation, and bedrest, 241
Thioridazine, 178
*Thirty-Six Hour Day* (Mace and Robins), 85
"Threshold" physiologic values, 240
Thyroid disease: clinical issues, 52–53; and delirium, 80
Tibialis anterior muscle, 244–45
"Tic douloureux," 124
Tidal volume, and inactivity, 246
Toris, 126
Tort liability, 344
Total blood volume, and bedrest, 243
Total body water, 120–21
Touch, and geriatric rehabilitation, 261–62
Toxic neuropathies, 41
Toxic organic brain dysfunction, 34–35. *See also* Delirium
"Toxic-to-therapeutic" dose ratio, 166
Trabecular bone, 42
Training programs, 435–37, 441–44
Transfer of assets, 343
Transient ischemic attacks, 82–83
Transluminal angioplasty, 56
Transluminal valvulotomy, 57
Transplanted fetal tissue, 40

Traumatic ulcer, 128
Trazodone, 176–77
Treatment refusal, ethics, 318
Triazolam, 171–72
Tricyclic antidepressants, 176
Trigeminal neuralgia, 124
Trypsin, 120
Tube feeding: legal aspects, 341; nutritional aspects, 220–21
Tufts Dental Pilot study, 115
Tufts Nutrition and Oral Health Study, 116

Ulcer disease, 59
Undernutrition, prevalence, 201–2
Unidisciplinary working relationships, 393–94
U.S. Healthcare, 383
"Use it or lose it" concept, 240

Values: and aging, 68; definition, 430–31. *See also* Attitudes, values, and ideologies
"Values history," 321
Valvular heart disease, 57–58
Vascular disease, 58–59
Vasodilator drugs, 180
Venice, California study, 304
Ventilation (pulmonary function), 246
Verapamil, 180
Very-low-density lipoprotein cholesterol, 204
Veterans Administration programs, 375
Vision: age-related changes, 32–33; environmental considerations, 273–74; evaluation of, 105; functional variability, 238
Vital capacity, inactivity effects, 246
Vitamin $B_{12}$, 60
Vitamin D nutrition, 216–17
Vitamin D supplements, 219
Vitamin supplements, 218–19
Vitamins, recommended allowances, 199
Volume of distribution, 147–53; drug selection factor, 163; and elimination half-life, 155–56
Vulnerability, 106

Walking aids, 266–67
Warfarin, 182
Water balance, 45–46
Water-soluble drugs: distribution, 147–49; and drug selection, 163
Weight reduction: hypertension benefit, 216; recommendations, 203
Weight shifting, 270–71
"Weighted" chairs, 260
Wheelchairs, 259–60; electric, 259–60
Women, caregiving responsibility, 290
Work, 294–309; definition, 295–96; as identity criterion, 69; leisure time continuum, 302; universal functions, 296–98; and worth, 302–9

Xerostomia, 121–22

Year 2000 goals, 193, 221–22
"Youngberg principle," 335